Essentials in
Medical Mycology
for Postgraduates

Essentials in Medical Mycology for Postgraduates

Editor-in-Chief

Vasant Baradkar
MBBS MD(Microbiology)
Additional Professor
Department of Microbiology
Seth GS Medical College and KEM Hospital
Mumbai, Maharashtra, India

Guest Editor

Ajit Damle
MBBS MD(Microbiology)
Emeritus Professor
Department of Microbiology, RK Damani Medical College
ShriRamchandra Institute of Medical Sciences (SRIMS)
Chhatrapati Sambhaji Nagar, Maharashtra, India

Editor

Simit Kumar
MBBS MD
Professor and Head
Department of Microbiology
Rampurhat Government Medical College and Hospital
Rampurhat, West Bengal, India

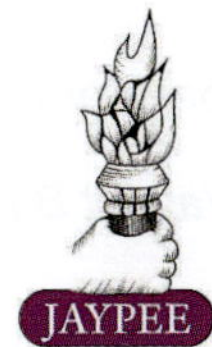

JAYPEE BROTHERS MEDICAL PUBLISHERS
The Health Sciences Publisher
New Delhi | London

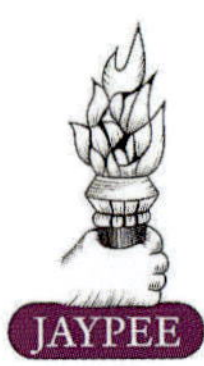

JAYPEE **Jaypee Brothers Medical Publishers (P) Ltd**

Headquarters
EMCA House, 23/23-B
Ansari Road, Daryaganj
New Delhi 110 002, India
Landline: +91-11-23272143, +91-11-23272703
+91-11-23282021, +91-11-23245672
e-mail: jaypee@jaypeebrothers.com

Corporate Office
4838/24, Ansari Road, Daryaganj
New Delhi 110 002, India
Phone: +91-11-43574357
Fax: +91-11-43574314
e-mail: jaypee@jaypeebrothers.com

Overseas Office
JP Medical Ltd.
83, Victoria Street, London
SW1H 0HW (UK)
Phone: +44-20 3170 8910
e-mail: info@jpmedpub.com

EU GPSR Authorised Representative
Logos Europe, 9 rue Nicolas Poussin
17000, La Rochelle, France
Phone: +33 (0) 6 67 93 73 78
e-mail: contact@logoseurope.eu

Website: www.jaypeebrothers.com

Website: www.jaypeedigital.com

Inquiries for bulk sales may be solicited at: jaypee@jaypeebrothers.com

***Essentials in Medical Mycology for Postgraduates* / Vasant Baradkar**

First Edition: **2026**

ISBN: 978-93-6616-116-7

Printed at: Samrat Offset Pvt. Ltd.

PREFACE

Medical mycology is probably one of the oldest branches of medical microbiology. It was considered "challenging" or "difficult". There are reasons for such views. One could be the long time required for the growth of the colonies. There are varying optimum temperatures for different fungi to grow, making it mandatory to utilize multiple culture plates/tubes to be inoculated. The identification is based mainly on colony characters and microscopic features, making it, so to say, tentative. Many saprophytes act as opportunistic pathogens. There may be cross reactions with serological and skin tests, thus making them worthless. All these factors hindered proper classification of fungi. New techniques for identification became available a few years ago. These include antigen detection and purification of antigens, which make antibody detection tests (serology) more specific. Molecular tests have revolutionized mycology.

An attempt has been made to make the text as simple and informative as possible. The book will be handy for graduate medical students; at the same time, it will be highly informative for postgraduates in microbiology.

This textbook is designed to meet that need, providing a comprehensive, clinically relevant, and academically rigorous resource for MD Microbiology postgraduate students in India. The curriculum for postgraduate medical microbiology has evolved to reflect both global scientific advancements and the specific epidemiological patterns observed in India. Fungal infections like mucormycosis, candidiasis, aspergillosis, and endemic mycoses, such as histoplasmosis and coccidioidomycosis, have become integral topics for clinical microbiologists. This textbook integrates these national concerns with foundational and advanced concepts in fungal biology, pathogenesis, diagnostics, antifungal resistance, and infection control.

The structure of this book mirrors the needs of students preparing for examinations, teaching assignments, and future clinical roles. Each chapter is written with clarity and depth, enriched with recent references, case-based discussions, and visuals that aid understanding. Emphasis has been placed on laboratory diagnosis, molecular tools, antifungal susceptibility testing, and quality control measures, all of which are essential for competent practice.

This textbook is the outcome of extensive collaboration between experienced academicians, clinicians, and researchers in the field of medical mycology. It is our hope that this work not only serves as a trusted academic resource but also inspires critical thinking, curiosity, and a lifelong interest in the fascinating world of fungi.

We welcome feedback and suggestions for future editions, as continuous learning and improvement are at the heart of both medical education and scientific progress.

Vasant Baradkar
Ajit Damle
Simit Kumar

ACKNOWLEDGMENTS

We thank M/s Jaypee Brothers Medical Publishers (P) Ltd., New Delhi, India, for giving us the opportunity to write this book. We express our gratitude to the publication team. Mr Ankit Vij (Managing Director), Mr Sabyasachi Hazra (Director–PG and PNR Content), Mrs Nedup Denka Bhutia (Publishing Manager) and Ms Kajal Keshri (Development Editor), for their professional approach and support in bringing out this publication.

CONTENTS

Section 5: Opportunistic Mycoses

Section 6: Miscellaneous Mycoses

Section 7: Pseudofungal Infections

Section 8: Annexures

SECTION

1

General Topics in Medical Mycology

Section Outline

CHAPTER 1

Introduction

The science that deals with the study of fungi is known as "mycology" [the name mycology is derived from two greek terms - mykes (fungus) + logos (study) = study of fungi]. Fungi are eukaryotic organisms placed in the kingdom "Fungi" which reproduce asexually and/or sexually by the formation of spores.

Agostino Bassi in 1835 prompted that the fungus *Beauveria bassiana* was the causative agent of silkworm disease. David Gruby (1842) suggested a fungal agent as the cause of "favus," infection of the scalp. Raymond Sabouraud studied extensively on dermatophytes. He laid down the foundation of medical mycology; hence, he is known as the "Father of Medical Mycology."

SIGNIFICANCE OF FUNGI

Some fungi are useful to human beings **(Table 1.1)** while some others are harmful, causing illnesses.

TABLE 1.1: Useful properties of fungi.

Fungus	*Uses*
Saccharomyces cerevisiae (Baker's yeast or Brewer's yeast)	• Used for baking • Used for the fermentation process to produce alcohols • Used as a cellular model to study many metabolic processes • Preparation of recombinant vaccine
Penicillium chrysogenum	Production of penicillin
Acremonium chrysogenum	Production of cephalosporins
Penicillium griseofulvin	Production of antifungal agent, griseofulvin
Aspergillus nidulans	Production of anidulafungin
Saccharomyces boulardii	Used as a probiotic
Endomyces	Production of fat
Claviceps purpurea	Ergot alkaloid production
Aspergillus terreus	Production of simvastatin

BURDEN OF FUNGAL INFECTIONS

An estimate in 2017 points out that about 1.5 million deaths and more than a billion infections occur due to to fungi worldwide. These figures underline the importance of medical mycolgy.

COMMON FUNGI AFFECTING HUMANS

- *Candida albicans* and other *Candida* species: Common infections include mucocutaneous infections such as oral thrush. Also, bloodstream infections are common.
- *Cryptococcus neoformans*: It causes meningitis in acquired immunodeficiency syndrome (AIDS) patients.
- *Aspergillus*: It causes pulmonary aspergillosis.
- Zygomycetes fungi such as *Rhizopus, Rhizomucor*, and *Absidia* may cause fungal rhinosinusitis.
- *Common dermatophytic fungi*: *Trichophyton rubrum, Trichophyton mentagrophyte*, and *Microsporum canis.*
- Pigmented fungi cause conditions such as chromoblastomycosis.
- *Deep fungi (endemic fungi)*: These fungi are also known as systemic fungi, and they can cause systemic infections even in immunocompetent individuals.

FUNGAL INFECTION BY ANATOMICAL SITE

- *Superficial mycoses*: Infection is limited to the upper (keratinized) layers of skin and its appendages.
- *Cutaneous mycosis*: Infection goes deeper to involve the epidermis. Hairs and nails may also get infected. Inflammation is expected.

- *Subcutaneous infections*: There is involvement of dermis and subcutaneous tissue; bone and muscles may be involved.
- *Systemic mycosis or deep mycosis*: The lung is the primary site of infection from where the fungus may disseminate to other sites of the body.

Fungal infection or disease is called mycosis (plural = mycoses). Some special mycoses are introduced here.

OPPORTUNISTIC MYCOSES

Fungi cause infections in immunocompromised patients. These infections are known as opportunistic mycoses. The following is the list of susceptible hosts:

- People living with human immunodeficiency virus (HIV)/AIDS
- Organ transplant patients
- Cancer patients
- Hospitalized patients
- Stem cell transplant patients
- People taking medicines that weaken the immunity, e.g., corticosteroids, immunosuppressants, or anti-metabolites
- Uncontrolled diabetes
- Renal failure patients

OPPORTUNISTIC INFECTIONS COMMON IN DIFFERENT POPULATIONS

Mucormycosis is common in diabetic patients. *Candida* and *Aspergillus* infections are common in solid organ transplant patients. *Candida, Cryptococcus,* and *Histoplasma* infections are seen in patients with long-term administration of antibiotics. Cytotoxic therapy leading to granulocytopenia makes the patient susceptible to *Candida* and *Aspergillus.* Chronic granulomatous disease patients are susceptible to *Aspergillus* and *Candida* infections. *Aspergillus* produces disease in graft-versus-host disease. Neutropenic patients may suffer from *Candida, Aspergillus, Fusarium, Allescheria boydii,* and *Trichosporon* infection, along with mucormycotic infections.

EMERGING AND REMERGING FUNGAL INFECTIONS

- An increasing number of cases of invasive candidiasis are caused by *Candida* species that are not albicans. There are increasing reports of a new species, i.e., *Candida auris*. This yeast does not respond to antifungals. It could be transmitted through healthcare facilities, which is a major concern because the disease is spreading fast globally.
- Patients with cancer or organ transplants are actually at a higher risk of acquiring fungal infections due to immunosuppression. However, nowadays they are less likely to experience invasive fungal illness, thanks to antifungal prophylaxis. The mold disease burden in these patients is now mostly caused by nonfumigatus *Aspergillus* species, Mucorales, and *Scedosporium/Lomentospora* species.
- The extensive use of topical antifungals in conjunction with corticosteroids has led to the development of resistant dermatophytosis caused by *Trichophyton mentagrophytes* genotype VIII in India. It has now spread beyond India. It has been named *Trichophyton indotineae.*
- Mycoses caused by the novel dimorphic fungal pathogen *Emergomyces* are common worldwide, especially in people with HIV.
- New blastomycosis pathogens, *Blastomyces helicus* in Western North America and *Blastomyces percursus* in Africa, were discovered recently.
- *Sporothrix* is a zoonotic sporotrichosis that has recently emerged as a major health concern in Brazil, affecting both cats and humans. Prior to genetic investigations, the only species known to be involved in the disease was *Sporothrix schenckii.* However, additional species such as *Sporothrix globosa, Sporothrix mexicana, Sporothrix luriei,* and *Sporothrix brasiliensis* have been described since the early 2000s. *Sporothrix brasiliensis* can cause severe inflammatory reactions. In addition, *S. brasiliensis* is linked to zoonotic (rather than sapronotic) transmission in cats, which is different from other sporotrichosis causes.
- Fungal infection risk categories for patients have changed. The B-cell cancer drug ibrutinib (that acts as Bruton's tyrosine kinase inhibitor) has been linked to the infection by *Aspergillus* and *Cryptococcus* in patients taking this drug. The relapsing-remitting multiple sclerosis drug fingolimod has been associated in certain patients with cryptococcosis and histoplasmosis.
- *New infections caused by yeasts*: *Candida glabrata* are currently responsible for more than 30% of candidemia infections in the United States. This is concerning because *C. glabrata* is associated with greater rates of antifungal resistance. Ten percent or more of *C. glabrata* strains in some environments have developed resistance to echinocandins due to mutations in the FKS1 hot spot. Also, a newly emerged species is *C. auris.*
- Due to a lack of data, the global distribution of *Cryptococcus bacillisporus* cannot be determined; however, it is known to mostly impact immunocompromised and HIV-positive hosts. There had been an earlier epidemic of *Cryptococcus deuterogattii*

in the Pacific Northwest and on Vancouver Island. *C. deuterogattii* has a higher isavuconazole minimum inhibitory concentration (MIC) than other species.

- *Mold infections other than Aspergillus*: Immunosuppressed hosts have also shown an upsurge in infections caused by *Fusarium* species and *Lomentospora prolificans*, the latter of which is more resistant to voriconazole and posaconazole. Isolates of *L. prolificans* show resistance to almost all systemically active antifungals, such as azoles, terbinafine, and amphotericin B.

NOSOCOMIAL FUNGAL INFECTIONS

Candida species cause nosocomial bloodstream infection. *Aspergillus* species, Mucorales, and *Fusarium* species are other fungi causing nosocomial infections. The risk factors are:

- Colonization
- Neutropenia
- Broad-spectrum antibiotics
- Corticosteroids
- Central venous catheter
- HIV
- Parenteral nutrition
- Diabetes mellitus
- Gastrointestinal or cardiac surgery
- Prolonged hospital and intensive care unit (ICU) stay
- Burns
- Premature neonate

ZOONOTIC FUNGAL INFECTIONS

Animals can act as a source of fungal infection to humans. Some examples are mentioned as follows:

- *Microsporum* species and *Trichophyton* species: Dermatophytosis can be caused by direct contact with sick animals on a global scale. Infectious agents can originate from any domestic mammal or even wild animals.
- *Sporothrix schenckii* and *S. brasiliensis*: Animal bites and scrapes can spread germs and infection. Alligators, pigs, horses, cows, camels, dolphins, goats, mules, armadillos, birds, and occasionally dogs can act as sources of infection.
- *Malassezia* species causing tinea versicolor infections can be transmitted from domestic animals such as dogs, cats, cows, sheep, pigs, horses, and wild animals kept in captivity or found in the wild.
- *Lacazia loboi*: Infection and the resulting granulomatous illness originate in dolphins.
- *Emmonsia species*: Adiaspiromycosis is caused by this fungus and spreads by rodents found in the wild. Infections in the lungs and other organs may spread.
- *Penicillium (Talaromyces) marneffei*: Potential vectors for infection include bamboo rats and domestic animals such as dogs and cats.
- *Cryptococcus neoformans and Cryptococcus gattii*: Fungus can infect a broad range of mammals, birds, reptiles, and amphibians all throughout the world, most commonly through inhalation but also through skin breaks on rare occasions.
- *Histoplasma capsulatum*: Inhaled fungal spores cause infection. An illness can spread from cattle, sheep, or horses.

Some fungi occur as filamentous as well as yeast forms (usually at different temperatures). Such thermally dimorphic fungi cause different infections. Their geographic distribution is specific. These points are shown in **Table 1.2**.

To summarize, with the increasing number of immunocompromised patients and the simultaneous development of resistance in the fungal population, fungal infections are becoming more common and difficult to treat.

TABLE 1.2: List of mycotic diseases caused by their corresponding dimorphic fungi.

Fungus	*Disease*	*Geographic distribution*
Histoplasma capsulatum	Histoplasmosis	North America, Central and South America
Blastomyces dermatitidis	Blastomycosis	North America, particularly the Mississippi and Ohio River valleys
Coccidioides immitis	Coccidioidomycosis (Valley fever)	Southwestern United States, Mexico, Central and South America
Paracoccidioides brasiliensis	Paracoccidioidomycosis	Central and South America, especially Brazil
Sporothrix schenckii	Sporotrichosis (rose gardener's disease)	Worldwide, particularly in tropical and subtropical regions
Talaromyces (Penicillium marneffei)	Talaromycosis (penicilliosis)	Southeast Asia, especially Thailand, Vietnam, and southern China
Emmonsia species	Emmonsiosis (adiaspiromycosis)	North America, Europe, Africa, and Asia
Emergomyces species	Emergomycosis	Africa, particularly South Africa; cases reported in Europe and North America

CHAPTER

2

Morphology of Fungi

INTRODUCTION

Fungi are eukaryotic organisms. They differ from bacteria in many aspects. They contain ergosterol in the cell membrane (cytoplasmic membrane) except *Pneumocystis*. They can produce sexual or asexual reproductive spores. A true nucleus with a nuclear membrane is present. Mitochondria and endoplasmic reticulum are present in their cytoplasm. Fungi may be unicellular or multicellular.

Morphologically, two basic units of fungi are yeasts and molds.

YEASTS

Yeasts are unicellular fungi. They divide by an asexual method called budding. The spores produced by budding are called blastopores, also known as blastoconidia. The daughter cell again divides to form blastoconidia of the next generation. Yeast colonies often have a smooth surface (pasty colonies) **(Fig. 2.1A)**. Yeast with a capsule such as *Cryptococcus neoformans* produces mucoid colony **(Fig. 2.1B)**. How yeast cells look like in a wet mount is shown in **Figure 2.2**. They appear gram positive, as shown in **Figure 2.3**.

Types of Budding

- *Narrow-based budding*: Most of the medically important yeasts (or yeast-like cells) divide by narrow base, e.g., *Candida*, *Cryptococcus*, *Rhodotorula*, and *Malassezia*.
- Broad-based budding is seen in *Blastomyces dermatitidis*, as shown in **Figure 2.4**.

Schizosaccharomyces also shows similar budding. In *Talaromyces marneffei* (previously *Penicillium marneffei*), there is a septum between yeast cells, and they appear as budding by a broad base **(Fig. 2.5)**.

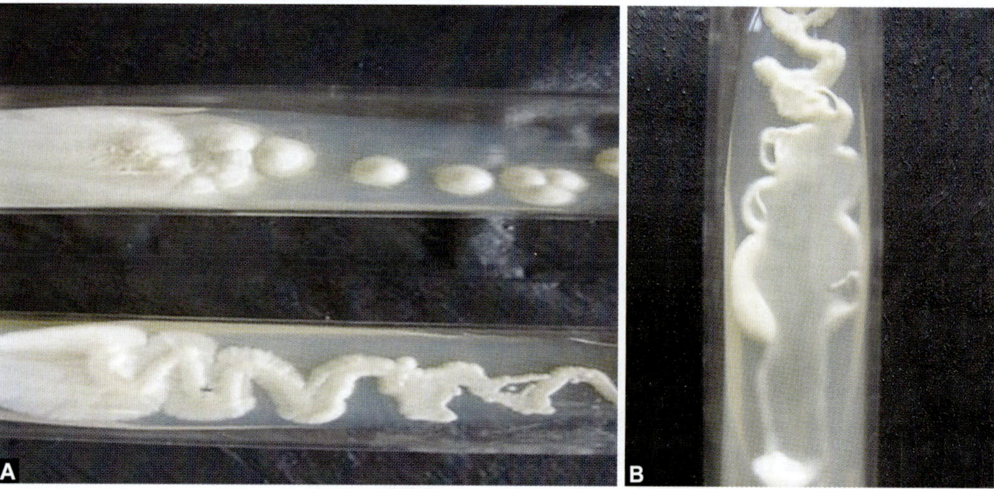

FIGS. 2.1A AND B: (A) Pasty colonies of yeasts on SDA; (B) Mucoid colonies of *Cryptococcus* species on SDA.
(SDA: Sabouraud Dextrose Agar)

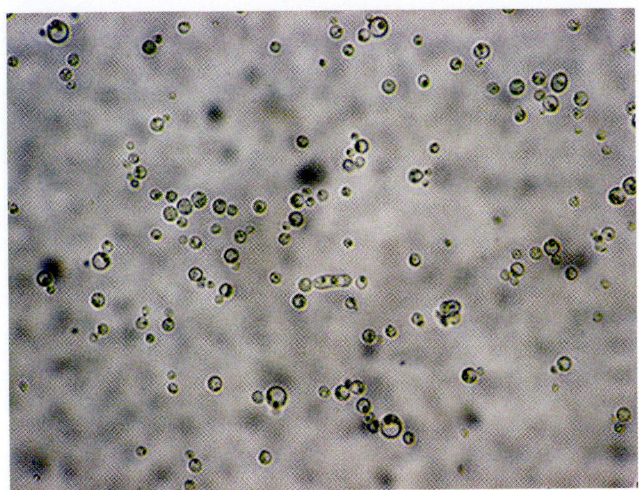

FIG. 2.2: Yeast cells in wet mount (400×).

Division by Fission or Transverse Septum Formation

The other method of division of yeast cells is fission (planate division) by formation of transverse septa. Examples are *Schizosaccharomyces* species, *Talaromyces marneffei* (previously *Penicillium marneffei*), and *Malassezia* species. Planate division is seen in the fungi causing chromoblastomycosis which gives rise to the formation of muriform bodies, as shown in **Figure 2.6**.

Exophiala werneckii is a dematiaceous fungus, yeast cells of which also show septum.

Single Bud versus Multiple Bud

Budding is also considered as either single bud formation or multiple bud formation from a parent yeast cell. Most

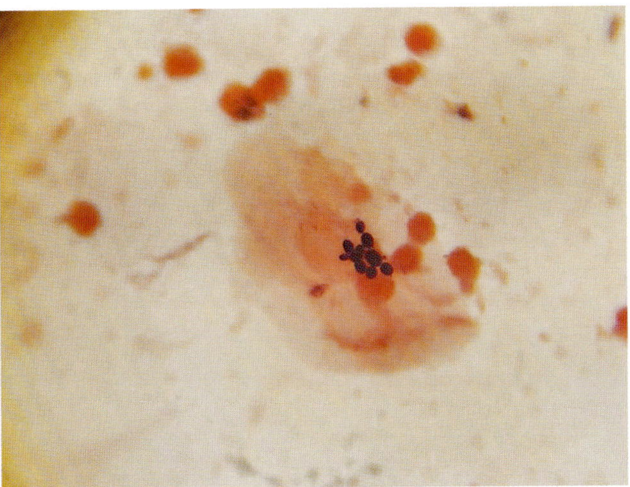

FIG. 2.3: Yeast cells in Gram-stained smear.

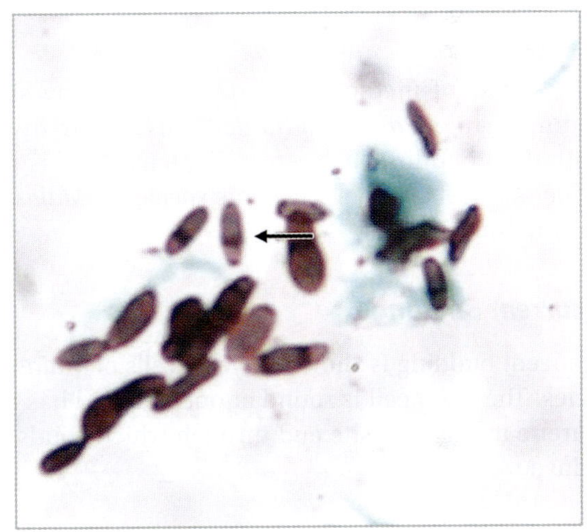

FIG. 2.5: Budding of *Talaromyces marneffei* (1,000×).
Note: Septum formation (arrow).

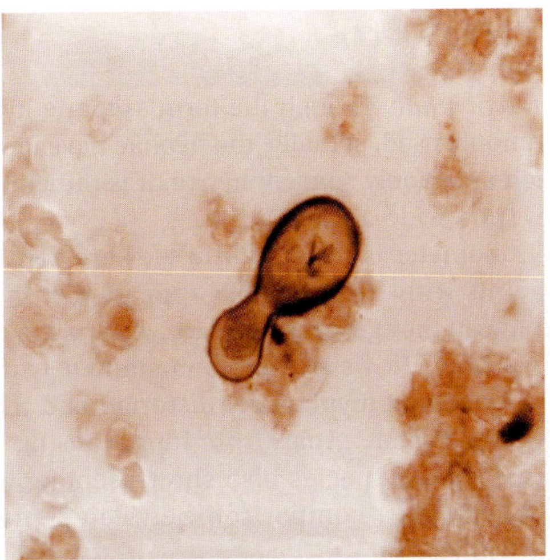

FIG. 2.4: Broad-based budding of *Blastomyces* species (1,000×).
Source: Public Health Image Library CDC.

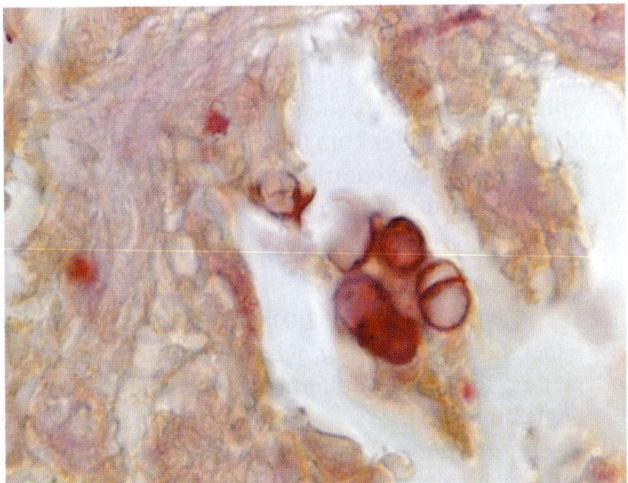

FIG. 2.6: Muriform cells seen in chromoblastomycosis (400×).
Source: Public Health Image Library CDC.

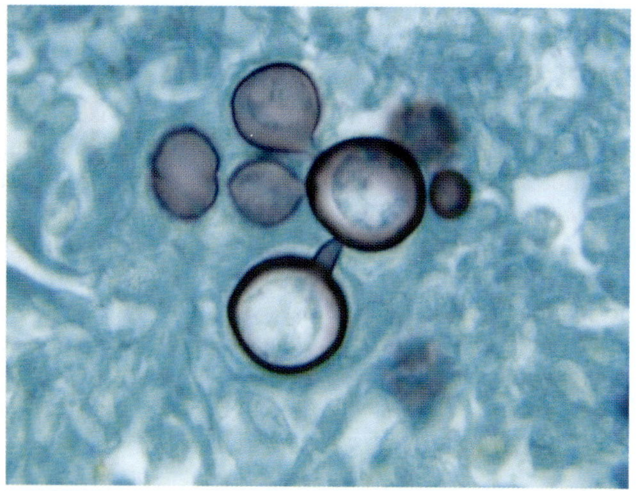

FIG. 2.7: Multiple budding shown by *Paracoccidioides brasiliensis* (1,000×).
Source: Public Health Image Library CDC.

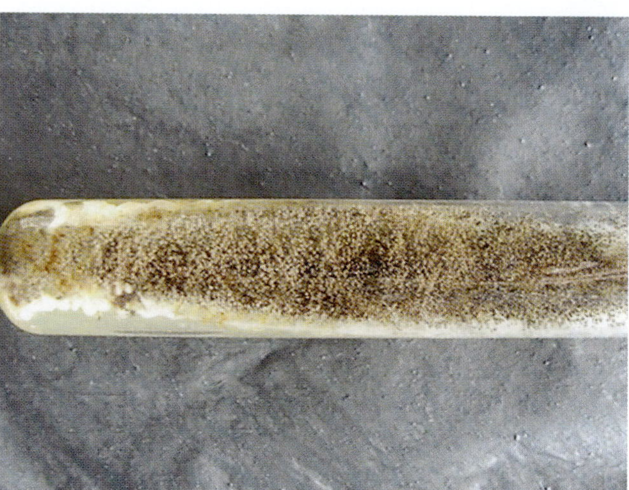

FIG. 2.8: Fluffy colonies of mold on SDA.
(SDA: Sabouraud Dextrose Agar)

of the yeasts of medical importance divide by single budding, while *Paracoccidioides brasiliensis* divides by multiple budding, as seen in **Figure 2.7**. This gives mariner's wheel appearance. Some species of *Malassezia* show multiple budding.

Percurrent Budding

Percurrent budding is shown by yeast cells of *Malassezia* species. The yeast cell is round at one end and has a flat collarette at the opposite end through which "buds" are produced.

MOLDS

Molds are multicellular fungi. They are made up of filament-like structures called hyphae. Hence, they are also called "filamentous fungi." They are formed by apical elongation. A group of hyphae or clusters is known as mycelium. Mycelium is seen in molds. The colonies of molds drastically differ from those of yeast cells.

Tube-like hyphae contribute to the fluffy appearance of macroscopic "mold" colonies **(Fig. 2.8)**.

There are two types of hyphae based on the presence or absence of septa:

1. *Septate hyphae* **(Fig. 2.9)** which are present in *Aspergillus, Penicillium, Fusarium,* and many other genera. They have a uniform diameter and show acute angle branching.
2. *Aseptate hyphae* ***(Fig. 2.10)***: *Mucor* and *Mucor*-like fungi (zygomycotic fungi) have *aseptate or sparsely septate hyphae.* Though the term aseptate hyphae is commonly used, actually, the hyphae have few septae which are widely spaced; hence, it is difficult to see. They show wide-angle branching.

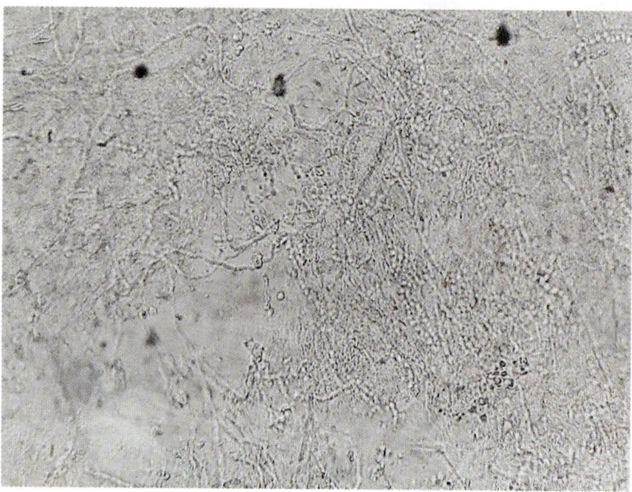

FIG. 2.9: Septate hyphae in KOH mount (400×).
(KOH: potassium hydroxide)

Their diameter is not uniform; they are collapsed at some points with "ribbon"-like appearance. In Gram-stained smear, they get easily decolorized and may appear Gram variable. In tissue sections stained with H&E, sometimes, septate hyphae get distorted and may look like aseptate hyphae. Apart from fungi causing mucormycosis, *Pythium* species also show aseptate hyphae. **Table 2.1** shows a comparison between septate and aseptate hyphae.

Hyaline Hyphae versus Dematiaceous Hyphae

Most of the fungi produce colorless hyphae, also known as hyaline hyphae. On the contrary, brown to black pigmented, i.e., dematiaceous hyphae, are seen in melanin (or melanin-like pigment) producing fungi. Such fungi are called dematiaceous fungi or melanoid fungi. The hyphae of dematiaceous fungi appear dark brown to black in wet mount, as shown in **Figure 2.11**. The presence of melanin on the cell wall causes dematiaceous fungi to display hyphae that are black in color. These fungi produce two types of infections: (1) Chromoblastomycosis and (2) phaeohyphomycosis. They have dematiaceous hyphae; hence, they are called "dematiaceous fungi" or melanoid fungi. Note that dematiaceous fungi show septate hyphae.

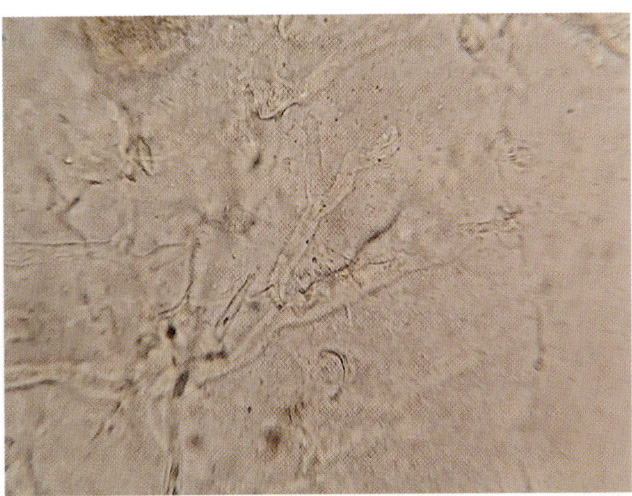

FIG. 2.10: Aseptate hyphae in KOH mount (400×). (KOH: potassium hydroxide)

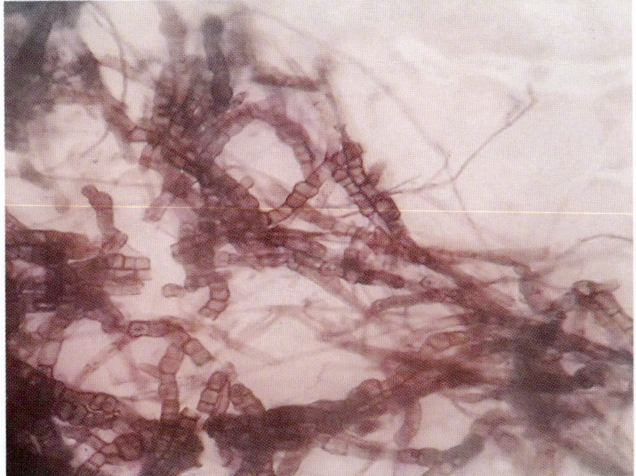

FIG. 2.11: Dematiaceous hyphae in wet mount (400×).

Pseudohyphae versus True Hyphae

Pseudohyphae: Yeast cells may elongate, without separating from each other and they may form a chain. These structures are called pseudohyphae. They differ from true hyphae in that there is constriction at the base and their diameter is not uniform. **Figure 2.12** shows pseudohyphae in a Gram-stained smear. Pseudohyphae are seen in *Candida* species. *Candida albicans* may show true hyphae and pseudohyphae along with budding yeast cells. Some other commonly isolated *Candida* species such as *Candida tropicalis, Candida parapsilosis, and Candida krusei* show pseudohyphae, while some of the species of *Candida* such as *Candida auris, Candida haemulonii, Candida glabrata*, and *Candida famata* do not show pseudohyphae; they appear as yeast cells only.

TABLE 2.1: Comparison between septate and aseptate hyphae.

Characteristics of aseptate hyphae of mucormycosis	*Septate hyphae of Aspergillosis*
• Broad hyphae (5–25 μm diameter), nonparallel walls • Sparsely septate hyphae • Characteristically twisted, collapsed, and folded in a ribbon-like fashion • Branching is irregularly spaced, nondichotomous, and at various angles (often at right angles) to the parent hypha	• Mostly 3–6 μm in diameter • Dichotomous branching (each branch is approximately equal in width to the originating parent hypha) at 45° angles

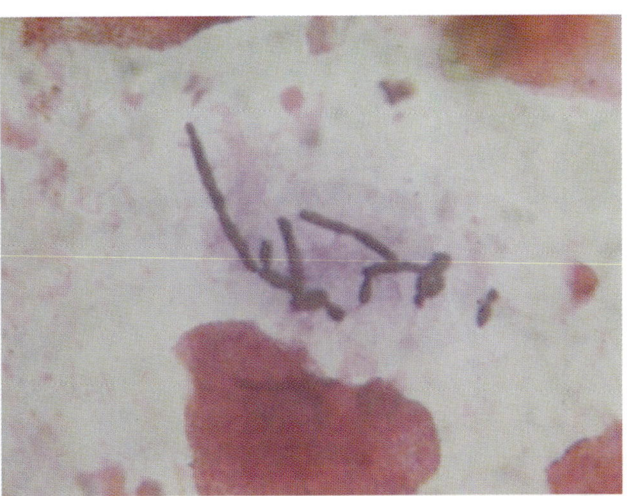

FIG. 2.12: Gram-stained smear showing yeast cells with pseudohyphae (1,000×).

Roughly depending upon morphology, fungi are classified into the following groups:

- *Yeasts*: These are spherical to oval unicellular fungi. These reproduce by budding, e.g., *Cryptococcus neoformans.*
- *Yeast-like fungi*: These are also spherical to oval unicellular fungi. They reproduce by budding and also show pseudohyphae. *Candida* species are yeast-like fungi.
- *Molds*: They have true hyphae. A group of hyphae is called mycelium. *Aspergillus, Penicillium, Mucor,* and fungi causing dermatophytosis are true molds.
- *Dimorphic fungi*: These fungi show two different morphological forms at two different temperatures. In host and culture at 37°C shows yeast forms, while in their natural habitat and in culture at room temperature (25°C) they are molds. The fungi causing systemic infections such as *Histoplasma* and *Blastomyces* are examples of dimorphic fungi. They are distributed in certain geographical areas and are also called "endemic fungi."

This classification is not foolproof. For practical purpose, we use the term yeast-like fungi of dimorphic fungi for the forms seen in tissues. Also, in the genus *Candida*, there are some species such as *C. glabrata, C. famata,* and *C. auris* that show only yeast cells without pseudohyphae.

Black yeasts: *Aureobasidium pullulans, Wangiella dermatitidis, Exophiala jeanselmei, Exophiala spinifera,* and *Hortaea werneckii* are the dematiaceous fungi which may show yeasts form at some stages, and they are called black yeasts. Their colonies initially may appear moist.

Based upon sexual spores produced by fungi, they are classified into Zygomycetes, Ascomycetes, Basidiomycetes, and Deuteromycetes. **Figure 2.13A** shows ascus produced by *Aspergillus nidulans* (ascomycete fungus) and **Figure 2.13B** shows zygospore produced by *Rhizopus* (zygomycotic fungus).

Vegetative Structures

Vegetative hyphae are useful in identifying and differentiating most of the fungi causing human infections.

Chlamydoconidium (Chlamydospores) (Fig. 2.14)

These asexual spores or conidia are thick walled and develop in nutritionally deficient media, e.g., cornmeal agar with Tween 80. They can sustain in adverse conditions. The word chlamydoconidia is now preferred over chlamydospores.

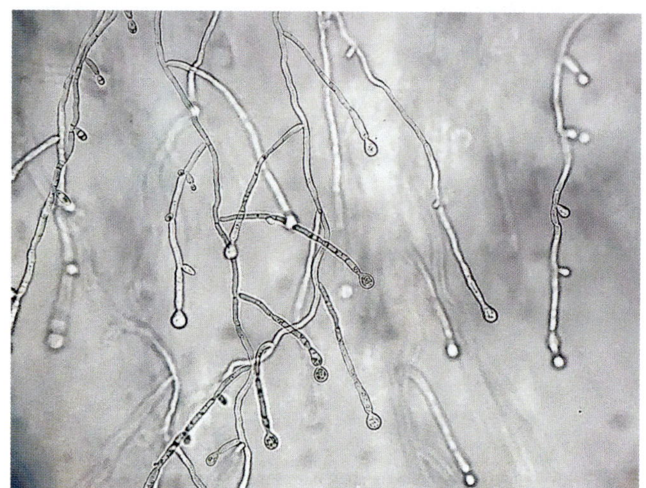

FIG. 2.14: Terminal chlamydoconidia of *Candida albicans*.

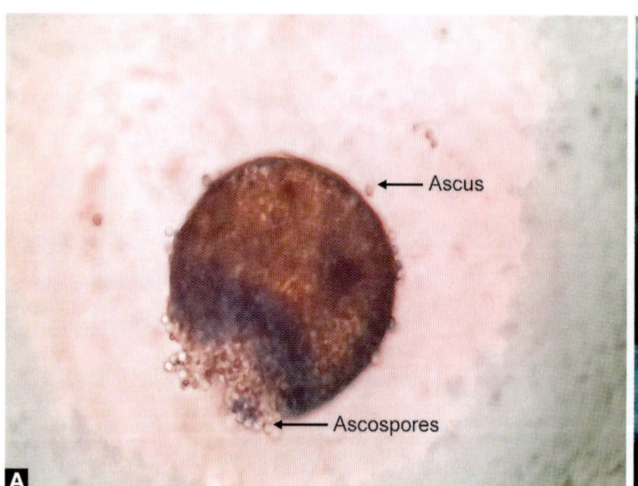

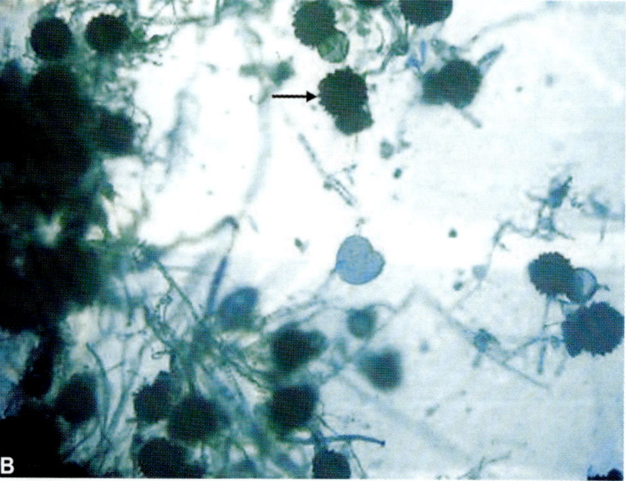

FIGS. 2.13A AND B: (A) Ascus with ascospores released; (B) Zygospores of *Rhizomucor* (mucormycosis).

Uses of chlamydoconidia in the identification of fungi:
- Among the *Candida* species, these are seen in *Candida albicans* and *Candida dubliniensis*. Other *Candida* species do not produce chlamydoconidia. Based on their position, they are classified as terminal or intercalary. *Candida dubliniensis* shows both terminal and intercalary chlamydoconidia. As other yeasts do not produce these conidia, their presence is one of the identification features. The production of these conidia may be common in some molds. **Figure 2.14** shows terminal chlamydoconidia produced by *C. albicans*.
- *Among molds*: Many fungi may show these spores. However, the presence of these spores predominantly in mounts from culture is seen in *Trichophyton violaceum*, *Trichophyton verrucosum*, and *Madurella mycetomatis*.

Arthroconidia (Arthrospores)

These rectangular cells are formed by fragmentation and separation of hyphal elements. The fungi which predominantly show the presence of arthroconidia in culture are *Geotrichum, Trichosporon, Coccidioidomyces, Neostylidium, Arthrographis*, and *Malbranchea*. **Figure 2.15** shows lactophenol cotton blue (LPCB) mount from culture of *Geotrichum* species showing arthroconidia. The presence of hyphae along with arthroconidia is a characteristic finding of potassium hydroxide (KOH) mount of dermatophytes (skin, nail, and hair infections). **Figure 2.16** shows arthroconidia in a direct KOH mount of skin scraping from a case of dermatophyte lesion.

Some morphological characteristics of hyphal types which help in identification of fungi are **(Fig. 2.17)** given as follows:
- *Spiral hyphae*: These are coiled hyphae. These are usually seen in *Trichophyton mentagrophytes.*
- *Nodular organ or knot body*: An enlarged part of hyphae in clusters gets twisted like a swelling. These may be seen in *T. mentagrophytes* and *Microsporum canis.*
- *Racquet hyphae*: There is regular enlargement of one end of each segment within hyphae. These are seen in *T. mentagrophytes* and *Epidermophyton floccosum.*
- *Pectinate hyphae*: One side of hyphae shows irregular perturbances giving a "comb"-like appearance, especially seen in *Microsporum audouinii.*
- *Favic chandeliers*: Terminally hyphae show many branches, and the whole structure resembles chandelier or reindeer horn. These are predominantly seen in *Trichophyton schoenleinii.*
- *Peridial hyphae*: The multiseptate hyphae are wide and indented which may end in a spiral structure. This may be seen in *Trichophyton mentagrophytes.*
- *Pycnidium*: It is a flask-shaped structure of hyphae inside which asexual conidia are produced. It resembles perithecium which is also a saclike structure, but it contains sexual spores.

REPRODUCTION IN FUNGI

Fungi may reproduce by sexual method or asexual method (or both). The asexual stage is called imperfect stage, while sexual stage is called perfect stage or

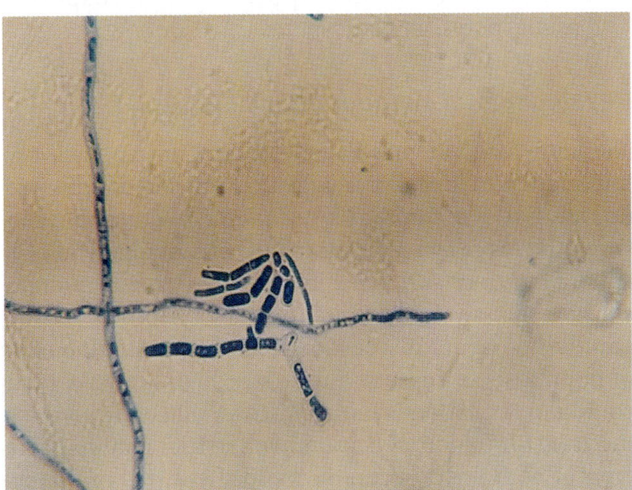

FIG. 2.15: LPCB mount from growth showing arthroconidia (400×). (LPCB: lactophenol cotton blue)

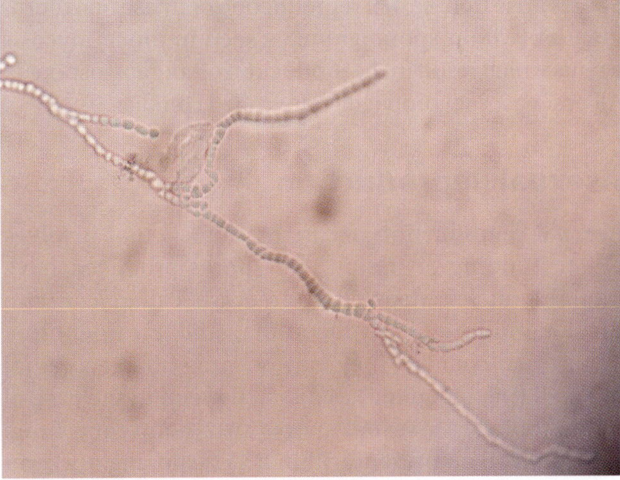

FIG. 2.16: KOH mount of skin scraping showing arthroconidia (400×). (KOH: potassium hydroxide)

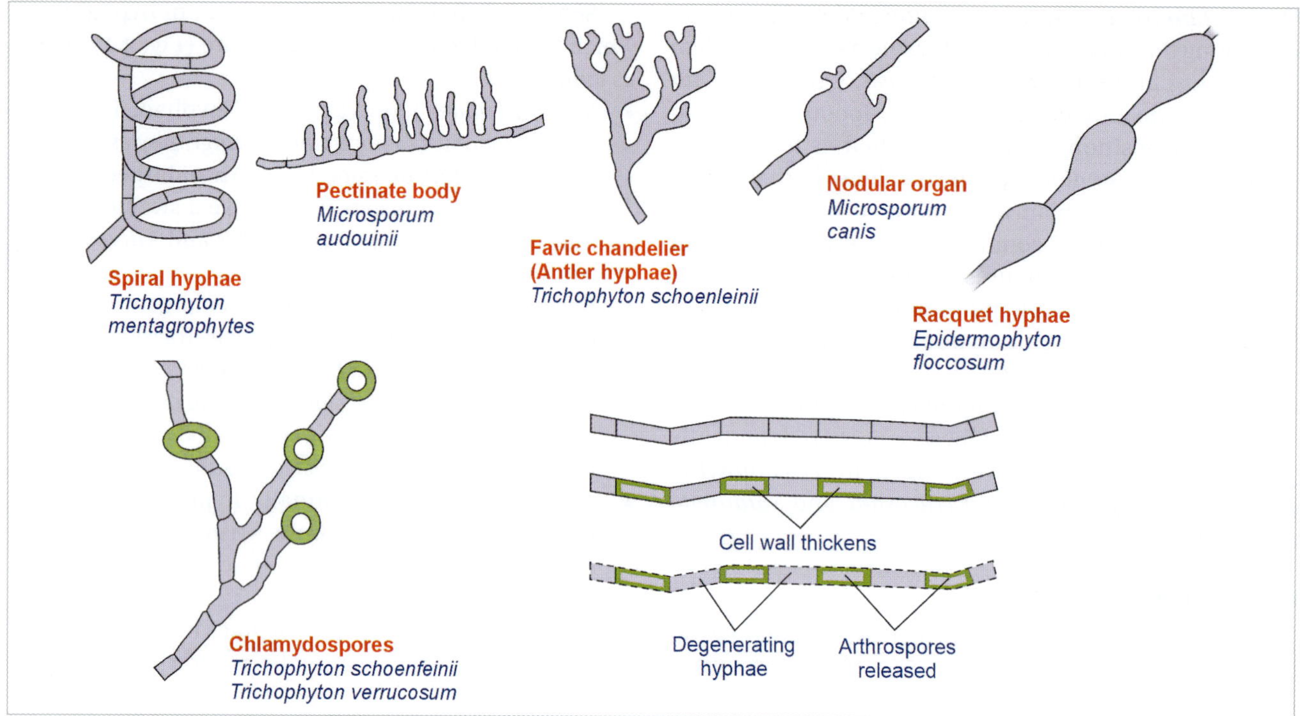

FIG. 2.17: Special types of hyphae.

teleomorphic stage. Usually, when grown on fungal culture media, mostly asexual spores are produced; the morphological features of these help in the identification of the fungus. Two terms are commonly used while describing units of reproduction of fungi: (1) Conidia and (2) Spores.

Terms Spores and Conidia

Spores arise from sexual reproduction or by asexual reproduction (within sporangium, as seen in mucormycosis agents which result in the production of sporangiospores). All other asexual propagules are called conidia.

Asexual Reproduction

Asexual reproduction occurs by mitosis that involves either budding or fission and spores produced have haploid nuclei. Asexual spores are called *conidia*. Blastoconidia, chlamydoconidia, and arthroconidia are asexual conidia. They may be large (macroconidia) or small (microconidia) as distinctly seen in the case of dermatophytes. Asexual spores in zygomycotic fungi (Mucorales) are present within a sac (sporangium) and are called sporangiospores. Exogenous spores are seen in *Aspergillus* and *Penicillium.*

Some arrangements of exogenous conidia are given as follows:

- *Acropetal*: Spores are in a chain, having the youngest spore at the top, e.g., *Alternaria* and *Cladosporium.*
- *Basipetal*: Youngest spore is at the base, e.g., *Aspergillus.*
- *Sympodial*: There is a zigzag pattern, e.g., *Bipolaris.*
- Examples of sexual spores are ascospores, basidiospores, and zygospores.

Developmental Methods of Conidia

The knowledge of conidiogenesis may not appear very important for clinical mycologists as they do not observe the methods of conidiosis on a light microscope, but knowledge is relevant for a mycologist. Conidiogenesis is either *blastic* or *thallic* type. In *blastic* type, new conidium starts which swells and is cut off by a septum. *Blastic* conidiosis occurs in yeasts and molds. In *thallic* type of conidiosis, a septum appears in hypha after which conidium formation is initiated. The thallic type involves the transformation of certain hyphae into conidia. This type of conidiosis occurs in molds. Arthric conidia as arthroconidia are specialized conidia formed from thallic conidiogenesis which disarticulate readily.

Holothallic and holoblastic conidiation: When the wall of the conidium is in continuation with the wall of cell which produced it, it is called holothallic (when thallic types) or holoblastic (when blastic).

Enterothallic and enteroblastic: In these types only the inner walls of conidium-bearing cell are involved in conidiogenesis.

Fungi showing different types of conidiogenesis are given as follows:
- *Holoblastic*: *Trichocladium* (not clinically significant)
- *Enteroblastic*: *Acremonium, Bipolaris,* and *Talaromyces*
- *Holothallic*: *Geotrichum*
- *Holoblastic*: *Coccidioides*

Arrangements of Conidia

Conidia may arise directly on hyphae or specialized hyphae called conidiophores. *Conidiophore, phialide, annelide.*

Sometimes, hyphae are the only source of conidia. However, annelide and phialide (specialized hyphae) are present in certain fungi and are responsible for bearing conidia. Specialized conidiophores may be either phialide or annelide (thus, while describing morphology, conidia are seen on conidiophore, annelide, or phialide).
- *Phialide*: Specialized conidiogenous cells called phialides produce conidia in a basipetal succession without the need for the conidiogenous cell's length to expand. In simple words, with progressive production of new conidia, the length of the phialide does not increase.
- *Annelide*: A specialized cell type that produces conidia in a basipetal succession through a series of brief *percurrent proliferations* is called an annelid. The annelid tip grows longer and narrower with each passing year.

Such changes can be observed when slide cultures made from fungal growth are regularly observed.

Some Definitions of Some Asexual Conidia

- *Blastoconidium*: Conidium is produced by budding from hyphae or a single yeast cell as seen in *Candida* species.
- *Aleurioconidium*: These are produced when a conidium expands directly from hyphae or conidiophores. They have a truncated base and fracture away from base.
- *Annelloconidium*: Conidia produced from annelid.
- *Phialoconidium*: Unlike annelloconidia, conidia made from phialide.
- Arthroconidium (described earlier)
- *Sporangiospores*: Asexual conidia produced inside a sac-like structure called sporangium. These are seen in the members of mucormycosis.
- *Adiaconidium (adiaspores)*: These are seen in *adiaspiromycosis* caused by *Emmonsia crescens* and *Emmonsia parva*. They are large, globular structures which enlarge to form a spherule.
- Chlamydoconidium (chlamydospores)

Sexual Reproduction

Sexual reproduction occurs with mating of compatible strains. Haploid strains fuse to form a diploid. The types of sexual spores produced are ascospores, basidiospores, and zygospores. This forms the basis on which fungi can be divided into Ascomycetes, Basidiomycetes, and Mucormycetes.

COMPOSITION AND STRUCTURE OF FUNGAL CELL WALL

Structural Organization and Cell Wall Layers (FIG. 2.18)

The basic framework of fungal walls is a strong scaffold made of carbohydrate polymers that are both fibrous and gel-like. The fungal cell wall can be tentatively divided into inner and outer cell walls.

Chitin (innermost, being near the cytoplasmic membrane also known as cell membrane) and covalently bound branching β-(1,3) glucan and β-(1,6) glucan make up the inner cell wall. These give the cell its strength and resilience against internal hydrostatic pressure.

Melanin is present in some fungal cell walls. It is an amorphous polymerized phenolic chemical. It may be present in the inner wall, outer wall, or throughout the cell wall. Melanin provides extra protection against harsh conditions such as temperature and osmotic pressure fluctuations.

Fungi can have different outer layers, but they often have gelatinous capsules, α-(1,3) glucan, or glycoproteins that are heavily mannosylated.

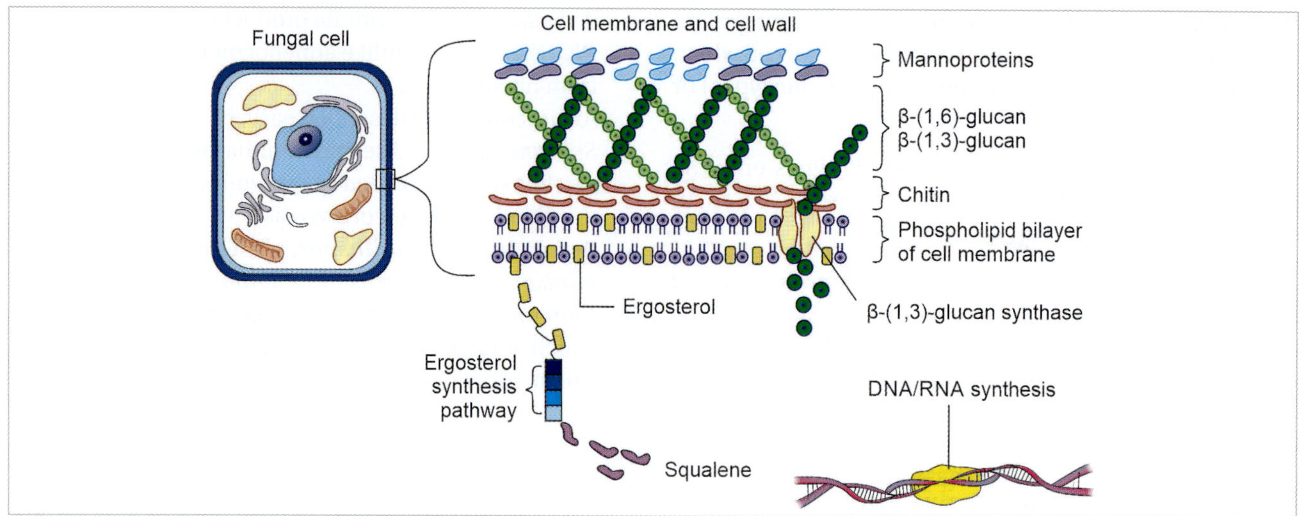

FIG. 2.18: Composition and structure of fungal cell wall.

Major Components of the Fungal Cell Wall

- *Branched β-(1,3) glucan and chitin*:
  - The central region of the inner cellular membrane
  - Supports the structure and prevents the buildup of internal hydrostatic pressure
  - A scaffold of fibrous microfibrils formed via covalent cross-linking
- *Mannoproteins*:
  - The inner cell wall is coated with glycoproteins that have been highly mannosylated.
  - Glucan and the chitin core in specific yeasts are connected through glycosylphosphatidylinositol remnants.
- *Capsules*: Glucuronoxylomannan (GXM) and galactoxylomannan (GalXM) are the components of the gelatinous capsules produced by *Cryptococcus neoformans*.
- *Hydrophobins*:
  - An extremely hydrophobic layer covers all filamentous fungi and their conidia.
  - The layer is made up of tightly packed fibrillar structures called "rodlets." They render the conidia resistant to wetting and desiccation.

DIMORPHISM IN FUNGI AND ITS RELEVANCE TO HUMAN HEALTH

Overview

Some fungi show different morphological forms when grown at different temperatures. These fungi grow as the yeast form when the culture medium is incubated at 37°C. On the culture medium incubated at 25°C (room temperature), their growth is like filamentous fungus. These dimorphic fungi occur as yeasts in the human body and filamentous form in the environment.

Types of Dimorphic Fungi

- *Thermally dimorphic fungi*:
  - The capacity to adjust its body temperature and transform into either yeast or a hypha makes it unique.
  - Anyone, even those with perfectly healthy immune systems, can get an infection.
  - As an example, there are sporotrichosis, blastomycosis, histoplasmosis, coccidioidomycosis, and paracoccidioidomycosis.
  - Those whose immune systems are already weak, including those with advanced HIV infection, are more likely to contract illnesses such as penicilliosis and emmonsiosis.
- *Nonthermal dimorphic fungi*:
  - This can also cause human infections (e.g., *Malassezia furfur*).
  - More commonly associated with phytopathogenic or entomopathogenic activities.

A unique class of Ascomycetes, thermally dimorphic fungi, can infect hosts with normal or compromised immune systems. A crucial factor in their pathogenicity is their ability to change morphologies from hyphae to yeast and adapt to the host's core body temperature of 37°C. During this transitional phase, several virulence factors are upregulated, which play a role in pathogenesis in multiple ways. These factors include the ability to adhere to tissues, survive and replicate within cells, avoid appropriate cytokine responses, and compromise cell-mediated immunity.

KEY INSIGHTS

- *Morphological phase transition*:
  - Dimorphic fungi's biology and way of life revolve around the reversible phase transition, which involves the transformation from hyphae to yeast.
  - These fungi develop as septate hyphae in soil between 22 and 25°C, but they transform into pathogenic yeast when breathed into the heated lungs of a mammalian host, which is 37°C, and cause pneumonia. The yeast can then spread to other parts of the body.
- *Factors influencing phase transition*:
  - Hyphae occur at 22–25°C and yeast occurs at 37°C, with temperature being the principal stimulus for the phase shift.
  - Besides estradiol and carbon dioxide tension, other variables influencing the dimorphic transition include exogenous cysteine.
  - Important factors that facilitate the morphologic transition include elevated CO_2 tension and the availability of exogenous cysteine.

The severity of infection is affected by the presence of 17β-estradiol, which regulates the growth and morphologic shift in certain dimorphic fungi, particularly in pregnant women.

CHAPTER 3

Taxonomy of Fungi

INTRODUCTION

Fungi share a common ancestor with animals. They form a diverse group characterized by a chitinous cell wall and osmotrophic nutrition. The estimated number of fungal species is 2.2–3.8 million. Some microbial groups, such as oomycota, have life forms similar to fungi. The term "fungi" is used broadly to encompass fungi, oomycota, and other fungus-like organisms. With the progress of molecular techniques, the International Code of Nomenclature for Algae, Fungi, and Plants (ICNafp) has changed over the years.

Dual nomenclature and "one fungus = one name": "Dual nomenclature" was an old practice of naming sexual and asexual morphs independently. Afterward, the idea of "one fungus = one name" is used so as to keep popular fungal names consistent.

EVOLVING LANDSCAPE OF FUNGAL TAXONOMY: BRIDGING OLD AND NEW

Before the late 20th century, fungal classification was based on observable characteristics and reproductive methods. While this system served as the foundation for fungal classification for many years, it has significant limitations. Heavy reliance on morphology may lead to the misclassification of unrelated fungi together. The absence of molecular data hinders accurate determination of true relationships between different fungal species.

Embracing the evolutionary tree: When molecular methods such as DNA sequencing became available in the late 20th century, there occurred a fungal taxonomy revolution.

Recently, names of many fungi have changed. These are given in **Table 3.1**.

TABLE 3.1: Old names versus new names of fungi.

Old name	***New name***
Zygomycetes	
Absidia ornata	*Lichtheimia ornata*
Mycocladus lutetiensis	*Lichtheimia ramosa*
Mycocladus (Absidia) corymbifera	*Lichtheimia corymbifera*
Rhizopus oryzae	*Rhizopus arrhizus*
Ascomycota	
Aspergillus fumigatus	*Neosartorya fumigata (teleomorph)*
Aspergillus fumigatus sl	*Aspergillus fumigatus ss*
Aspergillus fumigate affinis	*Aspergillus lentulus*
Clinical isolates of *Aspergillus ustus*	*Aspergillus calidoustus*
Aspergillus terreus sl	*Aspergillus terreus ss*
Candida albicans sl	*Candida albicans ss* (including *C. stellatoidea, C. africana*)
Candida glabrata sl	*Candida glabrata ss*
Candida parapsilosis sl	*Candida parapsilosis ss*
Coccidioides immitis sl	*Coccidioides immitis ss*
Fusarium oxysporum sl	*Fusarium oxysporum ss* and 257 sequence types
Fusarium solani sl	*Fusarium solani ss* and 44 phylogenetic species, including *Fusarium falciforme, Fusarium lichenicola,* and *Neocosmospora vasinfecta*
Exophiala jeanselmei sl	*Exophiala jeanselmei ss*

[*sl: sensu lato* (in the broad sense)*; ss: sensu stricto* (in the narrow sense)]

Most of the fungi are known by the anamorphic stage, and these terms are frequently used. Sometimes, it is reverse; e.g., *Pseudoallescheria boydii* is a telemorphic name which is commonly used more than the anamorphic stage, i.e., *Scedosporium apiospermum.*

The classification of fungi is based on phenotypic as well as genotypic characteristics. Some confusion regarding placing of some agents into fungi is solved by molecular characteristics. For example, *Pneumocystis* and *Microsporidium* are now considered as fungi; on the other hand, *Prototheca, Rhinosporidium,* and *Pythium* are no longer considered as fungi.

NOMENCLATURE

In medical mycology, *the binomial system* of nomenclature is followed in which the name of the genus and species is maintained. In the trinomial system, the third word may indicate subspecies, variety, forma (f.), or forma subspecies. In case of *Pneumocystis carinii*, the rat prototype was called *P. carinii* f. sp. *carinii* and human prototype was called *P. carinii* f. sp. *hominis* which is now known as *Pneumocystis jirovecii.*

The fungal species names are derived from the name of a scientist, city, country, or geographical area—*Talaromyces marneffei, Candida dubliniensis,* and *Paracoccidioides brasiliensis* in which *Marneff* is the name of a scientist, Dublin is the Capital city of Republic of Ireland, and Brazil is a country.

The ICNafp is based on rules or recommendations with formal botanical names given to plants, fungi, or few other organisms. ICN changed to International Code of Botanical Nomenclature (ICBN) at International Botanical Congress in Melbourne 2011 (known as the Melbourne code which replaced the previous Vienna code). The International Mycological Association (IMA) keeps on meeting regularly.

RECOGNIZED REPOSITORIES

For the new fungal descriptions, the use of identifiers from known repositories, i.e., *MycoBank* and *Index Fungorum,* is required. MycoBank is the online registry of IMA. It is a free service that provides new names, combinations, descriptions, and DNA barcoding. Index Fungorum is supported by the Index Fungorum partnership which has names of fungi. These two repositories provide a system to register new taxa, new names, and new combinations.

According to the Melbourne Code, the formal description of any newly published fungal name after January 1, 2013, must include an identification provided by a recognized repository. The DNA sequencing is a better identification method. The internal transcribed spacer (ITS) regions of ribosomal DNA are used for fungal species identification. This database is generated by the International Society for Human and Animal Mycology (ISHAM).

Species Complexes

Many fungi are genetically more complex, and species complexes include different strains which may not be differentiated by phenotypic characteristics. The various species complexes with the fungi included in them are shown in **Table 3.2**.

CLASSIFICATION OF FUNGI

Five-kingdom System

The five-kingdom system was suggested by Robert H Whittaker. The proposed kingdoms were Monera, Protista, Fungi, Plantae, and Animalia. It gave independent kingdom status for fungi. Monera contained prokaryotes and eukaryotes were classified into four remaining kingdoms. The kingdom Protista included unicellular eukaryotic organisms, i.e., Protozoa and unicellular eukaryotic algae. The kingdom Plantae included higher plants and multicellular algae. The kingdom Fungi included molds, yeasts, and mushrooms.

Six-kingdom Classification

The living world is divided into *two major groups*: (1) *Prokaryotes* and (2) *Eukaryotes*. The Prokaryote group includes two kingdoms (Archaebacteria and Eubacteria) and the Eukaryote group includes four kingdoms (Protista, Plantae, Eumycota, and Animalia).

Seven-kingdom System

With advances in taxonomy, the seven-kingdom system came into existence.

Archaebacteria, Eubacteria, Protista, Chromista, Plantae, Eumycota, and Animalia are the seven kingdoms. All members of the kingdom Eumycota are fungi, and two of the phyla in the kingdom Chromista are also treated as fungi.

All fungi reproduce by the asexual method but some of them also multiply by the sexual method. The word anamorphic stage indicates asexual stage, while the teleomorphic stage represents sexual stage. Mostly, the anamorphic state is usually isolated from clinical specimens. Hence, fungi are named according to the anamorphic stage.

TABLE 3.2: Various fungal species complexes.

Name of species complex	*Species included in this species complex*
Candida parapsilosis species complex	*Candida metapsilosis, Candida orthopsilosis,* and *Candida parapsilosis sensu stricto*
Candida rugosa species complex	*Candida mesorugosa, Candida neorugosa, Candida pararugosa, Candida pseudorugosa,* and *Candida rugosa sensu stricto*
Candida guilliermondii species complex	*Candida carpophila, Candida guilliermondii sensu stricto,* and *Candida fermentati*
Candida glabrata species complex	*Candida bracarensis, Candida glabrata sensu stricto,* and *Candida nivariensis*
Candida haemulonii species complex	*Candida duobushaemulonii, Candida haemulonii sensu stricto,* and *Candida haemulonii var. vulnera*
Cryptococcus neoformans species complex	*Cryptococcus neoformans sensu stricto* [formerly *Cryptococcus neoformans var. grubii* (serotype A)] and *Cryptococcus deneoformans* [formerly *Cryptococcus neoformans var. neoformans* (serotype D)]
Cryptococcus gattii species complex	*Cryptococcus bacillisporus, Cryptococcus decagattii, Cryptococcus deuterogattii, Cryptococcus gattii sensu stricto,* and *Cryptococcus tetragattii.* The complex encompasses serotypes B and C
Sporothrix schenckii species complex	*Sporothrix brasiliensis, Sporothrix globosa, Sporothrix luriei, Sporothrix mexicana,* and *Sporothrix schenckii sensu stricto*
Lichtheimia corymbifera species complex	*Lichtheimia corymbifera sensu stricto, Lichtheimia ornata, and Lichtheimia ramosa*
Apophysomyces elegans species complex	*Apophysomyces elegans sensu stricto, Apophysomyces ossiformis, Apophysomyces trapeziformis,* and *Apophysomyces variabilis*
Scedosporium apiospermum species complex	*Scedosporium apiospermum sensu stricto (teleomorph, Pseudallescheria apiospermum), Scedosporium boydii, Pseudallescheria ellipsoidea, Pseudallescheria fusoidium, Pseudallescheria angusta*
Exophiala jeanselmei species complex	*Exophiala heteromorpha, Exophiala lecanii-corni,* and *Exophiala jeanselmei sensu stricto*
Microsporum cookie species complex	*Paraphyton cookei sensu stricto, Paraphyton mirabile*
Nannizzia gypsea species complex	*Nannizzia duboisii, Nannizzia fulva, Nannizzia gypsea sensu stricto,* and *Nannizzia incurvate*
Trichophyton mentagrophytes species complex	*Trichophyton africanum, Trichophyton benhamiae var. benhamiae, Trichophyton benhamiae var. luteum, Trichophyton europaeum, Trichophyton eriotrephon, Trichophyton japonicum, Trichophyton mentagrophytes sensu stricto, Trichophyton indotineae, Trichophyton interdigitale,* and *Trichophyton quinckeanum*
Arthroderma terrestre species complex	*Arthroderma crocatum, Arthroderma eboreum, Arthroderma insingulare, Arthroderma lenticulare, Arthroderma melbournense, Arthroderma melis, Arthroderma thuringiense,* and *Arthroderma quadrifidum*
Aspergillus fumigatus species complex	*Aspergillus felis, Aspergillus fischeri (teleomorph, Neosartorya fischeri), Aspergillus fumigatiaffinis, Aspergillus fumigatus sensu stricto, Aspergillus fumisynnematus, Aspergillus hiratsukae, Aspergillus lentulus, Aspergillus novofumigatus, Aspergillus pseudoviridinutans, Aspergillus thermomutatus (teleomorph, Neosartorya pseudofischeri), Aspergillus udagawae (teleomorph, Neosartorya udagawae), Aspergillus viridinutans,* and *Aspergillus wyomingensis*
Aspergillus flavus species complex	*Aspergillus albertensis (teleomorph, Petromyces albertensis), Aspergillus alliaceus (teleomorph, Petromyces alliaceus), Aspergillus beijingensis, Aspergillus flavus sensu stricto, Aspergillus nomius, Aspergillus oryzae, Aspergillus parasiticus, Aspergillus qizutongi, Aspergillus sojae, Aspergillus tamarii, Aspergillus terricola,* and *Aspergillus toxicarius*
Aspergillus versicolor species complex	*Aspergillus creber, Aspergillus jensenii, Aspergillus protuberus, Aspergillus puulaauensis, Aspergillus sydowii, Aspergillus tabacinus,* and *Aspergillus versicolor sensu stricto*
Aspergillus nidulans species complex	*Aspergillus delacroxii, Aspergillus nidulans sensu stricto (teleomorph, Emericella nidulans), Aspergillus sublatus, Aspergillus tetrazonus,* and *Aspergillus unguis*
Aspergillus terreus species complex	*Aspergillus alabamensis, Aspergillus citrinoterreus, Aspergillus floccosus, Aspergillus hortai, Aspergillus neoafricanus,* and *Aspergillus terreus sensu stricto*

The teleomorphic states divide fungi into four phyla, i.e., (1) Glomeromycota, (2) Ascomycota, (3) Basidiomycota, and (4) Deuteromycota (fungi imperfecti).

Phylum Glomeromycotan

The name Zygomycota is eliminated. There are two subphyla in phylum Glomeromycota, Mucormycotina, and Entomophthormycota. The distribution of various species is given in the **Table 3.3**.

The characteristics of the members of subphylum Mucormycotina are given as follows:

- Members have broad, aseptate, or sparsely septate hyphae.
- Sexual spore formed by fusion of hyphae is known as zygote.
- Sporangiospores are asexual spores which are produced inside sporangium.

Phylum: Ascomycota

The basic characteristic of Ascomycota is sexual spores known as ascospores which are produced inside asci. Otherwise, ascomycetes can be identified by their bilayered hyphal walls with a thin electron-dense outer layer and a comparatively electron-transparent inner layer. Six classes are included in this phylum. These are (1) *Hemiascomycetes,* (2) *Plectomycetes,* (3) *Pyrenomycetes,* (4) *Discomycetes,* (5) *Laboulbeniomycetes,* and (6) *Loculoascomycetes*. Sexual fusion of hyphae forms a dense mass known as an *ascus* with ascospores inside. *Perithecium* is a group of asci. Asexual spores are produced outside and on hyphae. In the class *Plectomycetes*, it has more or less spherical fruiting bodies known as *Cleistothecia*, while *Pyrenomycetes* members have flask-shaped fruiting structures known as *perithecia* with cylindrical asci.

The distribution of important clinical species within *Ascomycota* is shown in **Table 3.4**.

Phylum: Basidiomycota

The sexual reproductive structure is known as basidium which is club-shaped organs. Tiny structures present on basidium are known as sterigmata, while each sterigmata holds haploid spores, i.e., basidiospores. The asexual

TABLE 3.3: Phylum Glomeromycotan.

Subphylum: Mucoromycotina	Order: Mucorales	Family: Mucoraceae	Genera: • *Lichtheimia* (formerly *Absidia)* • *Mucor* • *Rhizomucor* • *Rhizopus*
		Family: Cunninghamellaceae	*Cunninghamella*
		Family: Mortierellaceae	*Mortierella*
		Family: Saksenaeaceae	*Saksenaea*
		Family: Syncephalectraceae	*Syncephalestrum*
		Family: Thamnidiaceae	*Cokeromyces*
Subphylum: Entomophthoromycotina	Entomophthorales	Family: Ancylistaceae	Genus: *Conidiobolus*
		Family: Basidiobolacae	Genus: *Basidiobolus*

TABLE 3.4: Ascomycota.

Class	***Pneumocystidales***	***Genus: Pneumocystis jirovecii***	
Class	Pyrenomycetes	Family: Microascaceae	Genera: *Pseudallescheria, Scopulariopsis*
		Family: Ophiostomatales	Genus: *Sporothrix*
		Family: Sordariales	Genus: *Chaetomium*
		Family: Hypocreales	Genera: *Fusarium, Acremonium, Trichoderma*

Continued

Continued

Class	***Pneumocystidales***	***Genus: Pneumocystis jirovecii***	
Class	Loculoascomycetes	*Family*	*Genus*
		Mycosphaerellaceae	*Cladosporium*
		Herpotrichiellaceae	*Cladophialophora, Exophilia, Phialophora, Fonsecaea, Rhonocladiella, Ocroconis*
		Dothideaceae	*Hortaea werneckii, Aureobasidium pullulans*
		Piedraiaceae	*Piedraia hortae*
		Pleosporaceae	*Bipolaris, Excerohilum, Curvularia, Alternaria, Botryomyces*
Class	Plectomycetes	*Family*	*Genus*
		Tricomaceae	*Aspergillus, Penicillium*
		Thermoascaceae	*Paecilomyces*
		Onygenaceae	*Ajellomyces, Chrysosporium, Malbranchea*
		Arthrodermataceae	*Arthroderma*

TABLE 3.5: Phylum Basidiomycota.

Basidiomycetes	Agaricales	Genera *Hormographiella*
	Schiphyllales	*Schizophyllum commune*
	Stereales	*Sporotricum*
	Tremellales	*Filobasidiella, Trichosporon, Malassezia*
Ustomycetes	Ustilaginales	*Ustilago, Rhodotorula, Sporobolomyces*

spores are generally not found; if present, they are arranged externally at the tip of hyphae. Some fungi may show clamp connection before forming a fruiting body. Clamp connection is easily demonstrated microscopically as seen in *Schizophyllum commune*. **Table 3.5** includes fungi of phylum Basidiomycota.

Phylum: Deuteromycota

The sexual process is either absent or has not yet been observed; hence, fungi are temporarily placed in this phylum. These fungi are also known as "fungi imperfecti," "mitosporic fungi," or "anamorphic fungi." Various fungi are shown in **Table 3.6**. These fungi are further classified

TABLE 3.6: Phylum Deuteromycota.

Blastomycetes	Ascogenous		*Saccharomyces*
	Basidiogenous	Holobasid-iomycetes	*Filobasidia*
	Cryptococca-ceae		• *Candida* • *Malassezia* • *Trichosporon*
Hypomycetes	Moniliaceae	• *Acremonium* • *Arthrographis* • *Blastomyces* • *Aspergillus* • *Chrysosporium* • *Coccidioides* • *Epidermophyton* • *Fusarium* • *Histoplasma* • *Madurella* • *Microsporum* • *Paecilomyces* • *Paracoccidioides* • *Penicillium* • *Scropulariopsis* • *Sporothrix* • *Trichophyton*	

Continued

Continued

	Dematiaceae	• *Alternaria* • *Aureobasidium* • *Bipolaris* • *Cladosporium* • *Curvularia* • *Exophilia* • *Hortaea* • *Fonsecaea* • *Phialophora* • *Rhinocladiella* • *Wangiella*
Coelomyetes	*Phoma*	
	• *Nattrassia* • *Pyrenochaeta* • *Collectotricum dematium*	
Mycelia Sterilia	No sporulation	

considering the morphology and ontogeny of conidia and conidiogenous cells:

- Blastomycetes are asexual yeasts that produce spores following reproduction by budding.
- In Hyphomycetes, conidia are present on specialized conidiophores, and in many genera, the blastic process produces conidia.
- In Coelomycetes, spores are borne in pycnidium. Asexual fungi producing conidia are seen within fruiting bodies, pycnidia, which are spherical, and conidiogenous cells line inner cavity wall.

CHAPTER

4 Immunity in Fungal Infections

INTRODUCTION

Natural habitat of many fungi is environment. We are exposed to fungi on many occasions. Many of these fungi are pathogenic. But number of times we suffer from fungal infections is far less than those with viruses, bacteria, and parasites. The reasons are lower rates of exposure and our immune system. Both innate and adaptive immune systems are armed with weapons to prevent entry as well as fight the intruding fungi. This is appreciated when we see that fungal infections are quite common in immunosuppressed state. When we think of any host-parasite relationship we look at assets of the parasite that allow it not only to enter the body but survive. Then we see how our immune system tackles these assets and try to restrict or eliminate the agent. In this chapter we shall see all these aspects.

Some fungi or their products act as allergens—another aspect of immune system responding to fungal agents. Considering the scope of this aspect, it is covered in a separate chapter.

DETERMINANTS OF PATHOGENICITY OF FUNGI

- *Dimorphism*: While more virulent strains of *Histoplasma capsulatum* can change yeast to mycelium and mycelium to yeast forms more quickly, low-virulence strains take longer to go from mycelium to the yeast phase at 37°C. Even if small changes in temperature occur, it may affect a microorganism's capacity to cause disease and the type of illness the host presents.
- *Thermotolerance*: Pathogenic fungi can survive and multiply at 37°C. This property is known as thermotolerance. It is shown by *Cryptococcus neoformans, H. capsulatum*, and *Sporothrix schenckii.*
- *Capsule*: Fungi like *C. neoformans* have capsule that is antiphagocytic and hence a virulence factor. High levels of lung carbon dioxide promote capsule development in *C. neoformans.*
- *Intracellular survival*: Some fungi have developed characteristics to survive intracellularly inside phagocytes. *C. neoformans* may survive within soil amebae; thus, *C. neoformans* "learned how to become a pathogen" in that instance.
- *Adhesins*: Adherence to host tissues is an important step in the progression of microbial diseases, and receptor–ligand interaction plays a key role in this process. *Candida albicans* Als family of surface adhesins (membrane glycoproteins) and *Blastomyces dermatitidis* BAD-1 adhesin are two examples of these types of adhesins.
- *Role of enzymes*: Elastase degrades elastin and scleroproteins and enhances the invasion of elastin-containing tissues (e.g., lung, skin, and blood vessels). These are produced by *Aspergillus flavus, Aspergillus fumigatus*, and dermatophytes. Alkaline protease causes degradation of collagen and elastin and enhances the invasion of lung tissue. *A. flavus, A. fumigatus, Rhizopus* species, and dermatophytes produce this enzyme. Acid protease is responsible for the cleavage of immunoglobulin A1 and A2 (IgA1, and IgA2) and evades mucosal immunity which are produced by *Candida* species and *A. fumigatus.*
- Catalase production, as shown in *A. fumigatus* and *H. capsulatum*, breaks down hydrogen peroxide and blocks the oxidative microbicidal pathway of polymorphonuclear neutrophilic granulocytes.
- *Immune evasion*: Inhibiting phagolysosome fusion is one mechanism by which *H. capsulatum* is able to live in phagosomes. It is also able to scavenge iron from the host by secreting ferric reductase, transferrin, and siderophores.
- The cell wall components of *C. neoformans*, including melanin and glucuronoxylomannan (GXM) polysaccharide, make the fungus resistant to phagocytosis. *C. neoformans* is able to evade

TABLE 4.1: Immune components of fungi acting as antigens.

Category	Fungal agents	Immunogens
A. Yeast-like and opportunistic fungi	*Candida albicans*	Mannan, mannoprotein, and enolase
	Cryptococcus neoformans	Capsule, cell wall, and cell membrane components
	Pneumocystis jirovecii	Major surface glycoprotein (MSG) and p55
B. Dimorphic fungi	*Histoplasma capsulatum*	Cell wall, cell membrane proteins, and ribosomal–protein complex
	Blastomyces dermatitidis	BAD-1 (WI-1), a crucial virulence factor for immune system evasion
	Coccidioides immitis	C-antigenic spherule wall substance (C-ASWS), complement-fixing antigen, chitinase, antigen 2, and 33-kDa antigen
	Paracoccidioides brasiliensis	Glycoprotein gp43

(BAD1: *Blastomyces* adhesin-1)

immunological reactions, thanks to its melanin pigment.

- Resistance to microbiocidal products of neutrophils by neutralizing reactive oxygen species (ROS) (e.g., H_2O_2) and adapting to different tissue phases (yeast and spherule) acts as a virulence factor.
- *Melanin*: It protects against immunologically active cells, oxidative damage, and environmental stress.

There are some immune components of fungi which act as antigens and are exploited in serological tests. These are given in **Table 4.1**.

INNATE IMMUNITY AGAINST FUNGI

Epithelial surfaces have a protective role on the outside of the body and in the genitourinary, respiratory, and gastrointestinal systems. Biotherapy for candidiasis has demonstrated success with microbial antagonists, such as *Lactobacilli* and *Bifidobacteria.*

Complement

Fungi are able to evade the C5–C9 membrane assault complex because they have a strong cell wall. When a C3 fragment binds to a fungal cell, opsonization begins. The phagocytic cells, such as neutrophils, are attracted to chemotactic C3a, C4a, and strongest chemoattractant of all C5a—a complement activation factor. However, asthma symptoms manifest after an *Aspergillus* infection due to C3a, C4a, and C5a production during activation of complement. These factors are anaphylotoxins.

Toll-like Receptors

Where fungi are constantly interacting with humans, the body's inherent defense mechanisms kick in. These mechanisms include the barrier function of external surfaces as well as the mucosal epithelial surfaces of the respiratory, gastrointestinal, and genitourinary tracts. Unfortunately, majority of the host defense mechanisms can only be activated after infection. In order for these mechanisms to work, a group of pattern recognition receptors (PRRs), which includes toll-like receptors (TLRs), must identify certain invariant molecular structures that are shared by many different types of pathogens.

An immediate innate cellular immune response against intracellular fungi or the release of microbicidal chemicals against indigestible fungal components are the two primary means by which the innate response to fungi destroys pathogens. Additionally, the innate response instructs cells of the adaptive immune system by producing proinflammatory mediators such as chemokines and cytokines, inducing costimulatory activity in phagocytic cells, and presenting antigens via uptake and presentation.

Macrophages

While their antigen presentation is a secondary role, phagocytosis and fungal killing are the principal functions of macrophages, which are cells residing in tissues. When it comes to *A. fumigatus* and *Pneumocystis carinii*, alveolar macrophages are able to consume conidia or cysts into phagolysosomes, which allows them to eliminate fungal cells. There are oxidative and non-oxidative pathways to kill the phagocytosed fungal cells. In contrast to hyphae, conidia are susceptible to bronchoalveolar macrophages.

Fungal killing is triggered by reactive oxygen intermediates (ROIs) produced by phagocytic cells, which damage proteins and damage nucleic acids and lipids. Production of ROI is initiated by microbial products such as lipopolysaccharide (LPS) and is subsequently enhanced by opsonins and cytokines.

Dendritic Cells

In peripheral tissues, dendritic cells (DCs) act as antigen presenting cells (APCs). The main connection between the innate and adaptive immune systems is DCs, which express several TLRs. Lymphoid organs are the sites of development, cytokine release, and T-cell differentiation into TH1, TH2, or regulatory T cells following antigenic uptake and maturation. DCs along with macrophages and neutrophils are professional phagocytes. While macrophages and neutrophils completely destroy the ingested particle DCs aim at presenting the antigens to T-cells.

Neutrophils

Cells that express TLRs and dectin-1 are able to deactivate hyphae and spores of fungi. An example of a nonoxidative method would be the neutrophil-specific degradation enzymes, elastase, or cathepsin G. These act in combination with ROS produced inside phagolysosome to destroy the ingested fungus. As an additional means of killing, neutrophils can construct exterior lattices called neutrophil extracellular traps (NET) composed of DNA, histones, and antimicrobial proteins.

Patients suffering from chronic granulomatous disease are at a higher risk of developing invasive aspergillosis if their neutrophils are unable to produce ROS. The role of neutrophils in the fight against fungus is highlighted by the pathophysiology of a chronic granulomatous disease. When it comes to chronic granulomatous disease (CGD), neutrophils cannot handle catalase-positive microbes such as *Aspergillus* and *Candida* because they cannot generate oxidative bursts.

Natural Killer Cells

To combat *C. neoformans*, natural killer (NK) cells secrete interferon gamma (IFN-γ), which functions as a weak fungicide. IFN-γ stimulates macrophages. Evidence suggests that NK cells in people and mice can inhibit the growth of several fungal species, including *A. fumigatus, C. neoformans, and C. albicans.* To carry out their functions, NK cells release inflammatory cytokines, kill infected host cells, and use perforin to directly kill yeast.

Other Cells

Additionally, eosinophils, basophils, and mast cells are innate immune cells that help guard against fungi. Furthermore, epithelial cells are involved in antifungal action to a significant degree. One example is the mucosal epithelial surface, which is the initial point of contact between the host and *C. albicans*. To prevent *C. albicans*-induced tissue damage, epithelial cells upregulate TLR4.

There have been reports of endothelial cell interactions with fungi, such as *C. albicans*, in blood vessels. The exact nature of these interactions is unclear, but understanding them could lead to advances in both laboratory and clinical studies.

Innate-like Lymphocytes

Some lymphoid cells, such as γδ T cells, innate lymphoid cells (ILCs), and invariant natural killer (iNK) T cells, exhibit more innate-like traits. They are believed to have key functions in fungal allergic asthma and mucosal defenses in particular.

ADAPTIVE IMMUNE RESPONSES

Since opportunistic fungal infections are common in acquired immunodeficiency syndrome (AIDS) patients with low CD4+ counts, CD4+ T cells perform a crucial protective role against these infections. It is possible for some fungi to modify T-cell responses upon infection, allowing the fungus to thrive. Inducing a Th2-biased response and restricting Th1-biased responses may improve in vivo survival, e.g., through *C. neoformans* melanin synthesis.

Additionally, B cells are stimulated to produce antibodies by CD4 cells. Another way that CD4 T cells activate effector CD8 cells is via producing cytokines. By releasing proinflammatory cytokines, including IFN-γ, tumor necrosis factor alpha (TNF-α), and granulocyte-macrophage colony-stimulating factor (GM-CSF), Th1 cells guide antifungal immune responses. When an infection is present, the hallmark Th1 cytokine, IFN-γ, influences immune cells in many different ways. In order to stop the growth of intracellular fungal pathogens such as *H. capsulatum, B. dermatitidis, Paracoccidioides brasiliensis,* and *Coccidioides immitis*, it triggers typical macrophage activation.

T-cell and B-cell Immunity

Everyone agrees that in order to get rid of a fungal infection in the host, the adaptive arm of the immune system has to be activated. Diffuse cytoplasmic antigen presentation to CD4T cells occurs within the framework of class II major histocompatibility complex (MHC). This interaction first commits effector Th subsets. Additionally, DCs present antigen via class I MHC, which activates CD8T cells. To engage CD8+ cells, the immune system uses a process called cross-presentation, which involves the transfer of antigens from the exogenous pathway to the class I MHC pathway. While T cells must undergo Ag processing in order to become activated, B cells respond directly to fungal antigens and release immunoglobulins, which could impact the course of an infection.

Th1 Immunity

Antigen-presenting cells (APCs) activate type 1 helper T (Th1) cells by secreting interleukin-12 (IL-12) upon exposure. Among the proinflammatory cytokines secreted by Th1 are IFN-γ, TNF- α, and GM-CSF. In order to stop the growth of intracellular fungal pathogens, including *H. capsulatum, B. dermatitidis, P. brasiliensis,* and *C. immitis*, typical macrophage activation is caused by INF-γ. Activated phagocytes produce nitric oxide and ROIs, which are responsible for their fungicidal actions.

Th2 Immunity

In this context, "Th2 responses" refer to the production of cytokines such as interleukin-4 (IL-4), interleukin-5 (IL-5), and interleukin-13 (IL-13) by CD4+ T cells as well as the secretion of IgE by B cells. Multiple mechanisms are implicated in the weakening of host immunity by Th2 cytokines. IL-4 and IL-13 promote alternative macrophage activation, which is linked to uncontrolled fungal growth. *H. capsulatum* and *Cryptococcus neoformans* proliferate more robustly in IL-4-primed macrophages (called M2 macrophages) compared to conventionally activated macrophages. Contrary to these findings, Th2 mediated response is protective against *Pneumocystis*—probably related to production of IgG1 that helps in clearing the infection.

Th17 Immunity

Th17 cells secrete IL-17 and IL-22. People whose genes are defective in the IL-17 signaling pathway have a very reduced capacity to combat mycoses. Several experimental models of candidiasis are ideal for studying the function of IL-17 responses in antifungal immunity. Systemic and oral candidiasis can infect mice that do not have the IL-17 receptor.

Regulatory T Cells

The biology of regulatory T (Treg) cells refer to their capacity to encourage Th17 cell development and aid in host defenses against *C. albicans.* Oral candidiasis is more easily treated when a positive Th17 response is present.

HUMORAL IMMUNITY

This highlights the clinical significance of immunoglobulins in mycoses, as cryptococcosis can affect patients with B-cell abnormalities such as X-linked excess IgM, hypogammaglobulinemia, and IgG2 deficiency. Indirect effects of antibodies during infection include opsonization, complement pathway activation, and antibody-directed cell-mediated toxicity (ADCC). These processes are critical for the host's defense against fungal pathogens such as *C. albicans, C. neoformans,* and *H. capsulatum.*

Etiological Agents of Systemic Mycosis Associated with Specific Predisposing Factors

- *Ketoacidosis and deferoxamine therapy*: Agents of zygomycosis
- *Neutropenia*: *Candida* species, *Aspergillus* species, Mucorales, *Fusarium* species, and *Scedosporium* species
- *CGD*: *Aspergillus* species and *C. albicans*
- *Graft-versus-host reactions*: *Aspergillus* species
- *Impaired T-cell defects*: *Candida* species, *C. neoformans, H. capsulatum,* and *Penicillium marneffei*
- *Human immunodeficiency virus (HIV) and AIDS*: *C. neoformans, Candida* species, *H. capsulatum, C. immitis, P. marneffei,* and *Pneumocystis jirovecii*

Iatrogenic Factors Predisposing to Fungal Infections

There are many iatrogenic factors as long-term administration of antibiotics, corticosteroid therapy, cancer chemotherapy, and transplantation which predispose the patients to certain fungal infections.

VACCINATION AND IMMUNOTHERAPY

Because most serious fungal infections occur in immunocompromised hosts, it is possible that they will respond poorly to vaccination. That is a significant challenge in order to protect vulnerable patients. In experimental animals, a vaccine made of β-1,3-glucan conjugated with diphtheria toxin provided protection against candidiasis and aspergillosis.

One way to prevent infections caused by *C. albicans* is to inject heat-killed *Saccharomyces cerevisiae* yeasts (HKY).

In AIDS patients with low CD4+ T-cell counts, an attenuated strain of the endemic fungus *B. dermatitidis* has been investigated as a potential vaccine. BAD1 deletion makes the organism nonpathogenic in illness models in mice.

Immunizing mice with a strain of *C. neoformans* that has been modified to produce murine IFN-γ (H99γ) was another live vaccination method that was effective in a CD4+ T-cell-deficient mouse model.

The *anti-Candida vaccine*, NDV-3, protects endothelium and epithelial cells from yeast attachment and invasion with its formulation that includes the invasion protein agglutinin-like sequence 3 (Als3p) and alum. Inducing IgG and IgA antibodies against Als3p is the key to this strategy's effectiveness.

A vaccination that targets secreted aspartyl proteinase-2 (Sap2) is being developed by Pevion Biotech of Bern, Switzerland, to prevent recurrent vaginal candidiasis. *Candida* species found in vaginal mucosa express Sap2, a virulence factor, at high levels. GXM from *C. neoformans* was covalently bonded to tetanus toxoid (TT) in the conjugate vaccine against fungal infections. When administered with monophosphoryl lipid A (MPL) as an adjuvant, this antigen protected 70% of mice that were intravenously challenged and elicited high levels of IgG and IgA specific to GXM. Combined conjugated laminarin, a β-glucan polysaccharide sourced from brown algae, with inactivated diphtheria toxin [cross-reacting material (CRM)].

Researchers attempted amphotericin and recombinant antifungal monoclonal antibodies as passive treatments; these antibodies bind to the HS90 protein, which is present in *Candida* species. Adjuvant immunotherapy with IFN can stimulate Th1 responses in cases of certain systemic illnesses. In a limited number of patients afflicted with fungal disease, the use of IFN and colony-stimulating factors (CSFs) demonstrated encouraging outcomes.

CHAPTER

5 Laboratory Diagnosis of Fungal Infections

INTRODUCTION

As with any other infectious disease, the laboratory diagnosis deals with primarily demonstration and isolation of the organism from the site of infection. Other aspects like demonstration of antibodies or skin tests are secondary. Newer technologies like molecular diagnosis are gaining importance by the day.

The success of fungus diagnosis depends upon sample collection, as improper collection might lead to growth of a contaminant after all the efforts that go in for mycological processing.

- Appropriate sample collected aseptically and placed in labeled sterile containers (swabs are the least preferable sample, only to be taken when no better sample can be collected)
- Sample transportation to the laboratory at the earliest. If the samples need to be stored, then store them at room temperature, preferably in saline (do not accept samples in formalin)
- Proper specimen handling
- Sample inoculation onto culture media and subsequent temperature-controlled incubation

A valid sample requisition form must be submitted with the specimen; it must include the following information: Name, age, sex, unit number, date and time of specimen collection, source and nature, antimicrobial therapy, symptoms, preliminary diagnosis, and previous travel, housing, and employment experiences.

Various aspects of specimen collection are summarized in **Table 5.1**.

TABLE 5.1: Different specimens collected for fungal diagnosis.

Specimen	*Collection*	*Unacceptable specimen*
Pus	Aseptically with needle and syringe or expressed from opened abscess; transported in a sterile container/syringe and needle	Swab or materials from an open wound
Biopsy	Tissue between gauze pads, sterile Petri dish/tube	Swabs, thioglycolate broth, or normal saline
Grains	Collected from sinus, underneath pus, and removed bandages	
Cerebrospinal fluid	3 mL in a sterile tube	
Body fluids	Sterile tube or heparinized syringe	Swabs
Bone marrow	0.2–0.3 mL in a sterile heparinized syringe	Clotted bone marrow
Blood	5–10 mL in a syringe and transferred to a blood culture bottle of an automated system, biphasic medium, or BHI broth	
Urine	25–50 mL of clean catch or catheterized specimen	24-hour collection
Feces	Not usually acceptable; occasionally used for *Candida*	
Sputum	5–10 mL early morning, collected in a sterile container	Saliva, nasal secretion, throat swab, and 24-hour collection

Continued

Continued

Specimen	***Collection***	***Unacceptable specimen***
Bronchial brush/washing/ bronchoalveolar lavage	Collected in a sterile container using fiberoptic bronchoscopes	Dried specimen
Lung biopsy	Collected via a bronchoscope or fluoroscope-guided methods	Hazardous and dried specimens
Skin, hair, and nail (for dermatomycosis)	Skin scraping from the edges of ringworm lesions; hair plucked from the scalp—Wood's lamp may be useful for selection of hair (for piedra—piece of hair is acceptable); nail: whole thickness clipping of nail is needed. Discolored/brittle part preferred. Collect on paper (preferably black), fold it, and seal	
Corneal scraping (fungal corneal ulcer)	Best done by an ophthalmologist from the edge of the ulcer	Corneal/conjunctival swabs
Vaginal secretions	Aspirate in a syringe/swab	
Serology	*Serum*: 1–2 mL; 3–5 mL of spinal fluid	

(BHI: brain heart infusion)

SPECIMEN COLLECTION (TABLE 5.1)

Unsuitable specimens may still be processed after confirming that there was no other possible specimen that could be collected.

TRANSPORT

Container Requirements

A sterile, leak-proof container is required for the transportation of specimens. Always use a dry container when transporting specimens from the dermatology department. Avoid using transport medium unless the specimen can be easily retrieved. Anaerobic transport media are generally discouraged for fungal specimens.

- *Processing time*: Quickly, preferably within a few hours, process and inoculate specimens onto the main isolation media.
- *Storage in case of delay*: Specimens can be refrigerated at 4°C if processing is postponed for more than a few hours, with the following *exceptions*: Some delicate microbes might not make it past 4°C; therefore, it is best to keep blood and cerebrospinal fluid between 30 and 37°C. Because fungal elements become inactive when refrigerated, samples that may contain mucormycosis agents can be stored at room temperature. The ideal storage temperature for dermatophyte survival is 15–30°C, which is followed for dermatological specimens.

The processing of specimens and different methods used for the diagnosis are summarized in **Table 5.2**.

PROCESSING

There are specific protocols that must be followed when laboratory specimens are being prepared for testing for fungal infections:

- *Examination of specimens*: Give the specimen a thorough examination. On your search for the fungus, be on the lookout for any places that appear caseous, purulent, or bloody. Use a dissecting microscope to inspect mycetoma samples for granules prior to processing.
- *Handling biopsies*: For accurate representation of each tissue layer, separate the layers of punch biopsies vertically. Mucor agents become nonviable after crushing/grinding/vortexing. Hence, biopsies should be teased or cut finely for further processing.
- *Safety measures*: If a specimen is likely to contain fungus other than dermatophytes, it must be handled according to Biosafety Level 2 guidelines. For specimens likely to contain *Histoplasma* or *Coccidioides*—Biosafety Cabinet Class II, Type A2 or B2 *must* be used as they belong to the Biosafety Level 3 (BSL-3) category.
    1. **Gross examination:** In order to find mycetoma grains and other culture-friendly materials, a dissecting microscope is used to analyze a wide range of specimens, including sputum, abscess material, caseous material, aspirates, and drainage from the sinus system, among others.
    2. **Microscopic examination:** To determine if the fungus is yeast, mold, pseudohyphae, septate, or

TABLE 5.2: Outline of laboratory diagnosis.

Conventional diagnosis			
Processing of specimens	1	Gross examination	Gross examination of specimens,. For example look for the presence of granules in a suspected case of mycetoma
	2	Microscopic examination	• *Wet mounts*: ○ KOH mount (10–20%), KOH with DMSO ○ Calcofluor mount (KOH with calcofluor) ○ India ink or nigrosin staining • *Gram staining* • *Giemsa staining* • *Histopathological examination*: H&E staining, GMS, PAS, and Masson's staining
	3	Culture	• *For primary isolation*, SDA slants are used • For blood culture, BHI broth and automated culture bottles are used *Media used for identification*: • *Candida* chrome agar (for *Candida* species) • *Corn meal agar*: Dalmau culture (for identification of *Candida* species) • Niger seed agar/bird seed agar for *Cryptococcus neoformans* • Slide culture media for molds (SDA) and other media
	4	Nonculture methods for diagnosis	Detection of 1–3 β2 glucan: G test
			Detection of metabolites by GLC
	5	Serological tests	Antigen detection tests
			Antibody detection tests
Molecular tests			
	A	Hybridization tests	
	B	Amplification tests	
	C	Sequence-based tests	
Recently developed tests			
	I	Accuprobe	
	II	PNA FISH	
	III	MALDI-TOF	
	IV	T2 *Candida* panel	
	V	Biosensors	
Other tests: Skin test			
Epidemiological markers			

(BHI: brain heart infusion; DMSO: dimethyl sulfoxide; GLC: gas–liquid chromatography; GMS: Grocott–Gömöri's methenamine silver; H&E: hematoxylin and eosin; KOH: potassium hydroxide; MALDI-TOF: matrix-assisted laser desorption/ionization time-of-flight; PAS: periodic acid-Schiff; PNA FISH: peptide nucleic acid fluorescence in situ hybridization; SDA: Sabouraud Dextrose Agar)

nonseptate, a 40× objective primary microscopic examination is essential. Findings from preliminary experiments help choose the best culture medium and incubation temperature. Processing and plating specimens prior to microscopic examination is, however, a normal technique.

Wet Mounts: Potassium Hydroxide (10%) Mount (Figs. 5.1 and 5.2)

- *Purpose and composition*: Exudates, hair, nails, corneal scrapings, and skin scrapings are all examined using the conventional 10–20% potassium hydroxide (KOH) wet preparation. The fungal cell wall's glucan and chitin structure are unaffected by KOH, which dissolves cellular detritus and works as a cleansing agent.

- *Procedure*: After putting the specimen on a glass slide, add a drop of 10% KOH over it. Cover it and put it in the incubator after gently easing it apart if needed. In certain instances, the fluorescent brightener calcofluor white can improve the visibility of fungi.
- *Timing of examination*: Structures will be distorted if hairs are not checked early enough. Check the KOH mount as soon as possible but no later than 2 hours. Use 20% KOH and a tube of KOH to perform the procedure on an obtained biopsy (leave the specimen in the KOH overnight). It is important to distinguish between "mosaic fungus" and actual fungal components while analyzing dermatophyte specimens. The refractile margins of closely packed epithelioid cells produce this artifact. The findings of KOH preparation are summarized in **Table 5.3**.

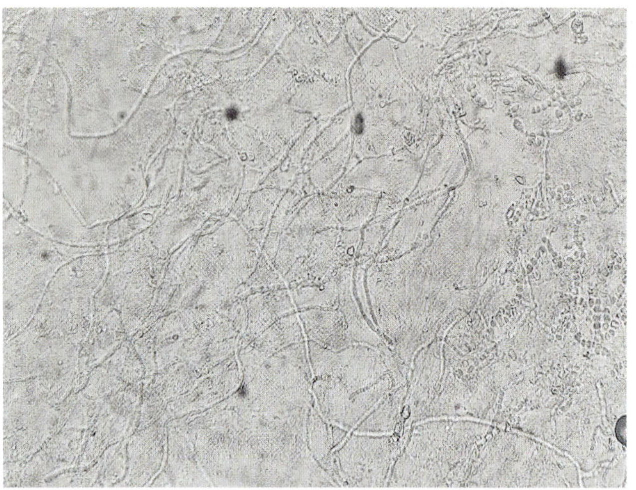

FIG. 5.1: 10% KOH mount showing septate hyphae (400×). (KOH: potassium hydroxide)

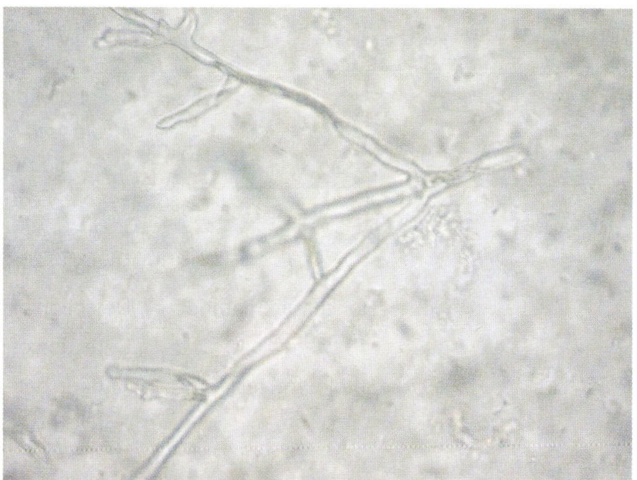

FIG. 5.2: KOH mount showing broad aseptate hyphae (400×). (KOH: potassium hydroxide)

TABLE 5.3: Findings of KOH mount.

Suspected condition	***Specimen***	***Diagnostic characteristics***
Aspergillus infection	Sputum	Septate hyphae (3–6 µm wide) with dichotomously branching (Y-shaped branching)
Candida infection	Skin scraping and nail clipping	Yeast (4–8 µm diameter) with or without pseudohyphae
Dermatophytes (ringworm fungi)	Skin scrapings, nails, or hair	Hyaline septate hyphae, arthroconidia, depending on the etiologic agents involved
Histoplasma capsulatum	Biopsy and sputum	Small (2–4 µm diameter) budding yeasts (mostly intracellular which are difficult to identify in KOH mount), some may be extracellular
Blastomyces dermatitidis	Pus, sputum, or skin specimens	Yeast cells (large budding yeast cells with a distinct broad base)
Coccidioides immitis	Biopsy, sputum, and BAL	Spherical, thick-walled spherules (20–200 µm diameter) with endospores
Mucormycosis	Tissue biopsy	Broad (6–25 µm wide), aseptate (or sparsely septate) hyphae without parallel walls with wide angle branching
Chromoblastomycosis	KOH preparation of scrapings from crusted lesions	Muriform cells (aggregation of dark brown cells resembling stones in a stone wall) or round and brown sclerotic bodies (4–10 µm diameter) with fission planes. They resemble copper pennies
Tinea versicolor	Skin scraping	Distorted hyphae and yeast cells give a "spaghetti meatball (or grapes and banana) appearance"
Phaeohyphomycosis	Specimens depending upon infection	Brownish or blackish, septate hyphae

(BAL: bronchoalveolar lavage; KOH: potassium hydroxide)

- *KOH glycerol or KOH dimethyl sulfoxide (DMSO)*: Addition of DMSO or glycerol prevents rapid drying of the fluid and permits observations of the slide for up to 48 hours. DMSO also acts as an excellent cleansing agent.
- *Calcofluor white*: This can be added to the KOH mount. A fluorescent microscope is required. Sparsely septate hyphae of mucormycosis can be easily made.
- *Gram staining* **(Figs. 5.3 to 5.6)**: Fungal elements appear gram positive. However, aseptate (or sparsely septate) hyphae may appear gram variable or gram negative.
- *Giemsa staining*: It is used to demonstrate intracellular yeast cells of *Histoplasma* and *Talaromyces* species *(within macrophages/neutrophils)*. It is also used for *Pneumocystis.*
- *Negative staining (India ink/Nigrosin)*: It is used to demonstrate capsule of *Cryptococcus neoformans* in CSF.

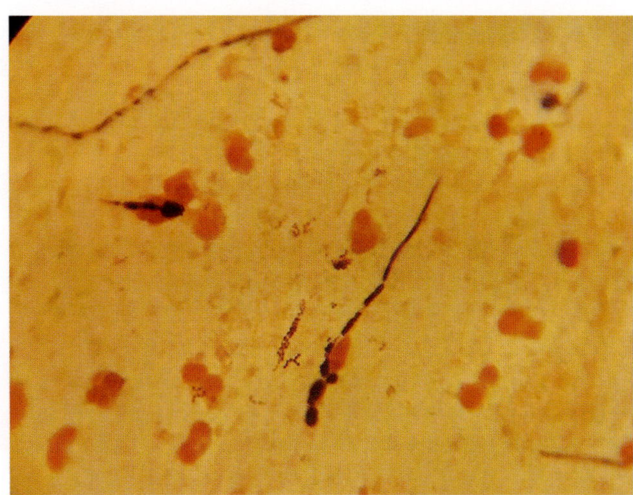

FIG. 5.3: Gram-stained smear showing gram-positive yeast cells with pseudohyphae along with pus cell (1,000×).

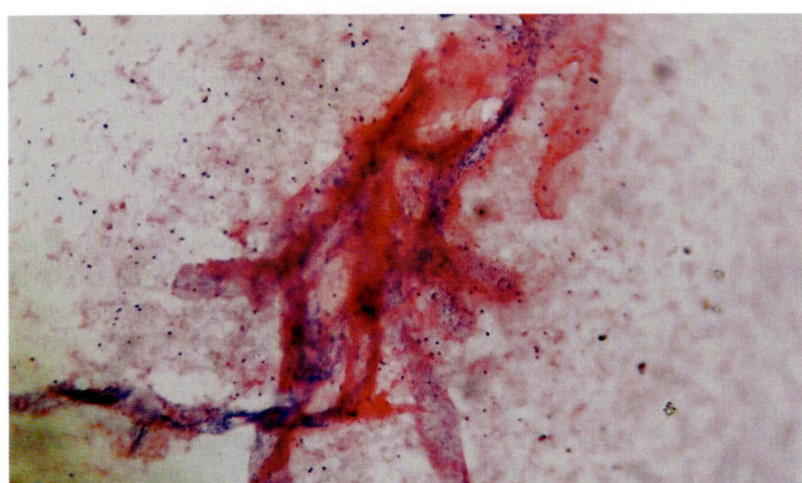

FIG. 5.4: Broad aseptate (ribbon-like, gram-variable) hyphae in Gram-stained smear (1,000×).

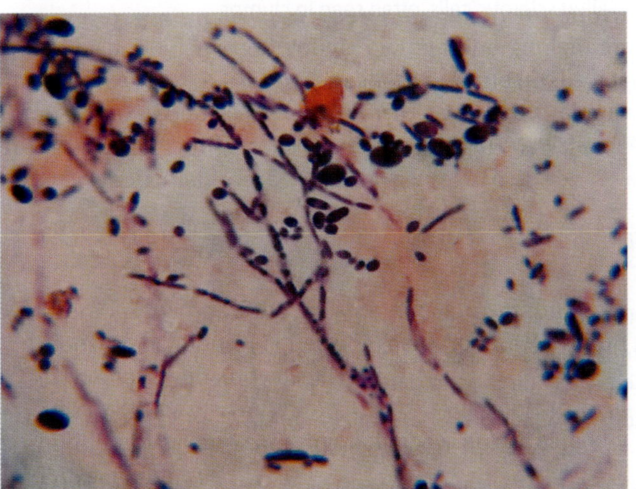

FIG. 5.5: Gram-stained smear on material taken from a suspected lesion of oral candidiasis showing yeast cells and pseudohyphae (1,000×).

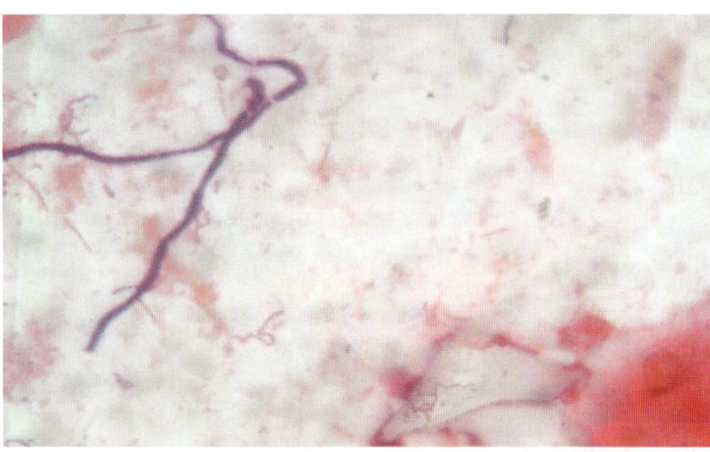

FIG. 5.6: Gram-stained smear showing septate hyphae (1,000×).

HISTOPATHOLOGY

Table 5.4 summarizes the histopathological features of different fungi. Various staining methods commonly used are H&E **(Figs. 5.7 and 5.8)**, Grocott-Gömöri's methenamine silver (GMS) **(Figs. 5.9 and 5.10)**, and periodic acid-Schiff (PAS).

TABLE 5.4: Histopathological appearance of different fungi.

Category	*Organism*	*Histopathological appearance*
A. Yeast-like appearance (Figures in µm indicate diameter)		
Histoplasma capsulatum	2–3 × 3–4 µm	Oval, narrow neck budding, uninucleate yeast cells, intracellular with granulomatous tissue reaction
Blastomyces dermatitidis	8–15 µm	Round, multinucleate, broad-based yeast cells with pyogenic and granulomatous tissue reaction
Paracoccidioides brasiliensis	2–30 µm	Multiple, budding, round cells with tiny pores between mother and daughter cells; daughter cells are small when released
Sporothrix schenckii	1–3 × 3–10 µm	Cigar-shaped cells or 2–10 µm round budding yeast cells with pyogenic and granulomatous tissue reaction
Candida albicans	3 × 5 µm	Oval, budding yeast cells with pseudohyphae; constriction is seen at point of septation; branching occurs only at septation; tissue reaction is usually neutrophilic and rarely granulomatous
Cryptococcus neoformans	4–6 µm	Round cells with a large capsule; narrow pores between mother and daughter cells; often neutrophilic tissue reaction but may be granulomatous in immunocompetent patients
Chromoblastomycosis	4–12 µm	Round or oval, brown, thick-walled sclerotic cells, often seen in clumps
B. Mold appearance (Figures in µm indicate width of hyphae)		
Aspergillus species	2–5 µm	Wide, frequently septate hyphae, even diameter, Y-shaped acute-angle branching; vascular invasion and necrosis. Hyaline fungi such as *Fusarium* and *Scedosporium/Pseudallescheria* species also have similar histopathological appearance
Mucormycosis agents	4–5 µm	• Wide, nonseptate hyphae, uneven diameter, often branch at wide angles; vascular invasion and necrosis • Differentiation from *Pythiosis insidiosum* is essential
C. Spherule-like appearance (Figures in µm indicate diameter)		
Coccidioides species	5–60 µm	Thick-walled spherules with endospores; granulomatous tissue reaction
Emmonsia species	50–500 µm	Large, thick-walled symmetrical, round to oval spherules; surrounded by fibrous granulomatous tissue reaction. Budding or endosporulation is never seen
Prototheca species	8–20 µm	Sporangia containing two to eight tightly packed sporangiospores, giving a "spoke-wheel" appearance
Rhinosporidium seeberi	200–300 µm	Sporangia with endospores about 6–9 µm; giant cells and lymphocytic reaction around mature sporangia

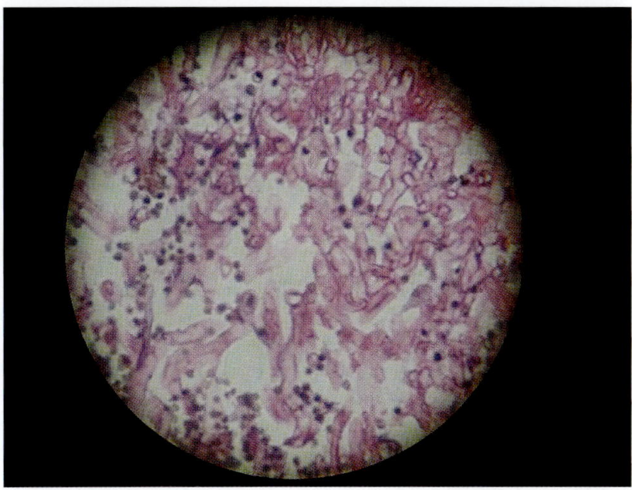

FIG. 5.7: H&E-stained slide showing septate hyphae (400×).
(H&E: hematoxylin and eosin)

CULTURE

Culture is the mainstay in the diagnosis of fungal diseases. Direct microscopy is useful for early reporting. The fungal elements of some agents have diagnostic importance. For example, correlating clinical features with microscopy findings can clinch the final diagnosis of tinea versicolor and oral thrush. This is possible because the causative agent has specific morphology in direct smear. However, microscopy is usually not sufficient for the identification of the causative agent in most other situations. Therefore, growing the fungi in the laboratory gives an opportunity to study the details of the isolate. The fungus can be identified up to the species level when cultured. Presently, many fungi are showing resistance to antifungals, even newer antifungals. For example, resistance among dermatophytes is on the rise. *Candida* species, *Aspergillus*

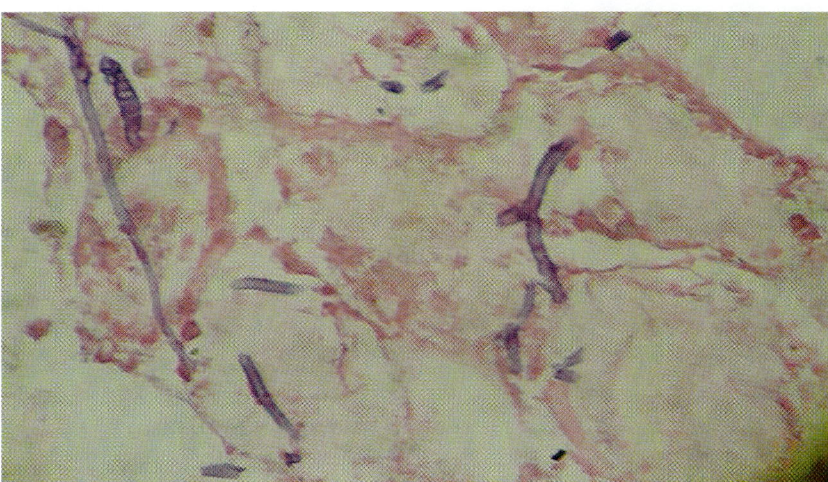

FIG. 5.8: H&E staining of biopsy showing aseptate hyphae (400×).
(H&E: hematoxylin and eosin)

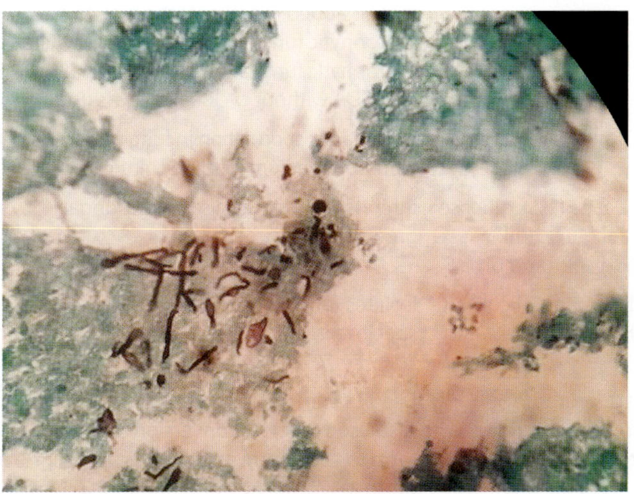

FIG. 5.9: GMS staining of biopsy showing black stained fungal elements against green background (400×).
(GMS: Grocott–Gömöri's methenamine silver)

species, and *Cryptococcus* species are showing resistance to echinocandin. When cultured, the fungus is available for susceptibility tests and further advanced techniques for identification.

Many culture media are available for culturing the fungi. Some media that were described about a century ago still continue to be useful. As bacteria grow faster than fungi, bacterial overgrowth in the fungal culture is one of the important issues. The addition of antibacterial agents to the culture media has overcome this problem. Some media are developed to enhance some property of the fungus under study. For example, corn meal agar favors sporulation in filamentous fungi and also development of chlamydospores of yeasts. Novel media such as the chromogenic media are now available that can identify an isolate just by looking at the color of its colonies. **Table 5.5** enlists some important and commonly used culture media for fungi.

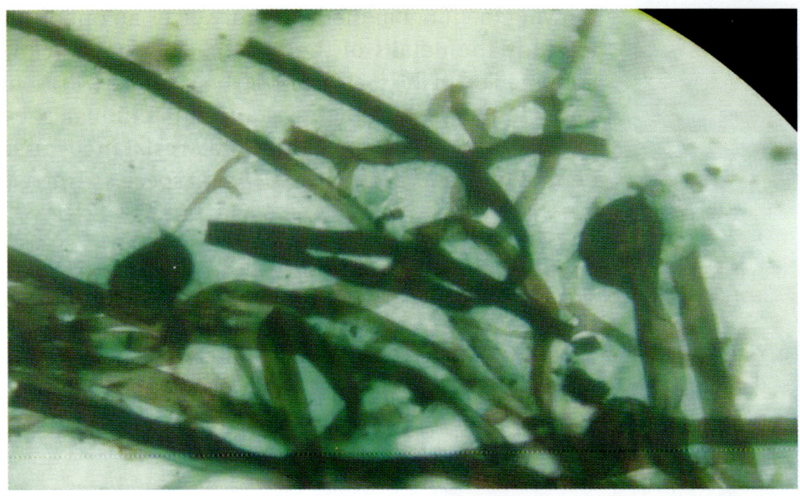

FIG. 5.10: Aseptate hyphae in GMS staining (1,000×).
(GMS: Grocott–Gömöri's methenamine silver)

TABLE 5.5: Important culture media for fungi.

Medium	*Purpose*	*Composition*	*Comment*
Sabouraud Dextrose Agar (SDA)	General fungal growth	Glucose (4%), peptone (1%), and agar pH 5.6	General purpose medium for fungi. Acidic pH inhibits growth of bacteria
SDA-Emmons modification	General fungal growth	Glucose (2%), peptone (1%), agar (with antibiotics), and with or without cycloheximide (actidione), antibiotics; pH 6.9	Most common medium for primary isolation of fungi. Higher pH and lower glucose encourage sporulation, while antibiotics prevent growth of bacteria. If cycloheximide is added, it prevents the growth of saprophytic fungi. However, in cases where saprophytic fungi are suspected as pathogen, SDA without cycloheximide is used
Potato Dextrose Agar (PDA)	Encourages sporulation	Potato starch (0.4%), glucose (1%), and pH 5.6	Encourages sporulation in fungi. Most common medium for slide culture of molds
Mycosel™	Inhibits bacteria and saprobic fungi	Papaic digest of soybeans (1%), glucose (1%), chloramphenicol (50 µg/mL), cycloheximide (400 µg/mL), and pH 6.9	Inhibits bacterial and saprobic fungal growth
Inhibitory Mold Agar	Isolates fungi from potentially contaminated specimens	Various nutrients, chloramphenicol (125 µg/mL), and pH 6.7	Isolates fungi in potentially contaminated specimens
Brain Heart Infusion Agar, ±5% sheep blood	Enriched medium to stimulate fungal growth	Calf brains, beef heart, proteose peptone, glucose, sodium chloride, disodium phosphate, and pH 7.4	Used to stimulate growth in certain fungi. Also used to show conversion of hyphal form to yeast form and vice versa (dimorphisms)

Continued

Continued

Medium	Purpose	Composition	Comment
• Sabouraud Brain Heart • Infusion (SABHI) Agar	Improved recovery of fungi	Brain heart digest, proteose peptone, enzymatic digest, dextrose, sodium chloride, disodium phosphate	Supplemented with sheep blood to increase the recovery of dimorphic fungi. It is also used to demonstrate dimorphism
Czapek–Dox medium	Used for sporulation of molds, especially *Aspergillus* species	Sucrose, sodium nitrite, dipotassium phosphate, magnesium sulfate, potassium chloride, ferrous sulfate, and agar	
Corn meal agar	Nutrition-deficient medium	Corn meal infusion, Tween 80, and agar	Various *Candida* species give a specific growth pattern which helps in the identification of *Candida* species. Also, chlamydospore formation is seen on this medium

Inoculation of Culture Plate/Tube

Specimens can be directly inoculated on media (up to 0.5 mL). This encompasses a wide range of sterile-site samples, such as aspirates from abscesses, body fluids, and swabs. To inoculate the media, pulverize the fluid if it contains a clot or membrane. Put three to five drops of fluid on the surface of the medium. Biopsies should be cut finely and then inoculate on media.

Concentration of fluids: Larger fluid volumes should be concentrated by centrifugation before inoculation on isolation media. This helps improve the detection and recovery of fungi.

Incubation: All fungi are strict aerobes. However, the optimum temperature for their growth differs. Incubation of two inoculated media at two different temperatures is required to demonstrate thermal dimorphism (when a dimorphic fungus is suspected to be the causative agent). For the identification of some species within a genus, temperature tolerance tests are used.

- Room temperature (25°C)—dermatophytes
- *37°C*: *Candida* and *Cryptococcus*
- *Both*: All systemic and subcutaneous fungi

Observe daily for 1 week. Then observe twice a week for at least for the next 3 weeks, before discarding as sterile. If a plate shows filamentous growth, immediately seal it so that it is not opened accidentally on an open bench. Such an incident might lead to dispersal of filaments, conidia, or spores in the laboratory, posing harm to the laboratory workers.

Some systemic fungi produce highly infectious spores during their mycelial form and might infect laboratory personnel. Therefore, cultures of all the molds *must* be handled *only* in biosafety cabinet class II (BSC II). The growths described as fuzzy, wooly, cottony, velvety, and powdery *should never* be opened on an open workstation, even if it has grown on a routine bacteriological culture plate. It is safe to open plates with a yeast-like colony on an open bench. However, if *Cryptococcus neoformans* is suspected, move the plate to BSCII A2.

Blood Cultures

Blood cultures are vital for detecting fungemia, a sign of invasive disease. Positive blood cultures indicate potential fungal infection, requiring prompt notification to physicians.

Types of Blood Culture Methods

- *Manual systems*: Manual blood cultures can be conducted in various ways:
  - *Brain Heart Infusion (BHI) broth*: Blood is inoculated in BHI broth. Periodic subcultures are done on solid media, i.e., Sabouraud Dextrose Agar (SDA) slants.
  - *Biphasic broth/agar combination system*: Examples include the Castaneda bottle and Septi-Chek®. This system uses agar overlaid with broth and slide agars for subculturing onto different media.
- *Lysis centrifugation system*: *The Isolator® solid medium system*: A lysis centrifugation phase is performed in the isolator system prior to plating on agar. In order to concentrate the samples and increase the likelihood of yeast growth, it utilizes ethylenediaminetetraacetic acid (EDTA) anticoagulant and saponin to lyse blood cells. The recovery of dimorphic pathogens is facilitated by this system.
- *Automated blood culture systems*:
  - *Continuous monitoring systems*: The use of a fluorescence sensor in automated systems that

provide continuous monitoring allows for the early detection of fungemia by detecting CO_2 generated by microbial growth.
  - *Mycosis IC/F medium and BACTEC® system*: The BACTEC system introduced the mycosis IC/F medium, a selective medium that outperforms conventional broth in terms of recovery rates. It speeds up the recovery of some yeasts while blocking the growth of rival bacterial flora.
  - *BacT/ALERT 3D®*: Using a broth that supports the growth of both bacteria and fungi, this is yet another continuously automated blood culture system. Compared to the BACTEC system, BacT/ALERT 3D in some studies was able to recover common yeasts and bacteria all at once, which saved money.

Observation of solid media: Colony characteristics are noted down which include growth rate, color, texture, diffusible pigment, exudates, aerial and submerged hyphae, and colony topography.

Identification of yeasts (refer to yeast identification chart in *Candida* chapter): Identification of yeasts is done by:
- Germ tube test
- Findings of Dalmau culture on corn meal agar which include noting down the presence or absence of pseudohyphae, true hyphae, and chlamydoconidia
- Sugar assimilation and sugar fermentation tests
- Color of colonies on Chrome agar
- Findings of India ink and growth on bird seed agar (for *Cryptococcus* species)
- Vitek test
- Matrix-assisted laser desorption/ionization time-of-flight (MALDI-TOF)
- Molecular methods

Identification of molds is done by:
- Lactophenol cotton blue (LPCB) mount from the colony **(Box 5.1)**
- Findings of the slide culture (microscopic findings) done on potato dextrose agar (PDA) or other media
- Biochemical tests for some fungi
- Temperature tolerance test for the identification of some species
- MALDI-TOF
- Molecular methods

Some additional tests may be required for some fungi:
- *Confirmation of thermally dimorphic fungi*:
  - Dimorphic fungi exhibit different forms at different temperatures.
  - Examples include *Blastomyces dermatitidis, Histoplasma capsulatum, Paracoccidioides brasiliensis, Penicillium marneffei*, and *Sporothrix schenckii.*
- *Cycloheximide resistance*:
  - Some fungi are resistant to cycloheximide at 30°C: *B. dermatitidis, S. schenckii, Coccidioides immitis, H. capsulatum,* and *P. brasiliensis.*
- *Temperature tolerance*:
  - Thermotolerance aids in the identification of medically important molds.
  - Examples include *Aspergillus fumigatus, Cladophialophora bantiana, Cladophialophora carrionii, Fonsecaea pedrosoi, Rhizomucor pusillus, Trichophyton mentagrophytes,* and *Exophiala dermatitidis.*

Box 5.1 | LPCB mount.

Standard tease mount:
- Place a small drop of lactophenol cotton blue on a clean microscope slide
- Aseptically remove a small portion of the fungal growth and place it on the slide
- Tease the fungus to create a thin spread
- Gently place a coverslip, avoiding air bubbles
- Seal the edges of the coverslip for preservation

Tape technique:
- Place a drop of mounting fluid on the slide
- Use tape to lightly touch the colony and then lay the tape onto the mounting medium
- Examine the mount directly

Techniques to enhance sporulation: Some fungi do not sporulate easily on routine culture media. Examples are *Saksenaea* species and *Apophysomyces* species. For this, the following methods are used:
- Microculture technique
- Water agar technique
- Dichloran Rose Bengal Chloramphenicol (DRBC) agar

SEROLOGICAL TESTS

Antigen detection tests are summarized in **Box 5.2**, and antibody detection tests are summarized in **Tables 5.6A and B**.

Exoantigen Tests

The various tests used for exoantigen detection are given in **Table 5.7**.

BOX 5.2 | Antigen detection tests for fungi.

- LA for detection of capsular antigen of *Cryptococcus neoformans* (serum and CSF)
- Lateral flow assay (point-of-care test, with low frequency of cross reactions)
- Detection of *Histoplasma* antigen from urine and serum: Immunoassay
- Detection of *Paracoccidioides brasiliensis* gp87 by immunoblot and ELISA—can be detected in urine
- Detection of cell wall mannoprotein enolase, HSP 90 for systemic candidiasis by ELISA, RIA, and CIE
- *Candida albicans* cytoplasmic antigen EIA (CACP EIA)
- Direct IF for PCP (false negative may occur)
- Direct IF for the detection of microsporidia
- Tests for *Talaromyces marneffei*: Dot blot ELISA and LA for detection of urinary antigen
- Use of FITC-based ELISA—quantification of antigen in urine is possible (1:40 titer)
- ELISA using nano protein 4D1—no cross-reaction with *Aspergillus fumigatus, Candia*, and *Cryptococcus*
- Tests for detection of *Aspergillus* antigen—LA, ELISA, and WB detection of galactomannan by ELISA
- Detection of *Pythiosis insidiosum* antigen: ELISA and WB

(CIE: counterimmunoelectrophoresis; CSF: cerebrospinal fluid; EIA: enzyme immunoassay; ELISA: enzyme-linked immunosorbent assay; FITC: fluorescein isothiocyanate; HSP 90: heat shock protein 90; IF: immunofluorescence; LA: latex agglutination; PCP: pneumocystis pneumonia; RIA: radioimmunoassay; WB: Western blot)

TABLE 5.6A: Antibody detection for diagnosis of aspergillosis.

Method	*Indication*
Aspergillus precipitins by ID or CIE	To diagnose chronic pulmonary aspergillosis (CPA)
Aspergillus-specific IgG EIA	To diagnose CPA, monitor treatment response, and diagnose allergic bronchopulmonary aspergillosis (ABPA)
Aspergillus Western blot IgG	To diagnose various forms of aspergillosis
Aspergillus-specific IgE (EIA or CIE)	To diagnose ABPA, detect *Aspergillus*

(CIE: counterimmunoelectrophoresis; EIA: enzyme immunoassay; ID: immunodiffusion)

TABLE 5.6B: Antibody tests for fungi other than *Aspergillus*.

EIA for *Blastomyces dermatitidis*, immunofluorescence, and Western blot	Antigen-A is used
ID, CFT and ELISA for *Coccidioidomycoses*	• These are useful in early diagnosis • Uses spherulin and coccidian antigens • ELISA is most sensitive and specific
Tests for *Paracoccidioides immitis*: CIE, CFT, and ELISA (using Gp43 antigen)	• Useful for diagnosis and prognosis • CIE (sensitivity—95% and specificity—100%) • CFT has low specificity
Indirect IF for *Encephalitozoon cuniculi*	
Latex agglutination	For the diagnosis of *Sporotrichosis*
Immunodiffusion, LA, and CFT for *Histoplasma capsulatum* antibodies	Histoplasmin antigen is used
MP1p-based ELISA and Western blot for *Talaromyces marneffei*	*Talaromyces marneffei* infection

(CFT: complement fixation test; CIE: counterimmunoelectrophoresis; EIA: enzyme immunoassay; ELISA: enzyme-linked immunosorbent assay; ID: immunodiffusion; IF: immunofluorescence)

TABLE 5.7: Exoantigen tests.

Hortaea werneckii	Rapid and specific identification of species
Exophiala jeanselmei and *Exophiala dermatitidis*	To differentiate among the two species and from other species
Histoplasma capsulatum	Species identificatio
Blastomyces dermatitidis	Identifies K antigen

The detection of biomarkers and their roles are summarized below.

Detection of Biomarkers

β-d-glucan (BDG)

β-d-glucan is a component of the cell wall of *Candida, Aspergillus*, and some other molds.

But it is present in a lesser amount in *Cryptococcus* and agents of mucormycosis. One way to identify invasive fungal infections produced by many pathogens is via the use of BDG, a panfungal marker. During invasive fungal infections, the fungal cell walls release BDG, a polysaccharide, into the bloodstream. Modification of the Limulus assay with a sensitivity of ~20 pg/L is used for the detection of BDG in serum. Different platforms and cutoff values are used for these methods. The sensitivity and specificity are high in febrile patients with fungal infections. Patients with hematological malignancies and those in intensive care with specified circumstances are the only ones allowed to use it up to specific thresholds (>80 pg/mL). *Pneumocystis* pneumonia, fungal meningitis, and intra-abdominal candidiasis with negative blood cultures are all conditions that BDG is expected to diagnose.

Limitations and considerations:

- *Cryptococcus* and *B. dermatitidis* are two examples of fungi that do not make BDG, which could result in false negatives.
- False positives may occur after blood transfusions. One limitation of using BDG levels to measure treatment response during antifungal treatment is how slowly they fall.

Galactomannan (GM)

It is a polysaccharide released by *Aspergillus*. The detection of GM in serum and bronchoalveolar lavage (BAL) is used for the diagnosis and monitoring invasive aspergillosis (IA).

The Platelia *Aspergillus enzyme immunoassay* (EIA) is used to detect GM. The galactomannan index (GMI) ≥0.5 is considered positive for IA. The EIA has excellent sensitivity and specificity in neutropenic patients. The decreasing levels are indicative of a favorable response to treatment. Though the role of the test in nonneutropenic patients is questionable, it has good negative predictive value. The detection of BDG in BAL is useful in cases of pulmonary infiltrates. A cutoff ≥1.0 is used for BAL, and the value ≥0.8 gives high sensitivity and specificity.

It is believed that measuring GM is a particular way to diagnose aspergillosis, although other filamentous fungi, such as *Paecilomyces* species, *Penicillium* species, and *Fusarium* species may also include GM in their cell walls but in lower quantities compared to *Aspergillus*. Possible causes of false-positive results include interactions with other types of fungi, some antibiotics (such as β-lactams), certain antibodies (such as IV immunoglobulins, hemosiderosis), and certain drugs (such as cyclophosphamide) that depress the immune system.

MOLECULAR TESTS

Uses of Molecular Methods

These tests are done for the detection of fungus in specimens or the identification of species. Other uses are for the detection of antifungal resistance and for epidemiology. **Table 5.8** shows the common targets used for the identification of fungal species.

Advantages

- Turnaround time (TAT) is less as compared to conventional methods.
- Early diagnosis is possible; hence, treatment can be started early.
- These tests are useful for nonculturable fungus such as *Pneumocystis.*
- These tests are highly sensitive and specific.
- Detection of genes responsible for drug resistance is possible.
- These tests are useful in epidemiology and in the detection of the source of infection in case of outbreaks.

Recently developed methods for fungal diagnosis are summarized in **Table 5.9**.

TABLE 5.8: Common targets for identification of fungal species.

Internal transcribed spacer regions (ITS1 and ITS2)	For the species identification of some fungi
Variable domains of 28S rRNA genes (D1/D2 domains)	For *Mucorales* identification
Beta tubulin II	*Aspergillus* species identification
Elongation factor α subunit	*Fusarium* species complex identification
Actin	Species differentiation of *Aspergillus* and *Cladosporium*
Chitin synthetase	Species differentiation of *Sporothrix*

TABLE 5.9: Some recent methods for fungal diagnosis.

Method	*Use*
Accuprobe	For rapid identification of *Candida albicans, Cryptococcus neoformans, Histoplasma capsulatum, Blastomyces dermatitidis,* and *Coccidioides immitis* from culture
PNA FISH	For the identification of *Candida* species
Quantamatrix Multiplexed Assay Platform (QMAP)	It is under evaluation for *Candida albicans, Candida glabrata, Candida tropicalis,* and *Candida parapsilosis*

(PNA FISH: peptide nucleic acid fluorescence in situ hybridization)

Anther recently developed method for fungal identification is MALDI-TOF.

MALDI-TOF-MS-based Fungal Identification

A small amount of fungal culture is applied to a target plate. The sample is overlaid with a matrix solution (usually an organic acid mixed with a solvent). The sample–matrix mixture dries, forming crystallized spots. The target plate is inserted into the MALDI-TOF-MS instrument. Laser irradiation causes ionization of the sample and matrix, producing charged particles. The ions are accelerated in an electric field and enter the flight tube. The time taken by ions to reach the detector is measured (flight time). Mass spectrum generation is done. The time-of-flight data is converted into a mass spectrum. Peaks in the spectrum represent ions of different masses. The mass spectrum is compared with a database which contains mass profiles of known fungal species.

Advantages of MALDI-TOF-MS for fungal identification:

- *Rapid identification*: Results can be obtained within minutes, faster than traditional methods.
- *High accuracy*: Provides accurate species-level identification.
- *Cost-effective*: Lower operational costs compared to some other identification methods.
- *Broad spectrum*: Capable of identifying a wide range of fungal species.
- *High throughput*: Suitable for processing a large number of samples simultaneously.
- It can be used for taxonomic and epidemiological studies.

Epidemiological Markers of Fungi

They are useful for epidemiological studies and are listed in **Table 5.10**.

SKIN TESTS

The various skin tests used in fungal diseases are summarized in **Table 5.11**.

TABLE 5.10: Epidemiological markers for fungi.

Marker	*Description*
Secreted lethal factor typing	Identifies fungal strains based on their production of specific toxic factors
Serotyping	Classifies fungi based on antigenic differences detected in their surface proteins
Morphotypin	Differentiates fungal strains based on morphological characteristics observed in culture
Mating typing	Identifies fungal strains based on their ability to mate and form hybrids
Resistotyping	Determines resistance profiles of fungal strains to various antifungal agents
Biotyping	Classifies fungi based on biochemical properties and metabolic activities
Protein electrophoresis (immunoblot)	Separates proteins based on size and charge, identifying specific proteins in fungal strain
Isoenzyme typing	Differentiates strains based on patterns of enzyme activity
Restriction fragment length polymorphism (RFLP)	Analyzes genetic variation by comparing DNA fragments produced by restriction enzyme digestion
Karyotyping	Identifies fungi based on chromosomal number and structure
Nucleic acid probes	Detects specific DNA or RNA sequences to identify and differentiate fungal strains

TABLE 5.11: Skin tests for fungi.

Fungal disease	*Antigen*	*Description*
Histoplasmosis	Histoplasmin	Detects delayed-type hypersensitivity to *Histoplasma capsulatum*. A positive test indicates previous exposure or active infection
Coccidioidomycosis	Coccidioidin	Assesses hypersensitivity to *Coccidioides immitis*. A positive result suggests exposure or active disease, often used to confirm diagnosis
Blastomycosis	Blastomycin	Measures hypersensitivity to *Blastomyces dermatitidis*. A positive reaction indicates exposure or ongoing infection with the fungus
Dermatophytoses	Trichophyton	Evaluates hypersensitivity to dermatophytes. Useful for diagnosing chronic dermatophyte infections by indicating prior or current exposure
Sporotrichosis	Sporotrichin	Detects hypersensitivity to *Sporothrix schenckii*. A positive test is indicative of exposure or active infection, helping to confirm sporotrichosis
Candidiasis	Candidin	Assesses hypersensitivity to *Candida* species. A positive result suggests prior exposure or current infection, aiding in diagnosing candidiasis

CHAPTER

6 Antifungal Therapy

INTRODUCTION

Antifungal agents can be considered in three groups: (1) Antifungal antibiotics, (2) synthetic antifungals, and (3) miscellaneous antifungals. Antifungal antibiotics include polyene antibiotics and other antibiotics **(Flowchart 6.1)**.

POLYENES

Amphotericin B

Amphotericin B (AmB) was made by Gold et al. using *Streptomyces nodosus* that was found in dirt in Venezuela. In order to kill fungal cells, AmB intercalates with ergosterol in their membranes, opening a hole that allows K^+ and other cell components to escape.

Polyenes also attach to cholesterol, albeit with a reduced affinity, and the cholesterol found in host cell membranes is quite similar to ergosterol. The result is that polyenes have poor selectivity. Compared to other polyenes, AmB's systemic toxicity is lower.

Cryptococcal meningitis is best treated with AmB in conjunction with flucytosine. It is the mainstay of treatment when treating rhino-orbito-cerebral mucormycosis. For this particular patient population, when severe neutropenia is present, the empiric treatment recommendation is AmB (in a lipid formulation). With the exception of *Candida lusitaniae*, it is effective against a wide variety of *Candida* species, including those with deep mycotic infections, sporotrichosis, and *Candida glabrata*. As far as aspergillosis and zygomycetes are concerned, its efficacy varies. AmB is not effective against *Fusarium*,

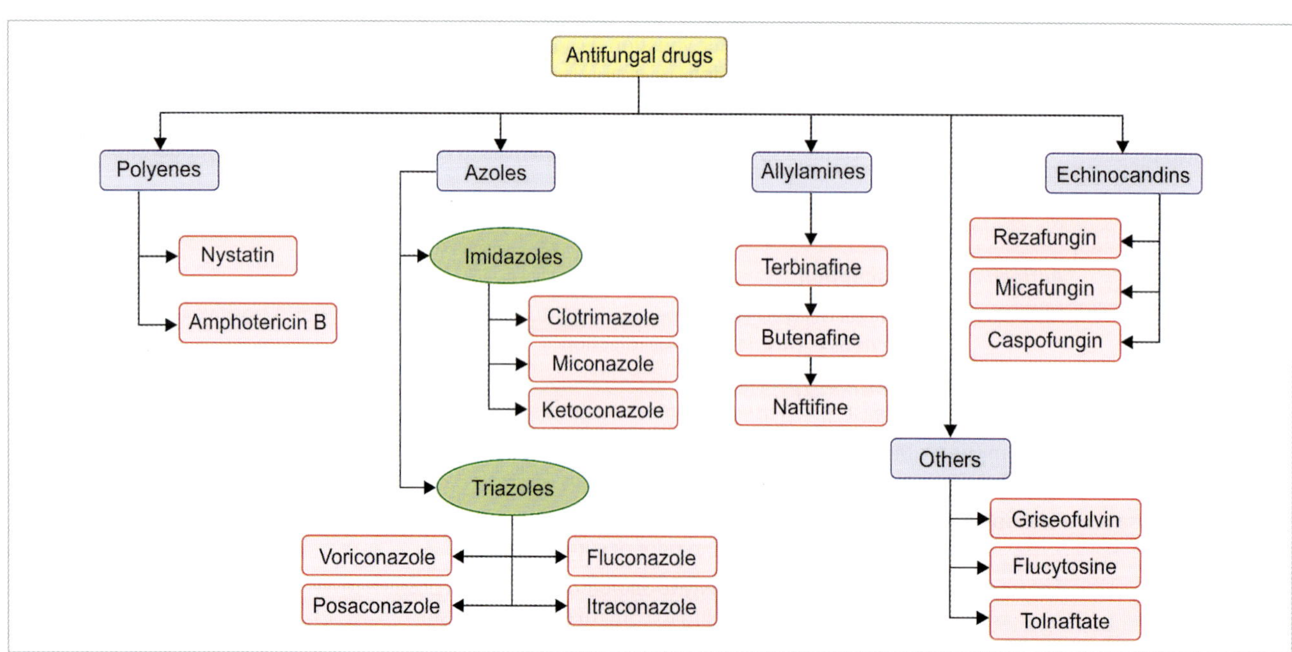

FLOWCHART 6.1: Antifungal antibiotics.

Trichosporon, and *Pseudallescheria boydii*. AmB is nephrotoxic. After voriconazole (VRC) demonstrated better survival than AmB, it was no longer the major treatment option for pulmonary aspergillosis. For salvage therapy of resistant aspergillosis, liposomal AmB is advised. When treating penicilliosis, AmB is a good first line of defense. Cerebrospinal fluid (CSF) concentrations are around 5% of serum.

By injecting AmB into the lumbar, cisternal, or ventricular CSF, higher quantities (0.5–0.8 μg/mL) can be achieved to treat cryptococcal meningitis and coccidioidal meningitis that refuse to respond to other treatments. Skin concentrations are too low to be effective against dermatophytes, even though they are sensitive in a laboratory setting.

Although it is not absorbed when taken orally, intestinal candidiasis can be safely treated with 50–100 mg taken orally four times a day (QID). For otomycosis, use 3% ear drops. Test dose: 1 mg in 20 mL dextrose, slow IV over 20-30 minutes, with monitoring for 2–4 hours afterward. If no adverse reactions occur, give 0.3 mg/kg body weight IV over 4–8 hours daily. Gradually increase dose to 0.7 mg/kg. Treatment of few weeks to months may be required depending on infective agent, severity of infection.

Note: AmB must be administered in dextrose solution.

Amphotericin B and its pharmacological and toxic effects differ in lipid formulations, also known as liposomal AmB. The spleen, liver, lungs, kidneys, bone marrow, and heart all absorb it.

There are a few different lipid formulations of AmB, including amphotericin B lipid complex (ABLC), amphotericin B colloidal dispersion (ABCD), and liposomal amphotericin B (LAmB), which stands for liposomal AmB.

Liposomal amphotericin B is composed of lecithin and other biodegradable phospholipids in uniformly sized unilamellar liposomes (60–80 nM) that contain 10% AmB. This preparation's unique qualities are as follows:

- It has milder infusion reactions.
- It is less nephrotoxic.
- It causes less anemia.
- It delivers AmB to reticuloendothelial cells in the liver and spleen—valuable for kala-azar.

Otomycosis, fungal corneal ulcers, oral and vaginal candidiasis, and other fungal infections can all be treated topically with AmB.

The renal toxicity of AmB can be worsened by cisplatin, nitrogen mustard chemicals, and antineoplastic medicines. AmB can make cyclosporine and aminoglycoside antibiotics more toxic to the kidneys.

Amphotericin B nephrotoxicity occurs when the protein binds to and blocks the lysosomal membranes of cells in the kidneys, which contain cholesterol, and when this lytic activity reduces blood flow to the glomeruli and renal tubules.

Patients with renal insufficiency and those undergoing stem cell transplants are at a greater risk of developing chronic kidney disease. A rise in blood urea nitrogen and serum creatinine and a fall in creatinine clearance, glomerular filtration rate, and renal plasma flow are common side effects of AmB treatment. Hypomagnesemia and hypokalemia can occur in many cases. Nephrocalcinosis and increased uric acid excretion are possible outcomes. There might be renal tubular acidosis. Nephrotoxicity can be lessened by preventing dehydration and prehydrating with intravenous normal saline.

Nystatin

Streptomyces noursei is the progenitor of this "New York State Institute" (or "NYSI") product. *Candida* infections of the skin, mucous membranes, and gastrointestinal tract can be effectively treated with nystatin. It is not recommended for invasive fungal infections since it cannot be absorbed orally. Tablets, troches, suspension powder, creams, ointments of nystatin in a range of concentrations (sometimes expressed as units) are all on the market. Oral suspension or tablets (dissolved in the mouth) of 500,000–1,000,000 units, taken three to five times daily for 1–2 weeks, is the recommended dose for oropharyngeal candidiasis. Side effects such as metallic taste, dry mouth, nausea, and anorexia are common.

Pimaricin

Five percent ophthalmic ointment is used for keratitis caused by *Fusarium solani* and *Aspergillus* species. It is produced from *Streptomyces natalensis*.

Hamycin

The suspension of hamycin contains 2,000,000 units/mL. It is used as a topical agent for oral thrush, cutaneous candidiasis, and otomycosis.

Other Antibiotics—Griseofulvin

When treating tinea capitis, the medicine of choice is griseofulvin, which has been approved by the Food and Drug Administration (FDA). Onychomycosis and other superficial fungal infections that do not respond to topical antifungal treatments are other indications.

The use of griseofulvin has declined in favor of itraconazole (ITC) and terbinafine (TRB) as treatments for adult tinea capitis. Because of its low price and ease of availability, it is the drug that doctors recommend to treat tinea capitis in youngsters. While newer antifungals such as TRB, ITC, and fluconazole (FLC) have mostly supplanted griseofulvin, it is still indicated for onychomycosis.

Griseofulvin blocks the assembly of microtubules. The mitotic spindle is shaped by its interactions with microtubules. In the end, this interference prevents dermatophyte mitosis. This is how griseofulvin blocks the growth of fungi such as *Trichophyton, Microsporum,* and *Epidermophyton.*

Noteworthy among its ineffectiveness is its treatment of chromomycosis, yeast (*Malassezia* and *Candida*), and dimorphic fungi. Griseofulvin needs to be taken for a long time to work because it is swiftly flushed out of the body. Since griseofulvin does not inhibit yeast growth, it will not alleviate infections caused by pityriasis versicolor or *Candida* species. Noncompliance may occur due to the lengthy therapy period (e.g., 6–12 weeks for tinea capitis).

On the whole, griseofulvin is safe to use. Nausea, vomiting, and diarrhea are the most typical gastrointestinal side effects, although headaches and allergic responses are also possible. Photosensitivity, petechiae, pruritus, urticaria, and fixed drug eruption are among the other side effects. Lupus or porphyria symptoms can get worse as a result.

Pradimicin: It has limited activity against *Candida albicans* and *Aspergillus* species.

SYNTHETIC ANTIFUNGALS

This group includes thiocarbamates, allylamines, benzylamines, and azoles.

Thiocarbamates

Tolnaftate

Tolnaftate is used in dermatophytes, especially in tinea corporis and tinea cruris. It is available as (1%) cream or lotion to be applied over the affected area for 1–3 weeks.

Allylamines and Benzylamines

Naftifine

This topical formulation is available in two concentrations: (1) 2% cream and (2) 1% gel, both of which are hydrochloride salts. Apply the 1% gel topically twice a day for 3–4 weeks to cure tinea pedis, tinea cruris, and tinea corporis caused by fungi such as *Trichophyton rubrum, Trichophyton mentagrophytes, Trichophyton tonsurans,* and *Epidermophyton floccosum.* The FDA has authorized the use of 2% naftifine cream for the treatment of interdigital tinea pedis, tinea cruris, and tinea corporis in adults for a period of 2 weeks.

Butenafine

Treatment of tinea pedis, tinea cruris, tinea corporis, tinea versicolor, and superficial candidal infections was initially authorized in Japan in 1992 with the use of 1% cream containing butenafine hydrochloride, a benzylamine derivative. The suggested course of treatment lasts for 7 days and involves applying the cream twice daily for tinea pedis and once daily for tinea cruris and corporis. Butenafine should be applied twice daily for 1 week or once daily for 2 weeks if the patient has tinea versicolor. This medicine has a fungicidal effect because it acts at an earlier stage of ergosterol production compared to azole.

Terbinafine

Onychomycosis caused by dermatophytes can be treated by terbinafine (TRB). While both TRB and griseofulvin are effective in treating pediatric tinea capitis, TRB has shown better results in treating infections caused by *Trichophyton* species and griseofulvin has shown better results in treating infections caused by *Microsporum* species in the hair shaft.

By acting as a noncompetitive inhibitor of the enzyme squalene epoxidase and the consequent conversion of squalene-to-squalene epoxide, the allylamine TRB acts early in the pathway. While squalene does not kill fungus in and of itself, it causes fungal cell death when it accumulates inside cells.

One of the first enzymes in the biosynthesis of ergosterol is squalene epoxidase, which TRB blocks. Fungi that have been treated build up squalene and lose ergosterol, which damages their cell membrane.

For toenail fungus, treating nail infections requires a 3-month oral prescription of tablet TRB, 250 mg daily. Onychomycosis of fingernails requires 6-week treatment

Refractory subcutaneous mycoses such as chromoblastomycosis, eumycetoma, phaeohyphomycotic cysts, and sporotrichosis can be treated with oral TRB as a main treatment, in combination with other therapies, or as an alternative treatment option.

Most people have no problems with TRB. Disturbances of the digestive tract and skin are the most often reported side effects. Some other possible side effects include increased levels of liver enzymes, problems with vision and taste, pancytopenia, rare cases of severe neutropenia, and allergic responses.

Azoles

Medications belonging to the class known as azole antifungals because they contain an azole ring. ITC, FLC, posaconazole (PSC), and VRC are examples of triazoles, while clotrimazole, econazole, ketoconazole, miconazole, and tioconazole are examples of imidazoles, which have two nitrogens in the azole ring.

Azole antifungals are effective because they block the enzyme lanosterol 14α-demethylase, which is dependent on cytochrome P450. This enzyme is responsible for converting lanosterol to ergosterol, the primary sterol found in fungal cell membranes. Ergosterol deficiency causes cell death by damaging the cell membrane.

Imidazoles

- *Miconazole*: It is available in topical (1% cream) and oral forms. Cream is used for superficial fungal infections—dermatophytosis, chronic mucocutaneous candidiasis, and pityriasis versicolor. Oral preparation may be used for *P. boydii* (300–600 mg in divided doses).
- *Clotrimazole*: It is used for candidiasis and for dermatophytosis. It is available as 1% cream, solution, or lotion for vaginal and cutaneous candidiasis.
- *Ketoconazole*: It used to be the drug of choice for chronic mucocutaneous candidiasis, pityriasis versicolor, tinea corporis, blastomycosis, histoplasmosis, and coccidioidomycosis. Ketoconazole shampoo is used for dandruff. It is not given in aspergillosis. Common side effects are anorexia, nausea, constipation, headache, hepatitis, and pruritus. This drug can cause adrenal gland disturbances. Hence, the use as a first line of treatment is stopped.
- *Econazole*: Econazole 1% cream is indicated for tinea pedis, tinea cruris, tinea corporis, and pityriasis versicolor.
- *Bifonazole*: It is used for vulvovaginal candidiasis and onychomycosis.
- *Tioconazole*: It is a topical agent available as a 6.5% cream.
- *Oxiconazole*: Oxiconazole lotion or cream (1%) is used for tinea pedis.

Triazoles

These drugs are safe to use in severe and systemic infections. Triazoles inhibit the cytochrome P450 enzyme lanosterol 14α-demethylase that is essential for the biosynthesis of ergosterol. As already noted, when ergosterol is not available, the fungal cell membrane is damaged and the fungus dies.

Fluconazole

Fluconazole has the narrowest antifungal spectrum among triazoles. It acts only against *Candida*, *Cryptococcus*, *Malassezia*, and a few dimorphic fungi.

Uses

- In immunosuppressed individuals [e.g., acquired immunodeficiency syndrome (AIDS) patients], oral once-daily FLC can be used to treat infections caused by *Candida species* and *Cryptococcus neoformans*. It can also be used to treat or prevent fungal infections in patients of neutropenia in cancer chemotherapy or stem cell transplant (SCT) recipients, depending on the severity of the illness.
- Infections caused by *Candida* in the throat and esophagus.
- *Candida krusei* and *C. glabrata* are naturally less vulnerable to FLC. For vulvovaginal candidiasis, a single oral dose of 150 mg of FLC is sufficient to cure over 90% of patients, and monthly doses of the same amount effectively prevent recurrences. The usual dose for mucosal candidiasis is 200 mg given as a loading dose followed by 100 mg daily for 2 weeks. If oropharyngeal candidiasis (OTC) becomes clinically resistant, larger dosages may be necessary.

Adult Dosing

It is necessary to administer FLC in multiple doses, with the exception of vaginal candidiasis, which only requires one oral dose of 150 mg. For candidiasis of the oropharynx and esophagus, the dosage is 200 mg on day one and 100 mg every day for 2–3 weeks. For candidiasis of the peritonitis and urinary tract infections, the dosage is 50–200 mg every day. It has been reported that dosages as high as 400 mg daily have been prescribed to those with systemic *Candida* infections or those undergoing bone marrow transplants in order to prevent candidiasis.

For cryptococcal meningitis 400 mg on first day, followed by 200 mg/day for 10–12 weeks is recommended. For HIV positive patients with CD4 count of less than 100 per cumm FLC is given as prophylactic dose of 100 mg daily; till the count rises above 100 per cumm. Higher doses of 600–1,200 mg daily are required for several endemic fungal infections, such as coccidioidomycosis, especially in situations with disseminated disorders.

Pediatric Patients

The following daily doses in adults (100, 200, and 400 mg) should be similar to the following doses (3, 6, and 12 mg/kg), respectively, in pediatric patients, although doses over 600 mg/day are not advised.

Itraconazole

- In patients with moderate symptoms of histoplasmosis, coccidioidomycosis, paracoccidioidomycosis, and sporotrichosis ITC can be used. In AIDS patients, ITC inhibits the recurrence of histoplasmosis.
- Compared to VRC, ITC has a lesser impact on aspergillosis.
- ITC may be preferred over AmB to treat aspergillosis due to its low toxicity.
- Systemic use of ITC effectively treats pityriasis versicolor, dermatophyte infections of skin and nails.
- When it comes to treating oral and esophageal candidiasis, ITC works wonders.
- Human immunodeficiency virus (HIV) patients, chemotherapy patients, and organ transplant recipients all benefit from ITC prophylaxis. Because of its wide-ranging effectiveness, lack of side effects, and low level of fungal resistance, ITC is a great preventative medication for these patients with impaired immune systems.
- Itraconazole is also an option for pulse therapy in cases of moderate-to-severe seborrheic dermatitis.
- Itraconazole is becoming more popular as a treatment for allergic bronchopulmonary aspergillosis (ABPA) and severe asthma with fungal sensitivity (SAFS). In patients with ABPA, ITC treatment enhances disease control and reduces corticosteroid prescriptions. When patients with SAFS are given ITC (200 mg twice a day), it tends to improve respiratory function and rhinitis symptoms. It also significantly improves their quality of life.

The active metabolite of ITC, hydroxyitraconazole has same spectrum as itraconazole. It is formed in liver. Its concentration in plasma is 2–3 times that of parent drug.

There are three formulations available: (1) Intravenous (10 mg/mL), (2) oral (10 mg/mL) in a solution, or (3) as a capsule (100 mg).

Onychomycosis of the Fingernails

200 mg of ITC orally twice a day for 7 days, followed by a three week break. Again 200 mg of ITC orally twice a day for a week. Immunocompromised patients should be given two courses.

Onychomycosis of the Toenails

Take 200 mg orally (capsules) each day for 12 weeks.

Candidiasis

- *Oropharyngeal*: 20 mL orally for 1–2 weeks; swish and swallow. Alternately, dose of 10 mL orally twice daily for 2–4 weeks
- *Esophageal*: 20 mL orally twice daily for 14–21 days

Note: Only oral solution is effective against oropharyngeal and esophageal candidiasis.

Blastomycosis

Loading dose 200 mg thrice a day orally for 3 days. Maintenance 200 mg once a day for 12 weeks. Dose may be increased to maximum 400 mg/day in divided doses. Note: Loading dose for life threatening infections.

Histoplasmosis

Loading dose 200 mg thrice a day orally for 3 days. Maintenance 200 mg once a day for 12 weeks. Dose may be increased to maximum 400 mg/day in divided doses. Note: Loading dose for life threatening infections.

Invasive Aspergillosis

Loading dose 200 mg thrice a day orally for 3 days. Maintenance 200 mg once a day for 12 weeks. Dose may be increased to maximum 400 mg/day in divided doses. Note: Loading dose for life threatening infections.

Cutaneous or Lymphocutaneous Sporotrichosis

200 mg orally once a day; if necessary, increase to 200 mg twice a day; keep taking the medication for at least 2 more weeks after lesions have healed. If you have to choose, go with the oral solution.

Gastrointestinal side effects include nausea, vomiting, mild diarrhea, and stomach discomfort that are the most commonly reported adverse effects. Cardiotoxicity and hepatotoxicity are rare side effects.

Comparing pulse therapy to continuous therapy, which involves taking 200 mg once a day with a 3-week break in between each pulse, the results suggest that pulse therapy is just as effective and has better tolerability. In most cases, treatment for fingernails often takes 2 months, while treatment for toenails typically takes 3 months.

Voriconazole

When it comes to killing *Aspergillus*, VRC is just as effective as AmB and much better than ITC. Voriconazole is a synthetic version of FLC. When compared to FLC, the activity was increased when one triazole ring was replaced with a fluorinated pyrimidine and an α-methyl group was added.

Voriconazole is effective against every kind of *Candida*, including the *C. krusei*, FLC-resistant *C. glabrata*, and FLC-resistant *C. albicans.*

It seems that VRC is effective against a wide variety of *Aspergillus* species, including the AmB-resistant *Aspergillus terreus.*

While many hyaline and dematiaceous molds are resistant to AmB, VRC has been shown to be effective against a number of these molds in laboratory tests. This encompasses a variety of species, including but not limited to *Scedosporium apiospermum*, an asexual form of *P. boydii*; *Fusarium*; *Paecilomyces*; *Bipolaris*; *Alternaria*; and a few more. VRC does not work against zygomycetes. Unfortunately, there is a lack of data from clinical studies for VRC, despite its great in vitro efficacy against *C. neoformans* and good CSF levels.

Posaconazole

Mucorales (e.g., *Rhizopus* species) and *Scedosporium apiospermum* are two examples of invasive molds that can be challenging to cure, but PSC, an extended range triazole antifungal drug, can help. Patients suffering from eumycetoma and chromoblastomycosis have found relief or an improvement in their clinical condition after undergoing PSC treatment. It has antifungal activities against several species of *Aspergillus*, *Fusarium*, and *Candida* (particularly *C. glabrata and C. krusei)* in vitro. This medication is also prescribed to bone marrow recipients and patients with neutropenia to prevent and treat fungal infections.

For invasive aspergillosis and candidiasis: Oral suspension 400 mg twice a day or 200 mg four times a day. Alternatively delayed-release tablet of IV formulation is given as 300 mg twice on day one followed by 300 mg once a day thereafter.

For oropharyngeal candidiasis: 100 mg twice a day on day one, followed by 100 mg once a day thereafter.

Isavuconazole

Isavuconazole is a new azole which is available as oral and intravenous formulations. It is effective against aspergillosis and mucormycosis.

MISCELLANEOUS ANTIFUNGALS

5-Fluorocytosine

Originally produced in 1957 as a cytosine analogue for the treatment of leukemia, the fungicidal action of 5-fluorocytosine was later discovered in animal experiments.

Due to the absence of cytosine permease in human cells, which prevents a significant amount from being converted to 5-fluorouracil, it is preferentially harmful to fungus. Systemic and severe *Cryptococcus* and *Candida* infections are treated with it. Due to the high possibility of drug resistance, it is not recommended to use flucytosine as a monotherapy. For nonsystemic and nonlife-threatening illnesses, including *Candida* infections of the lower urinary tract and vagina, it can be administered alone without a second medicine.

For systemic infections, the combination of flucytosine and AmB works synergistically. If patients are suffering from cryptococcosis meningitis or candidiasis that has spread to heart, eyes, peritonitis, cystitis, or rest of the body, a combined treatment may be able to help. Due to the drug's profound dependence on renal function, its administration must be done on a case-by-case basis. Because flucytosine does not undergo metabolism in humans, it remains unchanged in the urine for up to 95% of the time after administration.

When administering flucytosine to individuals with hepatic, renal, or hematopoietic impairment, close monitoring and extra caution are required. Nephrotoxicity, acute hepatitis, rash, stomach discomfort, diarrhea, emesis, and nausea are some of the side effects.

Flucytosine is not advised during first trimester of pregnancy and during breast-feeding.

As a monotherapy for candidiasis and *Cryptococcus*, flucytosine is not preferred due to the drug's inadequacy compared to AmB and the ease and speed with which secondary resistance can be developed during treatment.

If a patient experiences symptoms of candiduria or cystitis caused by a *Candida* species that is resistant to FLC, the alternate monotherapy indicated is flucytosine. When it comes to profound mycosis, it does not work.

When taken together, flucytosine and AmB inhibit the progression of flucytosine resistance and lower the dosage necessary to treat cryptococcal meningitis.

Flucytosine plasma concentrations are associated with bone marrow toxicity, which can manifest as reduction of bone marrow function. In most cases, moderate and reversible neutropenia and thrombocytopenia will ensue.

Since mucosal candidiasis often recurs quickly in AIDS patients without access to highly active antiretroviral therapy (HAART), secondary prophylaxis with 100 mg FLC/day is a recognized component of treatment for patients with severe or recurring candidiasis. Patients living with AIDS who also have cryptococcosis are good candidates for maintenance treatment with FLC.

Preventative Medicine

Patients at high risk of fungal infections during cytoreductive therapy, such as stem cell or solid organ transplantation, or cancer patients preparing to undergo chemotherapy may benefit from antifungal prophylaxis. Prophylactic agents such as FLC, AmB, ITC, micafungin (MCF), and PSC have all been proven to be efficacious through extensive research.

Echinocandins

The antifungal medicines stop the formation of β-(1→3)-d-glucan, which makes the fungal cells osmotically unstable. The action on β-(1→3)-d-glucan is comparable to how penicillin inhibits bacterial peptidoglycan formation.

One naturally occurring fungus that makes caspofungin (CASF) is *Glarea lozoyensis*. Micafungin MCF and anidulafungin (ANF) are two examples of semisynthetic lipopeptides that are derived from fermentation products produced by some *Aspergillus* species.

Echinocandins are effective in treating both invasive candidiasis and candidemia. The fungistatic effects of echinocandins against *Aspergillus* species make them a potential alternative to other therapies for invasive aspergillosis, especially if the side effects of these alternatives are too difficult to tolerate.

When it comes to FLC-resistant *Candida* species, echinocandins work moderately against *C. albicans, Candida guilliermondii*, and *C. lusitaniae*; nevertheless, they are effective against *C. glabrata* and *C. krusei*. When it comes to *Trichosporon* and *Cryptococcus*, these drugs work well. Echinocandins are effective against *Pneumocystis jirovecii* too.

Nonsusceptible

There are a number of fungi that are resistant to echinocandins, including *Blastomyces dermatitidis, Fusarium* species, *Histoplasma capsulatum, Mucorales, Scedosporium* species, *Paracoccidioides brasiliensis*, and *P. boydii*. Echinocandins are usually not effective against *Mucorales*.

The suggested administration of CASF is an intravenous loading dose of 70 mg followed by 50 mg daily doses. MCF is presently approved for the treatment of invasive candidiasis, esophageal candidiasis, candidemia, and fungal infections following a hematopoietic stem cell transplant. US FDA has approved ANF to treat invasive candidiasis, candidemia, and esophageal candidiasis.

Ciclopirox Olamine

The antifungal, antibacterial, and anti-inflammatory properties of this medicine make it a multipurpose treatment. By chelating polyvalent metal cations such as ferric (Fe^{3+}) and aluminum (Al^{3+}), it inhibits metal-dependent enzymes (cytochromes, catalase, and peroxidase), thereby interfering with cellular processes such as electron transport in mitochondria, energy production, and nutrient intake across cell membranes. It may also alter membrane permeability, which would prevent precursors from entering cells. Ciclopirox olamine is effective against virtually all clinically relevant yeasts, molds, and dermatophytes, including those species of *Candida* that are resistant to azoles, *Aspergillus, Penicillium* and *Saccharomyces cerevisiae*. Researchers have demonstrated that CPO can kill a broad range of bacteria in laboratory tests. These bacteria include gram positive (*Staphylococcus* species, *Streptococci, Micrococci*, and others), gram negative (*Proteus* species, *Pseudomonas aeruginosa*, and *Gardnerella vaginalis*). It has far more effective anti-inflammatory effects than other topical antifungals. It is available as shampoo (1% and 1.5%); topical cream (1% for yeast and dermatophytic infections) and an 8% nail lacquer (for onychomycosis) to be applied to affected nail/s every day.

Morpholines

A 0.25% cream formulation is available. This substance is highly effective against both phacoid fungus and dermatophytes. Enzymes reductase and isomerase, which are involved in the ergosterol synthesis pathway, are blocked from carrying out the activity.

Whitfield's Ointment

Whitfield's ointment contains benzoic acid (6%) and salicylic acid (3%) in a ratio of 2:1. These agents are effective against fungal infections and keratoses, respectively. This ointment can be used to cure pityriasis versicolor, tinea pedis, and other dermatophytes.

Castellani's Paint

In 1905, the Italian doctor and expert in tropical diseases Aldo Castellani (1878–1971) refined Castellani's paint. It treats tinea cruris and moniliasis in places between the trigonous bones. Pustular dermatoses of the feet and hands, as well as pruritus ani and pruritus vulvae, have all found relief with its use. To lessen the risk of secondary bacterial contamination in cases of onycholysis and chronic paronychia, colorless Castellani's paint can be applied.

The contents are:

- Basic fuchsin (0.3%)
- 95% ethyl alcohol (10.0%)
- Boric acid (1.0%)
- Phenol liquefaction (4.0%)
- Acetone (5.0%)
- Resorcinol (10.0%)
- Water (to 100%)

Use a cotton swab to apply it to the afflicted areas at night-time before sleeping.

There is a colorless variant that is apparently less effective but more aesthetically pleasing and less irritating

- Alcohol 90%
- Boric acid 0.8%
- Phenol 4.0%
- Acetone 4.0%
- Resorcinol 8.0%
- Water to 100.0%

Burrow's Solution

There are three different concentrations available: (1) 4%, (2) 8%, and (3) 13% of this acidic mixture that contains aluminum acetate. For a wide variety of skin issues, including stings and bites, swelling, allergies, and bruises, it is a go-to remedy. The most common usage, though, is in the treatment of otitis or ear infections, such as otomycosis.

Selenite Sulfide

Selenite sulfide is used as shampoo (2.5%) for pityriasis versicolor, dandruff, and white piedra.

- *Undecylenic acid*: It is available as an ointment for tinea pedis.
- *Haloprogin*: A 1% cream is used for athlete's foot.
- *Triacetin*: Both cream and ointment are used for tinea pedis.

Potassium Iodide

For sporotrichosis, basidiobolomycosis, and conidiobolomycosis, the medicine of choice is the saturated solution of potassium iodide (SSKI). It is also prescribed for pythiosis and cutaneous cryptococcosis. Nodular vasculitis, erythema multiforme, and erythema nodosum are among the other disorders that can be treated with it. The recommended dosage is 50 mg each drop. The potassium iodide (KI) solution can be mixed with milk, fruit juice, or water before drinking. Start with five drops three times a day, and after 6–12 weeks, increase the dose by five drops weekly until you are taking 25 to 40 drops three times a day.

Negative Consequences

The Wolff–Chaikoff effect occurs when the thyroid gland stops producing hormone. Therefore, it is important to keep an eye on how the thyroid gland is working.

SECTION

2

Superficial Cutaneous Mycoses

Section Outline

CHAPTER 7

Malassezia

INTRODUCTION

Pityriasis versicolor is a superficial mycosis that persists over time. The stratum corneum, which is present in smooth skin, is the main target. Most lesions manifest on the upper torso, particularly the arms, back, and chest. Spots of discoloration that grow and eventually blend into larger patches characterize their appearance. Lipophilic yeasts belonging to the genus *Malassezia* are responsible for the disease. The dimorphism of *Malassezia* yeasts allows them to thrive in two different forms: (1) Yeast and (2) mold. Humans and other animals normally have these yeasts in their skin microbiome. Tropical areas tend to have a higher prevalence of this illness, while temperate zones see a seasonal appearance. Additional clinical disorders linked to *Malassezia* include dandruff and seborrheic dermatitis. Fungal infections caused by *Malassezia* species can occur in certain people who take intralipid supplements.

HISTORY

The initial account of pityriasis versicolor was given by Eichstedt (1847). Isolation of the fungus was not possible. Isolating fungal components from lesions was first done by Robin in 1853. He observed that the fungus resembled the dermatophyte *Microsporum audouinii*, which led him to name the agent *Microsporum furfur*. Malassez (1874) observed budding "spores" in skin lesions. Baillon suggested the name *Malassezia* for the yeast in 1889. *Pityrosporum malassezia* was the term given to this organism by Sabouraud (1904), and it was recognized as the culprit responsible for dandruff. In 1951, Gordon discovered a new species, *Pityrosporum orbiculare*. In 1984, the genus name *Pityrosporum* was removed and the name *Malassezia* was approved.

TAXONOMIC AND PHYLOGENETIC EVOLUTION

Phylogenetic study has identified 15 distinct species of *Malassezia*. The *Malassezia* fungus belongs to the Malasseziomycetes class, within the Basidiomycota phylum, and the Malasseziaceae family within it.

MYCOLOGY AGENT

Lipophilic yeasts of the genus *Malassezia* are the culprits behind pityriasis versicolor. All humans and lower animals have these yeasts on their skin as part of their regular microbiome. They can change their development mode to become either short hyphae or monopolar budding yeasts.

Initially, seven species were included in the genus *Malassezia*. With advances in the taxonomy of *Malassezia* using DNA–DNA homology and 18S rDNA analysis, seven species of *Malassezia* were identified—(1) *Malassezia furfur*, (2) *Malassezia globosa*, (3) *Malassezia obtusa*, (4) *Malassezia pachydermatis*, (5) *Malassezia restricta*, (6) *Malassezia slooffiae, and* (7) *Malassezia sympodialis*. Afterward, four new species—(1) *Malassezia dermatis*, (2) *Malassezia japonica*, (3) *Malassezia yamatoensis, and* (4) *Malassezia arunalokei*—present on the skin were added to the genus. After the inclusion of four new species from animal skin, i.e., *Malassezia nana, Malassezia caprae, Malassezia equina, and Malassezia cuniculi*, the total number of species goes to 15. Differentiation among them is possible by morphology, G + C content, RNA/DNA sequences, requirement of long-chain fatty acids from C12 to C24 series, catalase activity, and temperature requirements. With the exception of *M. pachydermatis*, all other species are lipophilic. The names of many species have changed. Important physiological and biochemical

TABLE 7.1: Biochemical properties of *Malassezia* species.

Species	Lipid dependence	Growth at >37°C	Catalase	Esculin splitting	Cremophor (1–10%)	Tween 20 (high concentration)	Tween 40 (0.1–10%)	Tween 80 (low concentration)
Malassezia furfur	+	+	+	–	V	+	+	+
Malassezia pachydermatis	–	+	V	V	V	+	+	+
Malassezia sympodialis	+	+	+	+	–	–	+	+
Malassezia globosa	+	–	+	–	–	–	–	–
Malassezia obtusa	+	–	+	+	–	–	–	–
Malassezia restricta	+	–	–	–	–	–	–	–
Malassezia slooffiae	+	+	+	–	–	+	+	–

characteristics of common clinically isolated species are given in **Table 7.1**.

EPIDEMIOLOGY

As part of the typical microbiota found on the skin of humans and other animals, *Malassezia* species are thought of as commensal. They are present in every continent. There is some variation in the geographic distribution of different species.

Pityriasis versicolor tends to be more common in tropical regions, particularly during the warmer summer months with a prevalence of 30–40%. The occurrence often falls between the range of 1–4% in temperate zones. In Europe, the Southern area has a higher prevalence as compared to the Northern region. In Greek, Japanese, Indian, Iranian, Mexican, and Spanish population, the common species is *M. globosa*, while in Canada, *M. sympodialis* is isolated more frequently. Panama and Madagascar are the most common areas for *M. furfur* to be found.

As per as skin disorders are concerned, seborrheic dermatitis ranks high. For the first 3 months of life, many infants get cradle cap, which is a form of seborrheic dermatitis. It may get cleared when they become 1 year old. Seborrheic dermatitis affects 11.6% of adults; however, only 2.8% will encounter severe enough symptoms to seek medical advice. In acquired immunodeficiency syndrome (AIDS) patients, the disease is more common and worsens when the CD4+ T-lymphocyte count falls below 400/μL.

Risk Factors/Transmission

Although pityriasis versicolor can strike at any age, it is more common in younger individuals. Use of corticosteroids or oily tanning products is a risk factor. Pityriasis versicolor is often recurrent. Hence, the patient's past history is important. The fungus may be associated with catheter-related fungemia in preterm newborns. Colonization rates in hospitalized neonates are high (37–100%). Neonatal infections can occur in infants given intralipid supplementation by parenteral feeding. Infection in healthcare personnel may be associated with the handling of infected dogs. *M. pachydermatis* was initially found in rhinoceroses. Most cases of *M. sympodialis* infections happen when they form commensal flora. *Malassezia furfur, M. globosa,* and *M. restricta* often infect humans. *M. furfur* is seen in healthy as well as diseased conditions. *M. globosa* and *M. restricta* are the most common causes of pityriasis versicolor and seborrheic dermatitis, respectively. *Malassezia* infection or carriage is most common in the early 20s, when sebaceous gland activity is at its highest. Common areas of body where the fungi are most commonly present are scalp, face, and central chest. The reason behind this is the abundance of sebaceous glands.

The external ear and hair follicles are two other potential colonization sites. Colonization or sickness is rare in old age. How a disease manifests depends on the mechanisms that let the organism go from its saprophytic yeast phase to its mycelial phase. Conditions such as high sebum levels during adolescence, heavy perspiration, the warmer months (May to September), oil application, starvation, taking systemic steroids, having Cushing's disease, being pregnant, or taking antibiotics or oral contraceptives all increase the risk of acne. It is possible that some species found in normal flora are more harmful and can easily transform into mycelial form. There may be a family tendency.

CLINICAL FEATURES

Clinical forms of superficial mycoses caused by *Malassezia* species are as follows:

- *Pityriasis versicolor*: There are two types: One that is hypopigmented in people with dark skin and another that is hyperpigmented with lighter brown spots. The majority of patients are in good health and see their concerns primarily as aesthetic. The appearance of lesions as "tears of liquid gold" is considered as beauty spots. Wood's lamp examination is helpful to differentiate the condition from erythrasma. (Erythrasma is a bacterial infection of the skin. Wood's lamp examination shows coral red fluorescence with erythrasma. Pityriasis versicolor lesions give yellow-green fluorescence. Although *M. furfur* was formerly believed to be the culprit, the most common species linked to this illness is *M. globosa*. Humidity, heat, and starvation are the determinants of pityriasis versicolor. Vitiligo, pityriasis alba, tinea corporis, leprosy, and post-kala-azar cutaneous leishmaniasis are considered in the differential diagnosis.
- *Seborrheic dermatitis and dandruff*: There is some inflammation of the skin. Areas abundant in sebaceous glands, such as the scalp, face, upper chest, and back, are more commonly affected. It manifests as red, itchy, and greasy skin that is scaly. For newborns, it is called "cradle cap." There is some clinical evidence that the condition is associated with the fungus, as antifungal treatment relieves the symptoms. More cases of seborrheic dermatitis occur in people with AIDS. Many species of *Malassezia*, including *M. restricta*, *M. furfur*, *M. globosa*, *M. sympodialis*, and *M. slooffiae*, are commonly linked to this illness. A novel species, *M. arunalokei*, is reported from India. Other clinical conditions such as acne, atopic dermatitis, candidiasis, and dermatophytosis should be differentiated from seborrheic dermatitis. Scalp inflammation (seborrheic dermatitis) and scaling (mild form-dandruff) are both components of scalp diseases, and the phrase seborrheic dermatitis/dandruff complex is proposed to cover both. Emotional stress aggravates skin scaling. Compared to *M. furfur* strains isolated from healthy skin, those from seborrheic dermatitis lesions produce far more bioactive indolic compounds in vitro. The skin of a person with seborrheic dermatitis will also contain these chemicals, which are the most active aryl hydrocarbon receptor ligands. In addition to host immune status and the yeast's ability to produce secondary metabolites, they play a role in inducing and sustaining seborrheic dermatitis. The condition is more prevalent in neutropenic patients. Another piece of data points to a nonspecific immune response to *Malassezia* yeasts as the cause of seborrheic dermatitis. In addition to malassezin, oleic acid, arachidonic acid, and indole-3-carbaldehyde are directly irritating to the skin that the *Malassezia* fungus produces.
- *Folliculitis*: Pruritic red, follicular papules or pustules, commonly seen in regions with an abundance of sebaceous glands, are the hallmarks of folliculitis. Many patches are seen on the front of the chest, shoulders, and arms, as well as the upper back. It is more common in immunocompromised persons and diabetics. The yeast can be discovered in blocked hair follicles. *M. pachydermatis*, *M. globosa*, and *M. furfur* are species that can cause folliculitis.
- *Atopic eczema/dermatitis syndrome (AEDS)*: AEDS is a skin disorder characterized by chronic inflammation. *Malassezia* species act as aggravating factors as their antigens act like allergens. The lesions are seen on the scalp, face, and neck of adult patients. The lesions are pruritic. There is a genetic predisposition observed. Clinical features are erythema, papules, and pruritus, followed by scratching and rubbing, leading to secondary bacterial infections. Excoriations and lichenification are common findings. Skin samples taken from patients undergoing AEDs often include *Malassezia* species. Although healthy humans often have *Malassezia* species in their skin microbiome, certain people may be allergic to the allergens of these species. This can cause an inflammatory reaction. The skin barrier is disrupted by atopic diseases, which leads to the proliferation of *Malassezia* species. This, in turn, increases immune system exposure and elicits a humoral- and cell-mediated immune response in afflicted locations due to the high activity of sebaceous glands. While several *Malassezia* antigens (*M. globosa* 1304, *M. sympodialis* 8, and *M. restricta* r) have been extensively studied, others remain unidentified and have been found in patients' perspiration, which worsens their symptoms.
- *Head and neck dermatitis (HND)*: This may occur in patients with Alzheimer's disease, and there is a family history of the IgE-mediated form of the disease. The clinical features are pruritus, erythema, and erythematous plaques on the forehead, eyelids, perioral, neck, and upper trunk. The phrase "red face" comes from the fact that in extreme instances, the entire face could be affected.
- *Psoriasis*: Roughly 2% of American adults suffer from psoriasis vulgaris. It is a chronic inflammatory skin illness. It has a family tendency. The demonstration of *Malassezia* species in psoriatic lesions implies

that they may serve as external triggers that intensify inflammation, and the fungus does not directly cause psoriasis. Antifungal treatment improves the clinical condition of psoriasis scalp lesions, which may indicate that *Malassezia* is contributing to the worsening of the disease.

Clinical Form of Deep-seated *Malassezia* Mycosis: Fungemia

Systemic infection caused by *Malassezia* species is fungemia. As a deep-seated mycosis, fungemia caused by *Malassezia* species can be linked to a number of risk factors as follows:

- *Prolonged hospitalization*: Patients who have been in the hospital for a long time are more likely to get *Malassezia* fungemia. Colonization and bloodstream penetration of these yeasts that live on the skin are possible in hospital settings.
- *Central venous catheters*: *Malassezia* species can enter the bloodstream more easily when central venous catheters are in place. These catheters are used for a variety of medical purposes, including intravenous therapy and monitoring. These lipophilic yeasts can colonize catheters initially and then cause the disease.
- *Intralipid emulsions*: An increased likelihood of *Malassezia* fungemia is associated with nutritional assistance via intralipid emulsions. *Malassezia* is able to flourish in lipid-based nutritional supplements known as intralipid emulsions due to its lipophilic nature.

Thus, the pathogenesis of *Malassezia* fungemia is related to its ability to colonize catheters, intralipid emulsions, and the skin, subsequently entering the bloodstream. Clinical presentation of *Malassezia* fungemia can vary, with neonates often showing signs of sepsis and thrombocytopenia, while adults may present with fever as the primary symptom. Positive blood cultures are crucial for diagnosis, and treatment typically involves removing the colonized catheter and administering antifungal therapy, which may include medications such as amphotericin B (AmB) and flucytosine (5-FC) or fluconazole (FLC).

PATHOGENICITY

Several host and microbial variables are involved in the interactions between *Malassezia* species and their hosts, leading to the development of cutaneous and systemic infections.

Host Factors

- *Immunologic response*: In healthy human lymphocytes and mononuclear cells, *Malassezia* antigens can induce a marked reduction in leukocyte migration and a surge in lymphocyte blastogenesis. This shows that an immunologic response is established by the host immune system upon recognition of *Malassezia*.
- *Neutrophil phagocytosis*: In a complement-dependent process, white blood cells can be involved. *Malassezia* is much more resistant than *Candida albicans* to phagocytic attack.
- *Cytokine production*: Proinflammatory cytokines such as interleukin 8 (IL-8) and interleukin-1 alpha (IL-1α) can be released when *Malassezia* interacts with monocytes or granulocytes. These cytokines play a role in inflammation by activating neutrophils and lymphocytes and increasing their chemotaxis.

Microbial Factors

- *Lipases*: *Malassezia* species secrete three different lipases. One possible function of these lipases is to aid in the hydrolysis of host lipids on which the fungus survives.
- *Phospholipase*: In addition, *Malassezia* generates a phospholipase. It causes mammalian cells to release arachidonic acid, a building block of prostaglandins that are known to cause inflammation. Local inflammation in areas with infections may be exacerbated by this process.

Factors affecting depigmentation in pityriasis versicolor: In the case of pityriasis versicolor, *Malassezia* species can lead to skin depigmentation. Some factors contributing to this depigmentation include the following:

- *Azelaic acid*: Some species of *Malassezia* produce this substance that blocks the action of the enzyme tyrosinase, the one which is involved in the process of melanogenesis. Hypopigmented skin patches can be exacerbated by azelaic acid when exposed to sunlight. The medicinal use of azelaic acid includes the alleviation of skin hyperpigmentation.
- *Linoleic acid*: It stimulates *Malassezia* species to produce lipoperoxides. Reactive oxygen species are generated during this process; they have the potential to harm epithelial cells and play a role in depigmentation.
- *Tryptophan metabolites*: Pityriacitrin and pityrialactone are two examples of the tryptophan metabolites generated by *Malassezia*. These fungi have a powerful

broad-spectrum ultraviolet (UV) action and can lead to hypopigmentation in exposed skin by blocking out UV light.

Morphogenesis to Hyphal Forms

Species of *Malassezia* may adapt their shape to various environments. To induce the transformation of *Malassezia* yeast into hyphae, certain chemicals such as glycine, cholesterol, or squalene can be added to cultures. The pathophysiology of disorders connected to *Malassezia* is thought to include this morphological alteration.

LABORATORY DIAGNOSIS

- *Clinical diagnosis*: Typical microscopic features, discolored patches, and yellow-green fluorescence under Wood's light are the mainstays of a pityriasis versicolor diagnosis.
- *Collection of specimens*: Following a thorough cleaning of the area over the lesions with 70% alcohol, a sample is taken by scraping the active margins of the lesion using scalpel blade. Scales are easily collected using a blade or a glass slide.

Specimen in children can be taken with a piece of Scotch tape, with its adhesive side down. The tape is pressed over the lesion. It is then placed over one to two drops of potassium hydroxide (KOH) solution on the center of the glass slide for microscopic examination.

Direct Examination

KOH mount: Skin scrapings prepared with KOH allow for microscopic examination. It is possible to improve detection with the application of fluorescent brighteners, like Calcofluor-white or Parker ink. **Figure 7.1** shows clusters of spherical yeast cells (2–7 µm) with short, stumpy, slightly curved hyphae, giving the organism an appearance reminiscent of "spaghetti and meatballs" or "grapes and bananas." Yeasts showing "footprint" shape are seen by KOH mount or by staining. **Figure 7.2** shows these in Gram's stain.

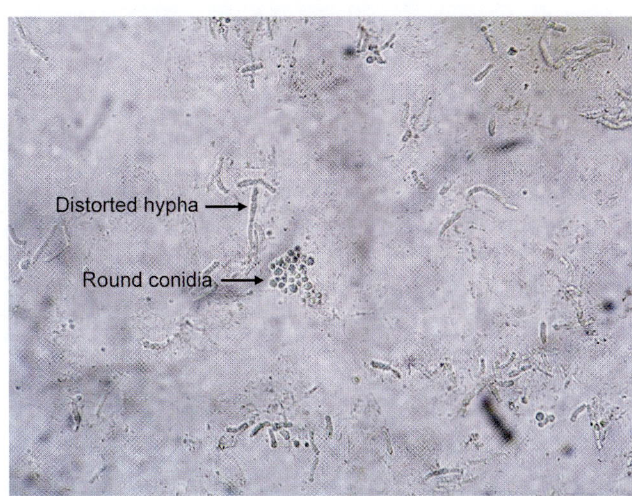

FIG. 7.1: KOH mount of a skin scraping from a case of tinea versicolor showing spaghetti (distorted hyphae) and meatballs (round conidia) appearance (400×).
(KOH: potassium hydroxide)

Histopathology

- There are two options for staining skin scrapings or biopsy specimens: (1) Periodic acid-Schiff (PAS) and (2) hematoxylin and eosin (H&E).
- *Specimens stained with PAS*: Clusters of round-to-oval budding yeast and short hyphal pieces are revealed by PAS staining.
- *Specimens stained with H&E*: Clusters of hematoxylinophilic yeasts and short hyphae are seen inside the hyperkeratotic layer in the H&E-stained biopsy specimens.
- Alcian blue and Masson-Fontana staining help to differentiate from *Candida*. It differs from *Cryptococcus* by staining positively for Congo red and negatively for mucicarmine.

Culture

- Species of *Malassezia* can be cultured for epidemiological studies or when a systemic infection is suspected, but it is typically not needed for diagnostic purposes.
- Media with lipids, such as oleic acid, olive oil, or Tweens, promote the fungus's growth since it is lipophilic.
- There are specialized media that can be used for recovery and speciation, such as Dixon's medium that contains glycerol monooleate and Tween 40. It aids in identification by showing colonies with typical morphology.
- Fungus growth is enhanced in the Leeming and Notman medium containing glycerol, full-fat cow's milk, and Tween 60.
- The use of GYP-S agar and the Datta and Dixit media allows for quick diagnostics. The ingredients in GYP-agar are olive oil, glycerol monostearate, glucose, yeast extract, peptone agar, and Tween 80. There is not a single growth medium that will reliably revive every species of *Malassezia*.

- Genus-level identification is performed by observation of lipid dependence, colony characteristics, and cell morphology. *Malassezia* species are urease positive.
- On Sabouraud dextrose agar (SDA) with actidione, chloramphenicol, and Tween 80 with olive oil, small (3–6 mm) cream-colored colonies with slightly raised irregular edges are developed in 5–7 days at 32–35°C. The colonies of *M. globosa* show "fried egg" colony morphology. On microscopy, it shows typical globose cells with a narrow budding base (bottle-shaped cells). Hyphae are occasionally seen in fungal cultures. *M. pachydermatis* can be grown on conventional culture media such as SDA.

Blood Cultures

Adding 3% wt/vol palmitic acid to the culture medium can improve the growth of lipid-dependent *Malassezia* species in blood culture bottles, which is useful for fungemia cases. *Malassezia* can be detected in blood cultures in this way.

Microscopic Morphology

- The yeast cells have a blunt end and are spherical with little collarettes, measuring 1.5–4.5 × 2–6 µm **(Figs. 7.2 to 7.5)**. By means of monopolar enteroblastic budding, they come into being.
- Although hyphal forms are infrequently formed in cultures, yeast cells are the most common.

IDENTIFICATION

The tests for sugar fermentation and sugar assimilation are useless for identification, making the task difficult.

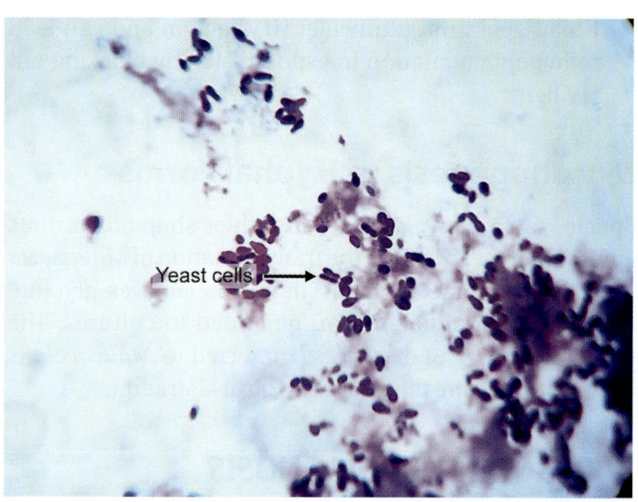

FIG. 7.3: Gram-stained smear of *Malassezia* (1,000×) (footprint shaped cells).

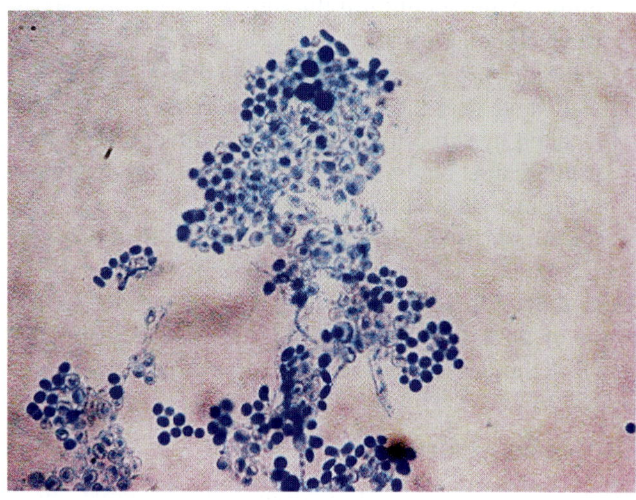

FIG. 7.4: LPCB mount showing yeast cells of *Malassezia* species. (LPCB: lactophenol cotton blue)

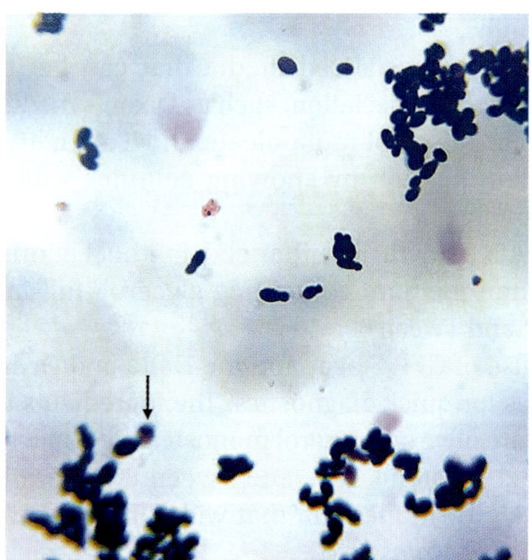

FIG. 7.2: Gram-stained smear showing "footprint"'-shaped yeast cells (1,000×).

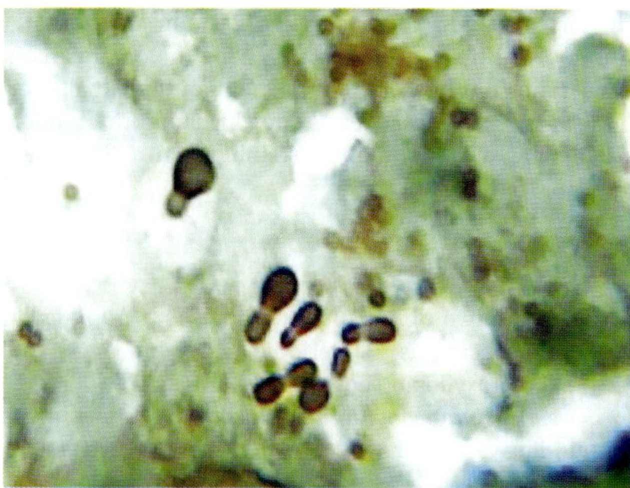

FIG. 7.5: GMS staining showing yeast cells (1,000×). (GMS: Grocott–Gömöri methenamine silver)

Urease is present in every single species. The **Table 7.1** provides a list of physiological and biochemical characteristics that can be used to identify species. Many laboratories now have matrix-assisted laser desorption ionization time-of-flight mass spectrometry (MALDI-TOF-MS) on hand for identifying different species of *Malassezia*.

Genetic Identification

- It is possible to genetically identify species of *Malassezia* using molecular techniques, such as polymerase chain reaction (PCR) and sequencing.
- An unknown yeast can be quickly identified as *Malassezia* species using DNA probes that target the D1/D2 (about 600 bp) and ITS (approximately 600–800 bp) sections of rDNA.
- For species-based identification using binding patterns, the Luminex detection method is utilized, which employs probes of different colors on beads. *Malassezia* and other pathogens can be identified at high throughput with this technique.

TREATMENT

Topical and systemic treatments are equally effective in addressing pityriasis versicolor. Patients should be aware that it may take a while for hypopigmented lesions to go away after treatment. Some therapy alternatives to consider are as follows:

- *Topical treatments*:
  - *Selenium sulfide shampoo*: It contains selenium sulfide (2.5%). It can be used topically, and recurrences can be prevented by periodic use.
  - *Topical ketoconazole (KTC) gel*: It is an effective topical treatment.
  - *Other topical agents*: Sodium thiosulfate (25%) with salicylic acid (1%), 50% aqueous propylene glycol, zinc pyrithione shampoo, ciclopirox (0.1% solution), and topical azoles such as clotrimazole (1%) or KTC (2%) as well as topical terbinafine (TRB) (1% solution).
- *Systemic treatments*:
  - *Oral KTC*: A single dose of 400 mg
  - *Oral itraconazole (ITC)*: At a daily dose of 200 mg for 5–7 days
  - *Oral FLC*: A single oral dose of 400 or 300 mg once a week for 2 weeks

It is advised to use suppressive medication to avoid the usual recurrences, which occur at a rate of 60% in the first year. A monthly dose of 400 mg of KTC, 200 mg for 3 days in a row once a month, or 400 mg of ITC once a month for 6 months are the options. A safer and more effective preventative measure is selenium sulfide shampoo.

Therapy for seborrheic dermatitis: Seborrheic dermatitis, often affecting the scalp, can be treated with the following approaches:

- *Scalp lesions*: To achieve remission, use KTC-containing shampoo twice a week for 1 month. After that, use it weekly or biweekly. Shampoos containing ciclopirox or selenium sulfide (2.5%) are two alternatives.
- *Facial lesions*: Optional but effective treatments include KTC foam or gel, ciclopirox cream, lithium salt ointment, or 0.1% methylprednisolone acetonate cream.

Therapy for fungemia: Some efficient ways to treat fungemia caused by *Malassezia* species, especially fungemia, connected to catheters are given as follows:

- *Catheter removal*: For majority of the time, all it takes to eradicate catheter-related fungemia is to remove the catheter and stop administering parenteral lipid emulsion.
- *Antifungal medications*: Most *Malassezia* species need oleic acid to develop, which makes susceptibility testing difficult. However, clinical isolates generally demonstrate in vitro susceptibility to AmB and triazoles.
- *Primary therapy*: The main options for treatment are FLC or voriconazole (VRC), and AmB is only used for infections that are recalcitrant or potentially fatal.
- *FLC dosage*: A regimen of 400 mg/day [oral or intravenous (IV)] is recommended.
- *AmB dosage*: A dose of 0.7 mg/kg of AmB-deoxycholate and 3 mg/kg of AmB formulations based on lipids is recommended. It is recommended to continue therapy for an additional 14 days after the last positive blood culture and catheter removal.

Clinical management: Premature infants and immunocompromised patients might greatly decrease attributed mortality from catheter-associated fungemia with proper therapeutic care.

CHAPTER

8 Piedra

INTRODUCTION

Superficial fungal infection of the hair shaft is known as piedra. "Piedra" means "stone" in Spanish. Along the hair shaft, irregular nodules appear. The nodules contain fungal mass attached to the hair shaft. These nodules resemble stones, hence, the name. Piedra is an asymptomatic illness that is often ignored. There are two varieties of piedra. *Piedraia hortae* causes black piedra, while *Trichosporon* species causes white piedra. Their geographical spread varies.

Both types have an effect on the hair shaft, which might lead to hair breakage. Cases of both black piedra and white piedra have been documented in India. Nodules on the hair shaft are white in white piedra and dark brown to black in black piedra. White piedra causes less hair damage, and hyphae and arthroconidia may be detected under the microscope. Microscopically, hyphae and sexual ascospores can be detected in black piedra.

WHITE PIEDRA

The genus *Trichosporon* is responsible for this superficial infection of hair. It can affect the beard, moustache, axillary hair, and groin hair. Nodules on the hair shafts vary in color from white to light brown **(Fig. 8.1)** and these are a telltale sign of mycosis. Nodules are fragile, irregular, and would not stay firmly in place on the hair. In most of the cases, there is just a single concretion in a shaft. *Trichosporon* shows true hyphae along with arthroconidia as well as blastoconidia (yeast cells). The fungal elements are present within and around the hair shaft. The other names for the clinical condition are white trichosporonosis nodosa, tinea blanca, Beigel's disease, and Chignon disease.

TAXONOMY

Trichosporon beigelii was the sole species in the genus. After taxonomical revisions and classifications, the

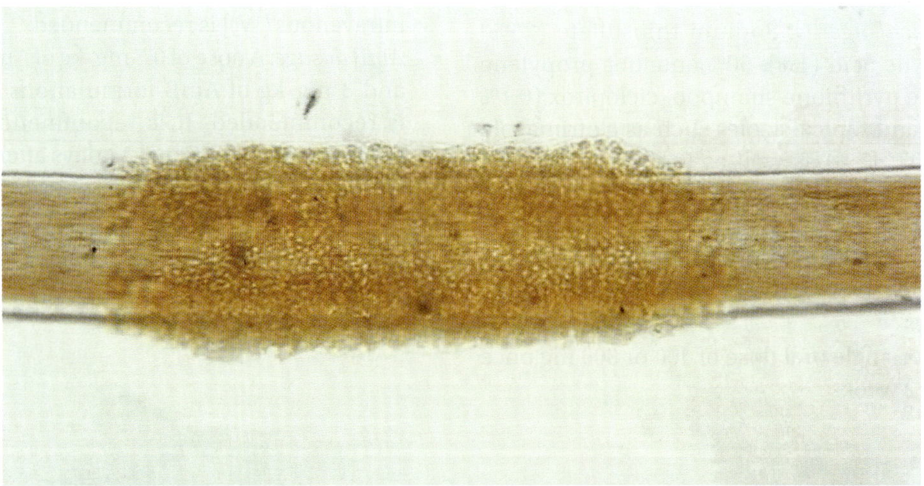

FIG. 8.1: Lesion of white piedra on hair (×100).
Source: Public Health Image Library CDC.

following six species of *Trichosporon* are identified. These include: (1) *Trichosporon ovoides*, (2) *Trichosporon inkins*, (3) *Trichosporon mucoides*, (4) *Trichosporon asahii*, (5) *Trichosporon asteroides*, and (6) *Trichosporon cutaneum*; their identifications are based on molecular characteristics, biochemical testing, and morphology. Although there is limited evidence that *T. mucoides* is involved in the production of white piedra, the majority of cases are produced by *T. ovoides* and *T. inkins*. *Trichosporon* is basidiomycetous yeast that is urease positive. Taxonomically, the genus is classified in the family Trichosporonaceae under the order Tremellales, class Tremellomycetes, and subphylum Agaricomycotina in the phylum Basidiomycota.

EPIDEMIOLOGY

Fungus *Trichosporon* looks like yeast. It is found in soil and also considered part of the natural skin flora. The most common species associated with white piedra of the scalp is *T. ovoides*, whereas *T. asahii* and *T. inkins* are found on pubic hair. Young Muslim women often have white piedra as a result of wearing the headscarf. Women who wear their hair in a ponytail before it dries often experience this as well. White piedra can occur after swimming or bathing in stagnant water, although the exact cause of infection is unclear. Sexual transmission may be associated with white piedra of pubic hair. Since *Trichosporon* species can infect human skin, nails, and mouth and spread by interpersonal contact, humans may also potentially contract white piedra from infected animals such as horses, monkeys, and dogs. White pebbles are found all over the globe, but they are more common in the areas with mild-to-moderate warm climates. This includes regions such as South America, the Middle East, India, Southeast Asia, Africa, Europe, Japan, and even some parts of the southern United States.

CLINICAL FEATURES

The soft nodules are seen on facial and axillary hair, beard, moustache, and pubic hair, whereas scalp, eyebrows, and eyelashes are occasionally involved. The nodules can be easily seen with naked eye and detached from hair. Hair shows break at the points of infection. The fungus is commonly seen in patients with acquired immunodeficiency syndrome (AIDS) and in those with neutropenia. There may be associated bacterial infection caused by *Corynebacterium* species.

PATHOGENESIS

There are gentle nodules that range in hue from white to light brown. Fungal infection begins just below the hair shaft's cuticle and progresses inward. At the sites of nodules, the hair becomes brittle and prone to breaking. The hyphae and arthroconidia are present in the nodule.

DIFFERENTIAL DIAGNOSIS

Both head lice (pediculosis capitis) and pubic lice (pediculosis pubis) can be identified. Phthiriasis pubis and trichomycosis axillaris, both caused by *Corynebacterium tenuis*, are other possible diagnoses. The agent can be better identified with the use of microscopic analysis and Wood's lamp testing.

LABORATORY DIAGNOSIS

Direct Examination

The specimen collected is epilated hairs. Nodules as little as 0.5 mm in diameter can be easily removed from the hair shaft. These are used for microscopy and culture. Hairs have soft, white to tan nodules.

Microscopy

Fungal elements are seen in and around the hair. Hyphae with oval to rectangular arthroconidia are the characteristic microscopic findings on a potassium hydroxide (KOH) mount or KOH with Parker blue-black ink. Perpendicular to the hair shaft, hyphae can be found. The nodule's periphery is a common place to find microorganisms that coexist. Neither locules nor asci are present as seen in cases of black Piedra.

Culture

At 25°C, Sabouraud dextrose agar (SDA) without cycloheximide, *Trichosporon* species grow quickly. The colonies are pasty and cream colored, but as they age, they become membranous, wrinkled with radial ridges and folds. After 2 or 3 weeks of maturation, the colony will be elevated, have a yellowish gray color, and be composed of emerging cells and arthroconidia.

Microscopic Morphology

The yeast cell cycle results in three distinct cell types: (1) Hyphae, (2) budding yeast cells, and (3) arthroconidia. *Trichosporon* species do not ferment carbohydrates.

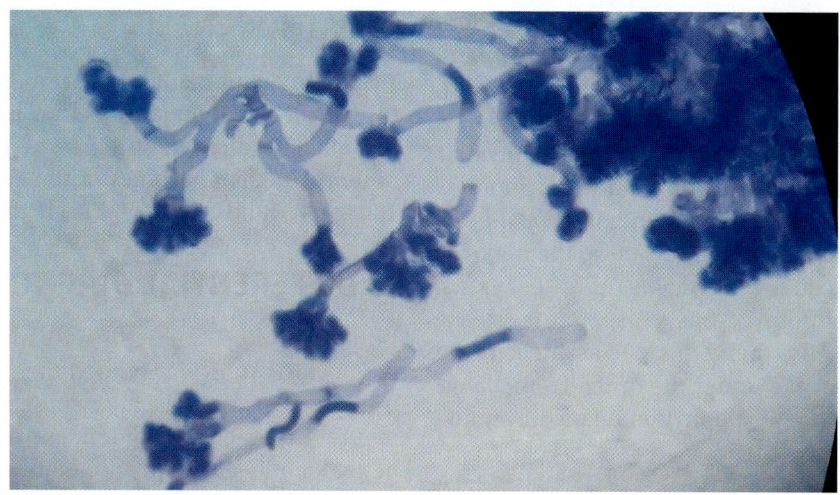

FIG. 8.2: *Trichosporon inkins* showing appressoria at the tip of hyphae (×400).

TABLE 8.1: Comparison of white piedra and black piedra.

Feature	***Black piedra***	***White piedra***
Causative agent	*Piedraia hortae* (a dematiaceous fungus, i.e., pigmented)	*Trichosporon* species (yeast-like fungi, non-pigmented)
Geographic distribution	More common in tropical regions of South America, Asia, and Africa	More common in temperate and subtropical climates (Europe, USA, Japan, etc.)
Hair affected	Primarily scalp hair	Beard, moustache, axilla, pubic hair (rarely scalp hair)
Appearance of nodules	Hard, black to dark brown, firmly attached nodules along hair shaft	Soft, white to light brown, loosely attached nodules along hair shaft
Consistency of nodules	Brittle, stone-like (hence "piedra")	Soft, easily detached
Effect on hair	Hair becomes brittle and may break	Usually no breakage, hair shaft remains intact
Microscopy (KOH prep)	Thick, pigmented, septate hyphae surrounding the hair shaft	Hyaline, septate hyphae with blastoconidia and arthroconidia
Culture	Black, slow-growing colonies	Creamy, yeast-like colonies
Clinical course	Chronic, often asymptomatic but cosmetically disturbing	Benign, asymptomatic, easily treated
Treatment	Cutting/shaving hair + topical antifungals (azole shampoos, keratolytics)	Shaving hair + azole antifungal shampoos or systemic azoles if extensive

Speciation can be achieved through the use of temperature tolerance and carbohydrate assimilation tests. The fungus is differentiated from *Geotrichum* by positive urease test, and no blastoconidia are seen in *Geotricum* species. Some species as *T. inkins* show appressoria at the hyphal tip, as shown in **Figure 8.2**. Using phenotypic techniques to precisely identify *Trichosporon* species is quite tough. The differentiating features of various species are given in **Table 8.1**. It is now advised to use genetic identification. The IGS1 region, which spans 26S and 5S rDNA, is an effective target within rDNA. Genomic sequence variations allow for the identification of species inside the IGS1 region, which ranges in size from 195 to 704 base pairs.

BLACK PIEDRA

The melanized mold *P. hortae* causes black piedra, a superficial fungal infection of hair. Melanized fungi are those that are pigmented or dematiaceous. The comparison between white piedra and black piedra is given in **Table 8.1**.

The scalp, beard, and moustache are all impacted by this disorder. Extremely seldom are pubic and axillary hair involved. Hard, gritty, and noticeable dark brown to black nodules that cling to the hair are developed when the fungus penetrates beneath the cuticle and spreads down the hair shaft. There are several nodules on a single shaft. The presence of ascoma and ascospores within the nodules is a defining feature of *P. hortae.* The mold *P. hortae* is a member of the Ascomycota phylum, class Dothideomycetes, and family Piedraiaceae.

Other melanogenic fungi or dematiaceous or pigmented fungi may produce other clinical conditions such as chromoblastomycosis, subcutaneous phaeohyphomycosis, and mycetoma.

EPIDEMIOLOGY

The natural habitat of black piedra is the humid tropical regions of the globe. Those indigenous peoples who live in the woods of South and Central America, Africa, and Southeast Asia are disproportionately likely to contract the disease.

Groups at Risk and Ways of Transmission

The exact cause of the infection is unknown, but it is believed to develop following exposure to certain environmental factors. When people in a household share tools such as combs and brushes, the disease can spread from person-to-person.

CLINICAL FEATURES

The hair follicles of the beard and scalp are impacted. A nodule's diameter might be anywhere from a few micrometers to 3 mm. Even on a single hair, several nodules can be seen. The infection starts just behind the hair's protective cuticle. Before infiltrating and disturbing the cuticle, the fungus only grows on the outer layer of the hair. Not all of the hairs are tangled up.

A cement-like substance or hyphae with many asci make up the nodules, which are packed with spores. Differentiating black piedra from pediculosis nits is important.

LABORATORY DIAGNOSIS

Direct Examination

Hairs are collected, and 20% KOH mount is done. Gentle warming of the slide facilitates the nodule's digestion. Microscopical findings are the presence of numerous thickened, brown-to-black septate hyphae and a large number of inflated intercalary cells that resemble chlamydospores. Additionally, ascus with as many as eight ascospores can be found. The ascospores are sexual spores produced by this fungus. They are fusiform, curved, and translucent, with projection on either side.

Culture

Sabouraud dextrose Agar slants with chloramphenicol as well as cycloheximide are used for the growth of fungus. The fungus is not lipophilic. The colony, which can be glabrous or coated with short aerial hyphae, grows slowly and is a dark brown to black in color. Brown to black pigment is seen on the reverse side of slant.

Lactophenol cotton blue (LPCB) mount from colonies shows only dematiaceous hyphae with chlamydoconidia and without sexual spores (ascospores). When culture is done on ascospore agar, asci with ascospores are seen.

TREATMENT

If left untreated, the disease may last for years. Shaving or trimming hairs contaminated with nodules is part of the treatment, followed by using an antifungal shampoo (ketoconazole). The effective topical applicants are imidazole, ciclopirox olamine, selenium sulfide (2.5%), precipitated sulfur in petroleum (6%), chlorhexidine solution, Castellani paint, zinc pyrithione, and amphotericin B lotion that can cause best cure. Orally terbinafine with dose of 250 mg daily for a period of 6 weeks is used along with topical agents.

CHAPTER

9 Tinea Nigra

INTRODUCTION

The stratum corneum becomes infected with the superficial yeast-like fungi *Hortaea werneckii* and *Stenella araguata* leading to the development of tinea nigra. A fungal infection can develop in the body after contact with infected dirt, sewage, wood, or compost. The condition was once called tinea nigra palmaris or tinea nigra plantaris because it develops on the palms or soles. The condition rarely affects other body parts. The lesions are in the form of brown to black pigmented nonscaly macules.

HISTORY

The first person to successfully isolate the fungus from human specimen was Paulo Parreiras Horta (1921). The fungus was given the name *Cladosporium werneckii* by him. In 1984, the genus name was revised by Nishimura et al. The genus *Hortaea* was established **(Fig. 9.1)**.

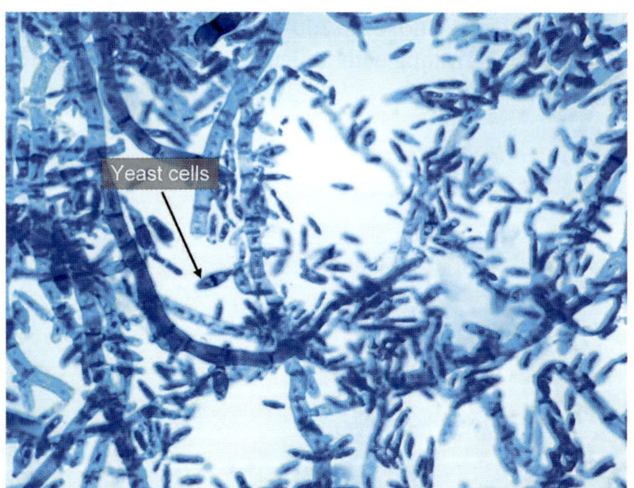

FIG. 9.1: LPCB mount of *Hortaea werneckii* (400×).
(LPCB: lactophenol cotton blue)

TAXONOMIC POSITION

Belonging to the class Dothideomycetes of the phylum Ascomycota, *H. werneckii* is a member of the family Teratosphaeriaceae and the order Capnodiales. The fungus was named "black yeast" because it looks like yeast and produces melanin. The genus *Hortaea* now has one more species, i.e., *Hortaea acidophila*, but this is not associated with tinea nigra. *S. araguata* is another fungus causing tinea nigra in Venezuela.

EPIDEMIOLOGY

Dirt, sewage, decaying plants, and spoiled, salted fish are all potential sites for this fungus. Commonly, this halophilic fungus is present on sandy beaches, where it thrives. Occasionally, the spread occurs by skin-to-skin contact. Hyperhidrosis is a condition that most people experience with their illness.

It was formerly believed that tinea nigra could only be found in the tropics of Asia, Africa, and Central and South America; however, it has now been discovered in North America and Europe as well.

PATHOGENESIS

No inflammatory response is observed since the infection is superficial. The infection is restricted within the stratum corneum without involving deeper tissue. The stratum corneum is packed with brown to black pigmented hyphae. Because the fungi causing infection are black pigmented (dematiaceous or melanized fungi), the lesions appear brown to black **(Fig. 9.2)**.

CLINICAL FEATURES

The macular lesion is asymptomatic. There is usually a single, well-circumscribed lesion of size 1–5 cm. It is pale

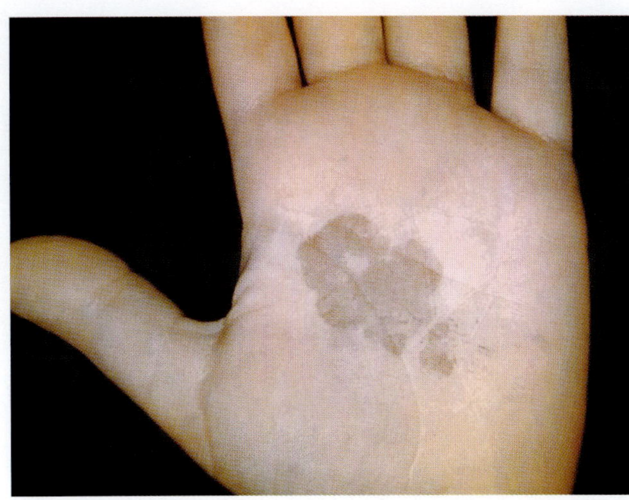

FIG. 9.2: Patch of tinea nigra on palm.
Source: Public Health Image Library CDC.

brown or black as the fungus has melanin on its cell wall. It expands slowly and causes cosmetic effects. The lesions are without redness and scaling. The clinical incubation period varies from 2 to 7 weeks. The color of skin differs from person to person, with darker patches at the edges. Infections typically manifest on the palmar or plantar side of the affected hand or foot. It is likely that hyperhidrosis, or excessive palm sweating, is a risk factor. Penis, interdigital web, wrist, forearm, trunk, or neck injuries are extremely uncommon sites which may be affected.

DIFFERENTIAL DIAGNOSIS

Additional illnesses that might be mistaken for tinea nigra include pityriasis versicolor, pina, syphilis, Addison's disease lesions, melanoma, chemical or dye staining, and malignant melanoma.

Dermoscopy

This may have some advantages to differentiate from other melanoid lesions.

LABORATORY DIAGNOSIS

Histopathology or KOH preparation of skin scrapings is used to get a diagnosis. To distinguish *H. werneckii* from other fungi that resemble black yeast, such as *Aureobasidium pullulans*, culture confirmation is required. To save the risk of scarring and excisional surgery, a proper diagnosis must be made. The active lesion margin is the site to take skin scrapings. In the KOH (20%) analysis, yeast-like cells measuring 2–8 µm in size and black-pigmented hyphae measuring 5–6 µm in diameter are observed.

Culture

Two Sabouraud Dextrose Agar (SDA) slants (with cycloheximide or actidione) are incubated at 25°C and 37°C, respectively. At 37°C, there is no growth.

Colony

Growth is slow, and maturation of the colony occurs in 3 weeks. Initially, the colonies are yeasty and brownish which become black with aerial hyphae after further incubation.

Microscopy from Colonies

The yeast cells (two to three celled) show transverse septae. The hyphae are septate, pigmented with thick walls. Intercalary annelids, the conidiogenous cells, are found in the hyphae. At their very ends, annellations can be seen. The production and discharge of hyaline annelloconidia result in the development of pale olive-colored yeast with one or two cells. After that, they develop into chlamydospore clusters or buds.

The fungus should be differentiated from other dematiaceous fungi such as *Aureobasidium* species and *Exophiala* species. *H. werneckii* hydrolyzes casein but does not decompose tyrosine. It is tolerant to 10% NaCl; absence of growth at 37°C and broad annellated zones are the characteristics used to differentiate it from various *Exophiala* species. There is an exoantigen test that is developed to differentiate the pathogen from other fungi.

HISTOPATHOLOGY

Mild acanthosis and hyperkeratosis are visible. Normal hematoxylin and eosin (H&E)-stained sections reveal *H. werneckii* due to their inherent pigment. Two-celled yeasts are seen in the tissue. The stratum corneum has red-stained septate hyphae when stained with periodic acid-Schiff (PAS).

Molecular Tests

Tests such as polymerase chain reaction (PCR) may be used for diagnosis but it is not cost-effective.

TREATMENT

Treatment includes the use of Whitfield's ointment, salicylic acid (5–10%), miconazole, clotrimazole, econazole, isoconazole, and thiabendazole (10%) for at least 2 weeks. Oral itraconazole, 200 mg BD, is given for 3 weeks with good success.

CHAPTER

10 Dermatophytosis

INTRODUCTION

Dermatophytosis is the fungal infection of skin, hairs, and nails caused by fungi of three genera, i.e., *Trichophyton*, *Microsporum*, and *Epidermophyton*. On the other hand dermatomycosis includes infections of skin, hair, and nails by yeasts, other molds in addition to dermatophytosis.

- *Trichophyton* species infect skin, hair, and nails.
- *Microsporum* species infect skin and hair but not nails.
- *Epidermophyton* species infect skin and nails but not hair.

HISTORY

In 1835, Remak made a groundbreaking discovery regarding crusts from favic lesions. He said that he could not identify the structures as fungal. It was Schönlein who, in 1839, described their mycotic nature. In 1841 David Gruby presented his paper at Academy of Science on isolation of fungus from favus. Raymond Sabouraud's renowned work, *Les Teignes*, was published in 1910 after he had begun scientifically studying dermatophytes from 1890. "Sabouraud glucose (dextrose) agar" is the name given to the medium he created, which is still used to cultivate fungus today under several formulations. In 1934, Chester Emmons established the current system of dermatophyte classification.

MYCOLOGY

Species of dermatophytes are classified into three genera according to their outward appearance:

1. *Trichophyton*: 24 species
2. *Microsporum*: 16 species
3. *Epidermophyton floccosum*

Arthroderma and *Nannizzia* were the original taxa used to classify teleomorphic dermatophyte stages. Anamorphs of *Arthroderma* belonged to the genus *Trichophyton* or *Chrysosporium*. Anamorphic members of *Nannizzia* belonged to the genus *Microsporum*.

Arthroderma is a genus of fungus that belongs to the Arthrodermataceae family, which is in the Onygenales order, Eurotiomycetes class, and Ascomycota phylum.

EPIDEMIOLOGY

There are three categories of dermatophytes distinguished by their environmental traits. The term "anthropophilic" describes fungi that exclusively infect humans. Host preferences for zoophilic fungi are birds and animals. Species that thrive in dirt or soil are called geophilic. The dermatophyte species belonging to each ecological group are listed in **Box 10.1**.

BOX 10.1 | Ecological classification of dermatophytes.

Anthropophilic:

- *Trichophyton rubrum*
- *Trichophyton mentagrophytes*
- *Trichophyton schoenleinii*
- *Trichophyton tonsurans*
- *Trichophyton violaceum*
- *Microsporum audouinii*
- *Epidermophyton floccosum*

Zoophilic:

- *Trichophyton equinum*
- *Trichophyton verrucosum*
- *Microsporum canis*
- *Trichophyton simii*
- *Microsporum gallinae*
- *Microsporum persicolor*

Geophilic:

- *Microsporum gypseum*
- *Trichophyton ajelloi*
- *Microsporum cookei*
- *Microsporum nanum*
- *Microsporum praecox*
- *Trichophyton terrestre*

Importance of Ecological Classification

Ecological classification aids in the identification of dermatophytes, which aids in the determination of the most likely source and therapy. In general, zoophilic and geophilic organisms develop lesions with greater inflammatory responses that respond quickly to therapy than anthropophilic species. Zoophilic and geophilic organisms are easier to treat, but anthropophilic species establish persistent infection. Infection is spread by direct touch or through fomites. Contact with contaminated fungus spores in soil, animals, or humans may spread the illness. Anthropophilic species are uniquely suited to man and are spread by desquamated skin and fomites such as combs, hair brushes, clothes, towels, and nail cutters but require intimate contact due to their low virulence and infectivity. The occurrence of dermatophytes varies from place to place and may be related to the environmental factors.

Risk Groups/Risk Factors

- *Age*: Kids of school age often get fungal infection of the scalp known as tinea capitis. Perhaps it is due to the fact that their stratum corneum is composed of fatty acids. After puberty, adolescent sebum contains medium-chain-length fatty acids, which inhibit dermatophyte growth.
- As a general indicator of immunodeficiency, dermatophytosis is prevalent in human immunodeficiency virus (HIV)-positive individuals.
- Smoking and peripheral artery disease may also act as predisposing factors.
- People who swim.
- *Gym participants*: There is a higher chance of exposure in gym and health club locker rooms and showers which is why the risk is higher.
- Dermatophytosis can progress to a more severe form in patients using immunosuppressive drugs. Among the medications that have been associated to dermatophytosis are cyclosporine, oral corticosteroids, prednisolone, and infliximab [a tumor necrosis factor (TNF)-inhibitor monoclonal antibody].
- *Professionals*: Dog and cat owners may be exposed to *Microsporum canis* that lives on their pets' fur. People who work with animals in laboratories, pet stores, zoos, stockmen, and veterinarians are more likely to get tinea corporis and tinea cruris. Also, agriculturists, farmers, athletes, and wrestlers are prone to infections.
- Maceration, little injuries, tight clothing, walking barefoot, and sharing the shaving equipment are all examples of personal behaviors and living situations that can increase the risk.
- The prevalence of dermatophytosis is determined by environmental conditions, personal hygiene, and individual's susceptibility from place to place and natural habitat.
- Excessive use of hair oil may have a protective role.

Infections

Infection spreads by fomites, and infective forms are the spores (arthroconidia) of the fungi. Some of the common geographical areas of dermatophytes are given in **Table 10.1**.

IMMUNITY

Antibody-mediated immunity (AMI), cell-mediated immunity (CMI), and innate responses try to restrict the growth of fungus in skin. The enzymes of fungi act as virulence factor. Some enzymes help to restrict the invasion by producing inflammation. Mannan produced by fungi may try to restrict CMI. The structure of nails is tough which acts as an innate mechanism of infection protection.

PATHOGENESIS AND PATHOLOGY

Skin lesion occurs when mild injured skin comes into touch with fungal arthrospores. Keratinase enzymes produced by fungi break down keratin which helps in the fungal entry into living cells. Fungi grow in dead, keratinized tissues. Fungus does not penetrate deeper skin layers. Invasion can develop up to the stratum corneum and progress laterally to cause a lesion.

Metabolic products generate inflammation in the epidermis, resulting in erythema, vesicles, and pruritus.

TABLE 10.1: Geographical distribution of dermatophytes.

Species of fungi	*Endemicity*
Trichophyton soudanense	Central and West Africa
Microsporum ferrugineum	Japan
Trichophyton concentricum	Restricted to islands in South Pacific and small areas in Central and South America
Trichophyton rubrum and *Microsporum canis*	Common agents in Western countries
Anthropophilic fungi have been replaced by zoonotic species such as *M. canis* and *Trichophyton mentagrophytes*	Southern and East European countries

They create ring-shaped pruritic scaly skin lesions with central clearing and elevated erythematous borders/edges with noticeable advancing margins. Multiple skin lesions merge to generate a unique geometric design. Older hyphae in the lesion split into arthrospores, which are eventually discharged. This is responsible for central clearing in ringworm lesions. Nail infection begins with darkening of subungual tissue, followed by hyperkeratosis and discoloration of the nail plate. This results in nail deformity. Hair infection begins as an erythematous papule around the hair shaft to discoloration and shaft breakage. Hair becomes brittle, and alopecia may develop. The hyphal tips that grow down within the hair shaft reach the borders of living keratinizing cells but finish above them in a fringe of hyphal endings known as Adam's fringe. Majocchi granuloma, a deep and chronic suppurative folliculitis, can also occur.

CLINICAL FEATURES

One definition of the Latin term tinea is "moth" or "gnawing worm." This term is used for the skin lesions as serpentine (snake-like) and circular or annular (ring-like) lesions **(Fig. 10.1)**. The moth-eaten appearance of ringworm lesions on the scalp reminded the ancient Romans of the Tineidae, a family of insects that cause damage to woollens. The word "Tinea," meaning dermatophytosis, was coined by Romans. Dermatophyte literally translates to "skin plant." Phytes is the scientific term for plants. Each lesion caused by dermatophytes has a specific name starting with tinea. It was formerly believed that the fungi were plants, but phylogenetic studies have proven otherwise, and they now have their own kingdom. The causative agents of various clinical types are summarized in **Table 10.2**.

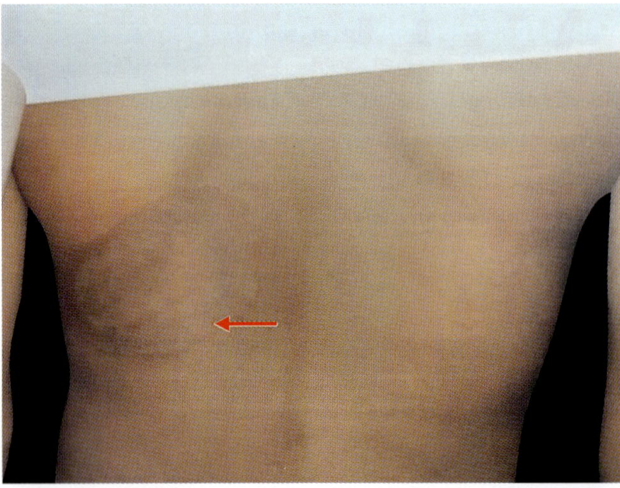

FIG. 10.1: Annular lesion of dermatophyte.

Tinea Capitis (Scalp Ringworm)

Tinea capitis is an infection of shaft of the scalp hairs and presents as the following clinical types:

- Inflammatory—kerion, favus, and agminate folliculitis (agminate = grouped or clustered together)
- Noninflammatory—black dot, seborrheic dermatitis-like, and gray patch

It affects the scalp, hair follicles, and hair shafts. Typically, the infection shows up in isolated areas, but it has the potential to spread throughout the entire scalp. The pathognomonic sign is hair loss. As a frequent childhood illness, tinea capitis is far less common in teenagers and extremely rare in adults.

Black Dot (Common)

There are areas of hair stubs that are not inflamed or scaling. As the fungus grows inside the hair shaft, it weakens and breaks at the scalp, leaving behind black spots of the remaining hair. The illness can persist for a long time if nothing is done about it. Occipital

TABLE 10.2: Clinical types with causative agents.

Clinical type	*Causative agents*	*Symptoms*
Tinea capitis	*Trichophyton* species, and *Microsporum* species	Scalp inflammation, hair loss, and scaling
Favus	*Trichophyton schoenleinii*, rarely *Trichophyton violaceum* and *Microsporum gypseum*	Yellow, cup-shaped crusts on the scalp, possible hair loss
Kerion	*Trichophyton verrucosum* and *Trichophyton mentagrophytes*	Inflamed, abscess-like lesions on the scalp
Tinea barbae	*Trichophyton rubrum*, *T. mentagrophytes*, and *T. verrucosum*	Itchy, inflamed lesions in the beard area
Tinea corporis	*T. rubrum* and other dermatophytes	Ring-shaped, itchy lesions on the body
Tinea imbricata	*Trichophyton concentricum*	Concentric rings of scaling on the skin
Tinea cruris	*Epidermophyton floccosum*, *T. rubrum*, and *T. mentagrophytes*	Itching, redness, and inflammation in the groin area
Tinea unguium	*T. rubrum*, *T. mentagrophytes*, and *E. floccosum*	Thickened, discolored, and brittle nails
Tinea manuum	*T. rubrum*, *E. floccosum*, and *T. mentagrophytes*	Itchy, scaling rash on the hands

lymphadenopathy affects around one third of all afflicted children.

Seborrheic (Most Common)

The scalp shows signs of redness. Hair loss that is either patchy or matted, as well as pustules, nodules, leaks, and crusting, may occur. The vast majority of affected youngsters will have occipital lymphadenopathy.

Kerion (Rare)

The lesion is also known as kerion celsi. It is common in children. This form is quite severe. It is purulent, boggy mass with a honeycomb appearance and pustules. The follicles discharge pus. It is possible to see pus escaping from multiple points. There is also the possibility of sinus formation. After severe crusting, scarring develops. Crusts formation occurs with matting of adjacent hairs. The lymph nodes are enlarged. There may be scar formation on the scalp. The lesions are sharply defined, painful edematous plaques in addition to pustules and abscesses that drain pus. **Figure 10.2** shows lesion of kerion.

Favus

This kind of tinea capitis is rare. Hyphae and keratin hair debris clump together to produce scutula (cup-like crusts around hair follicles). Minimal fungal growth occurs in hair. Scarring, skin shrinking, and cicatricial baldness are complications of favus that need medical attention. The condition is caused by *Trichophyton schoenleinii*, *Trichophyton violaceum*, or *Microsporum gypseum*. The South African word for favus is *witkop*, meaning "white head."

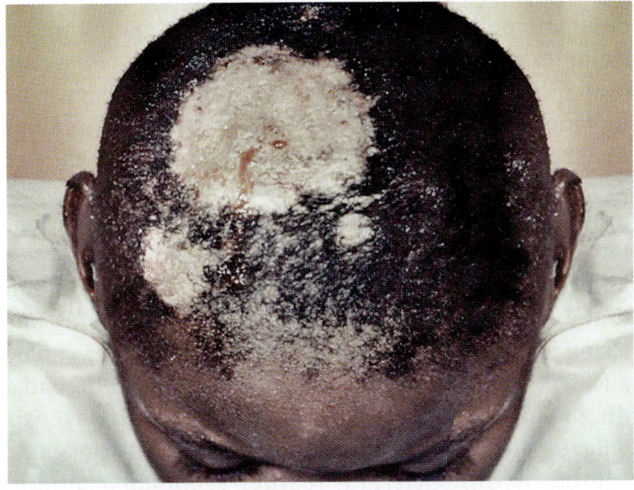

FIG. 10.2: Kerion.
Source: Public Health Image Library CDC.

Hair Invasion

Fungi invade the keratinized outer root sheath and the inner cortex of the hair follicle. They do not pass through the cuticle. They break down keratin in the hair shaft. Only above the zone of fresh keratinization do hyphae proliferate. Hyphae fracture into short arthrospores (3–4 μm) (infectious arthroconidia) as they grow inside the hair shaft.

Endothrix

Arthrospores and hyphae are located inside the hair shaft. The hair cuticle is typically destroyed and the hair shaft is weakened.

Ectothrix

Hyphae encase the hair shaft "like a sack full of marbles" with densely packed, spherical arthroconidia after penetrating the cuticle of the hair's outer layer. The fungi causing ectothrix and endothrix are given in **Table 10.3.** Some of the key differences between ectothrix and endothrix are given in **Table 10.4.**

Tinea Corporis (Tinea Glabrosa or Tinea Glabrata Circinata)

Infections caused by this sort of ringworm are the most prevalent. The smooth trunk skin is covered with well-defined patches or plaques that do not extend to the scalp, beard, groin, hands, or feet. Typical lesions of ringworm have a center clearing, a raised reddish-scaly border, and an oval or round shape (the "ring" form). The skin feels itchy. Flat, poorly-defined lesions might be erythematous, scaling, large, irregular, or psoriasiform in immunocompromised people. Because it can infect both smooth and glabrous skin types, tinea corporis

TABLE 10.3: Causative agents of ectothrix and endothrix.

Types of hair invasion	*Dermatophyte species*
Ectothrix	• *Trichophyton mentagrophytes* • *Microsporum canis* • *Microsporum gypseum* • *Microsporum audouinii* • *Trichophyton verrucosum* • *Trichophyton rubrum*
Endothrix	• *Trichophyton schoenleinii* • *Trichophyton tonsurans* • *Trichophyton violaceum* • *Trichophyton soudanense*

TABLE 10.4: Differences between ectothrix and endothrix.

Characteristics	*Ectothrix hair invasion*	*Endothrix hair invasion*
Location of fungal elements	Fungal spores (arthroconidia) are seen on the *outside* of the hair shaft	Fungal spores (arthroconidia) are located *inside* the hair shaft
Appearance under microscope	Hair shaft is coated by spores; the cuticle is often destroyed, leading to a rough and brittle appearance	Spores are within the hair shaft; the hair shaft may remain intact, appearing full of spores without external damage
Wood's lamp examination	May show fluorescence, particularly with *Microsporum* species	No fluorescence under Wood's lamp examination
Effect on hair	Hair becomes fragile and easily breaks off close to the scalp	Hair shaft may remain intact but is filled with fungal elements, leading to breakage within the hair shaft

is sometimes called tinea glabrosa or tinea glabrata circinata. In India, tinea corporis is a common infection caused by *Trichophyton rubrum.*

Majocchi's Granuloma (Nodular Granulomatous Perifolliculitis)

The lesions manifest as firm, violaceous perifollicular nodules, papules, or pustules. Infection of hair follicles with deep dermal inflammation is seen. This condition is common in women with tinea pedis or onychomycosis (cause by *T. rubrum*) who shave their legs.

Tinea Imbricata(Synonyms: Tokelau)

The causative agent is *Trichophyton concentricum.*

This condition is uncommonly seen. The lesions manifest as firm, violaceous nodules or papules. It is an unusual variant of tinea corporis. It has limited distribution in China, India, and particularly in Polynesian Islands (Tokelau, Fiji, Papua, Samoa, and Tamana), as well as Central and South America, including Mexico. There are concentric layers of scaly plaques. The lesions spread out over many years. Patient may have intense pruritus, and lichenification may occur.

Tinea Indecisiva (Tinea Pseudoimbricata)

Lesions caused by dermatophytes other than *T. concentricum* appear similar to tinea imbricata. Lesion appearances often resemble "rings within rings" or "double-edged tinea."

Tinea Gladiatorum

Wrestlers contract the disease through skin-to-skin contact. Symptoms manifest on the affected limbs, trunk, and neck. *Trichophyton tonsurans* is the causing agent.

Tinea Incognito

This type of tinea corporis involves the use of systemic or topical treatment of highly potent topical steroids to alter the lesion morphology. Papules, nodules, or pustules form the lesion's outward appearance. They are larger and more amorphous, though they may still look scaly. The face, trunk, or limbs can be affected by tinea incognito. There are similarities between pyoderma and eczema. While *T. rubrum* is the most common dermatophyte involved, other species are frequently isolated.

Tinea Faciei

The infection affects the skin of the face that is not bearded. Infections at different sites manifest clinically similarly.

Tinea Barbae (Barber's Itch or Tinea Sycosis)

Fungus affects the beard. It is common in men who work in close contact with animals. The most common clinical type is pustular folliculitis. There is minimum inflammation, and causative agents are *T. violaceum* and *T. rubrum.* Another presentation is the deep type in which nodular thickenings and kerion-like swellings are seen and it is usually caused by *T. verrucosum* and *T. mentagrophytes.* Alopecia results when hairs break at the skin's surface or when fungal masses block hair follicles. With severe inflammation, pustules, exudates, and crusts form. Tissues in the vicinity of keratoses and draining sinuses are severely affected. Mostly, only one lesion is apparent. However, the entire beard area can be affected, and alopecia can never go away. The differential diagnosis includes *Staphylococcus aureus,* sycosis vulgaris, furunculosis or carbuncles, and acne vulgaris, caused by *Cutibacterium* (earlier *Propionibacterium*) *acnes* and *Candida* folliculitis. Rarely, *E. floccosum* causes widespread verrucous lesions known as verrucous epidermophytosis.

Tinea Cruris (Synonyms: Jock Itch, Tinea Inguinalis)

Dermatophytes affect perianal, groin, and perineal areas. This variance is seen in those who wear clothing that is close to the body. The itching and discomfort of tinea cruris, sometimes known as jock itch, can last for a long time or come on suddenly. Lesion bases consist of small, spherical, and inflamed bumps with raised, red edges and dry, flaky skin. Thigh lesions can be symmetrical or asymmetrical, and they can be unilateral or bilateral. Babies can get nappy rash from tinea cruris, which is similar to nappy rash from *Candida albicans.* Transmission is possible through towels, beds, and garments.

Tinea Pedis

Figure 10.3 shows a clinical picture of tinea pedis. The webs between the toes and the bottoms of the feet are especially vulnerable to tinea pedis. The condition is also named "athlete foot" or "sandal ringworm," and it is more common in those who wear shoes for a long period of time. Toe webs might exhibit scaling, fissuring, maceration, redness, and cracking. Itching and burning sensations are present. Minor sacs develop into ruptured vesicles. Hyperkeratotic and microscopic scales appear on the infected feet over time. Common pathogens include *T. rubrum, T. mentagrophytes,* and *E. floccosum.* Various types are noted as follows:

Dry hyperkeratotic type: The hyperkeratotic, dry kind of infection that starts on the bottom of the foot and spreads up the side (moccasin or sandal ringworm). The scaling is incredibly fine and shiny. Normal skin tone is delicate. There may be significant redness. Many times, there is onychomycosis associated with this condition. *T. rubrum* is the causative agent.

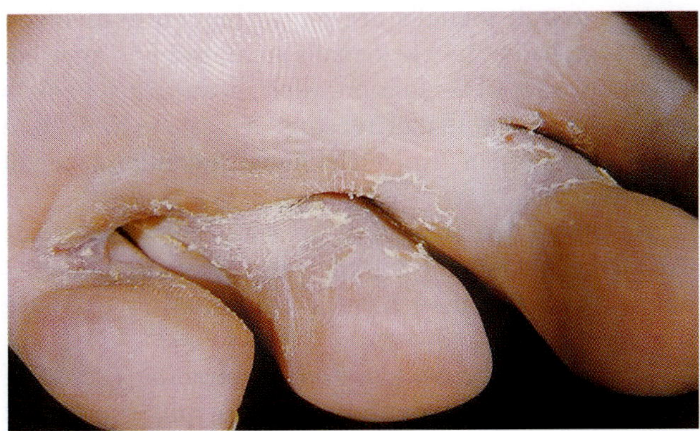

FIG. 10.3: Tinea pedis.

- *Vesicular type*: Infection becomes chronic tinea pedis. Lesions are pruritic, multilocular vesicles or bullae. They are initially filled with clear fluid. The lesions initially separated before coalescing into blisters. They may resolve or reoccur after rupturing. With secondary bacterial infection, pustules develop.
- *Ulcerative*: The presentation is ulcers with maceration affecting sole.
- *Type across digits*: It is interdigital infection. Clinical features are itching, peeling, maceration, and fissures in the toe webs. This illness may spread to toes.
- *Discomfort with just one hand*: Tinea pedis typically occurs 8–9 years earlier to tinea manuum. It mostly affects adult males. The feet are the first areas to get infected. According to patients, tinea manuum formed on the hand that picked at the itchy toenails or rubbed the painful bottoms of their feet.

Tinea Unguium

Tinea unguium is the dermatophyte infection of nail plates. Usually, adults are affected. The most common fungi which are responsible for this condition are *T. rubrum, T. mentagrophytes,* and *E. floccosum.* The infection starts under the edge of nail plate or lateral nail folds. It progresses to involve nail plate and nail bed. There is the formation of subungual debris. The nail thickens, chalks, and turns opaque as an infection of the nail plates starts under the free edge or laterally. Tinea unguium is a common complication of untreated tinea pedis. *T. rubrum, T. mentagrophytes,* and *E. floccosum* are the causative agents.

ONYCHOMYCOSIS

Onychomycosis is an infection of the nail unit caused by fungi (dermatophytes, nondermatophyte molds, and yeasts), presenting with discoloration of the nail **(***see* **Fig. 10.4)**, onycholysis, and nail plate thickening. Any component of the nail unit, including the nail plate, nail matrix, and nail bed, can be affected. The term "onychomycosis" is derived from the Greek words "onyx" meaning nail and "mykes" meaning fungus.

ETIOLOGY

The causative agents of this condition are mentioned in **Box 10.2**, and the predisposing factors for the development of onychomycoses are mentioned in **Box 10.3**.

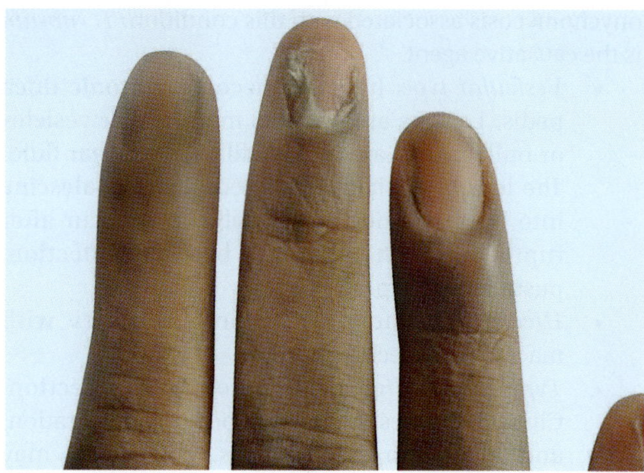

FIG. 10.4: Nail infection (onychomycosis).

BOX 10.2 Etiological agents of onychomycosis.

Dermatophyte molds:
- *Trichophyton mentagrophytes*
- *Trichophyton rubrum*
- *Epidermophyton floccosum*
- *Microsporum* species
- *Trichophyton verrucosum*
- *Trichophyton tonsurans*
- *Trichophyton violaceum*
- *Trichophyton soudanense*
- *Trichophyton equinum*
- *Arthroderma* species

Nondermatophyte molds:
- *Aspergillus* species
- *Scopulariopsis* species
- *Fusarium* species
- *Acremonium* species
- *Syncephalastrum* species
- *Paecilomyces* species
- *Neoscytalidium* species
- *Chaetomium* species
- *Onychocola* species
- *Alternaria* species

Yeasts:
- *Candida albicans*
- *Candida tropicalis*
- *Candida parapsilosis*

The condition is much more common in adults than in children, and the prevalence increases with age.

PATHOGENESIS

Infection is acquired through direct contact of the nail with fungi. As there is no immune response in the nails, they are susceptible to infection. Enzymes produced by fungi have proteolytic, keratinolytic, and lipolytic activities which degrade the keratin in the nail plate.

BOX 10.3 Predisposing factors for the development of onychomycosis.

- Chronic mucocutaneous candidiasis
- Use of occlusive modern footwear
- Obesity
- Fungal infection elsewhere on the body (in particular, tinea pedis), chronic paronychia, and previous onychomycosis
- Hyperhidrosis, participation in sports or fitness activities
- Nail trauma
- Poor nail grooming
- Use of commercial swimming pools
- Communal bathing
- Living with family members with fungal infection
- Poor health
- Genetic factors
- Immunodeficiency (in particular, acquired immunodeficiency syndrome and transplant patients)
- Diabetes mellitus
- Down syndrome
- Psoriasis
- Peripheral vascular disease, venous insufficiency

CLINICAL FEATURES

Discoloration of Nail Plates

Various shades of colors as white, green, and black discoloration of the nail plate have also been observed.

Other clinical manifestations include:
- Subungual hyperkeratosis
- Detachment of nail from the nail bed (onycholysis)
- Thickening of the nail plate (onychauxis)
- Linear, single, or multiple white, yellow, orange, or brown bands on the nail plate

In general, toenails are more frequently involved than fingernails. The big toenails are most often affected. Generally, several toenails are affected, and tinea pedis is often associated with nail infection. It is rare to have more than one fingernail involved without concomitant toenail involvement.

Based on the pattern of invasion, onychomycosis can be divided into the five clinical subtypes as described below (patients may have a combination of these subtypes):

1. *Distal lateral subungual onychomycosis (DLSO)*: It is the most common clinical subtype. The fungal infection starts at the hyponychium. It progresses to involve the distal nail bed and subsequently the nail

plate. The infection then spreads proximally through the nail plate, causing linear channels or "spikes." *T. rubrum* and *T. mentagrophytes* are the most common infective agents. There is yellowish, whitish, or brownish discoloration of a distal corner of a nail. Distal subungual hyperkeratosis, onycholysis, and/or onychauxis of the lateral and distal aspects of the nail plate are often present.

2. *White superficial onychomycosis*: The upper surface of the nail plate is involved. *T. mentagrophytes* is the most common pathogen. The lesions are white dots or patches on the surface of the nail plate. These can be easily scraped off.
3. *Proximal subungual onychomycosis*: The infection involves the undersurface of the proximal nail fold in the vicinity of the cuticle and then extends distally. The most common causes are *T. rubrum* and *Fusarium* species. Clinical presentation is an area of leukonychia in the proximal nail plate and moves distally with nail growth. The condition is commonly seen in patients with immunodeficiency, especially acquired immunodeficiency syndrome (AIDS).
4. *Endonyx onychomycosis*: It is the infection of the nail plate without infection of the nail bed. This condition is usually caused by *Trichophyton soudanense* and *T. violaceum*. Clinically, there are milky patches of the nail plate, indentations, and lamellar splitting. The nail plate is firmly attached to the nail bed, and subungual hyperkeratosis is absent.
5. *Total dystrophic onychomycosis*: There is total destruction of the entire nail apparatus and is usually the end stage of onychomycosis that may occur in any of the other subtypes. Clinically, it presents as severely dystrophic and crumbed nail plate which becomes yellowish, diffusely thickened, and friable.

DIAGNOSIS

Dermoscopy of the nails is a quick, noninvasive, and highly effective method that may help to differentiate onychomycosis from other nail disorders. The diagnosis methods are direct microscopic examination with a potassium hydroxide (KOH) wet-mount preparation, histopathological examination of the trimmed affected nail plate with a periodic acid-Schiff (PAS) stain, fungal culture, or polymerase chain reaction (PCR) assays.

Depending on the clinical presentation, nail clippings, nail plate scrapings, nail bed scrapings, and subungual scrapings are the samples collected for microscopy and culture. A sterile nail clipper is used to clip the full-thickness nail plate, and a sterile curette or blade should be used to obtain subungual debris. Nail plate dermoscopy is used to identify the best location to obtain adequate samples for mycological examination. In case of distal and lateral subungual onychomycosis, the sample is obtained from the most proximal area of involvement (the most active area of infection where the highest concentration of hyphae is located) after clipping the distal onycolytic nail plate. The hyphae at the distal end of the nail are mostly nonviable. In white superficial onychomycosis, the specimen is obtained by scraping the affected superficial aspect of the nail plate with a number 15 blade. In proximal subungual onychomycosis, the upper nail plate of the proximal nail is debrided and the underlying nail debris is collected with a curette. Before the sample collection, the nail plate and the surrounding soft tissue should be cleaned with 70% isopropyl or ethyl alcohol to prevent contamination. The samples should be collected in sterile paper for transport to the laboratory in a sterile container.

Complication of Onychomycosis

It acts as a source for cutaneous fungal infections such as tinea pedis, tinea corporis, and tinea cruris. The infection may also disseminate to other nails. There are also chances of bacterial infections such as cellulitis and paronychia, especially in immunocompromised individuals, including diabetics.

The condition may cause discomfort, pain, paresthesia, nail deformities, and difficulties in trimming thick nail plates and wearing shoes. It becomes unsightly and socially embarrassing (especially for females) and affects the quality of life.

Treatment modalities are oral antifungal therapy, topical antifungal therapy, laser therapy, photodynamic therapy, and surgical avulsion (e.g., very thick and chronic fungal nail).

Tinea Manuum

Hand skin on the palm side is affected. Palm and finger hyperkeratosis are seen. The pathogens include *T. rubrum*, *T. mentagrophytes*, and *E. floccosum*.

Id Reaction

Lesions are vesicles that develop at a location anatomically distant from the dermatophytosis site; they can be acute, localized, or widespread. When people are allergic to circulating fungal antigens, it can lead to dermatophytids. While the exact frequency is unknown, 4–5% of patients with dermatophytosis report experiencing id reactions. Id reaction is likely to to occur when a patient is put on systemic antifungals. It is easy to confuse drug reaction. Fungal antigens absorbed through the skin and circulatory system can trigger the id response. A list of symptoms that may accompany this reaction includes itching, fever, loss of appetite, splenomegaly, leukocytosis, and generalized lymphadenopathy. Two distinct "id" reactions are defined:

1. *Lichen scrofulosorum-like*: There are follicular lesions that are either clustered or dispersed all throughout the body.
2. *Pompholyx-like*: Examples of many kinds of lesions are pompholyx type, vesicular, bullous, and papular. Type III hypersensitivity reaction is the working definition of the reaction. In cases of tinea pedis, lesions can be seen on the palms and fingers.

Nondermatophytic Dermatomycosis

This is the infection of skin and nails caused by various fungi other than dermatophytes. These are *Candida* species, *Neoscytalidium dimidiatum*, *Fusarium oxysporum*, *Onychocola canadensis*, *Trichosporon* species, and *Lasiodiplodia* species. The details of these fungi are given in their respective chapters.

LABORATORY DIAGNOSIS

Wood's Lamp Examination

Cell wall fluorescence is caused by the presence of pteridine pigment in some fungi. When such fungi infect hair, the hair fluoresces under ultraviolet (UV) light. The fluorescence can be demonstrated when infected hair is seen using Wood's lamp. It utilizes "black light," a 365-nm wavelength filtered UV light source, to visualize the fluorescence of infected hairs. Wood's lamp is a handheld device. The patient sits in a dark room, and the doctor observes the scalp of patient for fluorescence of infected hair. The area of the scalp where the hair is infected will fluoresce. It helps to select hair for culture and microscopy. Hair infected with *T. schoenleinii* and several *Microsporum* species test positive. With an increasing number of cases involving diverse pathogenic species, the significance of Wood's lamp examination is diminishing. It is known that a false-positive result occurs while using some ointments. Numerous species' normal fluorescence is displayed in **Table 10.5**.

TABLE 10.5: Different colored fluorescence produced by different fungi.

Microorganisms	*Fluorescence color*
Microsporum audouinii	Bright green
Microsporum canis	Bright green
Microsporum ferrugineum	Blue green
Microsporum distortum	Blue green
Microsporum gypseum	Dull yellow
Trichophyton schoenleinii	Dull green
Malassezia furfur	Golden yellow

Specimen Collection

Skin, nails, and hairs are required for laboratory diagnosis of dermatophyte infection.

- *Skin*: Lesions should not be treated with topical antifungals for a minimum of 7 days. Thoroughly cleanse the area before collection by using sterile gauze squares soaked in 70% ethyl alcohol. If a cotton ball is used for cleaning, there may be a risk of introducing cotton filaments, which look like fungal elements. While center of the lesion has few and non-viable hyphae, a skin scraping taken from the lesion's edge reveals more and viable fungal hyphae. Choose epithelium from the roof if blisters or vesicles are seen.
- *Nails*: There are two types of specimens: (1) Nail clippings and (2) subungual detritus.
  Prior to collecting samples from the nail bed, the nail plate, and the deeper sections of nails that are discolored or dystrophic, it is recommended to wash and swab the nails with alcohol.
- *Hairs*: The method of gathering hair is plucking instead of cutting. Remove any stray hairs or stubs using sterile forceps. Collect hair samples and scrapings from scales for use in microscopy and culture.

The art of the toothbrush: A sterile, soft-headed toothbrush is used to massage the entire scalp in order to gather fungal materials. Then, the collected hair is promptly planted in solid culture medium. This method is very helpful when collecting hair from youngsters.

Transport: Samples are collected in a fold of black paper and transported at room temperature to the laboratory.

For microscopy, the following preparations are done:

- *KOH mount*: Use a glass slide to deposit a small portion of the specimen. Add one drop of 10% KOH (20% concentration for nails). Put a coverslip on it. Gently heat the slide at a temperature of 51–54°C (not boiling) and wait for 10–15 minutes. Fungal formations, such as endothrix and ectothrix, might disintegrate if kept longer; therefore, it is important to examine hairs promptly. If we are working with nails, we might have to leave the KOH mount in a moist chamber for a bit longer or soak the nail in a tube containing a small amount of 20% KOH overnight. Examine the specimen under both low and high magnification once it has cleared, meaning that the epithelial cells and debris have disappeared. Nails benefit from a mixture of KOH and dimethyl sulfoxide (DMSO).

- *KOH-permanent blue-black ink*: Place the specimen on a slide. Put a coverslip. Place a drop of ink-KOH at the edge of coverslip. Allow fluid to seep under it.
- KOH-calcofluor stain increases the sensitivity of the test.
- Nail clipping stained with PAS or Grocott-Gömöri's methenamine silver (GMS) is more sensitive method than KOH mount.
  The skin biopsy if taken is stained with GMS stain.

In cases of dermatophytosis:

- Microscopic characteristics such as arthrospores and hyaline septate hyphae are visible in KOH mount of skin or nail, as shown in **Figures 10.5 and 10.6**.

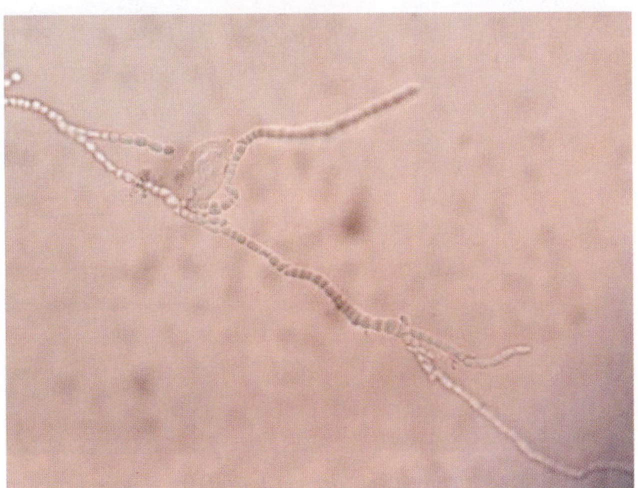

FIG. 10.5: KOH mount from skin scraping showing hyphae with arthroconidia (400×).
(KOH: potassium hydroxide)

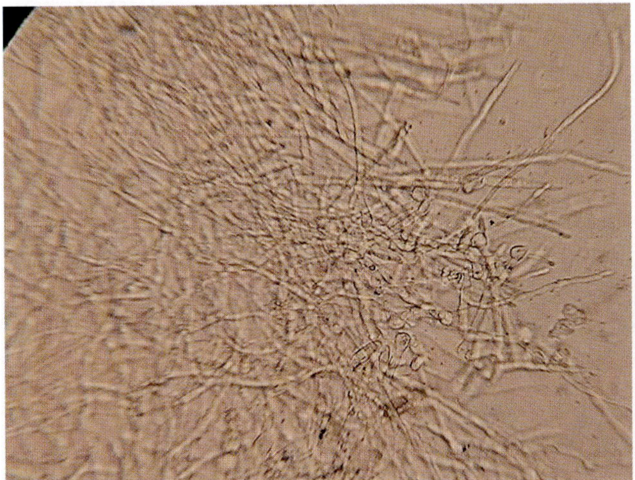

FIG. 10.6: KOH mount of skin with plenty of hyphae (400×).
(KOH: potassium hydroxide)

- Pigmented hyphae that can be observed in dermatomycosis caused by *Neoscytalidium* species. is a rare emerging fungal pathogen. It was traditionally considered a plant pathogen.
- Arthroconidia in the hair are ectothrix, which means that they are outside the hair shaft, or endothrix, meaning that they are inside the hair shaft **(Fig. 10.7)**.

Fungal Culture

Sabouraud Dextrose Agar (SDA)

Inoculated SDA slants containing antibiotics and cycloheximide are incubated at three different temperatures: (1) 25, (2) 37, and (3) 30°C, respectively. One more single SDA slant free of cycloheximide is also used at 25°C. Dermatophyte colonies grow slowly over a period of 10 days to 3 weeks. One way to identify a culture is by looking at it.

We take note of the surface and reverse colony colors, surface textures, presence of radiating hyphae in the media, and any other curious observations. Lactophenol cotton blue (LPCB) tease mount is prepared from the colony. Microconidia and macroconidia shapes, microconidia organization, and the presence of certain hyphae types (such as spiral, racquet, nodular, and favic chandelier) are used to identify an isolate. Microscopical results are analyzed after slide culture on cornmeal agar (CMA) and potato dextrose agar (PDA).

Dermatophyte Test Medium (DTM)

Dermatophytes are distinguished from other types of contaminants and bacteria by using this method. Phenol red indicator is present in the medium. The

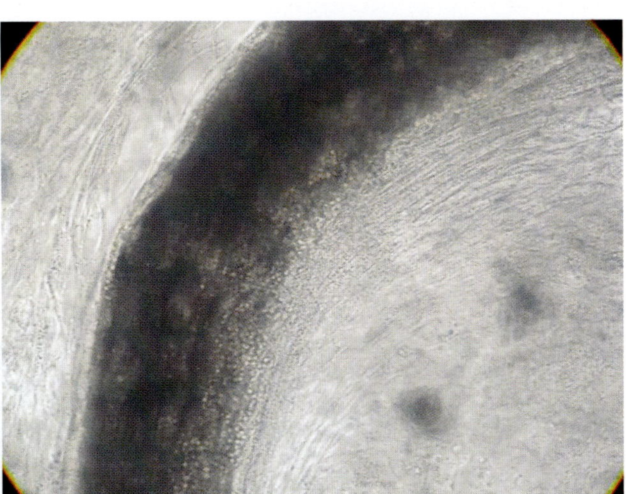

FIG. 10.7: KOH mount showing endothrix. Note abundant hyphae with arthroconidia within the hair shaft (400×).
(KOH: potassium hydroxide)

medium turns red as the fungus grows, since the fungus's metabolic products raise the pH of the medium. To reduce the possibility of false positives when utilizing DTM, presumptive identification is performed using dermatophyte identification medium (DIM). To further enhance sporulation, other media are used, such as SDA with yeast extract or SDA with 1% thiamine.

The type of sporulation seen in various genera of dermatophytes is shown in **Table 10.6**.

DESCRIPTION OF PATHOGENS

Trichophyton rubrum

- *Colony*: It may take 10 or more days for the colony to mature. The colony is usually cottony **(Fig. 10.8)** or granular. The surface is white or buff in color.
  The back side usually shows port wine red diffusible pigment, as shown in **Figure 10.9**. Even on flat, white colonies, the hue is visible through the medium. Growth on PDA or CMA may intensify the red pigment. There may be brown, yellow, orange, or pigment-free varieties. The pigment production is enhanced on corn Meal Dextrose Agar or PDA.
- *Microscopy*: The tear drop-shaped microconidia are shown in **Figure 10.10** which are borne on both sides of hyphae, often called "birds on fence or wire." The point to differentiate from *T. mentagrophyte* is that microconidia are not in clusters as seen in *T. mentagrophyte*. Some variants may show excess of microconidia. Macroconidia will be present or they will not. Their "pencil shape" (with 4–10 cells), and in some cases a "rat-tail" extension, is the defining feature. The granular variant shows more macroconidia, and microconidia are mostly round. Arthroconidia may be present.

TABLE 10.6: Characteristics of macroconidia and microconidia in dermatophyte species.

Dermatophyte genus	*Macroconidia*	*Microconidia*
Trichophyton	Rare, thin walled, and smooth	Abundant
Microsporum	Numerous, thick walled, and rough	Rare
Epidermophyton	Numerous and smooth walled	Absent

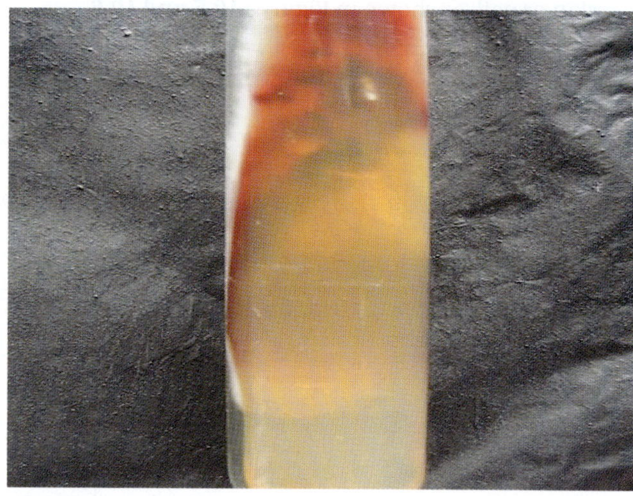

FIG. 10.9: SDA with growth of *Trichophyton rubrum*. Note red-colored pigment on the reverse side of slant.
(SDA: Sabouraud dextrose agar)

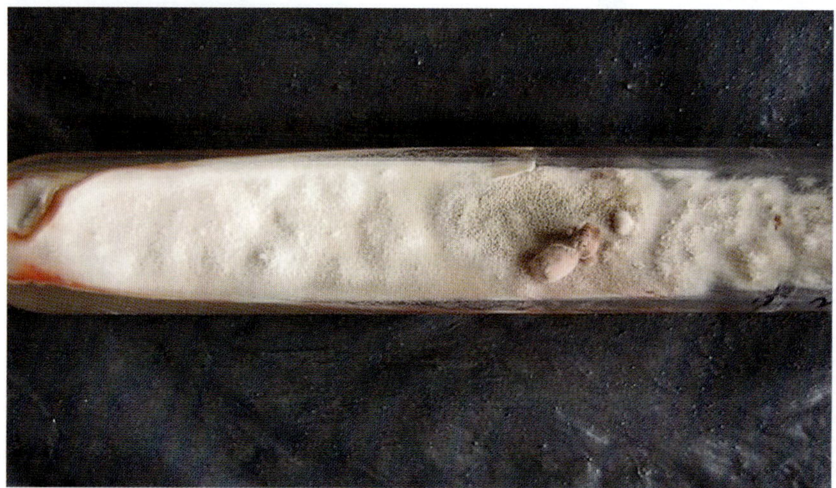

FIG. 10.8: SDA slant with growth of *Trichophyton rubrum* (obverse).
(SDA: Sabouraud dextrose agar)

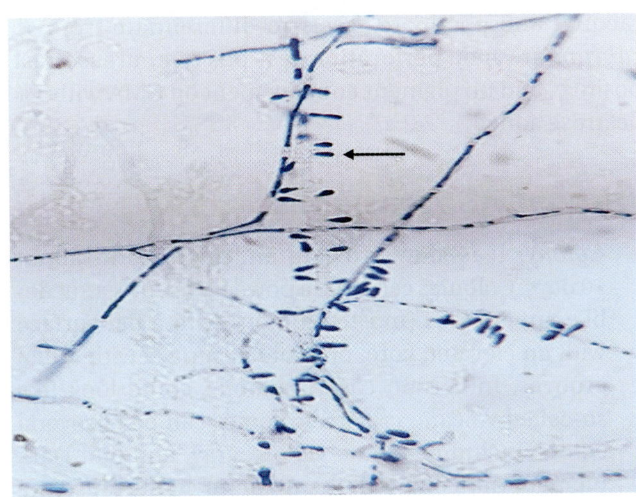

FIG. 10.10: LPCB mount of *Trichophyton rubrum* showing teardrop-shaped microconidia (400×).
(LPCB: lactophenol cotton blue)

Trichophyton mentagrophytes

The species complex includes *Trichophyton africanum, Trichophyton benhamiae var. benhamiae, Trichophyton benhamiae var. luteum, Trichophyton europaeum, Trichophyton eriotrephon, Trichophyton japonicum, T. mentagrophytes sensu stricto, Trichophyton indotineae, Trichophyton interdigitale,* and *Trichophyton quinckeanum.* These species are identified by molecular methods rather than phenotypic methods. Mostly, they are zoophilic, with the exception that *T. indotineae* and *T. interdigitale* are anthropophilic species.

- *Colony*: Growth rate is moderate (maturity takes 6–10 days). The colonies may have a cottony texture **(Fig. 10.11)** or a granular variety **(Fig. 10.12)**. Some strains have pigment, whereas others do not. Powdery colonies show concentric and radial folds. Pigment can be generated in a variety of colors,

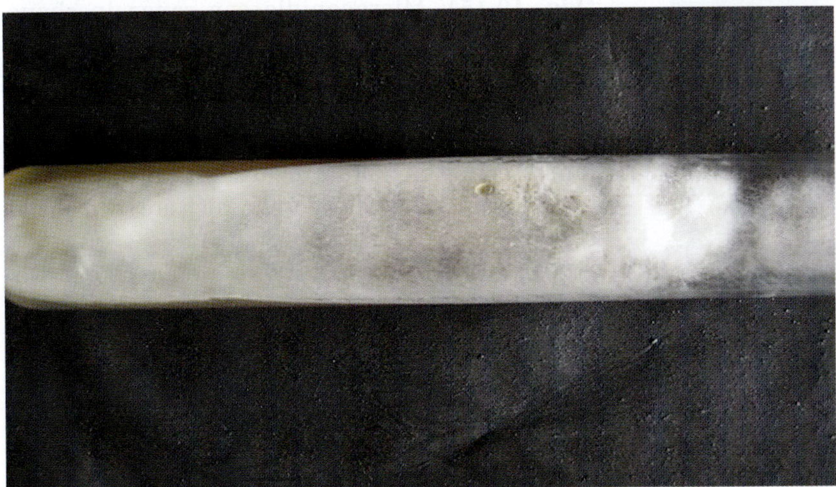

FIG. 10.11: SDA slant showing cottony growth of *Trichophyton mentagrophytes*.
(SDA: Sabouraud dextrose agar)

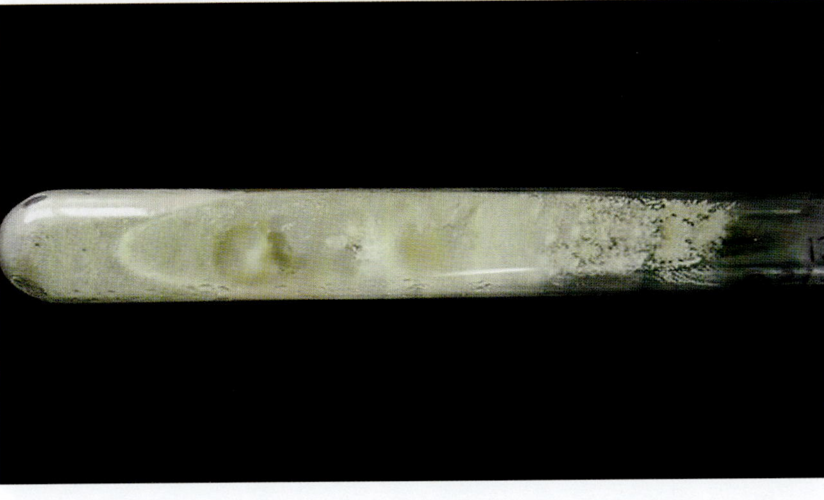

FIG. 10.12: SDA slant showing powdery growth of *Trichophyton mentagrophytes* (a rare variant).
(SDA: Sabouraud dextrose agar)

including red (like *T. rubrum*) or orange or even bright yellow.

- *Microscopy*: A typical isolate of *T. mentagrophytes* will have microconidia that are larger and more numerous, and they will be subspherical (may be even tear drop shaped) and clustered together like grapes. Especially powdery colonies have microconidia in clusters **(Fig. 10.13)** or on branched conidiophores.

Cottony (fluffy) colonies may show few microconidia which are "tear drop" shaped like *T. rubrum*. Macroconidia are "cigar shaped" or "pencil shaped." The hyphae of this species are characterized by their tightly coiled spirals **(Fig. 10.14)**. Other hyphae types include racquet and pectinate. Tests to differentiate from *T. rubrum* are hair perforation test positive, urease test positive, and no pigment enhancement on CMA with 1% dextrose added.

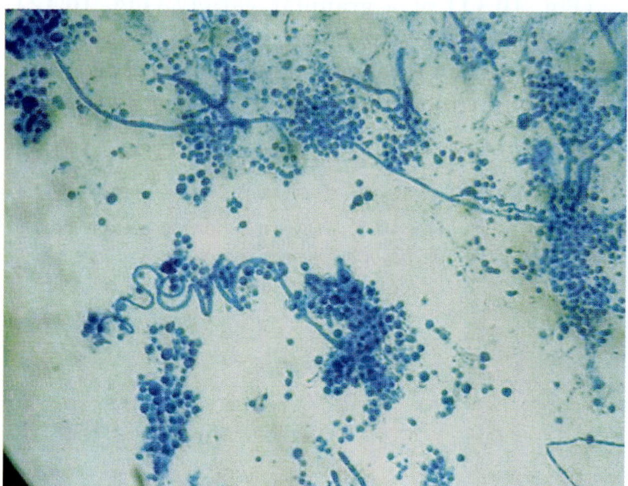

FIG. 10.13: LPCB mount of *Trichophyton mentagrophytes* showing microconidia in clusters (400×).
(LPCB: lactophenol cotton blue)

Trichophyton tonsurans

- *Colony*: It is slow growing and matures in about 10 days. Colonies can have a powdery texture, a suede-like appearance (most common) with a flat surface with an elevated core, or a folded surface with radial grooves. In certain cases, colonies could look like so-called volcano craters. Colonies can be of several colors, including white, yellow, gray, and tan. Dark pigment diffusing into the medium could cause the reverse to be reddish-brown, pale-yellow, or even look like the reverse of *T. rubrum.*
- *Microscopy*: Conidia are commonly found on hyphae or at the ends of short lateral "matchstick" stalks which are perpendicular to parent hyphae **(Fig. 10.15)**. Microconidia can range in shape from tear drop to club shaped and are arranged in open branching clusters. Excessive enlargement of microconidia, known as "balloon" cells, has been observed in older cultures. Macroconidia are rarely seen, which are irregular with thick surface. Common are chlamydospores, which are seen on old cultures.
- *Additional evaluations*: Endothrix invades hair in vivo. Thiamine is somewhat necessary for *T. tonsurans*. A thiamine supplement is quite effective in promoting growth. Some strains are urease positive.

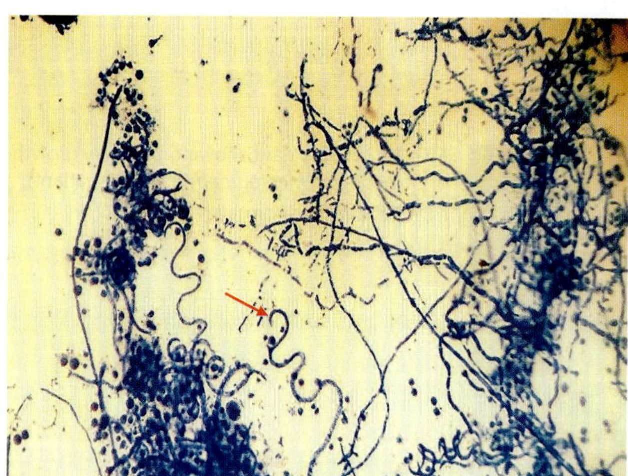

FIG. 10.14: LPCB mount from colony of *Trichophyton mentagrophytes* showing spiral hyphae (400×).
(LPCB: lactophenol cotton blue)

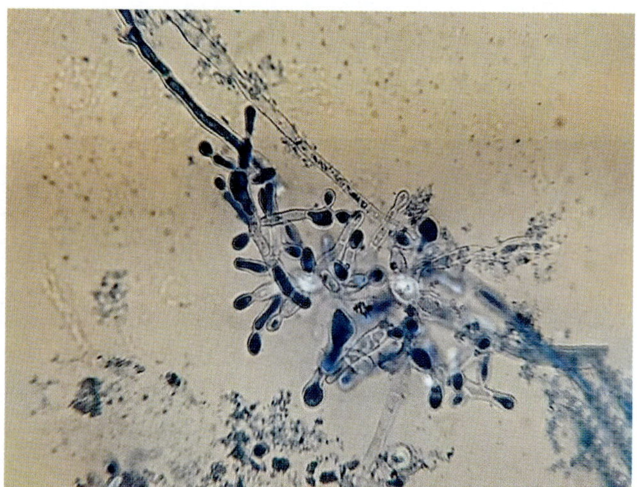

FIG. 10.15: LPCB mount of *Trichophyton tonsurans* with microconidia (400×).
(LPCB: lactophenol cotton blue)

Trichophyton verrucosum

- *Colony*: The development is either mostly subterranean or extremely sluggish, glabrous, piled up, and button-like. Flat or heaped-up growth may be seen. The rate of growth is accelerated at 37°C. This is an unusual feature for a dermatophyte. The color of the surface can range from white to ochre-brown. In most cases, the reverse is colorless, though it can range from pale brown to yellow.
- *Microscopy*: Some of the hyphae have a shape similar to antlers, and others are tortuous. When grown on SDA, they do not form microconidia. On special medium with addition of thiamine, they form tear drop microconidia and macroconidia with a rare "rat tail" or string bean shape. Chains of many intercalary chlamydoconidia are seen on SDA at 37°C, as shown in **Figure 10.16**.
- *Additional testing*: In vitro hair perforation is either very weak or negative. Trichophyton agar #3, which contains thiamine and inositol, is known to stimulate *T. verrucosum*. Most strains are urease negative.

Trichophyton violaceum

- *Colony*: Slow growing and matures in 10 days; velvety **(Fig. 10.17)** or heaped or wrinkled, and shiny colonies. Surface color is violet to deep purple.
- Reverse is deep purple.
- *Microscopy*: Branched hyphae, with no conidia produced on primary isolation. Cells with cytoplasmic inclusions are seen. Intercalary chlamydospores may be present. On an enriched medium (trichophyton agar #4), two- to eight-celled irregularly shaped macroconidia and pyriform microconidia are produced.
- *Further tests*: In vitro perforation is slow or negative. It does not grow at 37°C. Growth is stimulated by thiamine. *T. violaceum* is differentiated from atypical purple *T. rubrum*, which has no thiamine requirement. It is urease negative.

Trichophyton schoenleinii

- *Colony*: Growth rate is slow and matures in 10 days. Smooth, waxy, and whitish (or brownish) colonies are produced. Chlamydoconidia are plenty.
- *Microscopy*: Microconidia and macroconidia are not seen. The characteristic finding is presence of hyphae-like "favic chandelier" with swollen tips **(Fig. 10.18)**.

Trichophyton soudanense

- *Colony*: Growth rate is slow and matures after 10 days. Colonies are suede-like, flat to folded, which may show radiating fringe. Surface is yellow to orange. Purplish red variants exist. Reverse is similar in color to the surface.
- *Microscopy*: It shows hyphae with arthroconidia. The branched hyphae show "reflexive branching." Branches form at both forward and backward angles to the parent hypha. The adjacent hyphal branches are seen in the opposite directions, often with the appearance of barbed wire. Few tear drop shaped microconidia are formed along hyphae, but macroconidia are absent. There may be few chlamydoconidia.

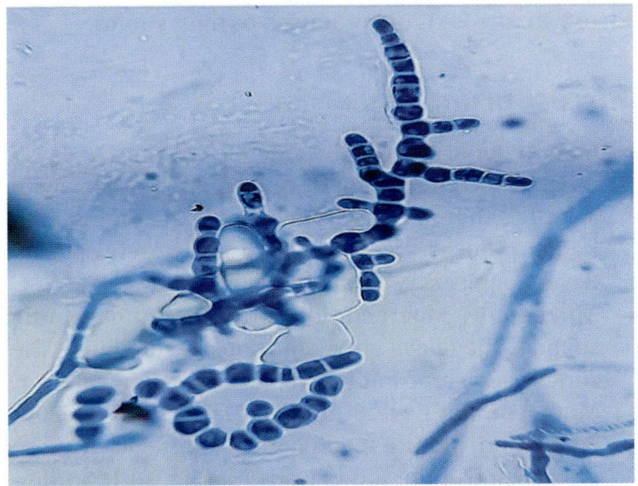

FIG. 10.16: LPCB mount of *Trichophyton verrucosum* showing chain of arthroconidia (400×).
(LPCB: lactophenol cotton blue)

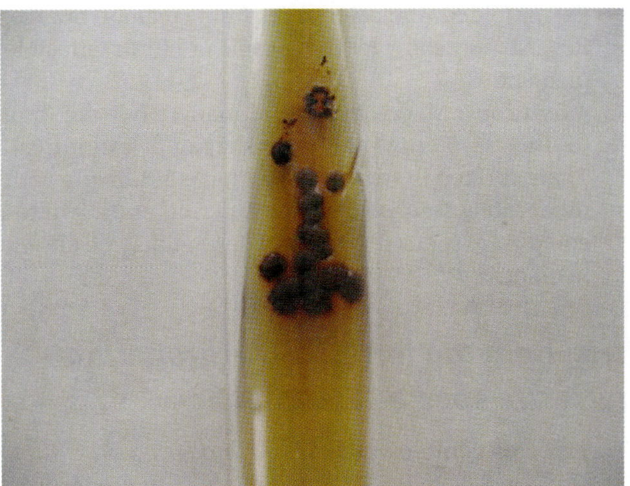

FIG. 10.17: SDA slant showing velvety colonies of *Trichophyton violaceum*.
(SDA: Sabouraud dextrose agar)

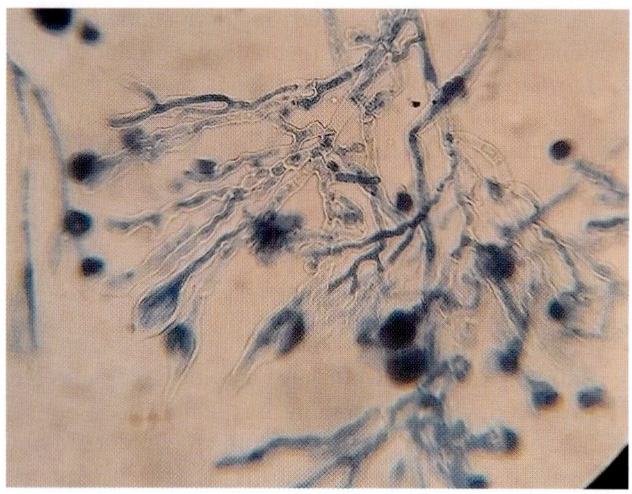

FIG. 10.18: LPCB mount of *Trichophyton schoenleinii* showing antler hyphae with swelling at the tip.
(LPCB: lactophenol cotton blue)

Trichophyton concentricum

- *Colony*: Delicately folded, glabrous, and slowly developing a velvety texture. The surface can be white, brown, or orange-brown in color. The back side has the same color as the front.
- *Microscopy*: No conidia or other distinguishing characteristics; instead, it is a complex web of hyphae that requires more testing. Thiamine has the potential to promote growth.

Trichophyton ajelloi (New Name: *Arthroderma uncinatum*)

- *Colony*: It matures in 8–10 days. Colonies are powdery, flat, or folded. The color varies from cream to orange. Reverse may show reddish purple or bluish diffusible pigment.
- *Microscopy*: Macroconidia are many. They are long (5–10 × 20–65 μm) and cigar shaped or cylindrical. Their surface is smooth. They have 5–12 cells with moderately thick walls with tapering ends. Microconidia are sparse in most isolates but may be absent in others.

Trichophyton terrestre (*Arthroderma terrestre* species Complex)

The species complex includes *Arthroderma crocatum, Arthroderma eboreum, Arthroderma insingulare, Arthroderma lenticulare, Arthroderma melbournense, Arthroderma melis, Arthroderma thuringiense,* and *Arthroderma quadrifidum.*

- *Colonies*: They are slow growing. Their surface is white to yellow and velvety or granular. Reverse is colorless, yellow, reddish, or brown.
- *Microscopy*: Club-shaped microconidia and many thin-walled macroconidia are seen.

Trichophyton megninii

- *Colony*: Growth rate is moderate; matures within 6–10 days. Surface is suede like, at first white and then pink to violet with widely spaced radial grooves. Reverse is red.
- *Microscopy*: Microscopic picture resembles *T. rubrum.* Microconidia are teardrop shaped. Macroconidia are pencil shaped. It gives urease test positive in 7 days. Initially, this species was suggested as a synonym of *T. rubrum.*

Microsporum audouinii

- *Colony*: It is glabrous to velvety. It shows wrinkles. Some examples of surface colors are brown, rust-buff, or white-gray. The back is a shade of peach to salmon (with reddish brown center).
- *Microscopy*: Macroconidia are rare and poorly developed. When seen, they are similar to those of *M. canis.* They have terminal spine-like projections. Additional findings are pectinate hyphae and terminal chlamydospores. *M. audouinii* is differentiated from other *Microsporum* species by its poor growth on rice grains.
- *Further tests*: In vitro hair perforation negative. No growth on polished rice grains; but turns grains brown. Urease is not produced by most strains.

Microsporum canis

- *Colony*: Rapid (5 days) to moderate growing (10 days); quickly becoming fluffy, woolly, hairy, or silky with a surface that ranges from white to pale yellow/buff. Radial grooves are seen which are closely spaced. Reverse appears yellow to brownish yellow.
- *Microscopy*: Macroconidia are large and spindle shaped. They have curved or hooked spiny tips. The surface of macroconidia is rough and walls are thick. Macroconidia have 8–15 cells. The size is 15–20 × 60–125 μm. Mature macroconidia, particularly those on the knob or tip, shows warts (*see* **Fig. 10.19**). Club-shaped microconidia may be present.

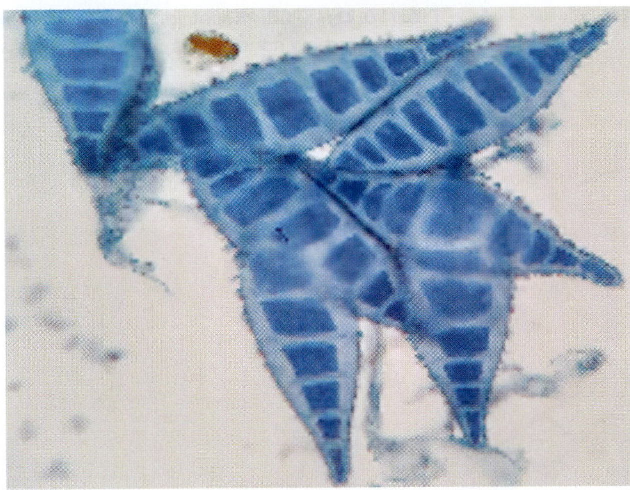

FIG. 10.19: LPCB mount of *Microsporum canis* showing macroconidia (1,000×).
(LPCB: lactophenol cotton blue)

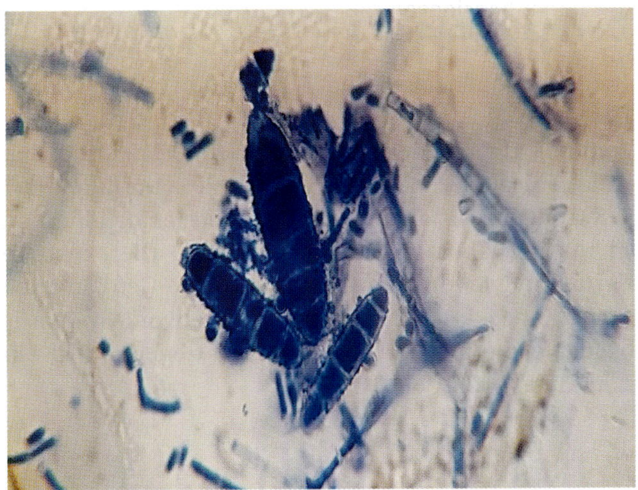

FIG. 10.20: Macroconidia of *Microsporum gypseum* (400×).

- *Other evaluations*: Good development, yellow color, and conidia are typical characteristics of growth on sterile-polished rice grains. *M. canis* is urease positive.

Microsporum gypseum (New Name: *Nannizzia gypsea* species Complex) (Fig. 10.20)

The species complex has *Nannizzia duboisii, Nannizzia fulva, Nannizzia gypsea sensu stricto*, and *Nannizzia incurvate* species.

- *Colony*: It has a moderate growth rate (6–10 days). The surface of colony is flat with floccose to powdery growth. The color of the colony is cinnamon to brown. The reverse side may show various shades—yellow, orange-tan, brownish red, or purplish red.
- *Microscopy*: A large number of club-shaped macroconidia with thin walls (7.5–11.5 × 25–60 µm) and unlike *M. canis*, four to six septa are produced **(Fig. 10.20)**. They have rough surface and they are symmetrical. There are two possible forms of hyphae: (1) Racquet and (2) pectinate. Macroconidia are easily identifiable by their rounded distal end and truncated bases.

Nannizzia nana (Previous Name: *Microsporum nanum*)

- *Colony*: Surface is initially first white and then becomes yellowish, peachy, or beige. The colony is downy or powdery, with fringed edges. Reverse is orange to reddish brown.
- *Microscopy*: Macroconidia (4–8 × 12–18 µm) have rough surface, with thin wall, and they are egg shaped with truncate base. The number of cells is one to three (usually two). Microconidia may be seen which are club shaped.

Paraphyton cookei (*Microsporum cookei*)

- *Colony*: It is powdery. Color is yellowish or dark tannish. Some aerial hyphae develop, under which there is a deep grape-red pigment. Reverse is deep purplish red.
- *Microscopy*: Macroconidia are oval (10–15 × 30–50 µm). Thay have thick wall with rough surface. The number of cells is five to eight. Club-shaped microconidia are usually plenty.

Epidermophyton floccosum

- *Colony*: Surface typically suede like, may have rough or grainy surface. Young colonies may produce subsurface-radiating hyphae. Color of primary colonies is a distinctive yellow-mustard green to olive-gray. Reverse of the mature colony is light-to-dark brown (typically described as *Khaki* colonies).
- *Microscopy*: Blunt and club-shaped macroconidia are formed singly or more commonly in pairs of "rabbit ears" or clusters **(Fig. 10.21)**. The macroconidia have thin, smooth walls, and two to five septa. Chlamydospores are present in old cultures.
- *Further tests*: In vivo hair invasion is negative. In vitro hair perforation is negative. It can grow at 37°C. It is a slow urease producer.

The other species of *Epidermophyton* as *Epidermophyton inguinale* and *Epidermophyton plicarum* are synonyms of *E. floccosum* and merged with it. However,

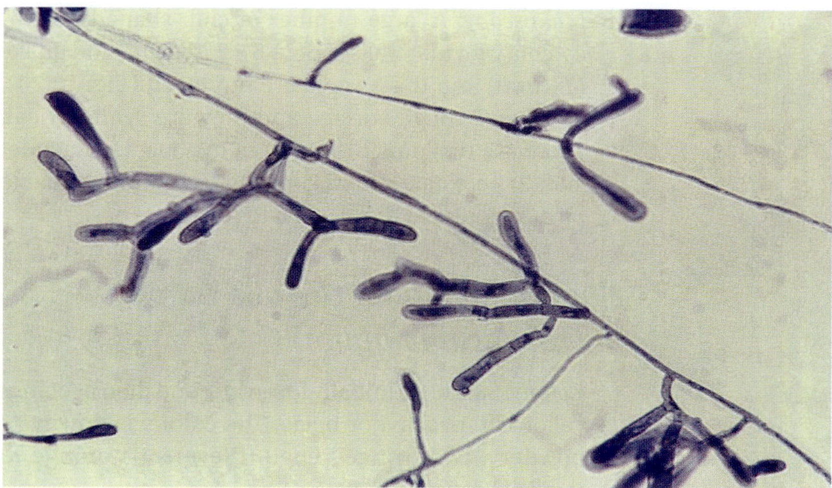

FIG. 10.21: LPCB mount of *Epidermophyton floccosum* showing club-shaped macroconidia (400×).
(LPCB: lactophenol cotton blue)
Source: Public Health Image Library CDC.

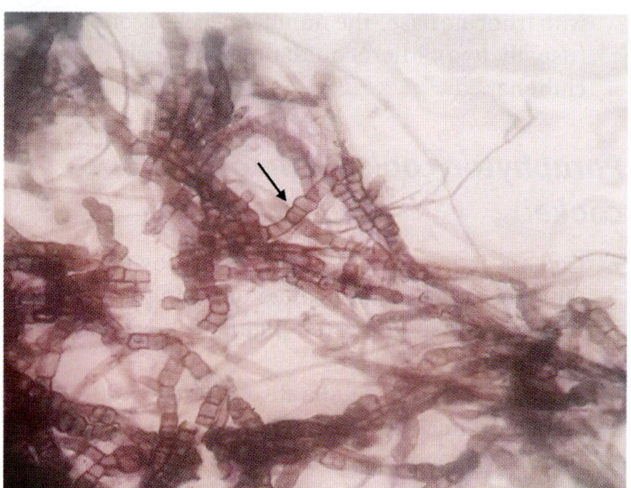

FIG. 10.22: LPCB mount showing pigmented hyphae with arthroconidia suggestive of *Neoscytalidium* species (400×).
(LPCB: lactophenol cotton blue)

Epidermophyton. stockdaleae is considered as a synonym of *Trichophyton ajelloi.*

Neoscytalidium dimidiatum

- *Colonies*: They are black colored.
- *Microscopy*: Microscopic findings are black hyphae with arthroconidia, as seen in **Figure 10.22**. *Scytalidium lignicola, Scytalidium dimidiatum,* and *Scytalidium hyalinum* were present in the genus *Scytalidium. Scytalidium* is now changed to *Neoscytalidium, N. dimidiatum* is phaeoid and *N. hyalinum* is hyaline. *N. hyalinum* is now considered to be a melanin-less hyaline mutant of *N. dimidiatum. N. dimidiatum* (previous name: *Hendersonula toruloidea*) is synanamorph of *Nattrassia mangiferae.*

Genetic Identification of Dermatophytes

Iterative sequencing of the ITS region of rDNA is considered the "gold standard" for the detection of troublesome or atypical dermatophytes. Direct identification from clinical specimens may be possible in the future, and ITS sequencing is already helpful for species identification in routine laboratories. In addition to the extensive dermatophyte identification database in GenBank, the SmartGene® Integrated Database Network System is available for purchase from the Smart Gene Company in Lausanne, Switzerland.

TREATMENT

- Topical antifungal preparations are useful in many cases.
- *Standard treatment for tinea corporis includes*:
    - *Terbinafine*: 250 mg/day for 1–2 weeks
    - *Itraconazole*: 200 mg/day for 1 week
    - *Fluconazole*: 150–200 mg once weekly for 2–4 weeks
    - *Griseofulvin*: Microsize 500–1,000 mg/day for 2–4 weeks
- Nondermatophytic fungi as *Aspergillus, Fusarium,* and *Scopulariopsis* are treated with itraconazole.

The summary of characteristics of various dermatophytes is given in **Table 10.7**.

Treatment

There is emergence of drug resistant strains of *T. mentagrophytes*. Treatment is summarized in **Table 10.8**.

TABLE 10.7: Summary of characteristics of different agents of dermatophytosis.

Organism	*Macroscopic*	*Microscopic*
Trichophyton rubrum	Cottony, with port wine red pigment on reverse side	Teardrop-shaped microconidia arranged along the hyphae giving "birds on fence" appearance, microconidia if present, they are pencil shaped
Trichophyton mentagrophyte	Cottony colony (powdery variant may occur)	Spiral hyphae common, microconidia in clusters, macroconidia present which are cigar shaped
Trichophyton violaceum	Waxy or velvety colonies with violet pigment on reverse side	Conidia rare, intercalary chlamydoconidia present, swollen cells with inclusion are present along hyphae
Trichophyton tonsurans	Powdery, cream to yellow having central furrows	Conidia on hyphae or at the ends of "short lateral" "matchstick" stalks Microconidia tear drop to club shaped, may be swollen macroconidia few irregular
Trichophyton schoenleinii	Smooth or waxy, brownish	Favic chandelier, swelling of hyphae at the tip, chlamydoconidia present
Microsporum audouinii	Velvety, brownish	Macroconidia are rare, with terminal spine-like projections, pectinate hyphae, and terminal chlamydospores
Microsporum canis	Cottony, reverse orange	Macroconidia curved or hooked spiny tips, rough surface, tick walls, with 8–15 cells. Club-shaped microconidia may be present
Microsporum gypseum	Powdery, buff to yellow-green	• Macroconidia club shaped with thin walls • Four to six septa rough surface and symmetrical
Epidermophyton floccosum	Surface suede-like, may have rough surface or grainy surface, yellow-mustard green to olive-gray color, reverse "khaki" colored	Blunt, club-shaped macroconidia, singly in pairs of "rabbit ears" or clusters, thin smooth wall

TABLE 10.8: Summary of treatment.

Diseases	*Treatment*
Tinea pedis	*Topical cream/ointment*: Terbinafine, imidazole (miconazole, econazole, clotrimazole, etc.), undecanoic acid, and tolnaftate
Tinea corporis	• *Oral*: ○ Terbinafine: 250 mg/day for 2 weeks ○ Itraconazole: 200 mg/day for 1 week ○ Fluconazole: 250 mg weekly for 2–4 weeks • *Topical cream/ointment*: Terbinafine and imidazole (e.g., miconazole, econazole, and clotrimazole)
Tinea capitis	• *Griseofulvin*: 10–20 mg/kg/day for minimum of 6 weeks • *Terbinafine*: ○ <20 kg: 62.5 mg/day ○ 20–40 kg: 125 mg/day ○ >40 kg: 250 mg/day • *Itraconazole*: 4–6 mg/kg pulsed dose weekly
Onychomycosis	• *Fluconazole*: 3–8 mg/kg pulsed dose weekly • *Fingernails terbinafine*: 250 mg daily for 6 weeks • *Itraconazole*: 400 mg/day for 1 week each month, repeated for 2–3 months • *Fluconazole*: 200 mg weekly for 8–16 weeks

Source: Adapted from Bennett JE, Dolin R, Blaser MJ. Mandell, Douglas, and Bennett's Principles and Practice of Infectious Diseases, 8th edition. Philadelphia: Saunders; 2014.

SECTION

3

Subcutaneous Mycoses

Section Outline

CHAPTER

11 Mycetoma

INTRODUCTION

Clinically, mycetoma is a skin and subcutaneous tissue infection which may also involve underlying tissue and bone with three important characteristics, i.e., (1) tumor-like swelling of the affected part, (2) formation of discharging sinuses, and (3) passage of granules or grains in the discharge. The granule or grain is a compact mass of the pathogen formed in the infected tissue. The color of granules varies with the etiological agent. **Figure 11.1** shows a typical presentation of mycetoma with swelling along with discharging sinuses.

The clinical signs are the same whether it is caused by bacteria (actinomycetoma) or fungus (eumycetoma). Differentiation between eumycotic mycetoma and actinomycetomas is essential from the treatment's point of view, progress of the disease, and extent of involvement of underlying bones. There is one more clinical condition which looks like mycetoma and is caused by bacteria known as botryomycosis.

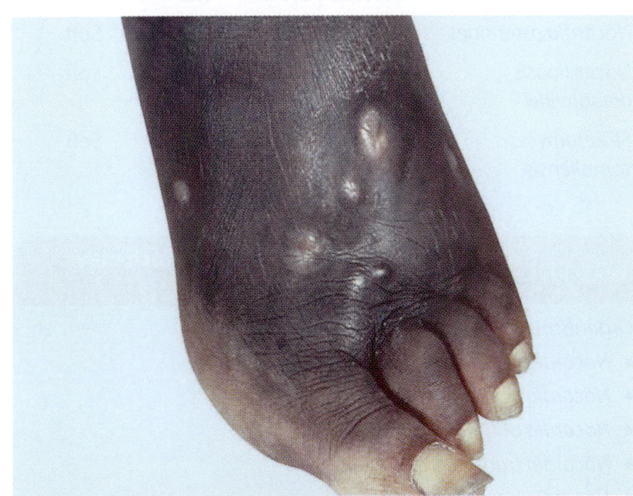

FIG. 11.1: Mycetoma of foot with draining sinuses.
Source: Public Health Image Library CDC.

HISTORY

An adult skeleton from the Byzantine era (300–600 AD) was the first to be associated with mycetoma infections due to its unusual bone structure. An old religious text from India, the Atharva Veda, recorded mycetoma under the name "Padavalmikam" or "anthill foot." Gill recorded the first cases of mycetoma in Madura, southern India, in 1842, and he came up with the name "Madura foot."

The name "mycetoma" was given by Carter to describe the disease. Pinoy could identify two distinct etiologic variables of the illness. He categorized the disease as either actinomycetoma (caused by bacteria) or eumycetoma (caused by fungus). In 1956, Abott made the initial effort to create a global map of mycetoma prevalence. He spent 2.5 years looking into 1,321 cases of mycetoma in Sudan. Mycetoma is the first fungal disease to be included in the list of neglected tropical diseases made by World Health Organization (WHO).

EPIDEMIOLOGY (FIG. 11.2)

Mycetoma cases are detected worldwide, but it is most common in tropical and subtropical regions, specifically in the "mycetoma belt" that extends from about 15° south to 30° north of the equator. India, Sudan, Mexico, and Venezuela have the highest rates of the disease. Many more countries that have reported the disease include—Somalia, Ethiopia, Senegal, Mauritania, Kenya, Niger, Nigeria, Chad, Cameroon, Djibouti, and Senegal.

The bacteria responsible for the condition thrive under extremely harsh environmental conditions. Whereas eumycetoma thrives in damp environments, actinomycetoma is more prevalent in arid regions. There are more eumycetomas (fungal agents) in Africa, whereas actinomycetomas (bacterial agents) are commonly found in South and Central America. Sudan appears to

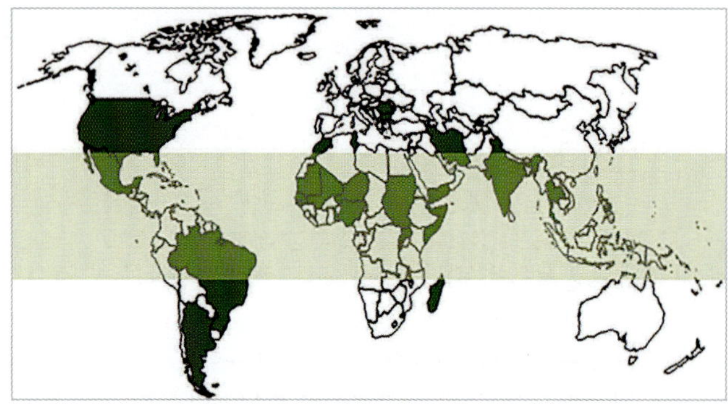

FIG. 11.2: Epidemiology of mycetoma (light green—endemic areas). *Source*: Centers for Disease Control and Prevention (CDC).

be the most mycetoma-endemic country in the world. In Khartoum, Sudan's capital, almost 7,000 people have received mycetoma treatment, and the most common pathogen was *Madurella mycetomatis*. *Nocardia brasiliensis* is the principal causative agent in Brazil and Mexico. In India, the southern and eastern regions are more affected by actinomycetoma, while the northern and western regions are more affected by eumycetoma. In India, a higher number of cases are seen in Tamil Nadu, the moist southern part, and Rajasthan, the dry western part of India.

Mode of infection: The causative agents live in the dirt and can enter the body through tiny punctures like those caused by thorns, wood splinters, or stone cuts.

Occupations susceptible to infection: These include farmers, shepherds, herders, carpenters, and builders.

Male-to-female distribution: Mycetomas are more common in men between the ages of 20 and 40 years, though they can affect anyone. The male-to-female ratio is 3.5:1, meaning that men are more likely to be affected than women, probably due to their outdoor activities. There are anti-infective mechanisms in women which is believed to be female hormones.

Animals do not serve as reservoirs for mycetoma, although a few cases come from dogs, horses, and goats.

ETIOLOGICAL AGENTS

Bacterial Agents

These bacteria are filamentous and gram positive. *Streptomyces somaliensis, Actinomadura (Actinomadura madurae* and *Actinomadura pelletieri), Nocardia (Nocardia brasiliensis, Nocardia asteroides, Nocardia otitidiscaviarum,* and *Nocardia transvalensis)*, and two more species of *Nocardia* (*Nocardia harenae and Nocardia takedensis*) are the most important agents of actinomycotic mycetoma. The list of bacterial agents along with the characteristics of their granules is given in **Table 11.1**. Some of the agents are weak acid-fast. **Box 11.1** mentions the bacteria which are weak acid-fast.

Fungal Agents

These are saprophytic environmental fungi. The most common causes of eumycotic mycetoma are *Madurella mycetomatis, Madurella grisea,* and *Scedosporium apiospermum*. Other causative agents include *Exophiala jeanselmei, Curvularia geniculata, Acremonium falciforme, Acremonium kiliense, Scytalidium dimidiatum, Aspergillus nidulans, Neotestudina rosatii, Leptosphaeria senegalensis, Pyrenochaeta romeroi,* and *Phialophora verrucosa*. The grains produced by various fungi may vary. This is shown in **Table 11.2. Table 11.3** shows differences between eumycotic mycetoma and actinomycotic mycetoma.

Biochemical tests which help to differentiate among various fungal agents are listed in **Table 11.4**. The differentiating characteristics of bacterial agents are given in **Table 11.5**.

TABLE 11.1: Bacterial agents with their characteristic grains.

Bacterial agents	*Color*	*Size (mm)*	*Texture*
Actinomadura madurae	White and yellow	2.0	Hard
Actinomadura pelletieri	Pink to red	0.5	Hard
Nocardia brasiliensis	Yellowish white	<0.5	Soft
Nocardia caviae	White to yellow	<0.5	Soft
Nocardia asteroides	White to yellow	<0.5	Soft
Nocardiopsis dassonvillei	Cream-colored	<0.5	Soft
Streptomyces somaliensis	Yellowish white	1.0	Soft

BOX 11.1 List of weak acid-fast agents which may cause mycetoma.

Organisms:
- *Nocardia brasiliensis*
- *Nocardia asteroides*
- *Nocardia otitidiscaviarum*
- *Nocardia transvalensis*
- *Nocardia harenae*
- *Nocardia takedensis*

TABLE 11.2: Some of the common causative agents of eumycetoma with characteristics of grains.

Causative fungal agents	*Texture*	*Size (mm)*	*Shape*	*Cement-like matrix*
A. Black grain eumycetoma				
Madurella mycetomatis	Hard	0.5–5.0	Oval to lobed	Present and homogeneous
Trematosphaeria grisea	Soft	0.3–0.6	Oval to lobed	Present and peripheral
Exophiala jeanselmei	Soft	0.2–0.3	Irregular	Absent
Curvularia geniculata	Hard	0.5–1.0	Oval	Present and peripheral
B. White grain eumycetoma				
Pseudallescheria boydii	Soft	0.5–1.0	Oval to lobed	Absent
Aspergillus nidulans	Soft	1.0–2.0	Oval	Absent
Acremonium falciforme	Soft	0.2–0.5	Oval	Absent
Fusarium species	Soft	0.2–0.6	Oval	Absent

PATHOLOGY AND PATHOGENICITY

Infections can develop after being pierced by thorns or splinters or from the use of wicks for removing wax from ears. For barefoot walkers, in particular, the foot is the most common area. Mycetoma of the back may develop in persons carrying heavy loads, such as grain and timber. In rare instances, the injury may occur on the head.

After the entry of the pathogen, inflammation starts. A small abscess forms with hyphae in the center surrounded by neutrophils. A small, painless nodule develops. To counterattack the pathogen, the immune system gets activated. Subcutaneous swelling along with digestion of subcutaneous tissues forms draining sinuses and leads to the discharge of grains.

Sometimes, pathogens are expelled, and healing of tissue starts. However, the remaining pathogens initiate new infections in nearby tissues. The cycle of recovery and reinfection occurs. The infective agent travels via the fascial planes to the muscles and bones underneath. This leads to the degeneration and deformation of both the osseous and muscular tissues. Histopathology shows epithelioid granuloma containing bacteria or fungi surrounded by chronic inflammation.

TABLE 11.3: Differences between actinomycetomas and eumycetoma.

Clinical features	*Actinomycetoma*	*Eumycetoma*
Causative organisms	Aerobic actinomycetes (e.g., *Actinomadura, Nocardia*, and *Streptomyces*)	Hyaline and phaeoid hyphomycetes (e.g., *Madurella mycetomatis, Fusarium*, and *Exophiala*)
Mass	Multiple, diffuse, with ill-defined margins	Usually single, with well-defined margins
Sinuses	Appear early and are numerous	Appear later and are relatively fewer in number
Opening of sinuses	Raised, inflamed, and flared up	Flat opening, not flared up
Flap of opening	Easily removed	Not easily removed
Discharge	Usually purulent (containing pus)	Serous or serosanguineous (containing fluid or blood)
Grains	White grains (except *Actinomadura pelletieri* which has red grains)	Black or white grains
Extent of involvement	More extensive and obliterative with hypertrophic, punched-out osteolytic lesions of bone	Less extensive, primarily osteosclerotic lesions
Diagnostic approach	Requires identification of aerobic actinomycetes and culture; PCR can aid in identification	Fungal culture and microscopic examination of grains for accurate identification
Histopathological findings	Presence of sulfur granules and chronic granulomatous inflammation	Presence of fungal grains, granulomatous inflammation, and tissue necrosis
Response to treatment	Generally responsive to antibiotics (e.g., sulfonamides and tetracyclines)	Typically requires antifungal therapy and may need surgical intervention
Common sites of infection	Extremities (e.g., limbs) and can involve deep tissues	Commonly affects the extremities but can also involve deeper tissues
Onset of symptoms	Gradual onset with chronic progression	May have a more gradual onset but tends to be more localized initially
Disease progression	Can lead to significant bone and tissue damage if untreated	Typically, less destructive to bone but can cause significant local tissue damage

(PCR: polymerase chain reaction)

TABLE 11.4: Biochemical features of agents of eumycetoma.

Fungal agent	*Utilization of glucose*	*Utilization of lactose*	*Utilization of maltose*	*Utilization of sucrose*	*Utilization of starch*	*Hydrolysis of starch*	*Proteas activity*
Madurella mycetomatis	+	+	+	–	+	+	+
Madurella grisea	+	–	+	+	+	+	+
Exophiala jeanselmei	+	+	+	+	+	–	–
Pseudallescheria boydii	+	–	+	+	+	–	–
Acremonium falciforme	+	–	–	+	+	–	–

TABLE 11.5: Characteristics of agents of actinomycetomas.

Filamentous bacteria	*Casein*	*Tyrosine*	*Xanthine*	*Urease*	*AFB*	*Growth in gelatin*
Acid-fast bacilli (AFB):						
Nocardia brasiliensis	+	+	–	+	+	+
Nocardia caviae	–	–	+	+	+	–
Nocardia asteroides	–	–	–	+	+	–
Nocardiopsis dassonvillei	+	+	+	±	+	–
Non-acid-fast bacilli (AFB):						
Actinomadura madurae	+	+	–	–	–	–
Actinomadura pelletieri	+	+	–	–	–	–
Streptomyces somaliensis	+	+	–	–	–	–

Classification of Mycetoma

Mycetoma can be classified into two categories based on the agents that cause them. Actinomycotic mycetoma is caused by *Actinomycetes*, whereas eumycotic mycetoma is caused by fungi. White or pale grain mycetoma and black grain mycetoma are two more ways to categorize them. With the exception of *Pseudallescheria boydii,* which has white granules, the majority of fungi produce black granules. The granules of most bacteria are white or yellow, while those of *Actinomadura pelletieri* are either pink or red. From a therapeutic standpoint and for gaining insight into prognosis, classification is crucial.

CLINICAL FEATURES OF MYCETOMA

Affected Areas

Most commonly involved areas are the feet, hands (more common on the right side), head, neck, chest, shoulder, and arms. There is a relation of site of infection with occupation. Any site may be prone to infection where there is trauma. Rarely, mycetoma can develop in unusual locations such as the abdominal wall, face (including bones), paranasal sinuses, orbit, or genitalia. In rare cases, mycetoma involving both limbs has been recorded.

The common sites for actinomycetomas are abdominal wall or chest instead of the extremities.

Typical Presentation

The duration between the history of trauma and the development of lesions varies, and it may even take 5–10 years. There is a painless, indurated subcutaneous mass with a woody hard feel. Numerous discharging sinuses are seen. Grains (microcolonies of pathogenic organisms) are present in the purulent or seropurulent discharge.

Variations in Presentation

- Soft, lobulated, or cystic swelling instead of the usual indurated mass
- Verrucous plaque or painless, hard swelling over the sole without draining sinuses

Progression of Lesions

- The initial lesion is often a papule at the site of injury, which becomes a painless nodule over time.
- Nodules and pustules enlarge, burst, and release grainy, purulent, or seropurulent discharge.
- Sinuses develop and may become interconnected as the disease progresses.

Skin Changes

- Areas of hypopigmentation surrounded by stretched-out and shiny skin
- Increased perspiration and local temperature due to sweat gland hyperplasia and inflammation

Grain Characteristics

- Grains are colonies of pathogenic organisms encased in a cement-like substance, usually visible to the naked eye.
- Grains are typically black or dark in eumycetoma and red or pink in actinomycetoma.
- Grain texture varies from smooth to firm or hard, depending on the species.

Pain and Discomfort

- Minimal discomfort was reported by most patients, likely due to anesthetic compounds produced by microbes.
- Discomfort may occur when new sinuses are about to break through the skin or due to the spread of infection.

Local Effects

- Typically, a localized condition affecting fascial planes initially. There is involvement of muscles and bones later. However, tendons and nerves are usually not involved. The bone involvement is more common with actinomycotic mycetoma, with both osteolytic and hypertrophic changes.
- Potential complications include osteomyelitis, compression of the spinal cord, and development of varicose veins.

Lymphatic and Hematological Spread

Most people do not have significantly enlarged regional lymph nodes. If they are involved, it is because of secondary bacterial infections. Occasionally, there is spread along the lymphatics with sporotrichosis-like lesions. The hematological spread is uncommon.

DIFFERENTIAL DIAGNOSIS

Differential diagnoses include botryomycosis, dermatophyte pseudomycetomas, chromoblastomycosis, hyalohyphomycosis, sporotrichosis, and cutaneous tuberculosis. Before anything else, in nonendemic areas, benign and malignant conditions such as fibroma, rheumatoid nodule, keloid, fibrolipoma, dermatofibroma, Kaposi's sarcoma, malignant melanoma, and verrucous carcinoma should be ruled out. A final diagnosis may be reached after microscopy, culture, histological evaluation, radiography, and molecular methods.

Botryomycosis

This is not a fungal disease in real sense. It is caused by bacteria, as listed in **Table 11.6**. The other names of this condition are schizomycosis and granular bacteriosis. It is a chronic granulomatous infection involving skin and subcutaneous tissue. There may be production of "sulfur" granules or grains. There is an inflammatory reaction with neutrophil proliferation which is uncommon in mycetoma. Patients with a deficiency of cell-mediated immunity are commonly involved. Clinically and histopathologically, it resembles mycetoma as well as actinomycosis.

Staphylococcus aureus, Escherichia coli, Actinobacillus lignieresii, Pseudomonas aeruginosa, nonhemolytic streptococci, *Proteus, Bacteroides,* and *Rhodococcus* species are the bacteria which cause this clinical condition.

Majocchi's dermatophytic granuloma or dermatophyte pseudomycetomas: This condition is caused by dermatophytes. Yellowish-white pseudograins without any cementing material are produced.

LABORATORY DIAGNOSIS

A detailed history regarding exposure history, geographical location, and duration of sickness must be taken. The specimens collected include granules, pus or exudate, and biopsy. After application of antiseptic, the site should be slightly pressed. Grains are collected by pushing the sinus outward from the edges into a sterile Petri dish. Another way to collect material is by delicately probing the sinus with a sterile loop. If granules are not seen in the collected material, dressings should be applied, and the

TABLE 11.6: Agents of botryomycosis.

Bacterial agents	*Color of granules*
Staphylococcus aureus	White
Pseudomonas aeruginosa	White
Coagulase-negative *Staphylococci*	White
Escherichia coli	White
Proteus vulgaris	White
Propionibacterium acnes	White
Streptococcus species	White
Peptostreptococcus species	White
Actinobacillus lignieresii	Yellow

patient should be called again in 48–72 hours. The grains then should be inspected. The characteristics such as color, size, shape, and texture of granules help in the diagnosis. The presence of granules on the dressing material should be observed. The grains are washed several times in a test tube with sterile normal saline. Granules are picked up with a sterile loop and pressed on sterile slides. Each granule is crushed between two slides.

Gross Examination

Observe size, shape and consistency of Granules.

Direct Microscopic Examination

For microscopic examination, potassium hydroxide (KOH) mount, Gram stain, and modified acid-fast staining (Kinyoun procedure with 1% H_2SO_4 as decolorizing solution) are performed. The acid-fast stain helps to demonstrate the acid-fast nature of some *Nocardia* species. The KOH mount should be observed after a few hours, so the material can dissolve. While observing the hyphae, their width, septation, pigmentation, cement material presence and color, and chlamydoconidia should be noted. Eumycotic filaments, especially those associated with chlamydoconidia, feature large swelling cells with a diameter of 2–4 µm. The findings of KOH mount of crushed eumycotic granule are shown in **Figures 11.3 and 11.4**. The filaments of actinomycotic grain can be either coccoid or bacillary, and their diameters range from 0.5 to 1 µm. Hyphae of eumycotic mycetoma are thick, 2–6 µm wide, and the large swollen cells are of size up to 15 µm which are present at the periphery. Gram stain findings in the case of actinomycetomas are gram-positive filaments, with bacillary and coccoid forms. The filaments of eumycetoma are gram positive but thicker. **Figure 11.5** shows gram-positive thick filaments of a eumycotic granule. **Figure 11.6** shows acid-fast filaments of *Nocardia* species. Staining procedures such as hematoxylin and eosin (H&E), Grocott-Gömöri's methenamine silver (GMS), and periodic acid-Schiff (PAS) are used on biopsy samples. **Figure 11.7** shows PAS-positive fungal material in a biopsy of a granule. In the PAS stain, fungi appear red. In the GMS stain, fungi appear black; in the H&E stain, sliced hyphae and cement substance are visible.

Culture

For culture, take two sterile test tubes. The first test tube contains normal saline, and the second test tube contains normal saline with antibiotics—streptomycin and penicillin. The material from the first tube is used for

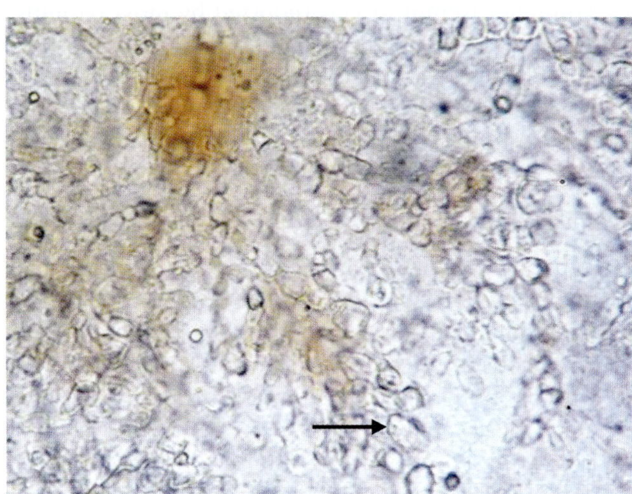

FIG. 11.3: KOH mount of crushed granule of eumycetoma showing hyphae with swollen cells (400×).
(KOH: potassium hydroxide)

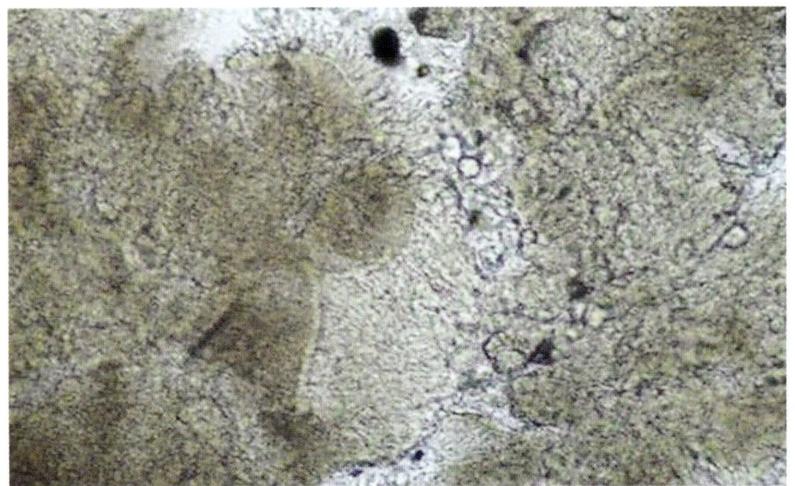

FIG. 11.4: KOH mount of crushed granule (400×).
(KOH: potassium hydroxide)

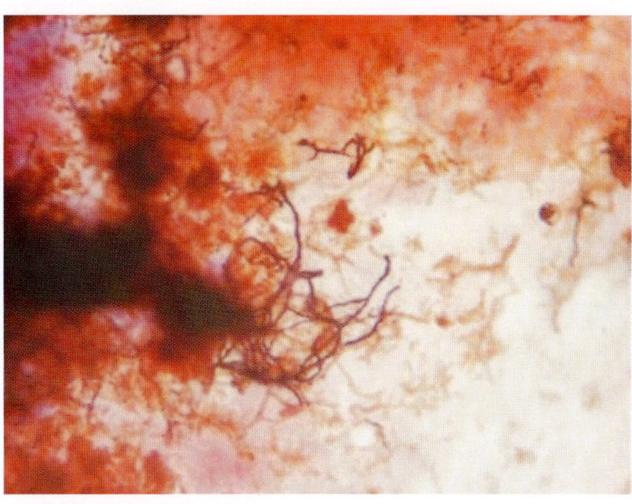

FIG. 11.5: Gram-stained smear of a crushed granule of actinomycotic mycetoma showing gram-positive filamentous bacteria (oil immersion).

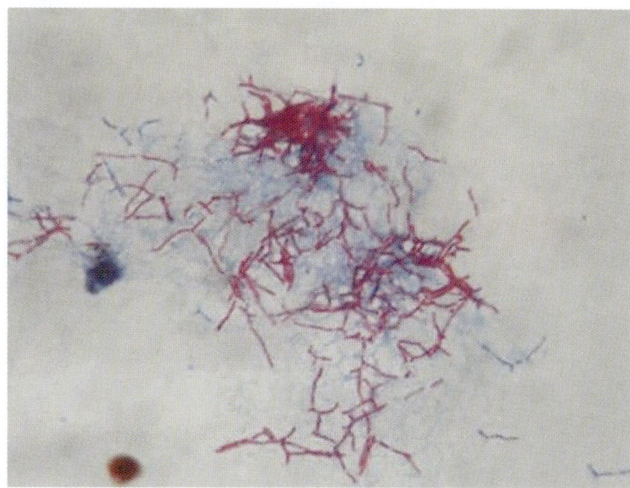

FIG. 11.6: Modified acid-fast staining showing acid-fast filaments of *Nocardia* species (1,000×).

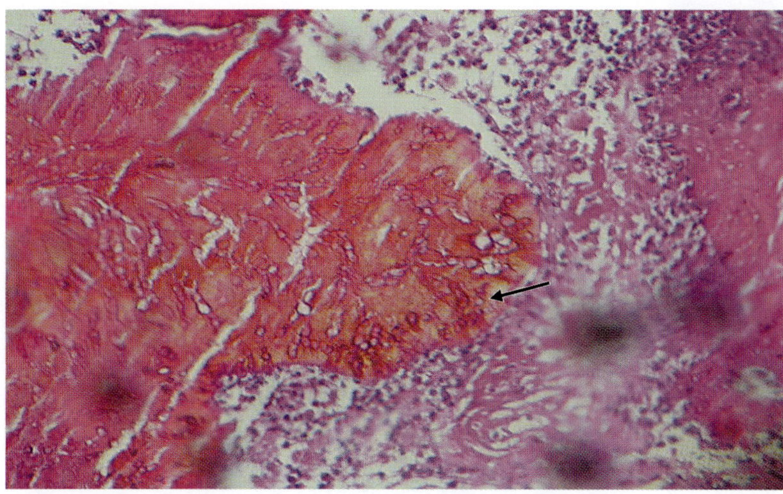

FIG. 11.7: PAS stain on biopsy of mycetoma showing granule (red) with fungal elements (400×).
(PAS: periodic acid–Schiff)

bacterial culture and the material from the second test tube is used for the fungal culture. Several sets of brain heart infusion broth, Löwenstein–Jensen (LJ) medium, Sabouraud dextrose agar (SDA) (free of cycloheximide), and brain heart infusion agar are used for the cultures. These are incubated at 25, 37, and 44°C as optimum temperature of growth for different organisms may vary.

Madurella mycetomatis

- *Granules*: They are <2 mm in diameter, black, brittle, and oblong to lobed. In rare cases, numerous big cysts are accompanied by vesicular open grain.
- *Colony morphology*: The colonies mature in 7–10 days. The colonies are either glabrous or powdery, usually folded (it may be smooth also). The color varies from white, yellow brown, olive brown, or dark gray. **Figure 11.8** shows the colonies of *M. mycetomatis* on an SDA slant. The reverse is dark brown with brown diffusible pigment.
- *Microscopy*: Lactophenol cotton blue (LPCB) mount prepared from SDA shows only septate hyphae with chlamydoconidia without development of spores, as shown in **Figure 11.9**. LPCB from cornmeal agar (CMA) produces pyriform conidia on simple or branched conidiophores or phialides with round conidia. These findings are shown in **Figure 11.10**. Otherwise, slide cultures done on SDA as well as PDA do not show spores.

The differentiation of *M. mycetomatis* from *M. grisea* is possible as the former grows at 37°C and develops brown diffusible pigment.

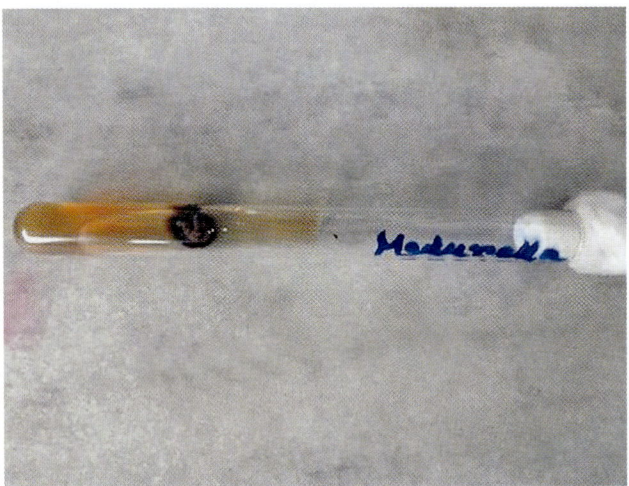

FIG. 11.8: SDA slant showing the growth of *Madurella mycetomatis*.
(SDA: Sabouraud Dextrose Agar)

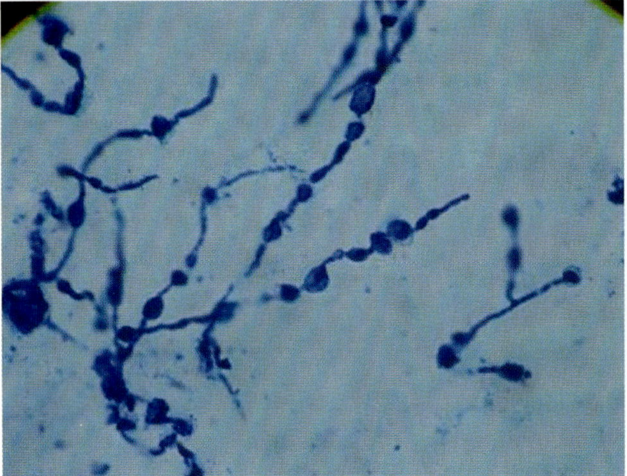

FIG. 11.9: LPCB mount of *Madurella mycetomatis* from PDA showing hyphae and chlamydoconidia of *M. mycetomatis* (400×).
(LPCB: lactophenol cotton blue; PDA: potato dextrose agar)

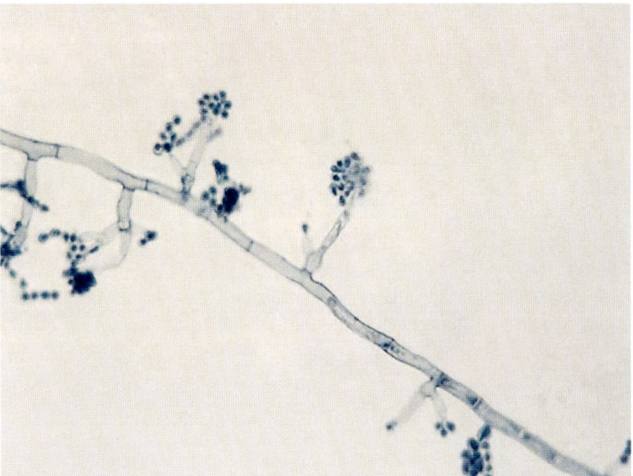

FIG. 11.10: LPCB mount of *Madurella mycetomatis* from growth on CMA (400×).
(CMA: cornmeal agar; LPCB: lactophenol cotton blue)
Source: Centers for Disease Control and Prevention (CDC).

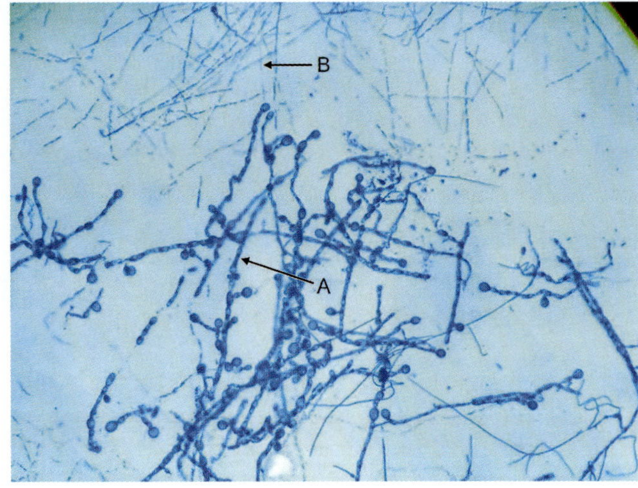

FIG. 11.11: LPCB mount of *Madurella grisea* showing hyphae of two widths: (A) Wide hyphae and (B) narrow hyphae (400×).
(LPCB: lactophenol cotton blue)

Madurella grisea (Trematosphaeria grisea)

Grain size is <1 mm; black colored; soft to firm.

- *Colony morphology*: Colonies mature in 10 days. It grows at 25–30°C but does not grow at 37°C. Colonies are leathery, folded, gray, or olive. The reverse is dark without diffusible pigment in most of the cases.
- *Microscopy*: Hyphae with two widths (some are thick and some are thin) are seen without conidia, as shown in **Figure 11.11**. Chlamydoconidia may be seen. There may be pycnidia.

Actinomadura madurae

Grain production is white and delicate. The dimensions range from 2 to 5 mm. It grows faster on LJ medium than on SDA. Growth is white to tan to somewhat orange. The colonies have wrinkles and are glabrous. Gram-positive filaments are seen in the Gram-stained smear. This bacterium is non-acid-fast.

Actinomadura pelletieri

A firm granule with a red color is formed. There are tiny, folded, dry colonies created. It starts off pink to peach and then turns cranberry red. It is a non-acid-fast, gram-positive filamentous bacillus.

Nocardia brasiliensis

Colonies take 7–9 days to mature, are chalky and dry, and expand slowly. The color varies from yellow to orange. The colonies on LJ medium and SDA are similar. They display filaments of gram-positive bacteria that split into coccoid and bacillary forms. This bacterium is acid-fast.

Nocardia caviae

Nocardia caviae grows fast. Similar to *N. brasiliensis*, colonies may have tufts of aerial hyphae. These bacteria are acid-fast.

Nocardia asteroides

Glabrous, chalky, folded, white to orange colonies with occasional aerial development are present.

Streptomyces somaliensis

On SDA and L-J media, wrinkled colonies with a cream color are formed. It displays spore-filled, nonfragmenting filaments that are gram positive.

The rest of the fungal agents of eumycetoma are discussed in subsequent chapters. Various biochemical tests used for the identification of bacterial agents and fungal agents are given in **Tables 11.4 and 11.5**.

Molecular identification helps to identify the fungi which do not produce spores easily on culture media.

TREATMENT

Curing eumycotic mycetoma is a difficult condition. Oral ketoconazole 200 mg twice a day and itraconazole 100 mg twice a day are given for a period of 12–24 months. Amphotericin B is a treatment for *Fusarium* and *Madurella*. Actinomycotic mycetoma is treated with antibiotics such as amikacin, tetracycline, cotrimoxazole, and streptomycin. A Welsh regimen consisting of amikacin and cotrimoxazole is recommended for 5 weeks. In some cases, surgery (debridement) is advised which enhances response to therapeutic interventions. Antimicrobials should be administered 3–6 months before surgery in order for the lesions to form a fibrous capsule that will facilitate easier surgical dissection and excision. The prognosis of actinomycetomas is good as compared to eumycetoma. Recurrences are known to occur in mycetoma cases.

CHAPTER 12

Sporotrichosis (Beurmann's Disease, Schenck's Disease, or Rose Gardener's Disease)

INTRODUCTION

Sporotrichosis is a human and animal fungal infection that affects the epidermis and subcutaneous tissues, caused by fungus of the genus *Sporothrix.* The infection generally takes place following traumatic inoculation of contaminated plant debris or through bites and scratches from infected animals. The disease can occur sporadically or in outbreaks. The initial lesion is usually restricted to the skin and subcutaneous tissue, but subsequently, the fungus can affect adjacent lymphatic vessels. Rarely, this fungus can disseminate through the blood or the lymphatic system with systemic infection. It is the most common subcutaneous mycosis worldwide, and in some regions, it is very endemic.

For the past 100 years, it has been believed that *Sporothrix schenckii* is the cause of the illness. Molecular studies reveal that *S. schenckii* is a species complex, comprising multiple cryptic species. Rose thorn sickness, rose handler's disease, rose gardener's disease, and Schenck's ailment are some of the other names for sporotrichosis. It is a fungus that changes into and thrives in the surroundings as mold. Once within the body, it exhibits temperature-dependent dimorphism, changing inside the tissues into a yeast form. This fungus shows thermal dimorphism, as is shown by systemic fungi. After the use of molecular studies, it has been reported that Indian isolates belong to *Sporothrix globosa.*

HISTORY

Benjamin Schenck, a medical student, first reported sporotrichosis in 1898 at the Johns Hopkins Hospital in Baltimore, United States. A sample taken from skin lesions on a patient's right upper leg grew fungus, and the patient received treatment. It was examined by pathologist Erwin F Smith, and he identified the fungus as *Sporotrichum* species.

Hektoen and Perkins reported the pathogen in Chicago in 1900. They named the fungus *S. schenckii.* For the first time, an "asteroid body" was found in a lesion specimen by Lutz and Splendore in 1907.

In 1914, the illness was initially reported in the Gauteng gold mines of South Africa. The first incidence in India was reported in 1932 from Kolkata by LM Ghosh. The two largest outbreaks happened: (1) One in the United States in 1988 and (2) the other in South Africa between 1941 and 1944. Australia reported a small outbreak between 2000 and 2003.

TAXONOMY

Sporothrix schenckii, with two variants: (1) *Sporothrix schenckii var schenckii* and (2) *Sporothrix schenckii var luriei,* causes the condition sporotrichosis. Later on, *S. schenckii* var *luriei* was considered a distinct species. Molecular studies demonstrated that *S. schenckii* is genetically a complex species. The clinically important species proposed by Marimon et al. in the year 2008 were *Sporothrix brasiliensis, S. globosa,* and *Sporothrix mexicana.* Atleast 51 species of *Sporothrix* were identified from the environment. But members of the *S. schenckii* complex are pathogenic and include the following species: *S. brasiliensis, Sporothrix schenckii sensu stricto (s.str.), S. globosa,* and *Sporothrix luriei.*

The causative agents of sporotrichosis are now named as *S. schenckii* species complex. Its gene sequencing has revealed the following species: *Sporothrix albicans, S. brasiliensis, S. globosa, S. luriei, S. mexicana, Sporothrix pallida,* and *S. schenckii* (both sensu stricto and sensu lato). The most common agents of human or animal diseases are *S. brasiliensis, S. schenckii,* and

S. globosa, while there are rare cases of infection caused by *S. mexicana, S. pallida,* and *S. luriei.*

Geographic dispersion also results in the division of the genus *Sporothrix* into five clades. Clinical isolates are included in clades I (*S. brasiliensis*), II (*S. schenckii*), and III (*S. globosa*). Environmental isolates are included in clade IV (*S. mexicana*) and clade V (*S. albicans*).

The genus *Sporothrix* is currently classified taxonomically as belonging to the class Pezizomycotina, phylum Ascomycota, family Ophiostomataceae, and order Ophiostomatales.

MYCOLOGY

Morphological Characteristics

S. schenckii usually looks hyaline (transparent) in tissue.

The Fontana–Masson stain can be used to show that the hyphal cell walls of *S. schenckii* contain melanin. Dimorphism in *S. schenckii* is temperature sensitive. At 25–30°C in a laboratory, soil, or the environment, it grows as a mold.

It becomes yeast in infected tissue or when grown at higher temperatures (35–37°C, as on Brain Heart Infusion Agar).

Because of pigmentation found in the sleeves of sessile conidia that form along hyphae, mature cultures of *S. schenckii* exhibit melanization.

EPIDEMIOLOGY

While some *S. schenckii* strains isolated from the environment can only grow at lower temperatures, others can grow at 35–37°C.

It is thought that the disease's lymphocutaneous or extracutaneous variants, which involve deeper tissue and lymphatic dissemination, are only caused by strains that can develop at temperatures between 35 and 37°C.

Geographic distribution: *S. schenckii* is found all over the world, in temperate, subtropical, and tropical climates. Sporotrichosis is very common in South America, Asia (India, China, Japan, and Malaysia). The fungus is more common in India's sub-Himalayan region, which stretches from Himachal Pradesh to Assam. The Kangra district of Himachal Pradesh looks to be a sporotrichosis hyperendemic location. There are three endemic zones in India: (1) Northern, (2) northeastern, and (3) southern states.

Ecological niche: *S. schenckii* is a saprobe, which means it can survive on both living and dead plants. In most cases, the fungus is transmitted to people by inoculation, which occurs when it comes into contact with the skin via dirt, wood splinters, prairie or salt marsh hay, straw, thorns, or sphagnum moss. Sphagnum moss is widely used in bonsai tree soil mixtures.

Risk groups: This sporotrichosis is more common in adults who work in outdoor environments or engage in activities that expose them to certain environmental factors. Some of the risk factors are given as follows:

- *Gardeners and forestry workers*: Individuals working with thorny plants, sphagnum moss, and decaying wood, such as floral and plant nursery workers, as well as forestry workers.
- *Agricultural laborers*: Individuals engaged in agricultural activities, where they may come into contact with thorny plants.
- *Transmission from infected cats*: There have been multiple incidences of sporotrichosis in people that have been traced back to diseased cats. Humans can contract the disease from cats by skin-to-skin contact, bites, or scratches caused by an infected cat.

S. brasiliensis infects cats and other mammals. It has ability to spread from cats to humans. Many outbreaks occurred within Brazil and several adjacent countries in South America due to zoonotic transmission.

Outbreaks of sporotrichosis also reported in China associated with flooding. There are localized areas of hyperendemicity in Guatemala, Mexico, Peru and South Africa. In South Africa, sporotrichosis has been associated with an outbreak of infection in miners following contact with contaminated wooden pit props.

Additional Risk Factors

Risk is further heightened when individuals in these occupational groups have compromised immune systems due to conditions such as alcoholism and diabetes. These underlying health issues can make them more susceptible to sporotrichosis.

In people with acquired immunodeficiency syndrome (AIDS), spread of sporotrichosis throughout the body is more common.

IMMUNITY

The immune response starts with the activation of macrophages by CD4+ T cells. Nitric oxide (NO) is a fungicidal agent and a component of innate immunity. The fungus cell wall antigen 70-kDa glycoprotein (gp70) boosts the adherence of conidia to the epithelium, enhancing fungal invasion, but they also have a protective impact on the host, which is mediated by T helper cells (Th1 in humans). It seems that cell-mediated immunity (CMI) is important in getting rid of the infection or for controlling infections. Humoral immune response results in the production of particular antibodies that target the *Sporothrix* cell wall. Sporotrichosis is commonly associated with cellular immunological deficiencies, including AIDS.

PATHOGENESIS

The spores (from environment) or yeasts (from animals) are the infective forms. The virulence factors of the fungus are thermotolerance, melanin production, ergosterol peroxide, and cell wall antigen. *S. schenckii* also produces two extracellular proteinases, namely proteinase I and proteinase II. In lymphocutaneous sporotrichosis lesions, antigen–antibody complexes encase individual yeast cells, resulting in star-shaped deposits called asteroid bodies. The radiating crown spikes of these asteroid bodies contain IgG and IgM antibodies. It could be a protective immune response to yeast. After incubation at 22°C, the yeast cells at the heart of these entities germinate, leading to the generation of conidia.

Histopathology

Hematoxylin and eosin (H&E) stain helps to see the inflammatory infiltration, while periodic acid-Schiff (PAS) or methenamine silver helps to identify the fungal forms. A persistent granulomatous dermatitis, often with a central abscess, is the key feature of the tissue reaction. Pathological changes include intraepidermal micro-abscesses, hyperkeratosis, or acanthosis. Granulomas can be found in skin lesions. Granuloma has a central region with neutrophils and eosinophils, an intermediate layer with mononuclear cells, and an outer area with lymphocytes and plasmacytes. Sporotrichosis could be indicated by the presence of asteroid bodies or the Splendore–Hoeppli occurrences. A probable immunoglobulin deposit attached to the microbe wall makes up the eosinophilic material surrounding the fungal cell.

The following three granulomatous patterns are described by Lurie:

1. *Sporotrichoid type*: Central necrotic material is surrounded by neutrophils, plasma cells, and lymphocytes. Histiocytes appear in concentric zones.
2. *Tuberculoid type*: The granuloma contains epithelioid cells mixed with fibroblasts, lymphocytes, and Langhans giant cells.
3. *Foreign body type*: In this type, a foreign body granuloma is seen.

CLINICAL FEATURES

- *Lymphocutaneous form or sporotrichoid pattern*: This is the most common clinical presentation. The fungus spreads through the lymphatic system. The most common presentation of sporotrichosis is the development of nontender, mobile nodules on affected limbs, which can later turn red and even ulcerate. The lymphatic vessels that drain the area take on a cord-like appearance. Successively, nodules and ulcers are formed that follow the path of lymphatic drainage from the original lesion, giving the area its characteristic "cording effect." It is possible for these nodules to suppurate or release pus.
- *Fixed cutaneous lesion*: Typically, the initial infection is limited to the site of inoculation without lymphatic or systemic spread. The lesions are infiltrating, plaque-like, verrucous, scaly, macular, or papular. The most common type, the fixed cutaneous variant, is sometimes called "plaque sporotrichosis." It is typical to see such lesions on the arms, chest, neck, and face. Individuals with this sort of presentation have a high level of immunity, most likely as a result of previous subclinical disease.
- *Extracutaneous and disseminated sporotrichosis*: Extracutaneous sporotrichosis is the second most frequent type of sporotrichosis after subcutaneous sporotrichosis. It is seen in patients with diabetes, chronic obstructive pulmonary disease (COPD), or human immunodeficiency virus (HIV) infection. It may also be seen in alcoholic patients. This clinical form presents in several categories as follows:
    - *Osteoarticular sporotrichosis*: It is due to result of direct inoculation, spread via skin lesions, or hematogenous transmission through the bloodstream. This condition can lead to bursitis and tenosynovitis, in addition to affecting bones and joints. The injured joint could be located at the site of an existing skin lesion, in bone structures far away from the original lesion, or a solitary finding. This form of sporotrichosis is associated with alcoholism. Disease at weight-bearing joints (such as the knee or the hip) can result from dissemination, although infections affecting the musculoskeletal system and spreading throughout the body are rare.

- *Pulmonary-systemic infection*: Inhalation of fungal conidia from the environment results in pulmonary-systemic infection caused by *S. schenckii*.
- *Mucocutaneous type*: The lesions are red, ulcerative, or suppurative initially and later become granulomatous, vegetative, or papillomatous. The regional lymph nodes are enlarged.
- *Ocular type*: Due to disseminated sporotrichosis in AIDS patients, choroiditis and dacryocystitis may occur.
- *Disseminated type*: Rarely, dissemination of fungus occurs to involve visceral organs (pyelonephritis, orchitis, mastitis, and meningitis).

DIFFERENTIAL DIAGNOSIS

Sporotrichosis should be differentiated from nocardiosis (lymphocutaneous), leishmaniasis, cutaneous tuberculosis (TB), chromoblastomycosis, cat scratch disease, cutaneous anthrax, and primary syphilis.

LABORATORY DIAGNOSIS

- *Collection of sample*: Biopsies of cutaneous or subcutaneous lesions, scrapings, or aspirated pus, curettage, swabbing from open lesions, sputum, cerebrospinal fluid (CSF), and synovial fluids are common specimens.
- *Direct examination*: As the concentration of yeast cells in the specimen is low, microscopic tests such as potassium hydroxide (KOH) mount and Gram staining have low sensitivity. Sensitivity can be increased by using a fluorescent stain as calcofluor stain. Gram-stained smear shows few gram-positive yeast cells with irregular staining.
- *Biopsy*: Granulomatous changes are more common with occasional fungal elements. Staining with PAS or Grocott-Gömöri's methenamine silver (GMS) reveals yeast forms. Yeast cells vary from round to oval to elongate (2–6 μm in diameter); sometimes the yeast cells may show budding with narrow base. Sometimes, yeast cells in the form of elongated "cigar bodies" (2 × 3–3 × 10 μm) may be seen. When diagnosing lymphocutaneous sporotrichosis, asteroid bodies—which are rare but noticeable—can be helpful. These formations may be seen with H&E staining and are indicative of sporotrichosis, albeit not pathognomonic. Immunoperoxidase stain is preferred over PAS or GMS.

  Fine-needle aspiration cytology (FNAC) can be done from lymph node which can be stained with GMS stain. Black-colored yeast cells (occasionally short pseudohyphal or hyphal form) are seen against a green background which can be easily confused with *Histoplasma capsulatum* and *Candida glabrata*.
- *Culture*: Culture is still the gold standard for diagnosis of sporotrichosis. The necessary material (e.g., tissue biopsy or drainage from skin lesions) is cultured on Sabouraud dextrose agar (SDA), brain heart infusion agar (BHIA), blood agar, chocolate agar, and Pine's medium. These media are inoculated in two sets, of which one set is incubated at 25°C and another at 37°C for up to 4 weeks. On the specified medium at 25°C, growth is often seen within 3–5 days. Isolates that can develop at 37°C are deemed pathogenic, whereas those that cannot grow at this temperature are classified as less pathogenic or nonpathogenic.

Colony Morphology

Colony matures in 6–10 days with a moderate growth rate. At 25°C, the colonies initially are small and white or pale orange to orange-gray with no cottony aerial hyphae. After further incubation, the colonies become moist, wrinkled, leathery, or velvety, brown or black with a narrow white border. The reverse is dark in the center and light at the periphery.

At 37°C, the colonies are cream or tan, smooth, and waxy.

Microscopic findings: At 25°C, the microscopic characteristics are better observed by putting the slide culture on cornmeal agar. The hyphae are very narrow (1–2 μm in diameter) and septate. The conidiophores are tapering, and they rise at right angles from the hyphae. This finding helps to differentiate from *Verticillium* species. At the tip of the conidiophore, many small, tear-shaped or almost round hyaline conidia (2–3 × 2–6 μm) are seen on delicate, thread-like denticles. They form a "rosette," "daisy" cluster, or "floret"-like arrangement of conidia in young cultures, as shown in **Figures 12.1 and 12.2**. Some sessile conidia may be found singly along the hyphae. Even a sympodial arrangement of conidia is seen. The conidia arranged along the hyphae produce a "sleeve"-like pattern.

At 37°C, round, oval, and fusiform budding cells of various sizes (1–3 × 3–10 μm), commonly called cigar bodies, are seen.

It is very important in the laboratory to demonstrate mycelial to yeast conversion and vice versa (dimorphism). It is done in a humid environment with 5–10% CO_2, BHI agar—a medium rich in vitamins and amino acids. The separate sets of media are incubated at 37°C and 25°C.

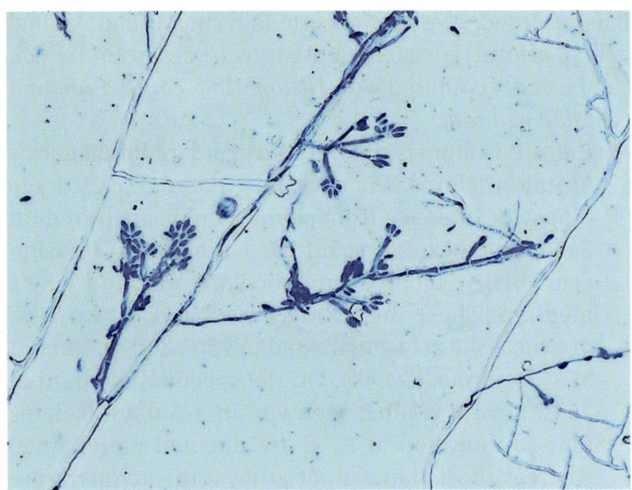

FIG. 12.1: LPCB mount showing floret-like arrangement of conidia of *Sporothrix* species.
(LPCB: lactophenol cotton blue)

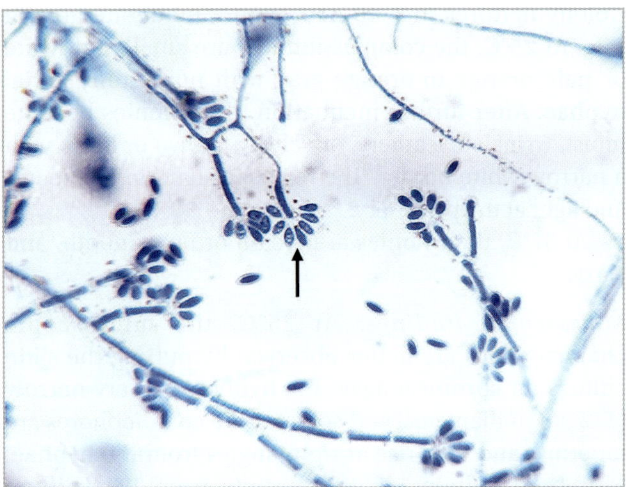

FIG. 12.2: PVA-LPCB mount under oil immersion showing floret-like arrangement of conidia of *Sporothrix* (1,000×).
(LPCB: lactophenol cotton blue; PVA: polyvinyl alcohol)

DIFFERENTIAL DIAGNOSIS

Sporothrix schenckii can be differentiated from other fungi such as *Ophiostoma stenoceras*, *Aureobasidium pullulans*, *Trichosporon* species, and other *Sporothrix* species based on growth characteristics and morphology.

Sporothrix globosa: The morphology is similar to other *Sporothrix* species; hence, the phenotypic tests are useless for identification purposes. The molecular techniques are required for species confirmation. However, some biochemical parameters help in species identification. One of them is the carbohydrate assimilation, such as sucrose, ribitol, and raffinose, which is different among the medically relevant *Sporothrix* species: *S. globosa* has positive assimilation to sucrose and ribitol and negative assimilation to raffinose, *S. schenckii* has positive assimilation for the three sugars, and *S. brasiliensis* has negative assimilation to sucrose and raffinose and positive assimilation to ribitol.

Serodiagnosis

Serological tests are used when yeast forms cannot be observed or when there is a delay in culture growth. Commercial tests such as latex agglutination can be employed to detect specific antibodies. Direct immunofluorescence (DIF) test, used to demonstrate antigen in tissue, is a highly specific method. Skin tests with yeast and mycelial phase antigen (sporotrichin) give variable results.

Genetic Identification

A nested polymerase chain reaction (PCR) assay using a target sequence in the 18S rDNA can be employed for genetic identification. This molecular approach can be used to confirm the presence of *S. schenckii*.

Animal Pathogenicity

Suspension of yeasts of filaments from culture is inoculated intraperitoneally in male Swiss albino mice. After 7–10 days orchitis occurs. Plenty of yeast cells are seen in testes. Only *S. schenckii* gives positive results. The test is not performed now.

TREATMENT

Treatment of different clinical types is summarized in **Table 12.1**.

TABLE 12.1: Summary of treatment of various clinical types.

Clinical form of sporotrichosis	***Treatment***
Cutaneous and lymphocutaneous sporotrichosis:	
First-line therapy	• Itraconazole (ITC) 200 mg/day (oral) until 2–4 weeks after all lesions resolve (usually 3–6 months) • Monitor serum concentrations to ensure proper absorption • Saturated Solution of Potassium Iodide (SSKI) as another cheap alternative for this type of infection
Second-line therapy (if needed)	Increase ITC to 200 mg twice a day. Terbinafine 500 mg twice a day
Other forms of sporotrichosis:	
Pulmonary	• Amphotericin B (AmB), lipid formulation (3–5 mg/kg/day IV), or AmB deoxycholate for severe cases • Step-down to ITC (200 mg twice a day, when patient responds to AmB). Surgery may be considered
Osteoarticular sporotrichosis	*Primary*: ITC (200 mg twice a day) for 12+ months or AmB (lipid formulation) for severe cases, followed by ITC
Meningeal	*Primary*: AmB lipid formulation (5 mg/kg/day, IV) for 4–6 weeks, then step-down to ITC (200 mg twice a day) for at least 12 months. Suppressive therapy with ITC is recommended for immunocompromised patients
Disseminated sporotrichosis	*Primary*: AmB lipid formulation (3–5 mg/kg/day, IV), followed by ITC 200 mg twice a day upon response, continuing for at least 12 months, or indefinitely for immunocompromised patients
Alternative therapy	Terbinafine (250 mg/day) is an alternative to ITC and has shown success

(IV: intravenous)

CHAPTER

13 Chromoblastomycosis

INTRODUCTION

The pigmented, melanogenic fungi called dematiaceous fungi produce chromoblastomycosis (CBM), a subcutaneous infection characterized by chronic granulomatous and suppurative symptoms. "Phaeohyphomycosis" is one more condition that is caused by chromogenic fungi. The main differentiating feature is the presence of pigmented hyphae in histopathology slides of phaeohyphomycosis, while in CBM, sclerotic bodies are seen in histopathology.

The condition is common in tropical and subtropical countries. The soil is home to these fungi, which can infect humans by traumatic inoculation. There are verrucous, crusted, or ulcerated lesions on exposed parts of the body without the tendency to spread. The most defining characteristic feature of the disease is the presence of sclerotic bodies in the lesions. This microscopic feature helps to differentiate the clinical condition from "phaeohyphomycosis" in which hyphae are seen in tissues instead of sclerotic bodies. The meaning of the term "chromoblastomycosis" is chromo = colored, blasto = budding, and mycosis = fungal infection. The old term "chromomycois" created a lot of confusion, and the term chromoblastomycosis is recommended for the disease.

Mycoses that spread by different kinds of transcutaneous damage are referred to as "plantation mycoses" or "subcutaneous mycoses." Endemic mycoses such as sporotrichosis, eumycetoma, lacaziosis (lobomycosis), and CBM are included in this group. One of the most prevalent implantation fungal diseases is CBM.

The disease is common in low-income persons living in tropical nations, and there are few treatment choices available. CBM was added to the World Health Organization's (WHO) list of neglected tropical illnesses in 2017.

HISTORICAL ASPECTS

In 1914, the Brazilian state of Minas Gerais was the site of the first description of CBM by Maximiliano Willibaldo Rudolph. Two of the four patients studied had pigmented fungus isolated, and Rudolph supplied all of the relevant disease-based data. In 1915, first case from Boston was reported by Lane and Medlar.

The initial American cases of CBM were reported by Lane and Medlar separately. The biopsy from the buttocks of the patient with the warty violet plaque grew *Phialophora verrucosa*.

In 1922, Terra and colleagues from Brazil used the name "chromoblastomycosis" CBM, which means "chromo-colored blossoms."

In 1975, Ajello came up with the term "phaeohyphomycosis" to characterize fungal diseases other than CBM that manifested on the skin and throughout the body. In order to distinguish between the various types of mycoses, it was necessary to look at the lesions' clinical and histopathological features. For example, in cases of phaeohyphomycosis, the histological section of the skin would show hyphae and yeast, whereas in situations of CBM, "muriform cells" would be seen. The muriform cells are known as sclerotic bodies, copper penne bodies, or Medlar bodies.

ETIOLOGIC AGENTS

At least 41 fungal species cause CBM in humans, which are arranged in the following families: Chaetomiaceae, Cladosporiaceae, Didymellaceae, Dothioraceae, Herpotrichiellaceae, Hysteriaceae, Microascaceae, Onygenaceae, Pleosporaceae, and Pleurostomataceae.

The most commonly identified agents are *Fonsecaea pedrosoi* and *Cladophialophora carrionii*. Sporadic cases have been caused by *P. verrucosa, Rhinocladiella aquaspersa, Botryomyces caespitosus, Exophiala jeanselmei, Exophiala spinifera, Aureobasidium pullulans,* and *Wangiella (Exophiala) dermatitidis.*

The characteristics of sclerotic bodies of fungi are given in **Table 13.1**.

The morphological characteristics of fungal genera causing CBM are summarized in **Table 13.2**.

EPIDEMIOLOGY

As saprophytes, these fungi inhabit soil and decomposing plant matter worldwide. The phaeoid fungus is introduced into the skin tissues through trauma, which is the way the infection is transmitted. This disease cannot be passed from one person to another or from animals to humans. People in their 30s–50s are the most common age group affected by the condition. Agricultural laborers, men, and people living in rural areas have a higher prevalence of this condition. A few cases have been reported in domestic animals such as dogs and horses, but they do not play a role in the transmission of disease to human beings.

TABLE 13.1: Characteristics of sclerotic bodies of fungi.

Fungal agent	*Characteristics*
Fonsecaea pedrosoi	Brown, thick-walled sclerotic bodies, often in clumps
Fonsecaea compacta	Brown, thick-walled sclerotic cells, usually smaller
Phialophora verrucosa	Brown, thick-walled sclerotic cells with a vase-like conidiophore
Cladophialophora carrionii	Brown, thick-walled sclerotic cells, often with a branching pattern
Rhinocladiella aquaspersa	Brown, thick-walled sclerotic cells with a dense, mat-like growth
Exophiala jeanselmei	Dark brown, thick-walled sclerotic cells with a soft texture

The condition is seen all over the world. Tropical and subtropical areas between 30°N and 30°S have a high incidence. Countries and areas with a higher prevalence are given as follows:

- *Western hemisphere*: Brazil (especially in the Amazon region), Mexico (in Oaxaca and Veracruz), Venezuela, the Dominican Republic, Cuba, and Colombia
- *Africa*: Madagascar, the Natal state of South Africa, Botswana, Cameroon, Nigeria, Rwanda, and Zambia
- *Asia*: Japan, China, and Malaysia

The country in Africa with the highest prevalence is Madagascar. The sub-Himalayan and Himalayan regions account for the bulk of cases in India. The first case in India was reported in the year 1957. This is more typical in warmer regions where people often go barefoot or wear very little clothing.

IMMUNITY

Purulent abscesses occur following a penetrating lesion with a thorn or splinter that harbors conidia. A papule forms, gradually increasing over weeks or months, and this is how purulent abscesses are born. There is no way that the PMNs can fight off the fungus. Copper-colored muriform cells that resist lysis in the host are seen in the lesions. A continuous antigenic stimulation may be the source of the extensive and increasing cutaneous fibrosis.

TABLE 13.2: Characteristics of fungal genera causing chromoblastomycosis.

Fungal genera	*Type of conidiogenous cells*	*Additional information*
Cladosporium	Blastoconidia in chains	Conidia are formed in chains, typically appearing as darkly pigmented, and are often described by their olive-green to black color
Phialophora	Phialides with collarettes	Conidia are produced in phialides that have a characteristic collar-like structure at the tip. The conidia are often flask shaped
Exophiala	Annellides	Conidia are formed in annellides, which are elongate, often tapering cells that produce conidia in a series
Rhinocladiella	Annellides and phialides	This genus produces conidia in both annellides and phialides. The annellides are conidiogenous cells with a tapering, elongated appearance, while the phialides resemble those of *Phialophora*
Fonsecaea	Sympodulae, also phialides and blastoconidia	Conidiogenesis occurs via sympodulae, which are branching conidiogenous cells, as well as phialides and blastoconidia. The sympodulae are characterized by their irregular branching pattern

HISTOPATHOLOGY

Pseudoepitheliomatous hyperplasia, fibrosis, pigmented sclerotic formations, and the development of microabscesses in the epidermis are the histopathological features of the disease. The cross-cell walls of mature cells meet at one point. These are dark brown cells with a size of 5–12 µm. Some younger muriform cells may show single septa. The presence of cross walls within round cells gives the typical "Mercedes Benz" sign appearance. The muriform bodies may be found single or multiple, within giant cells or extracellularly. It is believed that they are a hybrid of yeast cells and hyphae. The staining of histopathological sections with hematoxylin and eosin (H&E) results in a deep brown hue. The melanin pigmentation present on the cell wall of the phaeoid fungi can also be seen with the *Fontana-Masson stain.*

As time passes, the patients develop organized mixed mycotic granuloma (*OMMG*). There is fibrosis, increased cutaneous capillary vessels, pseudoepitheliomatous hyperplasia, and microabscesses with many fungi in suppurative granulomas. The multiplication of fungal cells is responsible for the formation of epithelial outgrowth. Typical "black dots" develop on the surface of the lesion. These are the sites through which inflammatory debris, blood, and fungal cells (Medlar bodies) come out. These sites are scraped which is the best specimen for microscopy and culture.

PATHOGENICITY

Melanin is the most important virulence factor, but other possible components of this disease include changes to cell surfaces, hydrophobicity, fungal cell wall remodeling, secretion of hydrolytic and proteolytic enzymes, adhesion molecules, aromatic hydrocarbon incorporation, and siderophores assembly. Cell adhesion, hydrophobicity, melanin, and muriform cells are important components of CBM that cause disease. The CMI response is not enough to restrict the infection.

CLINICAL FEATURES

A small, unilateral papular lesion with a smooth pink surface appears at the infection site. Papules may become larger and even develop a scaly appearance within a matter of weeks. The lesion has the potential to expand and develop into many lesions, leading to a variety of clinical manifestations.

The foot, ankle, and/or leg are the most typical areas affected. Other uncommon sites of infection are shoulders, arms, hands, and buttocks; ears, chest, face, and abdomen may also be involved. Rarely, there is invasion of muscle and bone. The margins of the feet are a common location to find verrucous lesions. These sores have a granulomatous appearance. When nodules enlarge, they can resemble cauliflowers of different colors and can develop into tumors. Untreated lesions spread over a greater region over the course of months or even years. We see five different clinical types. A single patient may exhibit symptoms of more than one kind:

1. Nodular lesions with a surface that is smooth or scaly.
2. Tumor-like masses, prominent, papillomatous, and sometimes lobulated or "cauliflower like."
3. *Verrucous*: Hyperkeratosis is the major feature of these warty, dry lesions.
4. *Cicatricial*: Flat lesions that enlarge by peripheral extension with atrophic scarring and healing at the center. They tend to cover extensive areas of the body.
5. *Plaque type*: Slightly elevated lesions of various sizes and shapes, reddish to violaceous in color, with a scaly surface.

Sequelae

The extensive fibrosis and chronic inflammatory infiltrate cause obstruction to lymphatic flow, forming lymphedema below the affected sites. Further deformity and ankylosis of joints lead to permanent disability. These lesions may get secondarily infected. Thus, sequelae common in long-standing lesions include scarring and deformity, lymphedema, elephantiasis, and recurrent bacterial infection.

DIFFERENTIAL DIAGNOSIS

Chromoblastomycosis should be differentiated from the following conditions: Blastomycosis, sporotrichosis, leprosy, leishmaniasis, syphilis, mycetoma, cutaneous tuberculosis, and phaeohyphomycosis.

LABORATORY DIAGNOSIS

Skin scrapings or biopsy from the edges of the lesion are the specimens collected for the diagnosis of infection. When *black dots* are seen, scrapings from these sites are good specimens for the demonstration of muriform bodies. Other samples to be collected are crusts, pus, and cyst fluid. Scotch tape or vinyl adhesive tape is also used for microscopic examination.

Microscopic Examination

The most useful test is the direct examination of a 10% potassium hydroxide (KOH) mount which is done to observe the presence of muriform bodies. Microscopic examination does not give any specific information about the infective agent. All of them give the same appearance in tissue, i.e., the presence of muriform bodies. A biopsy may be submitted. Various staining methods used for the demonstration of muriform cells include H&E stain, Giemsa stain, fluorescent stain, and Fontana-Masson stain.

Culture

Two sets of Sabouraud dextrose agars (SDAs) containing antibiotics and cycloheximide are inoculated with the specimens. A tube is kept at 37°C, while the other is kept at 25°C. Potato dextrose agar (PDA) medium is preferred over SDA, as the color of the colony precisely matches the description. Colonies, ranging in color from dark green to black, typically appear 10 days to 2 weeks later. Slide culture is done on PDA. Important phaeoid fungus taxa causing CBM are given below. They have the following pattern types of sporulation and conidiogenesis:

- *Cladosporium*: Blastoconidia in chains
- *Phialophora*: Phialides with collarettes
- *Exophiala*: Annellides
- *Fonsecaea*: Phialides and blastoconidia
- *Rhinocladiella*: Annellides and phialides
- *Fonsecaea*: Sympodulae, also phialides and blastoconidia

The fungi causing CBM may show more than one pattern of growth as seen in *Fonsecaea pedrosoi*; hence, they are pleomorphic.

Fonsecaea pedrosoi

Colonies might be brown-black, olive-brown to gray-black, with a black reverse; they develop slowly and have a downy surface. Colonies often develop a high convex protrusion at the site of initial inoculation, although they begin relatively flat. In just 14 days, colonies reach maturity.

Morphology: The following three types of sporulation are seen:

1. *Rhinocladiella like*: A "Rhinocladiella"-like *sympodial* arrangement of conidia is observed. On the upper part of the conidiophore which does not show branching, we can see conidia arranged at the tip of short denticles (single conidium on single denticle) which gives "bristles on bottle brush appearance."
2. *Cladosporium type*: This type of sporulation is predominant in *F. pedrosoi*. The upright conidiophores produce big primary conidia in the shape of a shield (*shield cells*). These conidia then spin out small, branching chains of oval conidia with *dark scars at the junctions*. The shield cells are seen at the intersection of various chains.
3. *Phialophora type*: The phialide (it is a special type of conidiophore)is like a *vase* and has collarettes at the end. The conidia are produced inside which come out through the apex of the phialide. Conidia are seen in clusters at the tip of phialide. Endogenously developing spherical or oval conidia swarm the apex of the phialide, which gives "flower in vase" appearance. This type of sporulation is very rare in *F. pedrosoi*, while such a type of spore formation is common in *P. verrucosa*. **Figure 13.1** shows the morphological features of *F. pedrosoi*.

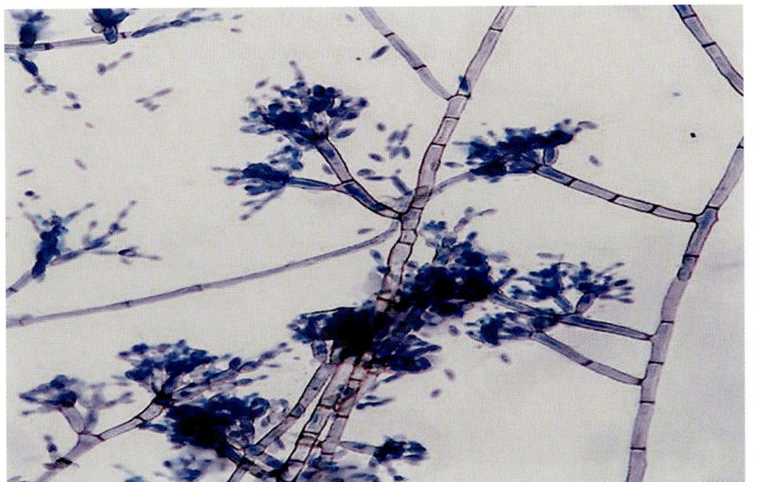

FIG. 13.1: LPCB mount of *Fonsecaea pedrosoi* (400×). (LPCB: lactophenol cotton blue)

Phialophora verrucosa

- *Colony morphology*: Slow-growing, gray-black, and velvety to woolly surface, with black reverse.
- *Microscopic morphology*: This fungus is characterized by brown, septate hyphae and (phialides) conidiophores which are in the shape of a *vase*. The conidia come out through the *funnel-shaped or cup-shaped collar (collarette)* of the phialide and are arranged in clusters (*vase of flowers arrangement*), as shown in **Figure 13.2**.

Cladophialophora carrionii

Colony: It matures in 10 days. The surface and reverse are olive-brown to brownish black.

The hyphae are brown and have septae. The morphological features are shown in **Figures 13.3A and B**. The conidiophores are arranged laterally or at the ends of hyphae. There are long, heavily branched chains of brown, smooth-walled, oval, or lemon-shaped conidia (~2.5 × 4.5–7 µm) arranged on conidiophores. The typical arrangement is disturbed easily when we try to prepare the LPCB mount. The conidia typically have relatively *pale scars* of attachment (not as dark and prominent as seen in *Cladosporium* species).

Rhinocladiella aquaspersa

The colony is olive-black in color, has a velvety surface, and a black reverse. It grows slowly to moderately.

Microscopic features: Denticles are densely packed with conidia that range in shape from ellipsoid to clavate and are pale brown in color. The conidiogenous cells are both terminal and intercalary.

Fonsecaea compacta

Colony: The rate of growth is low, and its reverse coloration is dark green or black. Conidia are round, 2–3 µm in size, and organized in a chain.

SEROLOGICAL TESTS

The immunoblotting technique employs a 54-kDa *F. pedrosoi* antigen, which could be useful for disease research. To determine when CBM caused by *C. carrionii* has progressed, an enzyme-linked immunosorbent assay (ELISA) could be helpful.

Molecular Methods

Fonsecaea isolates can be quickly and accurately identified using duplex polymerase chain reaction, which is especially useful for strains that defy morphological methods of identification. For the purpose of identifying harmful *Fonsecaea* species, rolling circle amplification (RCA) provides a sensitive and quick test that does not require sequencing.

Animal Pathogenicity

Intraperitoneal injection has been used to successfully produce the experimental infection in rats and mice.

TREATMENT

There is no satisfactory treatment for CBM. A variety of treatment methods are available, including surgery, laser

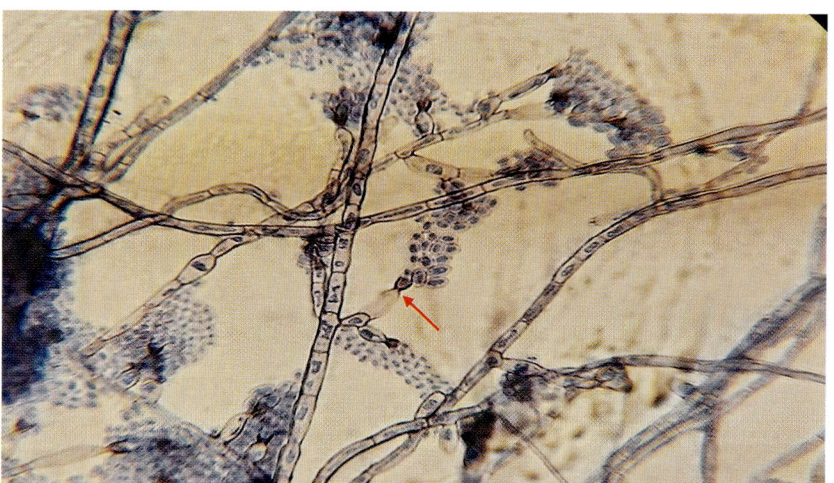

FIG. 13.2: LPCB mount of *Phialophora verrucosa* showing funnel-shaped collarettes (400×). (LPCB: lactophenol cotton blue)

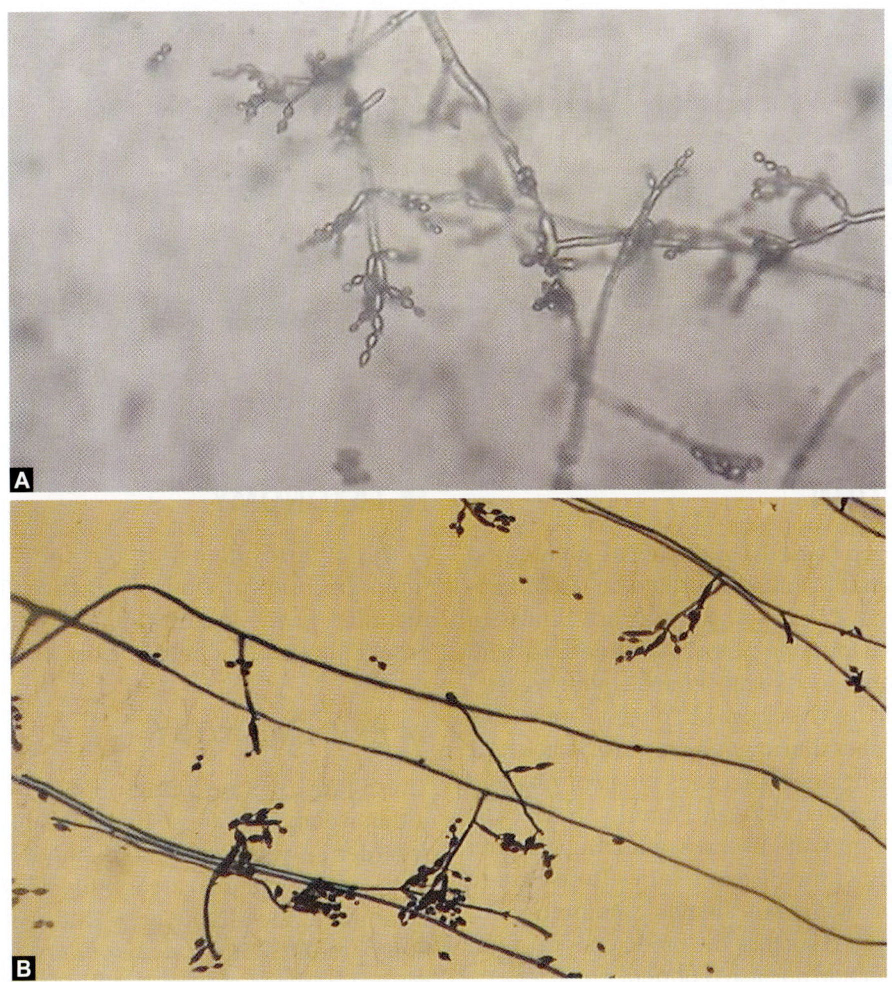

FIGS. 13.3A AND B: Microscopic morphology of *Cladophialophora carrionii* (400×).

therapy, cryosurgery, locally applied heat therapy, and combination therapy. If the lesion is small and detected early enough, it is best removed surgically. In such cases, itraconazole and 5-flucytosine work well.

Itraconazole, liquid nitrogen, flucytosine, and amphotericin B have all been successfully used together.

Another option is to take 500 mg of terbinafine once a day. The treatment and prognosis of the condition have been much improved by two antifungal medications—itraconazole and terbinafine—at present.

Photodynamic therapy has been found to be useful in some cases.

CHAPTER

14 Phaeohyphomycosis

INTRODUCTION

There is a large and varied collection of pigmented or phaeoid or dematiaceous fungi known as phaeohyphomycotic fungi. These fungi can cause illness in people with a normal immune system as well as those with a compromised immune system. "Phaeohyphomycosis" is a translation of the Greek word "phaios," meaning "dark," which describes the fungus's brownish-black hue. The melanogenic fungi, dematiaceous fungi, or phaeoid fungi have melanin on their cell wall. Phaeohyphomycosis includes various types of diseases affecting varying tissues. The severity of the diseases varies from case to case. Infection of skin and soft tissues is common, but infection of deep organs such as the brain, endocardium or disseminated infection are also reported.

The major difference between the clinical conditions chromoblastomycosis and phaeohyphomycosis is that in the case of former, muriform cells are present in tissues, while in later case, fungal hyphae are seen in the tissue which can be seen through histopathological examination.

Several hyaline fungi, including *Aspergillus niger*, *Aspergillus nidulans*, *Scedosporium* species, and *Scytalidium* species, can acquire a melanin pigment during their growth in culture media. Other fungi, such as *Cryptococcus neoformans*, have melanin pigment in their cell walls but are not pigmented. The term phaeohyphomycosis should probably be restricted to infection with fungi in which melanin is derived from the precursor *1,8-dihydroxynaphthalene (DHN)* in their cell wall and which have the pigment throughout their growth in both media and tissues.

HISTORY

Ajello et al. coined the term "phaeohyphomycosis" in 1974. However, Barsok had described the first case of *Alternaria* cutaneous infection in 1933.

TAXONOMY

Both the terms dematiaceous fungi and melanogenic fungi are used in clinical practice. The members are included in the family Dematiaceae of Hypomycetes, order Sphaeropsidales of Coelomycetes.

EPIDEMIOLOGY

These fungi can be found on decaying vegetation and rotten wood. They are so found in soil and are frequently regarded as laboratory contaminants. Few fungi are found in specific geographic areas. *Rhinocladiella mackenziei* is common in the Middle East. Outbreaks caused by these fungi are uncommon. *Exserohilum rostratum* caused a central nervous system (CNS) infection in the United States after epidural injections of methylprednisolone.

Some of the conidial morphological features are characteristic of some genera. Macroconidia with vertical as well as horizontal septae are called "muriform," which are seen in *Alternaria* species, *Ulocladium* species, and *Epicoccum* species. On the other hand, macroconidia with horizontal septae are present in *Curvularia* species and *Ochroconis*. The presence of small microconidia along with macroconidia is seen in *Cladosporium, Phialophora, Fonsecaea pedrosi*, and *Exophiala dermatitidis*.

PATHOGENESIS

Modes of infection are either inhalation of spores or inoculation through mild injuries. The patient may not notice the primary infection. Particularly in individuals who do not have impaired immune systems, very little is understood regarding the pathogenic pathways via which brown fungi cause illness.

The primary components of melanin in fungus are L-3,4-dihydroxyphenylalanine (L-DOPA) and dihydroxynaphthalene (DHN). Dematiaceous fungi only have DHN melanin. The melanin pigment acts as a virulence factor, as it is very resistant to a wide range of environmental stresses, including ionizing radiation, desiccation, toxic metals, and free radicals. The pigment also prevents the death of most organisms by removing hypochlorite and free radicals generated by phagocytic cells during an oxidative burst. Melanin also has the potential to attach to hydrolytic enzymes, blocking their ability to attack the plasma membrane. Chitin, which strengthens cell walls and makes them resistant to hydrolysis, has also been suggested as a potential virulence factor.

HISTOPATHOLOGY

Granulomatous inflammation is characteristic of cutaneous and subcutaneous phaeohyphomycosis. Epithelioid cells, macrophages, giant cells, and neutrophils surround the central area of subcutaneous abscess containing necrotic debris and polymorphonuclear neutrophils (PMNs). Layers of vascularized scar tissue are encased in a fibrotic capsule. A thick capsule encases a phaeomycotic abscess in the brain. Irregular, pale to medium-brown hyphae can be seen in infected tissue.

CLINICAL FEATURES

These saprophytic fungi are present in soil, dead and decaying vegetation. Some of these are plant pathogens. The following human infections are produced by them.

Central Nervous System Infection

This is one of the most common clinical presentations of phaeohyphomycosis, and it is seen in immunocompetent persons. These fungi spread through the bloodstream. The frontal lobe is frequently involved, and it is frequently misdiagnosed as meningitis, space-occupying lesion (SOL), or cerebral malaria. The patient has a headache and papilledema. The radiological finding is helpful in both diagnosis and follow-up. *Cladophialophora bantiana* was the most common species, accounting for half of the cases. *Rhinocladiella mackenziei, Ochroconis gallopava, Bipolaris spicifera, Exophiala dermatitidis*, and *Chaetomium strumarium* were among the other species.

Subcutaneous Phaeohyphomycosis

The symptoms are a subcutaneous nodule or cyst. The feet, legs, hands, arms, and back are all involved. The skin around the wound is normal. Infection occurs through deep fungal inoculation, and cases of intramuscular infections have been reported.

Pulmonary Infection

Pulmonary infection is usually seen in immunocompromised patients or in those with an underlying lung disease, and it may be due to a wide variety of species, including *C. bantiana, Chaetomium* species, *O. gallopava, Exophiala* species, *Alternaria, Cladophialophora boppii, Fonsecaea pedrosoi, L. theobromae, Aureobasidium pullulan, Curvularia* species, and *Pocillopora verrucosa.* Clinical manifestations include pneumonia, asymptomatic solitary pulmonary nodules, and endobronchial lesions which may cause hemoptysis.

Peritonitis

Peritonitis occurs essentially only in patients receiving peritoneal dialysis. The genera isolated included *Curvularia, Exophiala, Alternaria, Bipolaris, Aureobasidium*, and *Phialemonium.*

Allergic Fungal Sinusitis

The most common species isolated are *Alternaria, Bipolaris, Curvularia*, and *Epicoccum.*

Invasive Sinusitis

Immunocompromised patients are at an increased risk for this. As the infection progresses, it poses a threat to the sinuses and even the bone chambers that house the brain and eyes. Patients with impaired immune systems or diabetic ketoacidosis are at an increased risk for developing invasive sinusitis.

Invasive fungal sinusitis instances typically involve the following fungus species: *Alternaria, Bipolaris, Curvularia*, and *Exserohilum.*

Allergic Bronchopulmonary Mycosis

Patients with asthma or cystic fibrosis often get allergic bronchopulmonary aspergillosis (ABPA), which shares comparable symptoms. Most of the instances are caused by *Curvularia.*

Onychomycosis

Dematiaceous fungi are a rare cause of onychomycosis. *Alternaria, Scopulariopsis*, and *Neoscytalidium* have been reported.

Cutaneous Infection

Colonization of fungi over cracks of feet, ulcerations, or on eczematous skin is common.

RADIODIAGNOSIS

It is helpful for the diagnosis of brain abscess in which "double ring sign" may be evident.

DIFFERENTIAL DIAGNOSIS

The skin lesion should be differentiated from lipoma, fibroma, or ganglion. The brain abscess should be differentiated from bacterial infection and cryptococcal infection.

LABORATORY DIAGNOSIS

It is mainly based on microscopy and culture.

Microscopy

Potassium hydroxide (KOH) (10%) mount: The fungi appear dark brown. Sometimes, even hyaline fungal elements are seen; hence, Masson–Fontana stain that shows melanin is preferred. Other stains used are Giemsa [for fine-needle aspiration cytology (FNAC)], hematoxylin and eosin (H&E) stain, and Grocott's methenamine silver (GMS). Hyphae are 3–4 μm in diameter, short or elongated, branched or unbranched.

Culture

Various temperatures are used to incubate the Sabouraud dextrose agar (SDA) slants, including 37 and 27°C. Slow growth is typical for most of the fungi. The preferred medium is potato dextrose agar (PDA). The colony it generates has colors comparable to those mentioned, and it is typically enough for conidiation. Other plant-based media are also available, such as malt extract agar, V-8 juice agar, and cornmeal agar.

Cladosporium

This genus is ubiquitous and frequently found as a contaminant in laboratories. Some members are plant pathogens. These fungi rarely produce disease especially in immunocompromised individuals. There are three prominent species complexes in the genus: (1) *Cladosporium cladosporioides* species complex, (2) *Cladosporium herbarum* species complex, and (3) *Cladosporium sphaerospermum* species complex. Hyphae are dark and septate. The dark black conidiophores may be branched at the apex and usually produce two or more conidial chains. Round-to-oval conidia form branching tree-like chains. There are dark *spots (hila)* at the point where they were attached to the conidiophore or other conidia. The cells bearing the conidial chains are large, sometimes septate, and resemble shields (therefore called "shield cells"). **Figure 14.1** shows the *Cladosporium* type of sporulation.

Aureobasidium pullulans

It is a common laboratory contaminant which may enter by trauma and can rarely produce infections. There are reported cases which include corneal, peritoneal, cutaneous, pulmonary, and systemic infections, particularly as a result of traumatic implantation.

Colony characteristics: Initially, a moist, creamy colony is produced. Later, it becomes shiny, brown or black, with a shiny grayish fringe. Reverse is dark.

Lactophenol cotton blue (LPCB) mount from initial colonies shows unicellular, budding, yeast-like cells. Hyphae are hyaline and thin-walled which produce blastoconidia directly from the walls. Some hyphae are thick-walled and dark and produce chlamydoconidia **(Fig. 14.2)**.

Alternaria

This is a plant pathogen which causes opportunistic infection in human beings.

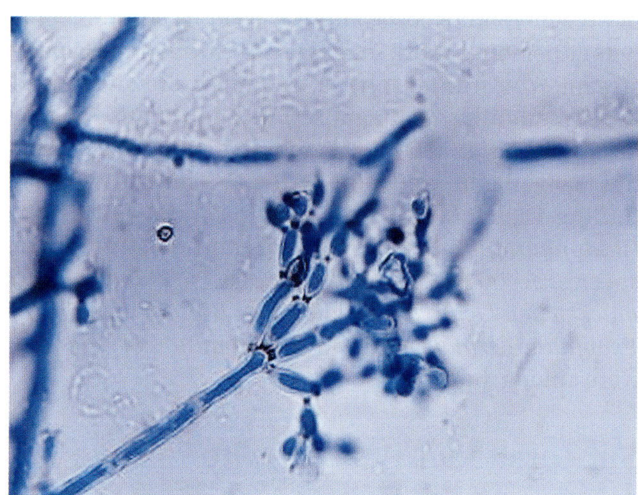

FIG. 14.1: *Cladosporium* type of sporulation (400×).

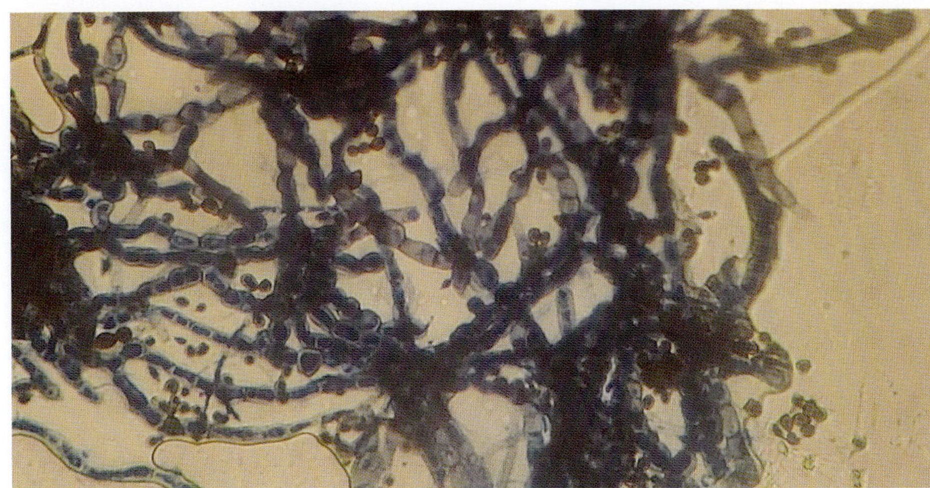

FIG. 14.2: LPCB mount of *Aureobasidium pullulans* (400×).
(LPCB: lactophenol cotton blue)

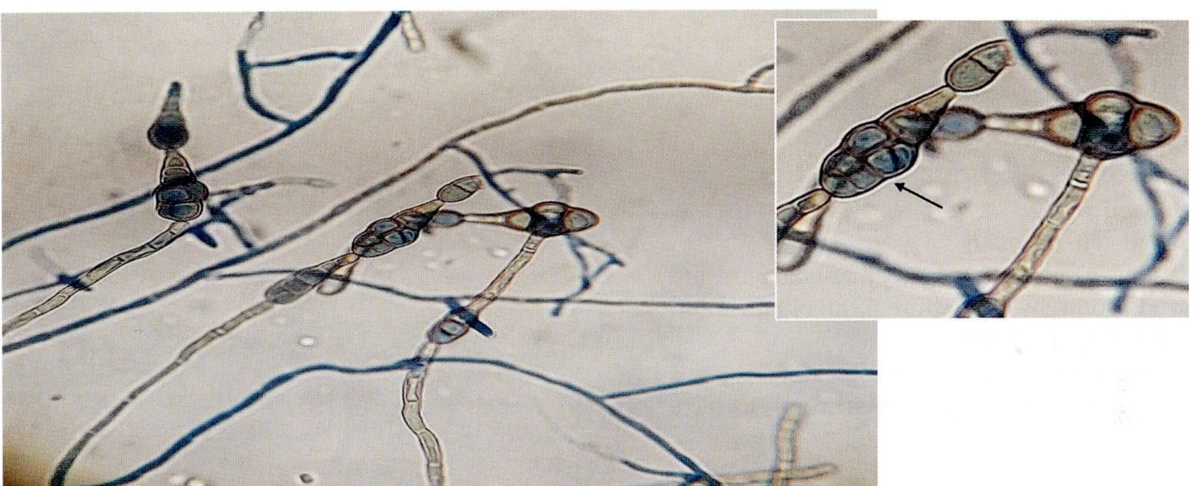

FIG. 14.3: LPCB mount showing macroconidia in a chain. Note down vertical as well as horizontal septae of macroconidia (400×).
(LPCB: lactophenol cotton blue)

- Cutaneous and subcutaneous infections in organ transplant recipients
- Sinusitis in patients with bone marrow transplant and Cushing's syndrome
- Mycotic keratitis
- Onychomycosis

The majority of clinical isolates are *Alternaria alternata* or *Alternaria infectoria*. The colonies are floccose with dematiaceous hyphae and have a black reverse. Conidiophore can be either simple or branched. This fungus is distinguished by the presence of macroconidia in chains with both transverse and vertical septae (muriform) **(Fig. 14.3)**.

Bipolaris

The microscopic picture is shown in **Figure 14.4**.

The *Bipolaris* species are now included in the genus *Curvularia.*

Curvularia (Including Previous *Bipolaris* Species)

With taxonomical revision and inclusion of *Bipolaris* species in the genus *Curvularia*, the following are the important pathogenic species:

- *Curvularia geniculata* and *Curvularia lunata*
- *Curvularia australiensis, Curvularia hawaiiensis*, and *Curvularia spicifera* (previously *Bipolaris* species).

Following infections are produced by *Curvularia* species:

- Onychomycosis
- Mycetoma
- Keratitis
- Sinusitis

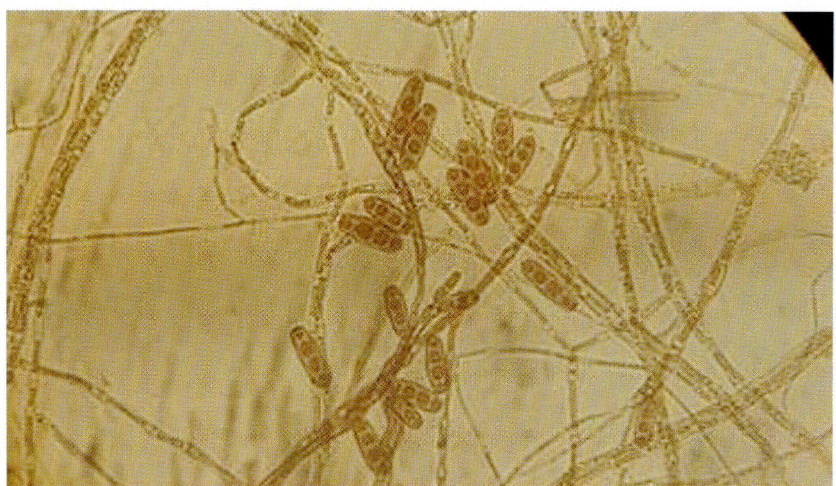

FIG. 14.4: LPCB mount of *Bipolaris* species (400×). (LPCB: lactophenol cotton blue)

- Cutaneous and subcutaneous infections
- Peritonitis
- Endocarditis
- Endophthalmitis
- Pneumonia
- Disseminated disease
- Dissemination to the brain

There is some association of heavy marijuana use and *Curvularia* infection, by inhalation of the organism on contaminated marijuana leaves.

Colony morphology of *Curvularia* species: Colony is flat, floccose to woolly with color ranges in from dark olive green to brown-to-gray black.

Microscopic characteristics of *C. geniculata and C. lunata*: Conidiophores are either simple or branched. They are bent or knobby at points of conidium formation (sympodial geniculate growth). Conidia are large (8–14 × 21–35 μm), usually contain four cells, curved with one bigger and darker swelling of a central cell (the curving may take 5 or more days to develop). The hilum is nonprotruding **(Fig. 14.5)**.

Microscopic characteristics of *C. australiensis, C. hawaiiensis*, and *C. spicifera* (previously *Bipolaris* species): *Curvularia* has dark, septate hyphae. Conidiophores show a bent at the point of attachment of conidia (sympodial geniculate growth), showing a knobby, zigzag appearance. Conidia are hyaline to brown when mature, oblong-to-cylindrical (6–13 × 14–39 μm). The conidia have thick walls and have three to five septa. They are rounded at both ends, with a slightly protruding hilum. As per the previous name, i.e., *Bipolaris*, it can produce *germ tubes at both the poles.* Differentiation from *E. rostratum* is done by number of septa, shape, and size of conidia.

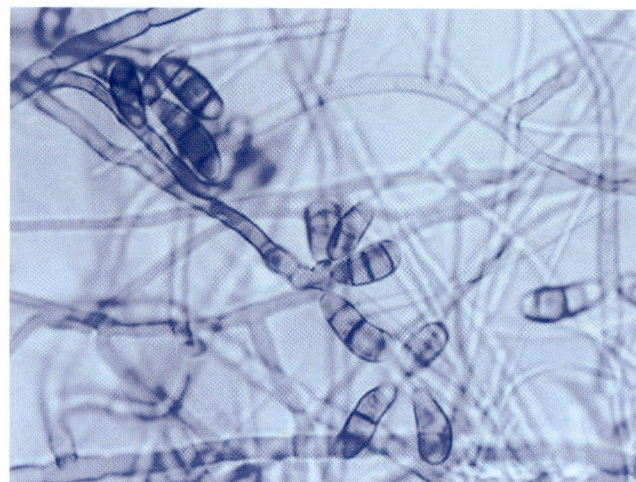

FIG. 14.5: LPCB mount of *Curvularia* species (400×). (LPCB: lactophenol cotton blue)

Exserohilum

Human pathogenic species are *Exserohilum rostratum* and *E. mcginnisii.* They are opportunistic and are etiologic agents of sinusitis, keratitis, cutaneous, subcutaneous mycoses, and rarely fatal disease in immunocompromised patients. The fungus may cause iatrogenic meningoencephalitis, meningoradiculitis, epidural abscesses, and vertebral osteomyelitis associated with intrathecal or lumbosacral injection of contaminated methylprednisolone solution.

Colony: A fuzzy brownish-black colony is swiftly expanding. Conidia of *E. mcginnisii* have warty projections on their exterior walls, while those of *E. rostratum* have darker basal and distal septa.

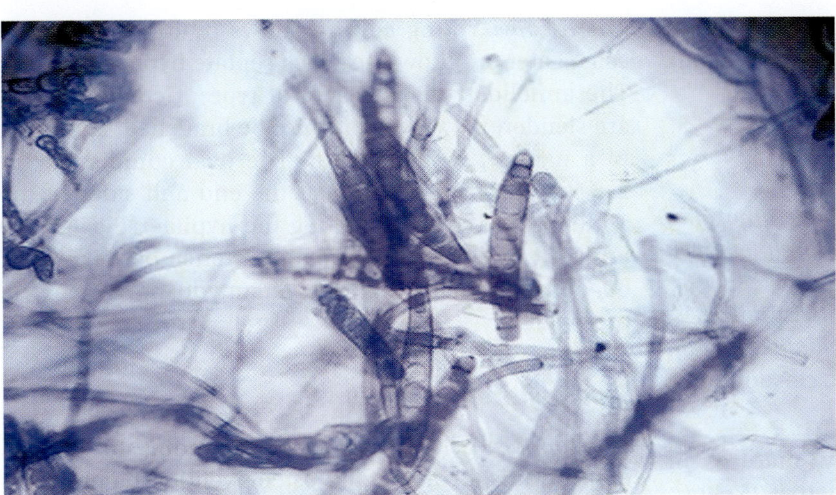

FIG. 14.6: LPCB mount of *Exserohilum* species (400×).
(LPCB: lactophenol cotton blue)

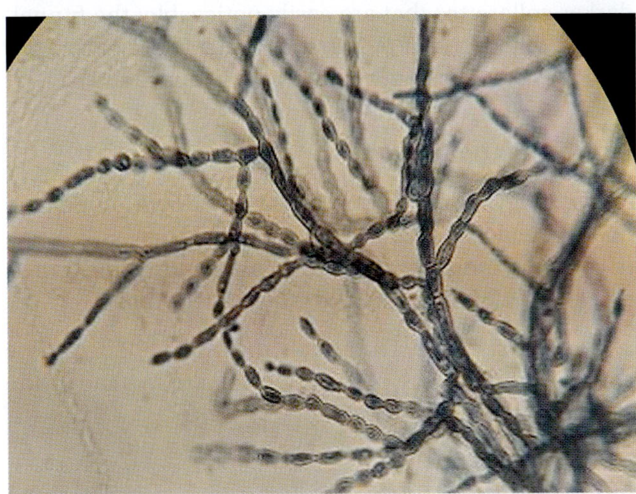

FIG. 14.7: LPCB mount of *Cladophialophora bantiana* conidia in chains (400×).
(LPCB: lactophenol cotton blue)

Microscopy: Sympodial conidiophores have a zigzag pattern. The conidia are long (average, 14 × 90 µm or greater), fusiform, and thick-walled, with 7–11 septa. The protruding square hilum (scar of attachment) on each conidium is dark and conspicuous **(Fig. 14.6)**. There is a distinctive dark band at both ends of the mature conidium.

Cladophialophora bantiana

The older names of the species are *Cladosporium trichoides, Cladosporium bantiana,* and *Xylohypa bantiana.* It causes brain abscess. It also causes subcutaneous infection and lung infection rarely. The mode of infection is inhalation, and it may cause infections in laboratory persons; hence, slide cultures should not be done. A biosafety cabinet is used while handling the cultures of this fungus.

The morphology of the colony is described as slow-growing, floccose, olive to gray to brown, and being reverse black. The optimal growth temperature for *C. bantiana* is 42–43°C; this characteristic helps to differentiate this species from similar fungi. The growth rate is slow, and colony matures in 10 days.

Conidiophores are long, sparsely branched. They produce wavy chains of smooth, oval lemon-shaped conidia (2.5–5 × 6–11 µm) **(Fig. 14.7)**. The scars of attachment are absent on conidia which are present in *Cladosporium* species. The youngest conidium is at the tip. The arrangement of conidiophore and conidia is not disturbed while performing wet mount from cultures.

Exophiala (Wangiella) dermatitidis

The organism has affinity for CNS. It causes infection of the brain, lungs (especially in cystic fibrosis patients) and cutaneous and subcutaneous tissue.

Colony morphology: Initially, for the first 10 days, the colony looks like yeast—black, wet, and shiny—but as it grows hyphae, in 2–3 weeks, it changes to velvety, olive-gray to dark. The temperature it can withstand is 42°C, and it evades cycloheximide.

Microscopic characteristics: LPCB mount from yeasty colony shows dark, oval-to-round, budding, yeast-like cells. Later on, dark septate hyphae are seen. The conidiophores are cylindrical to flask-shaped conidiogenous cells having a truncate apex without collarette. Round-to-oval, single-celled, pale brown conidia (2–3 × 3–6 µm) accumulate at the tip of the conidiophore. Some conidia slide down the sides of the conidiophore **(Figs. 14.8 and 14.9)**. Conidia may also be produced at projections along the hyphae.

Exophiala jeanselmei

The species complex includes *Exophiala heteromorpha, Exophiala lecanii-corni,* and *Exophiala jeanselmei sensu stricto.*

It causes black grain mycetoma, chromoblastomycosis, and phaeohyphomycosis. Species of *Exophiala* are often called "black yeasts" because some of them can develop a budding yeast-like shape.

Colony characteristics: It grows slowly, matures in 10 days. Growth occurs on media incubated at 25–30°C, but it does not grow at 37°C. Initial yeasty colonies convert velvety, olivaceous-black with a black reverse.

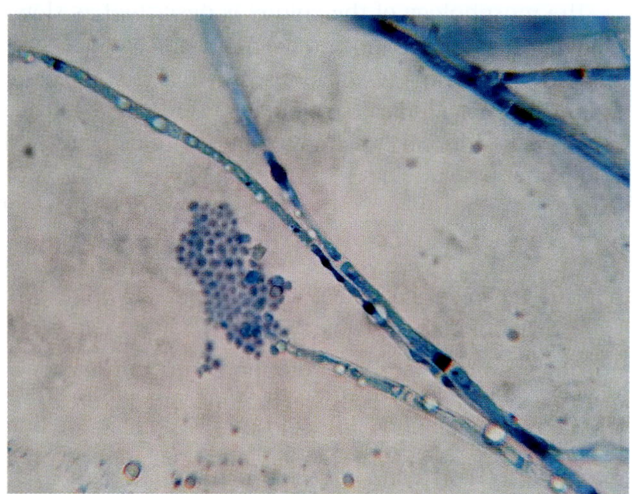

FIG. 14.8: LPCB mount of *Exophiala dermatitidis* (400×). (LPCB: lactophenol cotton blue)

Microscopy: Young culture shows budding yeast-like cells. Later on, brown-to-black septate hyphae develop. The annelids (this is a special type of conidiophore) are slender, may be or may not be branched, and taper to a narrow, elongated tip. The oval conidia (1–3 × 2–6 µm) occur in clusters at the end and sides of the annelids and at points along the hyphae **(Figs. 14.10 and 14.11)**. Conidium formation is often best exhibited on cornmeal agar or PDA. Chlamydospores may be present.

Phialophora

Phialophora verrucosa causes chromoblastomycosis, endocarditis, keratitis, and osteomyelitis. The phialides of both *Phialophora verrucosa* and *P. americana* have darker collarettes that are easily noticeable; the funnel-shaped phialides of *P. verrucosa* and the vase-shaped phialides of *P. americana* are similar in appearance.

Ochroconis gallopava

Morphology of colonies: Colony of brown, suedelike material which contains red pigment that may be diffused. It can withstand temperatures up to 45°C and grows quickly. Cycloheximide stops growth in its tracks.

Microscopic: Denticles attach the two-celled clavate conidia produced by pale brown septate hyphae to the supporting hyphae.

Ramichloridium mackenziei

Colony: Gradual change from lustrous dark brown-black colonies to fuzzy, dome-shaped colonies with a black reverse characterizes this slow-growing fungus. The fungus can grow in presence of cycloheximide. Though optimum temperature is 30°C, it can grow at 42°C.

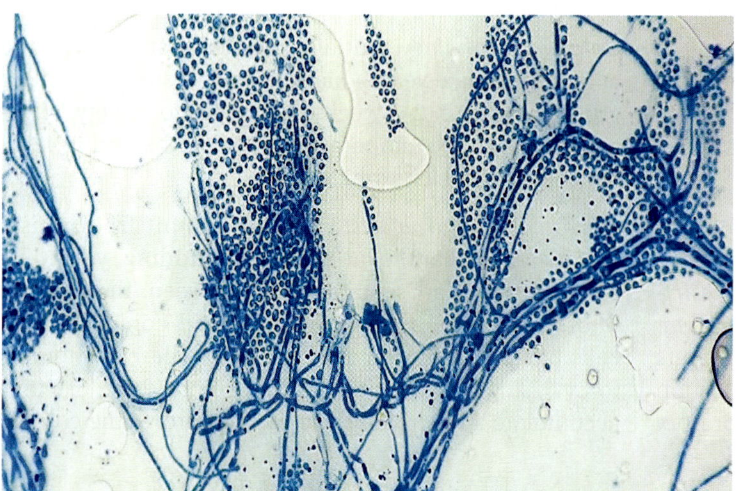

FIG. 14.9: LPCB mount of *Exophiala dermatitidis* (400×). (LPCB: lactophenol cotton blue)

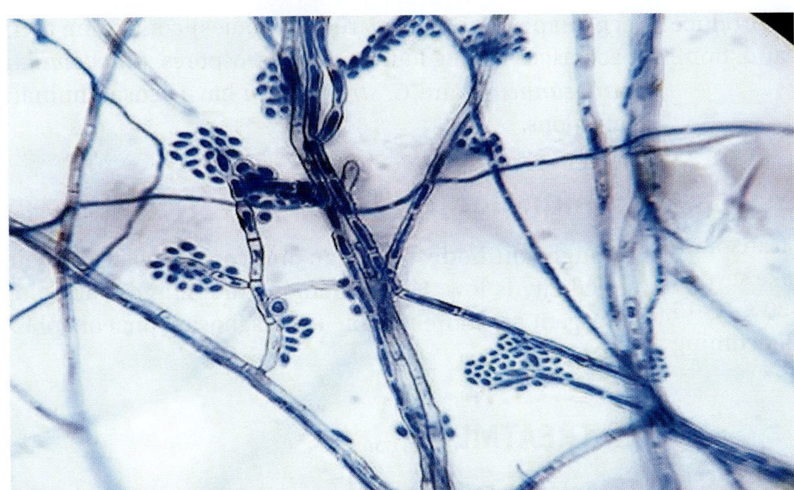

FIG. 14.10: LPCB mount of *Exophiala jeanselmei* (400×). (LPCB: lactophenol cotton blue)

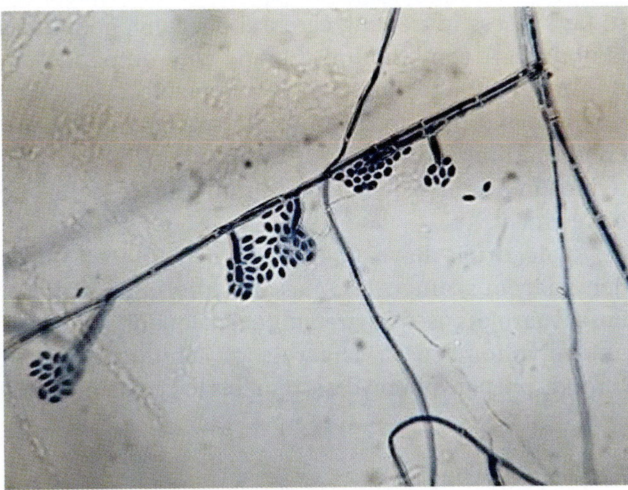

FIG. 14.11: LPCB mount of *Exophiala jeanselmei* (400×). (LPCB: lactophenol cotton blue)

Microscopy: Conidiophores rise at about right angles to the vegetative hyphae atop brown, septate hyphae. Two pale brown conidia with smooth walls protruded from either side of a rachis with thick walls, giving the impression of a "Mickey Mouse" shape.

Phaeoacremonium parasiticum

Subcutaneous abscesses, thorn-induced arthritis, and widespread infection are all infections that can be caused by *Phaeoacremonium parasiticum*. A variety of colony colors are possible, from brown to lavender to orange-brown.

Colonies, which are velvety and gray at first, turn brownish when aerial hyphae form after protracted incubation.

Microscopy: It shares characteristics of *Acremonium* and *Phialophora*. The hyphae are septate and pigmented, and the conidiophore is brown and tapered. Conidia are seen in clusters at the tip of conidiophore.

Scopulariopsis

The presence of both hyaline and dark species in the genus *Scopulariopsis* is quite remarkable. Although both *Scopulariopsis* and *Scedosporium* species use annelidic conidiogenesis, the production of conidia in chains rather than clumps distinguishes *Scopulariopsis* from *Scedosporium*.

Phialemonium

The infections produced in immunocompromised patients are given as follows:

- Subcutaneous infection
- Endocarditis
- Peritonitis
- Osteomyelitis
- Brain abscesses
- Fungemia (venous catheters related)

Although colonies frequently stay pale, the original description of the genus *Phialemonium* is similar to *Acremonium* species but show pigmentation. Colonies usually have a slightly filamentous texture.

Hyphae are septate and brownish. Phialides of varying sizes arise from hyphae. They are devoid of a basal septum, cylindrical in shape without collarette from which clusters of conidia arise.

Pleurostomophora

It incudes *Phialophora richardsiae* and the extinct *Panicum repens.*

Microscopically, *P. richardsiae* is identified by its conidia, which can be either globose or oval, and its characteristic flaring collarettes. Both species produce brown colonies. Subcutaneous infections and bone diseases are examples of human infections.

Lasiodiplodia

Lasiodiplodia theobromae is reported from cases of subcutaneous disease, pneumonia in a liver transplant recipient, and ocular infections. Conidia may take several weeks to mature and are distinctive, large (20–30 × 10–15 μm), and hyaline and single-celled initially, becoming dark, striated, and two-celled at maturity.

Leptosphaeria

Leptosphaeria senegalensis causes black grain mycetoma. In culture, colonies are slow growing and woolly, and black closed ascomata (cleistothecia) are immersed in the agar. Maturation of ascomata and ascospores is facilitated on plant-based media, and species are differentiated by ascospore features.

Chaetomium

These are soil saprophytes, ubiquitously distributed worldwide. Though they are considered common laboratory contaminants, rarely they cause subcutaneous infection, peritonitis, chromoblastomycosis, and onychomycosis. Microscopic findings include dense hairy, egg-shaped perithecia (fruiting bodies) containing asci, each ascus having four to eight ascospores. *Chaetomium atrobrunneum* and *C. strumarium* have caused human infections.

Immunological Tests

Though antibody tests can indicate exposure, their specificity is low. Hence demonstration and culture of the agent are more reliable for diagnosing phaeohyphomycosis.

TREATMENT

Complete surgical removal of the encapsulated abscess combined with antifungal therapy is recommended, but so far success in treating cerebral phaeohyphomycosis is limited. A combination therapy with amphotericin B (AmB), flucytosine, and itraconazole (ITC) may be lifesaving. In case of multiple cerebral abscesses, combination therapy with AmB, flucytosine, and terbinafine, or an extended-spectrum triazole is the line of treatment.

Azole drugs have good in vitro activity against dematiaceous fungi. ITC has had the most success. Posaconazole is useful in treating cutaneous disseminated phaeohyphomycosis. The role of echinocandins in cerebral phaeohyphomycosis remains to be determined.

CHAPTER

15 Lobomycosis Lacaziosis

INTRODUCTION

Lacaziosis (or Lobomycosis) is a chronic subcutaneous mycosis caused by *Lacazia loboi.* It is a keloid-like granulomatous lesion in the form of nodules or verrucose lesions on mucosa or in deep organs. The fungus causes infection in humans and dolphins. Other names have been used to describe this entity: Jorge Lobo's disease, Jorge Lobo mycosis, Jorge Lobo blastomycosis, amazonic pseudolepromatous blastomycosis, miraip or piraip (in the Tupi language), Caiabi leprosy (Caiabi Indians is an indigenous tribe located in the state of Mato Grosso of Brazil), and lacaziosis. Lobomycosis is the correct name for this disease.

This fungal infection is most common in the Americas, notably in the Amazon basin, and has a specific geographic distribution. While it has usually affected populations in localized endemic places, new instances in dolphins have broadened its reach to coastal areas.

HISTORY

A patient of sacral keloid-like lesions was the first case of lobomycosis that was documented in 1931 by the Brazilian doctor Jorge Lobo. "Blastomicose keloidiana" (keloid blastomycosis) was the name given to this "new" disease. In 1938, it was called Lombo's blastomycosis.

Borelli came up with the name "lobomycosis" for the disease and the fungus *Loboa loboi* as its causative agent.

TAXONOMY

The taxonomy of the causal fungus has been revised multiple times throughout the years, with *Lacazia loboi* being the most recent candidate.

Lacazia loboi is classified under the order Onygenales of the phylum Ascomycota based on molecular investigations.

MYCOLOGY

Lobomycosis is distinguished by the presence of lemon-shaped yeasts in tissues, either alone or in chains. These yeasts are generally *between 6 and 12* μm and have a birefringent membrane with a thick melanin-rich wall. The budding is connected by a tiny tubular connector or isthmus. There is a formation of blastoconidia and the unique rosary beadlike structures. Some yeast cells may exhibit secondary budding similar to the "mariner's wheel" of *Paracoccidioides brasiliensis.* The inability of *L. loboi* to be cultured in normal culture media is thought to be an adaptation to its parasitic lifestyle.

TRANSMISSION

An accidental trauma in association with plants, thorns, or insect bites probably acts as a precursor to skin lesions due to *L. loboi*, though not in all cases. The specific route of transmission is unknown, although it is thought to occur by implantation of the fungus into the skin. According to reports, transmission may occur via snakebites, stingray mishaps, or bug bites. There are a few case reports suggesting transmission of infections from dolphins to human beings. However, zoonotic transmission is rare. The potential of autoinoculation or reinfection as a result of recurrent trauma is still a worry, particularly for people living in endemic areas.

PATHOGENESIS

It is believed that trauma is the principal initiating event in lobomycosis, which mostly affects the skin of humans. It is believed that the saprophytic fungus *L. loboi*, which can be found in water, soil, and plants, infects the dermis through injection. Once inside the dermis, the fungus multiplies within macrophages. Transforming growth factor beta 1 (TGF-β1), a potent immunosuppressant, rises in concentration throughout this phase. There is a decrease in cell-mediated immunity (CMI) response.

Transforming growth factor beta 1 is released by T helper 3 (Th3) cells and macrophages; it does this by decreasing phagocytic activity, nitric oxide synthesis, and gamma interferon expression. It also makes the lesions look more keloid-like by increasing fibrosis, CD8 T-cell proliferation, and immunoglobulin A antibody production. Another cytokine seen in lobomycosis lesions is interleukin 10 (IL-10), which inhibits macrophage function and, by extension, cellular immunological responses. The absence of antigen responses suggests that this harmful effect on cellular immunity may cause localized immunodeficiency. Increased IL-4 and IL-6 production and decreased IL-2 production characterize the lesions' T helper 2 (Th2) cytokine profile.

A number of authorities have speculated that the fungal cell wall's melanin content serves as a defense mechanism. The processes behind the lysis of *L. loboi* cells are unknown, and fungal viability is very high (20–50%) despite the defensive measures. These pathways could be caused by complement system activation, cytotoxic effects of CD8 T lymphocytes or natural killer cells, or other factors that are currently unclear.

PATHOLOGY

A dense and dispersed histiocytic infiltration with an abundance of yeasts is present in the dermis. The infiltrate shows many epitheloid cells, Langhan's as well as foreign body giant cells and lymphocytes. Yeasts are seen inside phagocytic cells as well as in surrounding tissue. Typically the yeast cells are about 10 microns in size, seen as short chains having narrow tube-like connections between the cells. Fungal elements are best seen with GMS stain.

Atrophic areas are common features of the epidermis. Hyperkeratosis, spongiosis, and neutrophil accumulation may be seen in acanthotic areas.

The total number of lymphocytes might range from a few hundred to several thousand. It is not uncommon to see natural killer cells, plasma cells, and B lymphocytes. Rarely seen neutrophils are linked to fungal infections or ulcers in the skin. Notable features include fibrosis and the possibility of seeing asteroid bodies.

EPIDEMIOLOGY AND GEOGRAPHIC DISTRIBUTION

Lobomycosis is more common in areas with thick forests, considerable rainfall (>2,000 mm/year), average temperatures of 24°C, and 75% relative humidity. The Amazon basin in Latin America is an endemic area of lobomycosis, with the majority of cases being recorded from Brazil. Typically, vulnerable people are those living and working as forest workers, river dwellers, and Indigenous peoples. Furthermore, lobomycosis is seen as an occupational concern for those who work with dolphins, such as veterinarians, marine researchers, and personnel in the captive dolphin business. There has been an increase in both direct and indirect human-dolphin interaction due to the growing population of dolphins in managed care, commercial displays, and recreational activities.

Human cases of Jorge Lobo's disease have been documented in nine South American countries (Brazil, Colombia, Suriname, Venezuela, Guyana, French Guiana, Ecuador, Peru, and Bolivia), three Central American countries (Panama, Costa Rica, and Mexico), and other countries (the United States, Canada, France, the Netherlands, Germany, Greece, and South Africa) as imported cases.

CLINICAL FEATURES

The incubation time is likely to be 1–2 years. The illness affects mostly the exposed areas. The common sites of infection are pinna (38%), upper limbs (28%), and lower limbs (22%). It is commonly a localized illness. The other sites such as chest, scapula, lumbosacral area, buttocks, and scrotum may also be involved. The lesions may be hypo- or hyperpigmented. The mucous membrane or internal organs of the body are not affected. Regional lymph node involvement is seen in around 10–25% of cases. The older lesions typically become verrucoid and ulcerative with satellite lesions resulting from autoinoculation.

The lesion starts as a *papule* that can be superficial or deep. It is converted into a *plaque or nodule* over months to years. Smooth and glossy undamaged skin covers the lesion. The surface color ranges from erythematous brownish to red wine. It is with or without telangiectasia. This gives the lesions a fibrous look, similar to that of a *scar or keloid*. As a result, the clinical appearance might vary; there may be a shift from hyperpigmentation to hypopigmentation, and achromia may be common.

Ulcers can form during the rainy season, frequently as a result of trauma or maceration. Deeper lesions, known as infiltrative lesions, may be related to recent inoculations. In rare circumstances, continuous growth might result in an exophytic look. A *wartlike surface* may appear, primarily on the lower limbs, and can be misinterpreted as chromomycosis. *Gummalike lobomycosis* may develop in rare cases. These are macular lesions with turgid margins, pustules, and the exudation of thick yellow material, finally leading to scar tissue development. *In a few patients, all types of lesions such as macules, papules, keloidal nodules, and plaques to verrucous lesions and ulcers may be seen at a time.* Additional lesions in the vicinity of the index *may be seen probably due to autoinoculation* or local lymphatic spread. Autoinoculation can cause confluent lesions to create enormous plaques or hundreds of *lesions.* While most lobomycosis lesions are asymptomatic, itching and dysesthesia can develop in severe instances.

Lacaziosis-like Disease

The condition, similar to lacaziosis involves dolphins in some geographic areas. The exact etiology is not known. It is probably caused by a non-cultivable yeast and phylogenetic studies suggested a close relation between the lacaziosis-like disease (LLD) agent with paracoccidioidomycosis.

DIFFERENTIAL DIAGNOSIS

Chromoblastosis, sporotrichosis, cutaneous leishmaniasis, cutaneous psoriasis, lepromatous leprosy, cutaneous tuberculosis (TB), rheumatoid factor, and eumycetoma should be differentiated from lacaziosis. In a histopathological section, yeast cells of *L. loboi* should be differentiated from deep mycotic infections and *Sporothrix*. In *P. brasiliensis*, mother cell is large with multiple daughter cells. Also, as this fungus contains melanin, it is detected by Masson–Fontana stain. No chains of conidia are seen in other fungi.

LABORATORY DIAGNOSIS

The confirmation of the diagnosis should be achieved by identifying the fungal agents present within the lesion. Samples collected are mounting biopsy samples or curettage. Use of vinyl adhesive tape (VAT) preparation (Scotch test) is also useful for the direct microscopic examination. Various preparations are done such as potassium hydroxide (KOH) mount, calcofluor stain, and Grocott–Gömöri's methenamine silver (GMS) stain.

Characteristics of Yeast Cells

- *Type of budding*: Narrow-based budding
- *Shape*: Globose to elliptical or lemon shaped
- Doubly refractile, thick walled
- Multinucleate
- *Size*: 6–12 μm, with an average size of 10 μm
- *Number*: There may be chains of 20 or even more.
- Yeast cells are connected to each other by a large connecting isthmus.
- The organisms usually reproduce by budding at one or rarely.

The use of *calcofluor white stain* allows for easy demonstration. One simple way to see the fungus is to scrape the sores and examine them closely. It is also possible to use exfoliative cytology or vinyl sticky tape as alternate approaches.

Histopathological Findings (Hematoxylin and Eosin or Grocott–Gömöri's Methenamine Silver Stain)

- A deep and widespread histiocytic infiltration in the dermis
- Numerous fungal cells are seen inside macrophages; a few are also seen outside the cells
- Infiltration of lymphocytes, plasma cells, pseudo-Gaucher cells, and Langhans cells
- In H&E stain unstained fungal cells (intracellular and extracellular) look like vacuoles. Hence the complete granuloma gets a sieve-like appearance.
- Fibrosis

Culture

The fungus is non-cultivable.

TREATMENT

A broad surgical resection is the best course of treatment for lobomycosis. Care should be taken to avoid contamination of surrounding tissue during the excision of the lesion.

When surgery is not an option or when an infection has spread, there is currently no medicine that works as well as surgery. The outcomes of testing various antifungal medicines have typically been disappointing as follows:

- *Ketoconazole*: Ineffective
- *Amphotericin B*: Ineffective
- *Sulfa compounds*: Ineffective
- *5-Fluorocytosine*: Ineffective

The use of itraconazole as a follow-up treatment to prevent recurrence of surgically removed lesions has shown encouraging results. Treatment of lobomycosis relapses with itraconazole, and cryosurgery has demonstrated promising results. Several studies have tried clofazimine and found that it was ineffective when taken daily at doses of 100–300 mg for up to 2 years.

Lesion cure without remission was observed after 24 months of treatment with posaconazole, one of the more recent azoles with a wider spectrum, according to a 5-year follow-up. We need to follow up with patients for a long time after surgery to make sure that the disease has healed, since lesions could come back even after removal. Surgical removal is the most commonly used therapeutic procedure, and there is currently no highly effective pharmaceutical treatment.

SECTION

4

Systemic Mycoses

Section Outline

CHAPTER

16 Histoplasmosis

INTRODUCTION

Histoplasmosis is endemic in some parts of the world as well as some parts of India. It is a systemic granulomatous infection caused by thermally dimorphic fungus, *Histoplasma capsulatum* and other *Histoplasma* species. The fungus lives intracellularly in the cells of reticuloendothelial system. Primarily, there is infection of the lungs by inhalation of dust containing microconidia of the fungus, and the fungus may then disseminate to other sites, causing systemic illness. The clinical presentation varies from asymptomatic infection to disseminated infection. Soil contaminated with bat guano or bird droppings is a common habitat for this fungus, where it can survive for a long time. In particular, when repairing or demolishing old structures, the accumulation of bat guano or bird droppings in the attics and belfries can cause outbreaks.

This disease is also known by various other names as classic histoplasmosis, Caver's and Miner's disease, Cave disease, Bat disease, Ohio Valley disease, Tingo Maria fever, reticuloendotheliosis, and cytomycosis.

HISTORY

Samuel Taylor Darling (1905) documented the initial case of histoplasmosis. He performed an autopsy on the patient and believed that the illness is caused by an encapsulated *Plasmodium*. After observing two additional cases, he assumed that the infection was caused by *Leishmania donovani*. Hence, he suspected the pathogen as an encapsulated organism but without kinetoplasts in the cell. He renamed it *Histoplasma capsulate*, which is currently known as *Histoplasma capsulatum*. It seemed like the intracellular creature he saw in histiocytes had a "capsule" and looked like a "plasmodium." By showing it on a blood smear, Dr Edna H (1928) identified the first case of histoplasmosis. The first *H. capsulatum* was isolated and cultured from soil by Dr Chester W Emmons (1948). The illness was brought up by Johnny Cash, who correctly identified it in pigeon droppings. *Histoplasma capsulatum* var *duboisii* was the name given to a new variation identified by Drohet (1957). A subsequent discovery revealed a third variation, *H. capsulatum* var *farciminosum*.

TRANSMISSION AND RISK FACTORS

- Histoplasmosis primarily occurs due to the inhalation of dust particles containing *H. capsulatum* microconidia. Soil shows higher content of nitrogen associated with droppings of chickens, bats, and starlings. The fungus shows a high affinity for soil fertilized by bird's droppings or bat guano. Because of their high temperature, birds themselves are not infected with the fungus.
- People whose jobs or hobbies expose them to dust that is polluted with bat guano or bird droppings are at risk of developing histoplasmosis.
- While other systemic mycoses caused by dimorphic fungal infections can spread from person to person, histoplasmosis is not infectious.

Histoplasmosis is a significant fungal disease with distinct clinical presentations, varying levels of severity, and specific risk factors related to environmental exposure.

MYCOLOGY

The yeast cells of *Histoplasma* present inside macrophages were mistakenly thought to be a protozoan, which led to the organism's name *H. capsulatum*. It is not a protozoan or an encapsulated organism, despite its name, but rather a dimorphic noncapsulated fungus. Spores are present in the soil which is close to chicken coops, blackbird roosts, and caves or buildings where bats or pigeons reside. These are the places for the growth of *H. capsulatum*. Bats, with their lower body temperatures, can get infected and excrete the fungus in their droppings, while birds, with their high body temperatures, are not susceptible to infection. The primary route of infection is inhalation of microconidia from soil, which reach the alveoli and may germinate to cause pulmonary disease. *H. capsulatum* microconidia can infect humans when breathed in.

Histoplasma capsulatum is a mold that develops at room temperature in soil and on laboratory media incubated at 25°C. It shows the property of temperature-sensitive dimorphism. Within the human body, it replicates in the form of yeasts. Also, when the culture medium is incubated at 37°C, it changes into the disease-causing yeast type. Enriched media such as Brain Heart Infusion (BHI) agar with blood and cysteine are used to show conversion of yeast form to mycelial form and vice versa by incubating at 25 and 37°C, respectively.

Growth characteristics: Growth rate is slow. Usually, moldy or filamentous growth is seen at 25°C. Growth at 37°C is rare after primary isolation. Two colony morphotypes, albino (A) and brown (B), are shown on Sabouraud dextrose agar (SDA) at 25°C. Isolation of either variety from the same patient is possible; in some cases, the brown form can transform into the albino type. The albino-type growth is white with fine aerial hyphae, and brown-type colonies are flat with light tan or dark brown in color within 7 days. Later on, brown pigment diffuses into the medium. The albino-type colony may turn buff with the passage of time. At 37°C, colonies are granular to rough, cream-colored which later on become tan to brown.

Two types of unicellular asexual conidia are produced at 25°C: (1) Macroconidia and (2) microconidia. Macroconidia are thick-walled, plenty, and large (8–16 µm) and arise from short conidiophores, as shown in **Figures 16.1A and B**. They have projections on surface (tuberculate). Microconidia are small (2–4 µm) and arise from hyphae. The fungus comes in three varieties or strains:

1. *H. capsulatum var capsulatum* (classical histoplasmosis)
2. *H. capsulatum var duboisii* (African histoplasmosis)
3. *H. capsulatum var farciminosum* (epizootic histoplasmosis)

The first two are human pathogens, whereas the third is an animal pathogenic. Due to the size differences in yeast cells, human infections are sometimes known as "small-celled" and "large-celled" species for *H. capsulatum var* capsulatum and *H. capsulatum var duboisii*, respectively. In the mycelial phase, it is not possible to differentiate these two types. Differentiation is possible by DNA probe or by observing the morphology of yeasts. Differences between classical and African histoplasmosis are given in **Table 16.1**.

TAXONOMIC CLASSIFICATION

Histoplasma capsulatum belongs to the family Ajellomycetaceae, order Onygenales, within the Ascomycota phylum.

Varieties of *H. capsulatum* include the following:

- *Histoplasma capsulatum var. capsulatum*: Pulmonary histoplasmosis is most common. From this primary site of infection, the fungus may disseminate to other organs. The eastern and central parts of the United States are common places to see it.
- *Histoplasma capsulatum var. duboisii*: A systemic mycosis (fungal infection) is endemic to sub-Saharan,

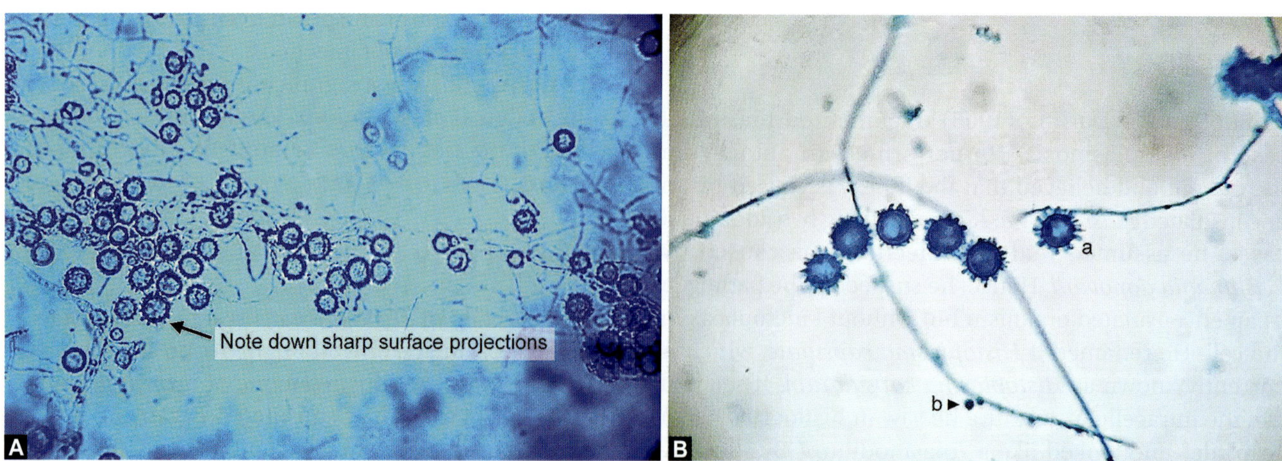

FIGS. 16.1A AND B: (A) LPCB mount of *Histoplasma capsulatum* showing circular macroconidia with tubercles (projections) (400×); (B) PVA-LPCB under oil immersion showing (a) tuberculate macroconidia and (b) microconidia (1,000×).
(LPCB: lactophenol cotton blue; PVA: polyvinyl alcohol)

TABLE 16.1: Differences between classical and African histoplasmosis.

Differentiating features	*African histoplasmosis*	*Classic histoplasmosis*
Areas of endemicity	Confined to the African subcontinent	Mainly Central and Eastern USA, isolated cases worldwide
Clinical presentations	Papules, nodules, and ulcerative lesions over skin, subcutaneous tissue, and bones	Systemic infection affecting the respiratory, cutaneous, mucocutaneous areas, and disseminated disease
Incidence of diseases	Rarely reported	Commonly reported
Association with AIDS	Rare	Common
Causative organisms	*Histoplasma capsulatum var. duboisii*	*Histoplasma capsulatum var. capsulatum*
Yeast morphology on HPE	Narrow-based, yeast cells of 7–15 µm found clustered in giant cells and histiocytes	Yeast cells 2–4 µm, scattered in the histiocytes
Differential diagnosis on HPE	Blastomycosis, lacaziosis, and emergomycosis (*Exserohilum orientalis*)	Leishmaniasis, toxoplasmosis, talaromycosis, and emergomycosis (*Exserohilum pasteurianus/Exserohilum africanus*)
Histopathological features	Larger yeast cells with thicker walls, less frequently seen in tissue compared to var. *capsulatum*	Smaller yeast cells with thinner walls, often more numerous in tissue samples
Immune response	Often presents with a more severe granulomatous response	Typically shows a more varied immune response, including granulomatous inflammation
Treatment response	May require more aggressive treatment approaches due to its rarity and presentation	Generally, responds well to conventional antifungal therapy

(AIDS: acquired immunodeficiency syndrome; HPE: histopathological examination)

western, and central Africa. Affected patients often experience a disorder marked by skin nodules, ulcers, and lesions that damage the bones, known as osteolysis.

- *Histoplasma capsulatum var. farciminosum*: It is pathogenic to animals and is responsible for a condition called epizootic lymphangitis, which affects horses. It is also endemic to Africa. This variety causes infections in equines, resulting in symptoms related to the lymphatic system, including nodules and lesions on the skin and lymphatic vessels.

There are at least eight clades within *H. capsulatum sensu lato* based on the phylogenetic studies and geographic distribution: North American classes 1 and 2 (NAm 1 and NAm 2), Latin American groups A and B (LAm A and LAm B), Australian, the Netherlands (Indonesian), Eurasian, and African clades. Except Eurasian clade, the other clades are considered phylogenetic species.

EPIDEMIOLOGY

Geographic Distribution

- *United States*: Central and southeastern United States, particularly those states bordering the river valleys of the Mississippi and Ohio, are the most common locations for *H. capsulatum* to be detected.
- *Worldwide*: Small endemic foci are present in Central America, Mexico, and Caribbean islands such as Jamaica and Puerto Rico. Thailand and India are among the several countries in South and Southeast Asia from where cases have been recorded.
- *Africa*: In the African continent, all three species of *H. capsulatum* are seen. Madagascar and most of the countries between the Tropic of Cancer and the Tropic of Capricorn are home to *var duboisii.*
- *Asia*: In Asia, there are many case reports. The fungus is not uncommon in India. However, there are no specific endemic zones across the country.

Ecologic Niche

Histoplasma capsulatum thrives in soil that has been contaminated with bird droppings or bat guano. Common environments where the fungus can be found include:

- *Chicken house litter*: Soil in chicken coops and poultry houses where bird droppings accumulate.
- *Blackbird roosting sites*: Locations where blackbirds gather, potentially leading to soil contamination with their droppings.
- *Pigeon- or bat-occupied buildings*: Caves, pigeonholes, and attics that pigeons and bats use as homes can contaminate the ground around them.

Individuals become exposed to the fungal spores when they disturb these settings, which results in aerosolization of fungal microconidia. Construction, restoration, demolition, and operations using contaminated soil can all raise the risk of exposure. There is no person-to-person transmission of the fungus. Preventive measures, such as proper respiratory protection and avoidance of activities that disturb contaminated soil, can help lower the risk of histoplasmosis in endemic areas.

Occupational Risk

- *Farming and gardening*: Workers involved in farming or gardening activities, especially in areas with contaminated soil, are at risk.
- *Roofing*: The droppings of pigeons and bats in caves, roosts, and attics enrich the soil with organic matter, creating a favorable environment for fungal growth and subsequent contamination.
- *Cleaning chimneys*: Chimney cleaners working in buildings with bird or bat infestations can be exposed.
- *Demolition and construction*: Individuals involved in demolishing old structures or constructing new ones in endemic areas face a risk of exposure.
- *Installation or maintenance of heating, ventilation, and air conditioning (HVAC) systems*: Workers installing or maintaining HVAC systems in contaminated areas may be exposed.
- *Building restoration*: Restoration workers dealing with old or abandoned buildings, particularly those with bird roosting sites, can be exposed to *Histoplasma.*
- *Cave exploring*: Cave explorers, especially in regions where bats reside, are at risk of inhaling airborne microconidia.
- *Very young and elderly*: Serious symptoms can manifest more quickly in newborns, toddlers, and the elderly.
- *Preexisting lung disease*: Individuals with preexisting lung conditions, such as chronic obstructive pulmonary disease (COPD), are at a greater risk of developing severe forms of histoplasmosis.
- *Smoking*: Heavy smokers are also at an increased risk of severe disease.

Immunocompromised Individuals

People living with acquired immunodeficiency syndrome (AIDS) (PLWAs): Individuals with human immunodeficiency virus (HIV)/AIDS have a higher likelihood of developing chronic or disseminated histoplasmosis. People with leukemia are more susceptible to severe histoplasmosis. Cancer patients and those with autoimmune disorders who are undergoing cytotoxic chemotherapy or systemic corticosteroids are at risk of disease.

IMMUNITY AND PATHOGENICITY

Host Factors

- *Intracellular pathogen*: An intracellular pathogen, *H. capsulatum,* causes a granulomatous reaction in the host. Once inhaled, they undergo germination into yeast forms that are resistant to lysis by immune cells.
- *Immune response*: Effective immune response relies on effective T-cell-mediated immunity. By activating macrophages to eliminate yeast forms, T-cell immunity, which is developed approximately 10–14 days after infection, limits the infection.
- *Granulomatous response*: Granulomatous reaction is seen in the lungs. At some point, pulmonary granulomas may calcify.
- *Delayed-type hypersensitivity (DTH)*: Histoplasmin skin testing can evoke a classic DTH reaction in individuals exposed to *Histoplasma.*
- *Immunoprotection*: Immunoprotection is partially restored during histoplasmosis recovery. Later on, nevertheless, there is a chance of reinfection or endogenous reactivation.

Fungal Virulence Factors

- *α-(1 → 3)-D-Glucan*: This is a cell wall component, a ligand for dectin-1, preventing phagocytosis. Dectin-1, seen on human dendritic cells, acts as a receptor for β-D-glucan, thereby promoting phagocytosis. *H. capsulatum* produces α-D-glucan that can mask β-D-glucan. This prevents Dectin-1 from recognizing β-D-glucan, in turn preventing phagocytosis.
- *Adherence to monocytes*: Heat shock protein 60 (Hsp60) on the yeast cell surface acts as an adhesin, binding to integrins on monocytes.
- *Calcium-binding protein 1 (Cbp1)*: It is secreted only by yeast forms and is essential for their survival inside macrophages.
- *Catalase*: *H. capsulatum* secretes catalase (M antigen) as a defensive agent against effective phagocytosis.
- *DRK1*: Histidine kinase gene (*DRK1*) is involved in pathogenicity and morphogenesis. The gene controls dimorphism and ensures the conversion to infectious yeast form when in the host tissue
- *Iron acquisition*: The ability to extract iron with siderophores and reductases acts as a virulence factor.
- *pH modulation*: *H. capsulatum* yeast forms change the pH of the phagolysosome (pH 6), promoting iron release from transferrin.

- *Restriction fragment length polymorphism (RFLP) class*: Isolates of *H. capsulatum* can be classified into three RFLP classes based on genetic markers. These classes show varying degrees of pathogenicity, with class 2 being the most pathogenic and expressing Yps3.

After inhalation, microconidia reach lungs and develop into yeast cells within the alveoli. The organism is attempted to be killed by phagocytosis by neutrophils and alveolar macrophages. Yeast cells proliferate inside the macrophages. Infectious organisms can go from the lungs to other organs via the regional lymph nodes. Granulomas can develop in immunocompetent individuals and then recover with fibrosis and calcification.

PATHOLOGY

A preliminary diagnosis of histoplasmosis can be made by looking for distinctive, narrow-based budding yeasts that are 2–4 µm diameter.

Histoplasmosis is not easily clinically differentiated from other infections like leishmaniasis. In most instances leishmaniasis may be identified histopathologically. *L. donovani* looks like *H. capsulatum* in tissues. However, the parasite has kinetoplasts in its cytoplasm (seen by Giemsa stain). On histological examination, other yeasts that produce symptoms comparable to histoplasmosis appear differently. Although the tiny yeasts will not be visible with standard hematoxylin and eosin (H&E) stains, a high concentration of organisms gives the impression that the macrophages are carrying something, though the exact nature of this something remains unknown. Staining tissue with periodic acid–Schiff (PAS) or Grocott–Gömöri's methenamine silver (GMS) helps to better see *H. capsulatum.* Most of the yeast cells are seen intracellularly within macrophages and some are seen extracellularly. It is possible to demonstrate yeast cells in various biopsies from various sites such as lymph nodes, liver, bone marrow, skin, or mucous membrane lesions. Although histoplasmosis is one of many diseases characterized by granulomatous inflammation, the most prevalent kind of tissue reaction is caseation necrosis.

CLINICAL FEATURES

Most of the infections are asymptomatic. Clinically, the illness will manifest a few years after primary infection. The factors which define the type of illness are infective dose, immunity of patients, and underlying predisposing factors. Various clinical types of classical histoplasmosis are given in the following text.

Acute Pulmonary Histoplasmosis

This variety is characterized by moderate, nonspecific symptoms similar to self-limiting influenza-like illnesses (cave disease). Fever, lethargy, headache, chills, dry cough, dyspnea, and chest pain are some of the symptoms. Occasionally, patients may develop arthritis, lymphadenopathy, skin rashes, or pericarditis. Individuals exposed to large amounts of *Histoplasma* spores may develop moderate-to-severe disease with more prominent respiratory symptoms.

Findings of chest imaging are given as follows:

- Characteristic patterns such as the "snowstorm" appearance
- Swollen lymph nodes in the mediastinum and hilar region
- Patchy pneumonia

A few atypical cases of erythema nodosum and erythema multiforme may affect young women. Myalgias and arthralgias are common symptoms of an acute infection, but in rare cases, a small number of people may develop symmetrical arthritis that is self-limiting and affects several joints.

In severe cases, the infection can spread to many lobes in patients without cell-mediated immunity, and symptoms are dyspnea, chills, cough, and fever. Adults may develop respiratory distress syndrome if chest X-rays show diffuse reticulonodular infiltrates on both sides.

Chronic Pulmonary Histoplasmosis

This form affects individuals with preexisting *COPD.* There may be progressive lung disease, cavitation, and other respiratory symptoms.

Pulmonary lesions may get calcified along with fibrosis leading to the formation of "histoplasmoma." Necrosis of enlarged mediastinal lymph nodes may occur along with fibrosis of mediastinal structures. The so-called marching cavity is unique to chronic cavitary histoplasmosis, in which ongoing necrosis expands the cavity, eventually consuming a whole lobe. While pleural effusions are extremely unusual, pleural thickening around apical cavitary lesions is common. The clinical features of chronic histoplasmosis are lethargy, fever, night sweats, loss of appetite, exhaustion, blood in sputum, and shortness of breath. Typical lesion in the lung is the development of histoplasmoma in which the lesion gets calcified, surrounded by fibrous tissue.

Cutaneous or Mucocutaneous

This may follow a pulmonary infection. Petechial lesions are seen on the chest or abdomen. In the mouth, lesions can form. Oral mucosa is the common site for mucosal infection. The fungus can be isolated from oral lesions.

Progressive Disseminated Histoplasmosis

People with impaired immune systems, including those with AIDS or who have received organ transplants, are more likely to develop this severe version, which can harm several organs such as the spleen, liver, bone marrow, and gastrointestinal system. This sort is common in children younger than 2 years old. Immunosuppressive drugs, corticosteroids, congenital T-cell deficits, hematologic malignancies, and hematopoietic stem cell transplant are other predisposing factors. The central nervous system (CNS) manifestation is rare, in the form of a spinal cord abscess. The gastrointestinal histoplasmosis has nonspecific symptoms; it can present with bloody diarrhea. Rarely, intestinal obstruction, perforation, and gastrointestinal bleeding are the complications of histoplasmosis.

Presumed Ocular Histoplasmosis Syndrome

This is primarily seen in regions endemic for histoplasmosis, characterized by multifocal choroiditis, peripapillary atrophy, and choroid neovascular membrane formation.

LABORATORY DIAGNOSIS

Specimens collected include sputum, bone marrow aspiration, lymph node aspiration or biopsy, peripheral blood, and biopsies from cutaneous and mucosal lesions.

Direct Examination

Histoplasma capsulatum, a tiny ovoid yeast, is seen in bronchial washings and sputum in cases of acute pulmonary histoplasmosis. Due to its diminutive size, it frequently goes unnoticed in potassium hydroxide (KOH) mount. It is better to use staining techniques such as Wright's, GMS , PAS , Giemsa, or calcofluor stain for various specimens.

Giemsa **(Figs. 16.2A and B)** or Wright's stains are used for peripheral blood smear or bone marrow aspirate. Intracellularly in monocytes and neutrophils and occasionally outside of cells, one can see oval yeast forms, 2–4 µm in size, as shown in **Figure 16.2**. A blue cell wall and a dark blue protoplasm are visible in a Giemsa stain, with white space between them which may give the appearance of halo or capsule, but it is an artifact produced when protoplasm slightly retracts from the wall. In PAS stain, fungus appears pink. In GMS stain, yeasts are uniformly black colored. One more method for detecting fungus in tissues is the direct immunofluorescence test.

Histopathology

Yeast cells are seen within macrophages in granulomas. Histopathology revealed small clusters of neutrophils, many macrophages, and multinucleate giant cells (both Langhans and foreign body giant cells).

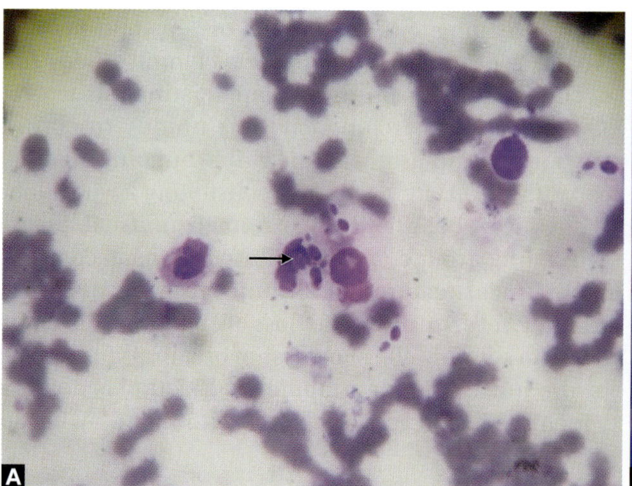

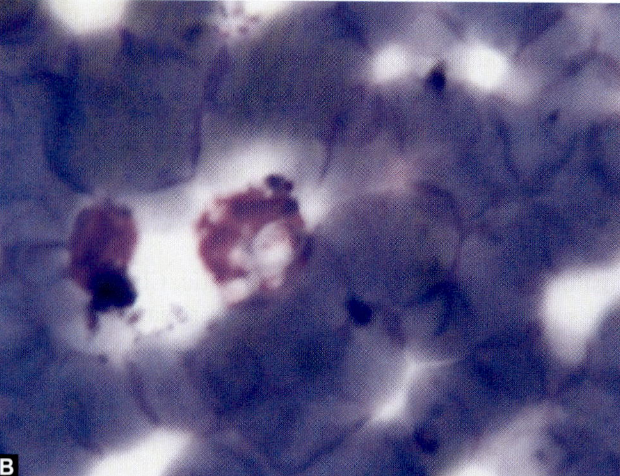

FIGS. 16.2A AND B: Giemsa-stained smear showing yeast cells of *Histoplasma capsulatum* (1,000×).

DIFFERENTIAL DIAGNOSIS

When distinguishing *H. capsulatum var. duboisii* from other fungal infections with similar histopathological features, consider the following points:

- *H. capsulatum var. capsulatum*: This variant of *H. capsulatum* has smaller yeast forms (2–4 µm in diameter) compared to *H. capsulatum var. duboisii*. The yeast forms of *H. capsulatum var. capsulatum* typically lack the distinctive large size and thick walls as seen in *H. capsulatum var. duboisii*.
- *Cryptococcus neoformans*: The yeast cells of *Cryptococcus neoformans* are slightly smaller than those of *H. capsulatum var. duboisii* and have a distinctive thin cell wall. *Cryptococcus neoformans* cells are frequently enclosed by a broad, clear, unstained capsule that stains positively with the mucicarmine stain, but *H. capsulatum var. duboisii* does not.
- *Coccidioides* species: Spherules are bigger in size.
- *Blastomyces dermatitidis*: Although it resembles *H. capsulatum* var. *duboisii* in size and shape, the yeast form of *B. dermatitidis* shows broad-based budding.
- In clinical specimens, other fungi that look like *H. capsulatum* include *Candida glabrata, Pneumocystis jirovecii*, and yeast form of *Penicillium marneffei*. These fungi can be distinguished by their microscopic morphology. *C. glabrata* does not have halo; absence of budding in *P. jirovecii* and presence of transverse septum in *P. marneffei* are the differentiating features.

Culture

Biohazard Safety Level 3 infrastructure is recommended for handling cultures of *Histoplasma*. Positivity of cultures from sputum cultures can vary widely across cases of histoplasmosis; nevertheless, in case of self-limited acute pulmonary histoplasmosis, they tend to be minimal. In order to get a positive result, it may be necessary to collect many sputum samples. Two sets of SDAs (without actidione) and BHI blood agar are inoculated. One set of each medium is incubated at 25°C, while the other set is incubated at 37°C. For conversion to yeast form, blood-glucose-cysteine (BGC) agar is also recommended. *H. capsulatum* requires the presence of a reducing substance in the form of a free thiol group provided from cysteine.

During the first week, cultures should be observed daily. After that, they should be observed twice a week until the fourth week. Phase conversion is accomplished using specialized media such as BHIB, BHI agar, Kelley's medium, and Pine's medium. The exoantigens H and M detection can be performed on colonies. Phase conversions in the laboratory often fail. Nucleic acid probe tests, such as AccuProbe, can be used to identify young mycelial cultures.

Conidiation (Production of Conidia)

Colonies of *H. capsulatum* usually produce tuberculate macroconidia and few microconidia (asexual spores), as shown in **Figures 16.1A and B**. The fungus should be differentiated from saprophytic fungi such as *Sepedonium* and *Chrysosporium*. In *Sepedonium*, tubercles on the surface of macroconidia are blunt, and microconidia are not seen. DNA probes are used in many laboratories for identification.

Conversion to Yeast Form in Vitro

Confirmatory testing with in vitro yeast conversion can be helpful in detecting *H. capsulatum*. It should be kept in mind that some strains may be stubborn, so that mycelial to yeast conversion cannot be demonstrated.

Histoplasma must be demonstrated to possess H and M exoantigens in order to be identified at the genus level. In terms of identification, they are dependable markers.

Serology

Serology is used to demonstrate antibodies in a patient's serum.

The antigens used for the test are derived from either (1) sterile culture filtrate (*histoplasmin*) of 3–6 months' old culture on asparagine-glucose broth or (2) merthiolate suspension of *whole yeast* cells in saline.

Histoplasmin contains two antigens: (1) H antigen and (2) M antigen. The antibodies against "H" are formed during active histoplasmosis. "M" band is seen in either acute infection or chronic infection or in a person in whom prior skin testing with Histoplasmin was performed. "M" antigen is abundant in mycelial form. Both H and M antigens are regarded as being species-specific proteins. They are used in immunodiffusion (ID) and complement fixation tests (CFTs). Antibodies to H antigens and M antigens, respectively, provide the two main bands seen in an ID test. "M" band is thicker and is near to the antigen well as compared to "H" band which is thinner and near to antibody wells of ID test. In <20% of instances, the presence of the H band establishes the presence of an acute infection; it is uncommon to find the H band alone. The M band is far more prevalent and frequently remains even after the illness has gone away.

Immunoblotting test: A monoclonal antibody is used to detect 80 kDa by the immunoblotting method.

Tests used to confirm the fungus grown as Histoplasma is done by:

- Mycelial to yeast conversion on BHIA blood agar incubated at 37°C
- Exoantigen testing
- AccuProbe which targets rDNA

Antigen Detection Tests

Urine antigen tests are useful in disseminated histoplasmosis and sometimes in early acute pulmonary cases. It is a usual practice to combine ID with latex agglutination and CFT (titer 1:32). EIA tests are also available. Antigen detection might be better for diagnosis in immunocompromised persons.

Histoplasmin Skin Tests

The histoplasmin intradermal test is used in epidemiological studies. It is capable of locating endemic areas. It is ineffective for detecting infections. It involves injecting 0.1 mL of antigen into the forearm. The test is read after 48 hours and is termed positive with induration of 5 mm. Because of a present or past infection, the test is positive. Skin testing done prior to antibody detection test gives a false-positive antibody test.

Importance of Histoplasmin Skin Test

The *histoplasmin skin test* evaluates DTH to *H. capsulatum* antigens, helping in the identification of exposure to the fungus. Its key points are as follows:

- *Diagnostic role*:
  - Detects *prior exposure* to *H. capsulatum*, especially in endemic areas.
  - Helps in *epidemiological studies* to determine the prevalence of histoplasmosis in populations.
- *Epidemiological significance*:
  - Useful in mapping the geographic distribution of histoplasmosis, as endemicity varies significantly worldwide.
  - Allows assessment of high-risk areas or populations frequently exposed to *H. capsulatum* (e.g., farmers, cave explorers).
- *Limited role in active disease*:
  - *Does not confirm active disease*: A positive test indicates exposure but not necessarily current infection.
  - May have *limited utility in immunocompromised individuals* (e.g., HIV/AIDS), as they may not mount a sufficient immune response for positivity.
- *Interpretation*:
  - A *positive reaction* (induration at the injection site) suggests prior exposure or infection with *H. capsulatum.*
  - A *negative test* does not exclude histoplasmosis, especially in individuals with compromised immune systems.
- *Obsolete in certain regions*:
  - Largely replaced by more specific diagnostic methods [e.g., antigen detection, serology, polymerase chain reaction (PCR)] in clinical practice.
  - Can lead to *cross-reactivity* with other fungal infections, such as blastomycosis, reducing its specificity.

Histoplasma duboisii

This is also called "African histoplasmosis" and is caused by *H. capsulatum var. duboisii* . Yeast cells have a pear shape and are found in large numbers in giant cells. It is largely a disease of the cutaneous, subcutaneous, and osseous tissues, with limited evidence of lesions in internal organs and reticuloendothelial cell involvement. Inhalation is thought to be the mode of infection.

The disease differs from classical histoplasmosis in the distribution of lesions and the morphological features of fungus. The skin lesions manifest as papules that progress into nodules, ulcers, and abscesses with draining sinuses. Bony lesions are well-defined and osteolytic. Despite the fact that the respiratory system is considered the site of entrance, there are relatively few indications of pulmonary illness. Lymph nodes are more likely to be involved.

The mycelial form is similar to *H. capsulatum var capsulatum.* The yeast cells have thick walls and a size of 7–15 μm. Histopathological examination is important in diagnosis.

Because of the huge size of the yeast cells, it is sometimes mistaken with *Blastomyces.* The difference is that *Blastomyces* yeast cells have a broad base and do not develop intracellularly.

Differentiating features of *H. capsulatum var. duboisii* are as follows:

- Its area of endemicity is the African subcontinent.
- Higher chances of involvement of lymph nodes, skin, and bones with granulomatous lesions but systemic disease is uncommon.
- The yeast cells have thick walls, 7–15 μm (large size).
- Giant cell formation is common.
- It is infrequently associated with AIDS.
- It shows different results in multilocus sequence analysis.

Histoplasma farciminosum

Animal histoplasmosis is caused by *Histoplasma capsulatum var. farciminosum*. It is host specific, and the disease has been observed in horses, mules, and dogs and is extremely rarely in humans. The four clinical manifestations are asymptomatic, cutaneous, respiratory, and disseminated disease. It is common in Africa, Japan, and the far East. Yeast cells resemble *H. capsulatum*. The fungus grows exceedingly slowly, taking 3 months to create colonies. Lactophenol cotton blue (LPCB) analysis of the mycelial colony reveals short, irregularly curved aerial hyphae with round-to-oval conidia. In animals, a PCR-based test is utilized to diagnose the ailment.

TREATMENT

The treatment part of various clinical types is summarized in **Table 16.2**.

TABLE 16.2: Treatment options for various clinical types.

Clinical presentation	***Treatment options***
Acute pulmonary histoplasmosis	• *Mil-to-moderate*: Typically, no specific antifungal therapy required • *Moderately severe*: Itraconazole (ITC) 200 mg three times a day for 3 days, followed by 200 mg once or twice a day for 6–12 weeks. Add methylprednisolone for severe cases
Complications of acute pulmonary histoplasmosis	• *Pericarditis*: Nonsteroidal anti-inflammatory medicines and steroids if needed, along with ITC • *Mediastinal granuloma*: Consider amphotericin B before surgery • *Pulmonary nodules (Histoplasmosis)*: Typically, no antifungal therapy is needed
Chronic cavitary histoplasmosis	• Long-term oral ITC 200 mg three times a day for at least 1 year, possibly more for reduced relapse risk • Amphotericin B (AmB) for nonresponders
Progressive	*Severe cases*: Liposomal AmB for 1–2 weeks
Disseminated histoplasmosis	Therapy is followed by itraconazole (ITC) for at least 12 months. Amphotericin B deoxycholate may be considered in patients with low renal risk. • Prolonged suppressive therapy with lower-dose ITC for certain patients
Other special categories	*Pregnant patients or children*: Refer to specific therapy recommendations as needed

CHAPTER

17 Blastomycosis

INTRODUCTION

Members of the genus *Blastomyces* which is a thermally dimorphic fungus produce the disease known as blastomycosis. It is a chronic granulomatous disease which primarily infects lungs, and the fungus may spread to skin, bones, and genitourinary system.

The fungus occurs as mold in the environment, whereas yeast is the form seen in a human host. The geographic distribution of each species of *Blastomyces* is unique. The name "North American blastomycosis" comes from the fact that fungi are common throughout the United States. Another name for the disease is Gilchrist's disease, as he is the discoverer of the disease.

HISTORY

Blastomycosis was originally believed to be a protozoan infection when Thomas Gilchrist initially identified the illness as a skin disease in 1894. The causative agent was tentatively identified as Oidium. He and Stokes in 1898 finally isolated and identified the pathogen and named it *Blastomyces dermatitidis*. This fungus was first reported in 1902 by Walker and Montgomery as a systemic infection. The word "dermatitidis" is acknowledged due to the high proportion of cases, including skin involvement. "Chicago illness", "North American blastomycosis" and "Gilchrist disease" are different names of the illness caused by *B. dermatitidis*.

In the year 2013, another species of the genus, i.e., *Blastomyces gilchristii*, got recognition, while in 2017, a third species, i.e., *Blastomyces percursus*, was identified. *Blastomyces helicus* (Western USA and Canada) is one more species. *Emmonsia parva* is renamed *Blastomyces parvus*.

MYCOLOGY

Three distinct species of fungus—(1) *B. dermatitidis*, (2) *B. gilchristii*, and (3) *B. percursus*—cause the illness. Blastomyces is a thermally dimorphic fungus. The fungus is present in the environment as the mycelial form. The yeast cells seen in tissue display a "figure of eight" due to their 8–15 µm size and "broad base" (bud with a wide orifice) budding. The two cells stay connected until the daughter cell, which has a thinner wall, grows to be almost as big as the parent cell, at which point it is freed (dehiscence), and the cell wall thickens. Hence, the yeast has a *doubly refractile wall*. Size, shape, and thickness could vary. Yeast cells can have multiple nuclei as seen in well-fixed tissue. The exoantigen test is a tool for identifying isolates. The AK and K serotypes are present. The "K" serotype is more common in Africa, whereas "AK" is present all over the world.

TAXONOMY

The telemorphic stage of the fungus is *Ajellomyces dermatitidis*, in the family Onygenaceae, order Onygenales, class Plectomycetes, phylum Ascomycota.

EPIDEMIOLOGY

Fungal spores, or conidia, can be inhaled and enter the lungs, making this the principal route of transmission. The clinical presentation varies widely from asymptomatic cases to an active disease which has the ability to spread to other areas of the body. So far, neither the native habitat nor the reservoir has been located. Soil that is damp is likely to be home to the fungus. Person-to-person transmission is not observed. The fungus is more common in men because they are more prone to engage in outdoor activities. The fungus can infect people with normally functioning immune systems if they engage in certain hobbies or work in rural areas where the fungus grows in the soil.

Geographic Distribution

The Mississippi and Ohio river basins, along with Canada, are among the places where blastomycosis is endemic. The eastern part of Canada and the eastern, central, and midwestern states of the United States are also endemic areas. It is found only in the Great Lakes, the river basins of the Ohio and Mississippi, and elsewhere in the United States. Middle Eastern countries (Saudi Arabia, Israel, and Lebanon) and African countries also have small blastomycosis foci. Zimbabwe accounts for the bulk of the cases reported in the African zone. Very few instances of infection in humans have been recorded in India. In 1983, a patient from Uttar Pradesh, close to New Delhi, was the first case documented by Randhawa et al. Few reports came from Mumbai, Bengaluru, and Vellore. Soil disturbance by construction, excavation, or outdoor recreational activities such as camping, fishing, or hunting is usually associated with blastomycosis epidemics. Dogs, especially those used for hunting, are at a great risk of contracting blastomycosis in areas where the disease is prevalent and it can be fatal.

Just a few northern US states and Canadian provinces—Alberta, Saskatchewan, British Columbia, Ontario, New York, Minnesota, and Wisconsin—are home to *Blastomyces gilchristii*. A new species of *Blastomyces*, *B. helicus*, was described by Schwartz et al. (2019), in the American West and Western Canada.

IMMUNITY

Assuming that host responses to *B. dermatitidis* are similar to those induced by *Histoplasma capsulatum* and *Coccidioides* species, much of what is known about cellular immune responses to *B. dermatitidis* comes from animal models. Blastomycosis also indicates a critical cellular immune response since yeast cells are either inside or in contact with monocytes, macrophages, and giant cells. When protecting oneself from *B. dermatitidis*, humoral immune responses serve no purpose. Neutrophils, macrophages (innate immunity), and activated T lymphocytes (adaptive immunity) appear to play an important role in immunity against *Blastomyces*. There is no reliable skin test as of now.

PATHOGENESIS

The conidia, which are infectious and can become aerosolized, are produced by *B. dermatitidis*. The next step is to transfer the conidia to the lower respiratory system. Many conidia are phagocytized and subsequently destroyed by neutrophils and alveolar macrophages. In such persons, the infection remains asymptomatic. In a symptomatic case of lung infection, conidia undergo phase transition to the yeast form. The yeast form has a thick cell wall that resists phagocytosis. A characteristic of blastomycosis is the pyogranulomatous inflammatory response. It begins with the accumulation of neutrophils followed by macrophages. Eventually, this progresses to the formation of a granuloma. Blastomyces adhesion-1 (BAD-1) is a predominant antigen present on the fungus.

PATHOLOGY

A suppurative and granulomatous reaction forms in the host in response to the fungus (pyogranuloma). Caseous necrosis is not present in the granuloma. Some cases may resolve on their own. Both pulmonary and extrapulmonary diseases are known to cause endogenous reactivation of the main focus.

CLINICAL FORMS OF BLASTOMYCOSIS

- *Pulmonary blastomycosis*: Subclinical infections are common. Various clinical symptoms might be observed in cases of acute pulmonary blastomycosis. Flu-like illness with fever, chills, myalgia, and productive cough may occur.

  Some patients may have mild pulmonary infiltrates even when they show no outward signs of illness. A small proportion of cases suffer from self-resolving pneumonia. Rarely, it is a life-threatening event. Even in some cases, routine chest radiographs can raise suspicion that a patient has pulmonary infiltrates even though they are symptom-free. Acute pulmonary blastomycosis can be visible on computed tomography (CT) and radiographs as patchy infiltrates; however, consolidation with air bronchograms can also be observed. Cavitary illness similar to reactivation tuberculosis and miliary disease patterns have also been observed; imaging can show mass-like lesions resembling cancer or nodules of varying sizes in less severe infections. After a particularly severe first infection, adults could develop acute respiratory distress syndrome (ARDS) and diffuse pneumonitis. Fever, cough, and dyspnea typically appear suddenly in those patients of pulmonary blastomycosis who develop ARDS.

As soon as hypoxemia develops, intubation and mechanical breathing are required. There have been reports of mortality rates ranging from 40 to 80%.

- *Cutaneous blastomycosis*: Most cases of cutaneous blastomycosis are actually symptoms of a systemic disease, either active or dormant at the time. The dermatitis is secondary to disseminated disease. The lesions are observed on the face, neck, and hands. Papules and small, perhaps ruptured nodules are the outward signs of a lesion. Lesions may ulcerate. Primary cutaneous disease is rare. It may be present among mycologists, pathologists, and veterinarians as an occupational hazard following accidental inoculation. Whether or not lymphangitis or regional lymphadenopathy is present, the lesion often starts as a papule and rapidly develops into a pustule. Pustule may rupture to produce a discharging ulcer. The discharge is foul smelling. Cutaneous disease should be differentiated from many conditions such as atypical tuberculosis, histoplasmosis, coccidioidomycosis, and basal cell carcinoma, etc.
- *Osseous blastomycosis*: Osteomyelitis is common and arthritis is rare. The vertebra, pelvis, sacrum, skull, and ribs are the bones involved. Paravertebral abscess should be kept in the differential diagnosis of vertebral tuberculosis (TB) in endemic areas.
- *Disseminated disease*: It occurs by hematogenous dissemination from the primary focus in lung. Abscess and granuloma formation take place at various sites including bones, breast, genitourinary system, and central nervous system (CNS).
- *Genitourinary blastomycosis*: It appears that blastomycosis predominates in the male genital system, which includes the kidneys, prostate (which is among the most frequently affected areas), testes, epididymis, and seminal vesicles.
- *CNS blastomycosis*: A higher frequency of CNS involvement is seen in immunocompromised patients, such as those with acquired immunodeficiency syndrome (AIDS), and occurs in 5–10% of instances with disseminated blastomycosis.
- *Laryngitis*: The involvement is rare.

LABORATORY DIAGNOSIS

To make a tentative diagnosis of blastomycosis, it is common to use the patient's medical history, symptoms, microscopy, culture, and serology.

Specimens: Depending upon the suspected site of involvement, the following specimens are collected: Sputum, bronchoalveolar lavage (BAL), biopsy, pus, urine (after prostatic massage), skin scraping, blood, and aspirates.

Direct Examination

Potassium hydroxide (KOH) mount: It is performed on suitable specimens. *B. dermatitidis* is seen as big yeast cells (10–15 μm), with thick refractile walls, and a characteristic figure-of-eight shape, with single broad-based budding **(Fig. 17.1)**. To improve detection, add *calcofluor white* to KOH.

Histopathology

Periodic acid-Schiff (PAS) and Grocott-Gömöri's methenamine silver (GMS) stains are preferred for the demonstration of yeast forms in tissue. In PAS stain, yeast are pink, while in GMS, they are black. It is difficult to note down the classic morphology in hematoxylin and eosin (H&E) stain. The fungus needs differentiation from *Cryptococcus neoformans* or immature *Cryptococcus immitis*/*Coccidioides posadasii* spherules. *Blastomyces dermatitidis* often has weakly mucicarmine-positive cell walls; mucicarmine staining is utilized to differentiate encapsulated *C. neoformans* strains from *B. dermatitidis* (*C. neoformans* capsule is strongly mucicarmine positive. Noncapsulated *C. neoformans* can be differentiated by melanin stain—*C. neoformans* being melanin positive and *B. dermatitidis* being melanin negative). While

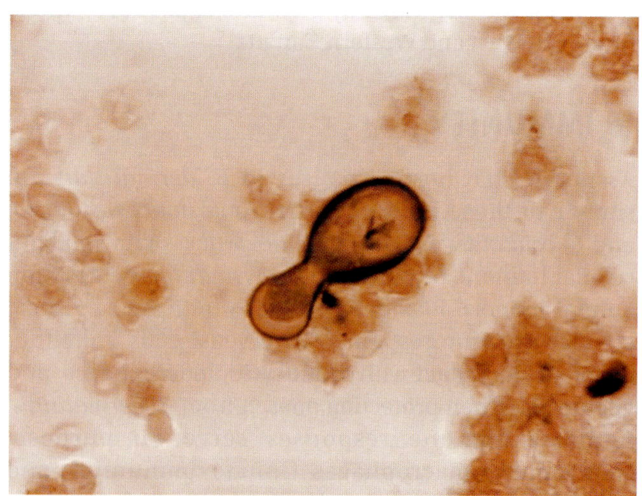

FIG. 17.1: Broad-based budding of *Blastomyces dermatitidis*.
Source: Public Health Image Library CDC.

C. immitis and *C. posadasii* are negative by Alcian blue (pH 2.5) and acid-fast stains, *B. dermatitidis* is weakly positive.

It is rare to find atypical strains of *B. dermatitidis* in tissues. These yeast cells are extremely tiny, measuring 2–4 μm in diameter, and they can be mistaken for *H. capsulatum*. Congo red staining to differentiate between microforms of *B. dermatitidis* (positive) and *H. capsulatum* (negative) is one method that could be useful for identifying unusual forms.

Culture

At room temperature, *B. dermatitidis* grows in a mycelial (mold) form; when incubated at 37°C on enriched media, it transforms into yeast. Growth can take anywhere from 5 to 30 days on average. Two sets of media, incubated at 25 and 37°C, are utilized for culture. The media comprise Sabouraud Dextrose Agar (SDA) slants, brain heart infusion (BHI) agar, blood agar, and blood glucose cysteine agar. It takes about 2–4 weeks for the fungus to start growing and form colonies.

Colony characteristics: At 25°C after 14 days, the colonies' yeast-like texture turns into a downy, fluffy white. As colonies mature, their color may lighten to a tan, and sporulation is more common in tan colonies compared to white ones.

Microscopic findings: When looking at *B. dermatitidis* under a microscope, one can see small, septate hyphae that are 1–2 μm in diameter. The most diagnostic feature is the presence of oval or pyriform single-celled conidia that are 2–4 μm in diameter. These can be seen singly at the ends of short or long conidiophores and look like *lollipops* **(Fig. 17.2)**. It looks like other fungi such as *Chrysosporium* species and *Pseudallescheria boydii*. *B. dermatitidis* grows on cycloheximide-containing media, whereas *P. boydii* and other *Chrysosporium* species do not.

Dimorphism: The transformation of mold into yeast and vice-versa is a practical test for medical diagnosis. A mycelial colony is transferred to enriched media which are incubated at 37°C. Wrinkled yeast-like colonies, characteristic of *B. dermatitidis*, develop within 3–4 days. The conversion is carried out using BHI agar and cysteine heart hemoglobin agar.

Serotyping

African isolates are differentiated from North American ones by detecting "K" and "A" antigens on yeast form of *B. dermatitidis*.

The African isolates share a common "K" antigen and form different serotypes. However, antigen "A" is present on most of the fungus isolates, including North American isolates. Serotyping of the mycelial fungal isolates is possible by detecting these antigens. The mycelial form of the dimorphic fungus *B. dermatitidis* can be identified with this test. Serotype of the isolate can be identified by exoantigen analysis test of the yeast phase (antigen-A) of fungus.

The procedure comprises a two-step immunodiffusion reaction in agar with a known, standardized antigen and an unknown antigen (an aqueous extract of a mycelial culture that is 7–10 days old).

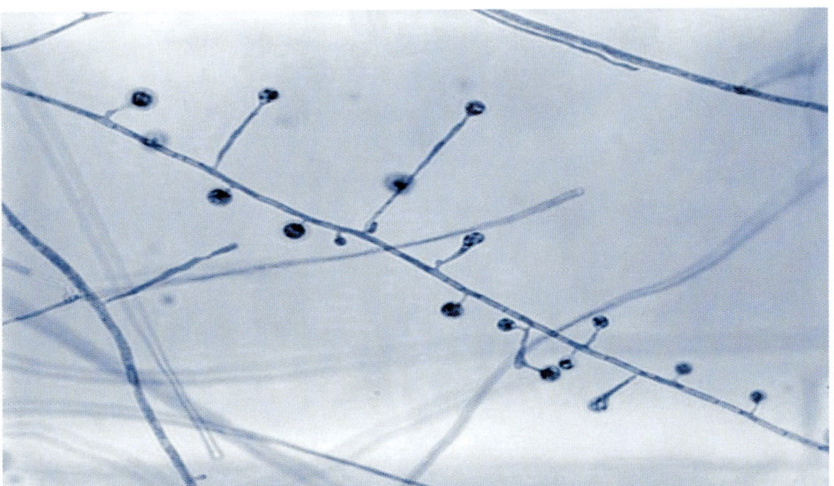

FIG. 17.2: LPCB mount of (mycelial phase) of Blastomyces dermatitidis (400×).

(LPCB: lactophenol cotton blue)

Source: Public Health Image Library CDC.

Serodiagnosis

The serological tests that can be used to diagnose blastomycosis include the immunodiffusion (ID) precipitin test, complement fixation (CF) test, and radioimmunoassay. These tests have low sensitivity. Enzyme immunoassay (EIA) test uses antibodies against "A" antigen that has improved the sensitivity.

Newer tests for the diagnosis of blastomycosis include DNA probes, Western blotting, and indirect immunofluorescence tests.

TREATMENT

Fluconazole, itraconazole, and amphotericin B are the drugs utilized in the treatment. Itraconazole is given to patients who have healthy immune systems, while amphotericin B is given to those who do not. The dose of itraconazole is 200–400 mg daily for 6 months. The dose of amphotericin B is intravenous (IV) 0.7 mg/kg/day for 8–12 weeks. In case of severe disease such as CNS involvement, amphotericin B is used.

CHAPTER

18 Coccidioidomycosis

INTRODUCTION

Soil molds, such as *Coccidioides immitis* and *Coccidioides posadasii*, cause coccidioidomycosis, an infection of the respiratory tract. Inhaled arthroconidia of the fungus are infective forms. Within the host (human or animals), the infective forms get converted into spherules containing endospores. The severity of the illness varies from subclinical infection which clears up on their own to severe disease. Extrapulmonary spread affects the skin, meninges, bones, and joints. Some persons have persistent fibrocavitary sickness that requires therapy. The other names of the disease are valley fever, desert rheumatism, desert fever, desert pimples, Posadas-Wernicke sickness. Coccidioidin skin test conversion is often sufficient to detect subclinical illness in about 60% of infected individuals. Some people, particularly those with impaired immune systems [acquired immunodeficiency syndrome (AIDS) patients and solid organ transplant recipients], may be at risk of fatal disease. Differences between species and similar looking fungi are given in **Table 18.1**.

HISTORY

The first description of the illness was made in 1892 by Alejandro Posadas in a patient who was a soldier and was suffering from a suspected tumor, i.e., mycosis fungoides. The newly-discovered illness was thought to be parasitic since a biopsy had found organisms that looked like the protozoan Coccidia meaning a cyst with endocystic cells.

TABLE 18.1: Differences between different species of the fungus and similar fungi.

Morphological features	*Coccidioides immitis*	*Emmonsia crescens*	*Prototheca wickerhamii*	*Rhinosporidium seeberi*
Taxonomic status	Fungus	Fungus	Protista	Protista
Size of spherules/sporangia	60–100 µm	50–500 µm	7–13 µm	10–450 µm
Thickness of spherule walls	1–2 µm	10–70 µm	–	3–5 µm
Size of endospores	2–5 µm	Not applicable	2–11 µm	6–10 µm
Maximum number of endospores	200–300	Not applicable	50	16,000
Arthroconidia/hyphae	Present	Not applicable	Not applicable	Not applicable
Pathological reaction of host	Necrotic granuloma	Fibrotic granuloma	Necrotizing epithelioid granuloma	Acute/chronic inflammatory
Growth on artificial media	Mycelial	Mycelial	Yeast-like	Noncultivable
Special fungal stain				
GMS	Positive	Positive	Positive	Positive
PAS	Positive	Positive	Positive	Positive
Mucicarmine	Negative	Negative	Negative	Positive

(GMS: Grocott–Gömöri's methenamine silver; PAS: periodic acid-Schiff)

As the pathogen had resemblance with protozoan coccidia and severity of disease caused by it, the pathogen received a new name—*Coccidioides immitis* (coccidia-like; im—not; mitis—mild). In Latin, "immitis" is also used for "harsh" describing the clinical course. William Ophüls and Herbet Moffitt demonstrated that *C. immitis* is actually a dimorphic fungus and not a protozoan. Stewart and Mayer (1932) isolated the fungus from soil. In 2002, *C. immitis* was separated into two species: (1) *C. posadasii*, named after the disease's first describer, and (2) *C. immitis*, continuing the evolution of coccidioidomycosis with two distinct species.

EPIDEMIOLOGY

Contaminated soil or fomites can infect humans in endemic areas whether they live, work, visit, or come into contact with them. Commonly referred to as "valley fever," the disease is most prevalent in the Central Valley (San Joaquin Valley) in California, where it is endemic.

The seasonality of coccidioidomycosis depends on the weather factors. Rainfall supports the growth of hyphae in soil at places such as Kern County, California, and Southern Arizona. After this phase, dry interval is needed to desiccate and produce arthroconidia, which are infective forms of the fungus. Wind, earthquakes, and dust storms disperse the arthroconidia in the environment. Such an epidemic occurred in the San Joaquin Valley in 1978 as a result of dust storm. The Northridge earthquake in California (1994) resulted in landslides that discharged dust carrying arthroconidia, resulting in an outbreak of coccidioidomycosis in which 203 cases were identified in a span of approximately 2 months.

The following human activities help to spread the disease:

- Sites of possible archaeological work
- Agricultural work, since arthroconidia can be released when soil is cultivated
- Training in land warfare
- Recreational events, such as model aeroplane-flying contests, held in desert regions

Laboratory Exposures

Laboratory personnel who do not follow sufficient safety precautions when handling cultures risk get exposed.

ETIOLOGICAL AGENTS

Coccidioidomycosis is caused by two closely related fungus species, (1) *C. immitis* and (2) *C. posadasii*. There are genetic and epidemiological differences between two species. *C. immitis* from California and *C. posadasii* from other parts of the world are known as "Californian" and "non-Californian species", respectively These two species share common morphology, clinical characteristics, and treatment.

CLASSIFICATION

The fungus belongs to the Onygenaceae family within the order Onygenales and phylum Ascomycota (anamorphic species).

Epidemiological features of the etiological agents are as follows:

- *C immitis—Geographic distribution*: *C. immitis* is primarily found in the California endemic area, particularly in the Central Valley of California.
- *C. posadasii*: *Geographic distribution*—parts of Mexico, the Arizona-Phoenix region, and smaller areas in Central and South America are among the most common places.

Phenotypic and Genotypic Similarity

Because of their striking phenotypic similarity, it is difficult to tell *C. immitis* and *C. posadasii* apart from one another. Both types of molds are filamentous and produce white and fluffy hyphae that break into arthroconidia that resemble barrels. These arthroconidia are important for the infectious propagation of the fungus.

Dimorphism

The life cycle of *Coccidioides* species is dimorphic. When propagules are inhaled by a host, they undergo morphogenesis, commonly within the lungs, and transform into spherules, which are spherical structures ranging in size from 10 to 80 µm. These spherules are densely packed with endospores.

Development of the Spherule Form

Several phases of nuclear division and segmentation take place during the transition of arthroconidia to spherules. The released endospores grow in size and form new spherules, which give rise to second-generation 200–300 new endospores. As spherule grows, its size increases. It is segmented to develop peripheral compartments that surround the core cavity. Endospores grow in these periphery compartments. When the spherules rupture, uninucleate endospores are released, which might migrate to other regions of the body and potentially produce new spherules.

The fungus is less temperature sensitive than other dimorphic fungi. The mycelial to spherule conversion occurs in a glucose salt medium at 37°C in the presence of 5–10% CO_2. They form spherules on glucose yeast extract agar.

IMMUNITY

The pathogenesis and immune response to *Coccidioides* infection involve various components of the immune system.

Innate Immunity

- *Polymorphonuclear leukocytes (PMNs)*: While they can destroy some arthroconidia, they struggle with larger spherules.
- *Monocytes/macrophages*: Alveolar macrophages typically struggle to eliminate arthroconidia and endospores.
- *Natural killer (NK) cells*: They migrate to infection sites and act by producing cytokines to activate other cells as well as directly kill the fungus by release of enzymes such as perforins and granzyme.
- *Cytokine activation of monocytes*: Interferon gamma (IFN-γ) and tumor necrosis factor alpha (TNF-α) activation enhances phagosome–lysosome fusion, improving the killing of *Coccidioides* arthroconidia and endospores and generating reactive nitrogen/ intermediates.

Humoral Immunity

Antibodies

Elevated levels of immunoglobulins G, A, and E (IgG, IgA, and IgE) are associated with polyclonal B-lymphocyte activation indicating a complex interplay between innate and adaptive immunity.

Immune Evasion

Outer wall glycoprotein misleads the host immune response; they can suppress the synthesis of some cytokines required for inflammation and macrophage-mediated immunity.

Pathogenesis

The pathogenesis of *Coccidioides* infection involves various stages of morphogenesis and immune evasion. A summary of the key points mentioned in the text is as follows:

- *Arthroconidia*: Tiny arthroconidia are inhaled and reach the lungs' alveoli. These arthroconidia contain a hydrophobic layer and withstand the first host reaction, including phagocyte assault.
- *Morphogenesis to spherules*: Arthroconidia convert into spherules as the partial pressure of CO_2 in the host tissues increases. Spherules develop glycoprotein called spherule outer wall glycoprotein (SOWgp) along with a lipid-rich outer wall layer called the spherule outer wall (SOW) as they enlarge.
- *Maturation of spherules*: After enlarging, the spherule becomes multinucleate and measures 40–80 μm in diameter. New cell wall synthesis occurs, and plasma membrane invagination separates it. Chitinase breaks down the extracellular matrix in spherules, which helps them mature.
- *Endospore formation*: Endospores, which are produced by the developing spherule, have a thin cell wall and a single nucleus. These endospores are released when the spherule ruptures, which again can initiate the infection.
    - *Vaccine development*: Researchers are hard at work on a *Coccidioides* vaccine. A fusion protein comprising Ag2/Pra and Csa, an aspartyl proteinase, a T27K subcellular antigenic complex, and live-attenuated chitinase mutants are all promising vaccine candidates. These vaccinations are designed to elicit protective immunological responses in animal models.

PATHOLOGY

Lung is usually the affected organ. There may be reactivation or new infection. The host responses may be pyogenic (neutrophil proliferation) and granulomatous (lymphocytes, plasma cells, epithelioid cells, and giant cells). Calcification can occur in lung lesions.

CLINICAL FEATURES

Coccidioidomycosis can manifest in various clinical forms in humans, and these are often categorized based on the severity and location of the infection.

Pulmonary Coccidioidomycosis

Acute Primary Pulmonary Coccidioidomycosis

The incubation period is 2–3 weeks. In mild infection, the only finding is a positive skin test. In minority of cases, mild, influenza-like infection occurs. There may be headache, fever, cough, myalgia, and malaise which are self-limiting. In some patients, an allergic reaction develops in the form of pain in the joints, toxic erythema, erythema nodosum, erythema multiforme, and peripheral eosinophilia. In an endemic area, the primary infection occurs in the form of atypical pneumonia along with arthralgia (known as "desert rheumatism") or erythema nodosum. Pleural effusion may be the sole sign of an early infection.

Progressive or Persistent Pneumonia

Diffuse pulmonary or miliary disease can be caused by coccidioidomycosis in certain cases. Acute respiratory failure and persistent pneumonia lasting > 2 months are possible outcomes of this sickness.

Chronic Fibrocavitary Pneumonia

About 5% of patients with symptomatic coccidioidomycosis may develop chronic pneumonia with lung infiltrates and thin-walled cavities. Systemic symptoms, including night sweats and weight loss, can be caused by this, which is often associated with pulmonary fibrosis and type 2 diabetes.

In coccidioidomycosis, various allergic skin findings and other symptoms can occur as part of the primary illness. These manifestations can include:

- *Toxic erythema*: This is the most prevalent coccidioidomycosis cutaneous manifestation. It often manifests as a nonpruritic small papular rash during the first 48 hours after a patient has their initial symptoms. The rash usually goes away on its own. The acute exanthem refers to this early cutaneous response.
- *Erythema multiforme*: It manifests itself in a variety of ways, including target-like skin lesions, mouth involvement, pruritus, and palmar desquamation. This cutaneous response's clinical signs can be similar to those of an acute exanthem in the early phases of an infection. When many allergic skin signs are present, the result is toxic erythema.
- *Erythema nodosum*: The characteristic rash known as erythema nodosum can occur anywhere from 1 to 3 weeks into the course of the disease in some people. Most cases of this rash manifest on the front of the legs, specifically the shins, and they are marked by red nodules that are sensitive and located subcutaneously (under the skin).

  Within the endemic area, residents refer to this condition as "the bumps." Strangely, the prevalence of erythema nodosum in coccidioidomycosis can be affected by gender and ethnicity. White women may, for instance, experience it at a higher rate than women of other races.

  The development of delayed hypersensitivity in coccidioidin skin tests is often associated with erythema nodosum, suggesting that it might be a marker of a robust and protective cell-mediated immune (CMI) response. Erythema nodosum is connected with a positive result in certain instances, notably in pregnant women.
- *Migratory arthralgias*: It is another typical symptom of coccidioidomycosis arthralgia. The local populace refers it "desert rheumatism" when patients encounter a mix of fever, erythema nodosum, and arthralgias.

Disseminated Coccidioidomycosis

Although uncommon (affecting just around 0.5% of individuals infected), this variant includes the illness spreading beyond the lungs and lymph nodes to other organs. Hematogenous spread occurs from pulmonary foci (active, latent, or residual illness). Granuloma in the skin is the most prevalent manifestation. Abscesses can arise when subcutaneous tissue is involved.

Osteomyelitis and synovitis are the second most prevalent types of spread. Long bones, vertebrae, the skull, and the ribs may all be affected. Bones may have osteolytic and sclerotic foci. Several joints, including the knee, elbow, wrist, and ankle, may be implicated. Meningitis can occur in some situations of disseminated illness.

Chronic Cutaneous Coccidioidomycosis

On the skin, verrucous ulcers, surface maculopapular lesions, and subcutaneous fluctuant abscesses are formed. It is possible to misdiagnose squamous cell or basal cell carcinoma in some skin lesions.

Osteoarticular Disease

Common sites of spread include joints and bones, particularly weight-bearing joints and vertebrae. Synovitis and effusion are common symptoms of joint infections, which can spread to the underlying bone.

Meningitis

Coccidioidomycosis can induce meningitis, which is frequently associated with granuloma development or coccidioidoma. Headache, vomiting, and altered mental state are all possible symptoms.

Coccidioidomycosis in Acquired Immunodeficiency Syndrome Patients

Disseminated and severe form of disease is seen in AIDS and other immunocompromised conditions as those undergoing solid organ transplants, diabetes, Hodgkin's disease, or other immune system disorders. In 1987, it became a part of the AIDS monitoring case definition. There may be reactivation of previous focus.

Lesions in AIDS patients are as follows:

- *Cervical lymphadenopathy*: Lymph nodes may suppurate and discharge pus outside through sinuses.
- There may be primary cutaneous lesions in the form of plaque, nodules, and ulcers.
- Lymphangitis
- Allergic reaction with erythema (desert bumps)

Coccidioidomycosis is transmissible not only to humans but also to a wide variety of animals, including pigs, llamas, sheep, tigers, coyotes, nonhuman primates, rodents, sea otters, snakes, and horses.

Radiodiagnosis

X-ray chest shows lung infiltrates. Hilar or mediastinal lymphadenopathy is common. Cavity formation or coin-like lesions appear in lungs. The bones may show osteolytic lesions.

DIFFERENTIAL DIAGNOSIS

The pulmonary form of the disease resembles influenza, primary atypical pneumonia, and tuberculosis. Pulmonary infiltrates in an AIDS patient may be confused with infection with *Pneumocystis* pneumonia. Other forms of the disease should be differentiated from neoplasia, syphilis, tularemia, Glander's disease, bacterial osteomyelitis, and pyogenic meningitis.

LABORATORY DIAGNOSIS

Clinical specimens collected are sputum, bronchoalveolar lavage (BAL), cerebrospinal fluid (CSF), exudate, skin scrapings, pus, and biopsy.

Specimens and cultures should be handled using "Biohazard Safety Level 3" precautions.

Direct Examination

Clinical specimens should be examined under a microscope for quick diagnosis. Coccidioides tissue types are recognized by thick-walled spherules containing endospores.

Potassium hydroxide (KOH) mount, Gram stain, calcofluor white (CFW), and Papanicolaou stains: Clinical specimens reveal 20–80 µm thick-walled, doubly refractile spherules containing endospores. Some of the free endospores may be seen outside the spherule.

When endospores are expelled, they might be confused for yeast cells. Spherules and endospores are revealed in histopathological examinations of tissue samples stained with hematoxylin and eosin (H&E), periodic acid-Schiff (PAS), and Grocott–Gömöri's methenamine silver (GMS). Inflammatory cells surround the spherules. Young spherules or endospores should be differentiated from other fungi as *Blastomyces*, *Emmonsia* species, *Prototheca*, *Rhinosporidium seeberi*, and *Cryptococcus*.

Hyphal forms of the fungus may be rarely found in the clinical specimens. Immunofluorescent staining is a useful tool.

Culture

Specimens can be cultured on various media such as brain heart agar (BHIA), Sabouraud dextrose agar (SDA), or potato dextrose agar (PDA) at 25°C and 37°C. SDA at 25°C shows growth within 3–5 days. Colonies are initially smooth and moist and become suede-like to downy grayish white. They appear tan to brown on the reverse side. The fungus develops as mold at both incubation temperatures, which is unusual for fungi of deep mycotic infections. Arthroconidia with barrel shapes and sizes ranging from 2 to 4 µm are generated, and their morphology varies in color and appearance. Autolysis occurs in the alternate cells between arthroconidia. Hence, empty cells appear between arthroconidia. Other fungi which predominantly show arthroconidia are *Malbranchea* species and *Geotrichum candidum* which do not show "empty cells" between arthroconidia. All cultures are formalin-fixed before lactophenol cotton blue (LPCB) mounting. This is the only dimorphic fungus with quick growth and shows hyphal forms at both incubation temperatures.

The *exoantigen test*, which employs heat stable (HS) and heat labile (HL or F) antigens, can be utilized for identification. The test is highly sensitive and specific.

Genetic Identification

The AccuProbe test is used for definitive identification. It relies on a specific DNA probe that hybridizes to target rRNA of *Coccidioides* species, emitting a chemiluminescent signal for detection. Nucleic acid amplification tests (NAATs) are highly sensitive and can detect fungal DNA in clinical specimens like sputum.

Serology

Serological tests, such as complement fixation (CF) and immunodiffusion for CF (IDCF), latex agglutination (LA), and precipitation tests, are used for diagnosis and prognosis. The precipitin antibodies appear in 1-3 weeks and disappear in 2-3 weeks. Complement fixation test (CFT) that detects antibodies against the *Coccidioides* "F" antigen (chitinase-1) is strongly positive in disseminated cases. As antigen cross-reacts with *Histoplasma, Histoplasma* tests can be useful for diagnosis in an endemic area.

Skin Test

Coccidioidin skin tests are used to determine *Coccidioides* exposure or immunity. Asymptomatic lung infection produces a substantial positive response, although asymptomatic exposure can also provide a favorable consequence over time.

Cutaneous Anergy

Some people with active pulmonary illness may develop *C. immitis*-specific anergy, in which the skin test result turns negative. Following effective medication, a positive skin test response is commonly returned.

Animal Pathogenicity

Mice are infected through various routes such as intraperitoneal, intravenous, and intrathecal. Fatal disease is produced in animal within 3–4 weeks.

Because *Coccidioides* cultures are contagious, they must be handled with caution. Furthermore, genetic and serological tests are crucial in detecting infection.

TREATMENT

Various treatment options are summarized in **Table 18.2.**

TABLE 18.2: Treatment options for coccidioidomycosis.

Clinical form	*Antifungal treatment options*	*Indications for specific treatment*
Acute primary pulmonary coccidioidomycosis	• Supportive therapy • Azoles	• Weight loss > 10% • Intense night sweats > 1–2 weeks • Pleural effusions • Infiltration involving more than one half of both lungs • Prominent or persistent adenopathy • CF antibody titer > 1:16 • Symptoms persisting > 2 months • Ethnicity or medical condition predisposing to dissemination
Progressive or persistent pneumonia	• Amphotericin B (AmB) • High-dose azoles	• Hypoxia • Rapid disease progression
Chronic fibrocavitary pneumonia	• Oral azoles • Consider AmB	• Patients with type 2 diabetes or pulmonary fibrosis • Involvement of more than one lobe • Night sweats and weight loss • Persistent thin-walled cavities > 2.5 cm
Extrapulmonary coccidioidomycosis	• Oral azoles • Consider AmB	• Dissemination beyond the lungs and lymph nodes • Involvement of skin, bones, joints, and meninges

(CF: complement fixation)

CHAPTER

19

Paracoccidioidomycosis

INTRODUCTION

Paracoccidioidomycosis (PCM) is caused by a thermally dimorphic fungus of the genus *Paracoccidioides*. It may present as acute, subacute, or chronic granulomatous disease. Lungs are the primary target of the disease, and fungus may disseminate to other parts of the body. Although it is native to South and Central America, imported cases are reported from North America, Europe, Africa, and Asia. As a soil saprophyte, this fungus typically infects people when they work in the fields. *South American blastomycosis* is the name given to the disease since it is prevalent over the South American continent. *Paracoccidioidal granuloma, Lutz' mycosis, Brazilian blastomycosis*, and *Paracoccidioidal* blastomycosis are some of the alternative names for this condition.

HISTORY

Paracoccidioidomycosis was first described from Brazil in 1908 by Adolpho Lutz from cervical lymph node specimens of patients. In 1930, Floriano Paulo de Almeida named the genus *Paracoccidioides* and proposed the name of the species as *P. brasiliensis*. A new species was identified as *Paracoccidioides lutzii* by Teixeira et al. in 2014.

MYCOLOGY

In host tissues and on culture at 37°C, yeast form is present. At lower temperatures, it takes the moldy form. Yeast colonies appear after 10–15 days of incubation; the colonies are soft, wrinkled, and cream-colored. The yeast cells in the colonies range in size from 4 to 30 μm. They have a thick, refractile cell wall and a cytoplasm with noticeable lipid droplets. Yeast cells can be oval or elongated in shape with multipolar budding. The "pilot's wheel appearance" or "mariner's wheel appearance" is the most distinctive feature of yeast **(Figs. 19.1A and B)**. This form is characterized by mother cells encircled by a variety of peripheral daughter cells of size 2–10 μm in

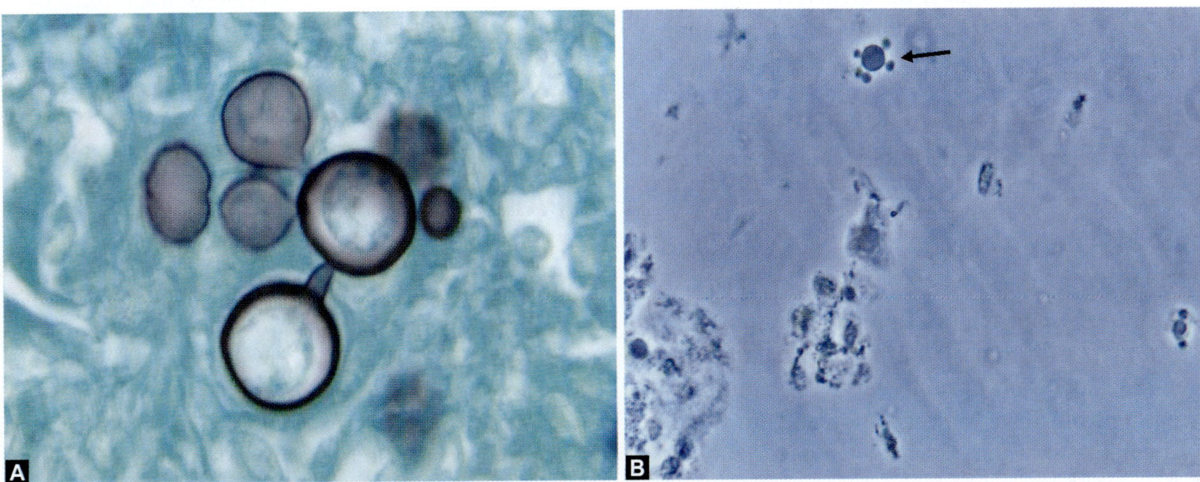

FIGS. 19.1A AND B: Multipolar budding of *Paracoccidioides brasiliensis*.
Source: Public Health Image Library CDC.

diameter. Few larger buds present along with smaller buds on the mother cell gives "Mickey Mouse" appearance. Additionally, cells with a single bud or a few blastoconidia chains can be seen.

During its 20–30-day growth phase at 20–26°C, the mold phase produces small colonies that range in color from white to tan. These colonies are encased in short aerial mycelia that frequently cling to the agar, eventually breaking its surface. Some of these isolates create a pigment that is rather brown in color.

Thin septate hyphae and single-celled conidia are seen on microscopic examination. Intercalary chlamydospores may be seen. Some strains can produce bulging arthroconidia along with conidia, when cultivated in an environment of nutritional deficiency. Also, conidia are contagious, and the yeast cells that develop from them cause a persistent, progressive illness. Yeast form to mycelial form (Y-M) conversion takes around 4–6 days on appropriate culture media. The conidia of *P. lutzii* appear elongated.

PHYLOGENETIC ANALYSIS AND GENETIC ANALYSIS

Using molecular techniques, *Paracoccidioides brasiliensis* has been classified as a member of family Onygenaceae, under order Onygenales and phylum Ascomycota.

EPIDEMIOLOGY

Geographic Distribution

Mexico, Central America, and South America are the main endemic regions of the fungus. Men in their 20s and 30s are the most common victims from rural communities. Brazil, South Paraguay, northeastern Argentina, Colombia, and Venezuela (especially the southern states) have the most cases documented. It is believed that there are between one and three cases per 100,000 people in Brazil. Few imported cases are reported outside of endemic countries such as the United States, Europe, and Japan.

Climate

The average temperature in these regions is between 18 and 23°C, and the subtropical forests are cold and humid. They get 800–2,000 mm of rain every year. Habitats in these areas typically have wet vegetation and are situated close to the bodies of water.

Uncertain Ecological Niche

There is no exact information about ecological nitche of the fungus since it is rarely found in soil alone. On rare occasions, nevertheless, the fungus has been isolated from Brazil's wild nine-banded armadillos (*Dasypus novemcinctus*).

Risk Factors For Paracoccidioidomycosis

- *Gender*: PCM predominantly affects male (10–100 times more than females) which is due to the interaction between estrogen receptors on *P. brasiliensis*, the presence of estrogens in the female body. The transformation of fungal mycelia into yeast forms is inhibited when estrogens bind to estrogen receptors in women. As a result of estrogen binding, females are less likely to develop disease after being infected. Males and females have identical infection rates before puberty, but the gender gap widens thereafter.
- *Occupational exposure*: Young- and middle-aged men working in farming, coffee cultivation, and lumber-related work are more likely to be exposed to fungal spores.
- *Nutritional status*: Poor nutritional status can weaken the immune system, making the individuals more susceptible to fungal infections, including PCM.

  Malnutrition and inadequate dietary intake can compromise the body's ability to mount an effective immune response against the fungus.
- *Alcoholism*: Chronic alcoholism can suppress the immune system, making individuals more vulnerable to fungal infections.

Modes of Transmission

Inhalation of mold spores (conidia) of the fungus causes infection. The conidia can infect the lungs once they are breathed in. PCM is not a contagious disease because it cannot be passed from one person to another or from animals to humans.

PATHOGENICITY

The development of PCM involves several factors, including host factors and microbial factors.

Host Factors

- *Protective T helper 1 (Th1) immunity*: A strong Th1 immune response is an important part of the host's

defense mechanism against PCM. Important effector cells in this reaction are macrophages.
- *Neutrophils [polymorphonuclear neutrophils (PMNs)]*: They also play a role in the host defense against PCM, and their fungistatic effect is enhanced by interferon gamma (IFN-γ) and granulocyte-macrophage colony-stimulating factor (GM-CSF).
- *Th1 versus T helper 2 (Th2) response*: People who suffer from PCM have unique immunological responses. A Th2-polarized response, marked by elevated levels of interleukin-4 (IL-4), interleukin-5 (IL-5), and interleukin-10 (IL-10), is linked to PCM.
- *CD4+/CD8+ T-lymphocyte ratio*: A decreased CD4+/CD8+ T-lymphocyte ratio is associated with the severity of PCM.

Microbial Factors

- *α-(1 → 3)-d-Glucan*: The level of pathogenicity is inversely proportional to the amount of this layer present in the cell wall. Macrophages are unable to break down the α-(1 → 3)-d-glucan outer layers.
- *Glycoprotein 43 (gp43)*: *This glycoprotein is strongly immunogenic*. Both diagnostic and prognostic applications rely on antibody titers to gp43.
- *Adhesin*: gp43 also acts as an adhesin, binding to laminin in the extracellular matrix of mammalian tissues.
- *Glyceraldehyde-3-phosphate dehydrogenase (GAPDH)*: This enzyme, found in the cell wall and cytoplasm of yeast forms, can bind to extracellular matrix proteins and promoting adherence to host tissues.

PATHOLOGY

Infection occurs by inhalation. In the lung the fungus transforms into yeast form. This induces non-specific inflammatory response in the acute phase. Granuloma formation, severe fibrosis of the interstitial spaces, necrosis, characterize the chronic progressive type.

Typically, lesions may spread to other parts of the body, such as the oropharyngeal mucosa, larynx, trachea, skin, lymph nodes, liver, spleen, adrenal glands, gut, and kidneys.

Pleomorphic yeast-like cells predominate in tissue sections. Finding the distinctive multiple budding cells that look like a "mariner's wheel appearance" is the final step in making a histopathological diagnosis of PCM.

Additional research demonstrated that the gp43-derived peptide P10 showed great promise as a vaccine candidate.

DIFFERENTIAL DIAGNOSIS

The list of diseases which should be differentiated from PCM is large. It includes pulmonary tuberculosis, cryptococcosis, leishmaniasis, leprosy, sporotrichosis, chromoblastomycosis, actinomycosis, and syphilis (skin eruptions).

The summary of clinical features is given in **Box 19.1**.

CLINICAL FEATURES

The disease may have acute presentation (Juvenile form). It is rare and seen in children and adolescents. It could affect lymph nodes, liver, spleen, and bone marrow.

Chronic form is seen in adults > 30 years. Lungs are affected predominantly. Spread may occur to lymph nodes, mucous membranes, etc. A third form called quiescent or latent form may also occur. Primary lesion of lung becomes a chronic granuloma that stays latent.

Clinical signs and symptoms depend on site of affection. Mucous membranes show ulceration, skin shows warty lesions. Lymph nodes get enlarged when infection spreads. When infection spreads to visceral organs it may present as cough and dyspnea. Other symptoms depend on site of affection—GI tract, CNS or musculoskeletal.

LABORATORY DIAGNOSIS

Specimens

The most common samples taken include mucocutaneous scrapings, sputum, cerebrospinal fluid (CSF), lymph node aspirate, biopsy, and tissue samples. Centrifugation [for sputum, bronchoalveolar lavage (BAL), CSF, and lymph node aspirate] and maceration of fragmented, biopsied tissues are examples of prior processing. Prior to being added to an appropriate culture medium at 25°C, the

BOX 19.1 Clinical forms of paracoccidioidomycosis.

- *Paracoccidioidomycosis*: Infection
- *Paracoccidioidomycosis*: Disease (duration based):
  - Acute or subacute forms (juvenile type): Severe
  - Chronic form (adult type):
    - Unifocal
    - Multifocal
  - Quiescent or sequelae (latent form)
- *Paracoccidioidomycosis: Disease (sites based)*:
  - Mucocutaneous lesions
  - Lymphatic lesions
  - Visceral lesions

sputum sample should be prepared using potassium hydroxide (KOH), sodium hydroxide, and N-acetyl L-cysteine.

Direct Examination

It is done by KOH mount/calcofluor stain and direct immunofluorescence (DIF). *Paracoccidioides* cells have a thick mucopolysaccharide wall and are birefringent under light microscopy in the 10% KOH mount (20–40% for biopsy). Characteristic morphological form of fungus resembles a "mariner's wheel appearance" or "Mickey Mouse" which are considered diagnostic findings. They are easily identifiable from other fungus by their size (from 10 to 30 μm) and the presence of multiple budding. Using calcofluor white makes direct microscopy more sensitive in general. The specificity and sensitivity of a DIF test are high.

Histopathology

Staining is done using hematoxylin and eosin (H&E) stains or special stains such as Grocott–Gömöri's methenamine silver (GMS) and periodic acid–Schiff (PAS). *P. brasiliensis* yeast forms appear as large cells with multiple small peripheral buds connected by narrow necks. Giant cells along with other inflammatory cells are seen in the granuloma. Immunohistochemical method is highly sensitive and specific. Other fungi such as *Histoplasma capsulatum*, *Cryptococcus*, and *Coccidioides imitis* should be ruled out. Due to multiple budding, the fungus may be confused with *Cokeromyces recurvatus* and *Mucor circinelloides*.

Culture

Sabouraud dextrose agar (SDA) slants are (with antibiotics and actidione) incubated at 25 and 37°C.

- *Growth at 37°C*: White to cream colored, wrinkled, and pasty colonies are produced within a week.
    - Lactophenol cotton blue (LPCB) mount: It shows oval or globose multiple budding yeast cells with daughter cells attached.
- *Growth at 25°C*: SDA slant shows flat to wrinkled, leathery colonies initially, which later on get covered with mycelium. The reverse side is brown to tan.
    - LPCB mount: Thin, hyaline, septate, and branched hyphae are produced with two types of conidia: (1) intercalary and (2) terminal bulging arthroconidia, which later differentiate into small aleurioconidia and single-celled sessile conidia, pear-shaped, formed randomly along fertile hyphae.
- *Conversion to yeast form in vitro*: Yeast extract agar or enriched medium such as brain heart infusion (BHI) agar with 5% sheep blood and glutamine are used to demonstrate mycelial to yeast transformation.
- *Exoantigens test* using antigens 1, 2, and 3 is used for identification of the fungus.

Serodiagnosis

Antibody Detection Tests

- *ID test*: Immunodiffusion assay is performed that relies on a standardized yeast culture filtrate antigen that primarily contains gp43. The specificity of the test is 98.9% and sensitivity is 84.3%.
- *Counterimmunoelectrophoresis (CIE)*: CIE has sensitivity comparable to or higher than ID test.
- *Complement fixation (CF)*: It uses an antigen derived from yeast and yields a positive result in 80–90% of patients experiencing active illness.
- *Enzyme immunoassay (EIA)*: It uses *P. brasiliensis* gp43 antigen and can eliminate cross-reactions with proper serum adsorption. Specificity can be increased by deglycosylation of gp43.

Antigen Detection Tests

One way to identify antigen in a patient's serum is to use the species-specific monoclonal antibody against gp43. Immunoblotting and EIA test are used. The test is highly sensitive. The advantage of antigen detection test can be seen in the diagnosis of infection in immunosuppressed patients in which there is poor antibody response. EIA is also available for the detection of antigen in urine.

- *Paracoccidioides skin test*: It is commonly used as for epidemiology purpose. The antigen is produced from *P. brasiliensis* strains and contains gp43 as a major active component. It is used to elicit delayed cutaneous hypersensitivity. A positive test cannot differentiate between previous exposure and recent active disease and the test is not suitable for immunocompromised patients.
- *Genetic identification*: Polymerase chain reaction (PCR) methods target PbGP43 exon 2 or universal fungal primers [internal transcribed spacer 4 and 5 (ITS4 and ITS5)] for amplifying ITS1, 5.8S, and ITS2. Sequencing ITS regions can confirm the genetic similarity of *P. brasiliensis* isolates.

TREATMENT

Treatment options for PCM are given in **Table 19.1**.

TABLE 19.1: Treatment options for paracoccidioidomycosis (PCM).

Treatment	*Descriptions*	*Indications*	*Duration*
Sulfonamides (e.g., sulfadiazine)	Effective for nonlife-threatening PCM	Moderate-to-severe nondisseminated PCM, primarily oral and mucosal lesions	• 6–12 months (induction) • 12–24 months (maintenance)
Amphotericin B (AmB)	Reserved for severe cases unresponsive to other therapies	Severe disseminated PCM or patients unresponsive to other therapies	30–60 days (induction)
Azoles (e.g., ketoconazole, itraconazole, voriconazole)	Effective for most PCM cases with lower relapse rates compared to other treatments	Various forms of PCM, including pulmonary, mucocutaneous, and disseminated	6–24 months, depending on patient's response

SECTION

5

Opportunistic Mycoses

Section Outline

CHAPTER

20 Candidiasis

INTRODUCTION

Candidiasis is caused by Candida species. *Candida* is a yeast-like fungus that occurs as commensal in the human body in some persons. The common sites of its location are mouth, vagina, and intestinal tract. Even at these sites, it can produce symptoms when the numbers increase to a great extent. It is therefore challenging to know whether the agent is occurring as a commensal or it is responsible for infection. When the immunity is compromised it can produce invasive disease. Chronic illnesses, malignancy, anti-cancer drugs, immunosuppressants, acquired immunodeficiency disease (AIDS) are some predisposing causes of invasive candidiasis. *Candida* is probably one of the commonest opportunistic fungi causing human infections. Though *Candida albicans* is the commonest species seen in humans, there are many other species that cause illness in humans. These are referred to as non-albicans *Candida*. They are reported in increasing numbers in recent years. Their speciation is essential as many are showing drug resistance. Some species recognized in last few years like *C. auris* are even showing multi-drug resistance. Newer technologies are available for rapid and accurate identification of *Candida* species. These aspects are covered in this chapter.

HISTORY

For ages, the presence of clinical symptom "thrush" or "moniliasis" has been known as a "clinical entity." In the year 1844, Bennett firmly showed fungal etiology of thrush. The developing yeast-like fungus was termed *Odium albicans* by Robin in 1853. Earlier, Hill (1751) misclassified *Candida* as *Monilia*, a genus that contains fungi that grow on plants. Berkhout (1923) established the genus *Candida* for asporogenous yeasts with few hyphae that lie flat and crumble apart into longer or shorter pieces.

COMMON *CANDIDA* SPECIES

There are 163 species of *Candida*. The common species which produce human infections include:

- *Candida albicans*
- *Candida tropicalis*
- *Candida parapsilosis*
- *Candida glabrata*
- *Candida krusei*
- *Candida guilliermondii*
- *Candida kefyr (previously known as pseudotropicalis)*
- *Candida dubliniensis*
- *Candida auris*
- *Candida haemulonii*
- *Candida rugosa*
- *Candida famata*
- *Candida lusitaniae*
- *Candida viswanathii*

Candida stellatoidea is now included in *C. albicans*.

TAXONOMY

The genus *Candida* is included in the phylum Fungi Imperfecti, order Moniliales, and family Cryptococcaceae. Serotype A and serotype B are the two varieties of *C. albicans*. The areas in which they are found differ. India is home to both serotypes. When it comes to antigens, *C. tropicalis* and serotype A are very similar.

Candida species are common in human gut, vagina, and skin flora. Even at these locations, they may infect whenever they get an opportunity. More and more cases of infection have been documented in the recent years due to *Candida* species other than *albicans*.

EPIDEMIOLOGY

In humans, *Candida* species occur as commensals. Common sites of their presence include the skin, the digestive system, and the female reproductive system. The majority of cases of candidiasis is endogenous, meaning they originate within or on human tissues.

It is known that strains can be transmitted in hospitals and communities through direct contact between people or through fomites.

As the third most common cause of bloodstream infections (BSIs) contracted while receiving medical treatment, *Candida* species are serious disease-causing microorganisms. In intensive care units, it has the potential to spread like wildfire. Nonalbicans *Candida* species have recently become more common than *C. albicans*. Species such as *C. auris* and the *C. haemulonii* complex show remarkable resistance to therapy.

IMMUNITY

The immune system's ability to fight candidiasis depends on both innate and adaptive responses. *Candida* infections affect a large number of people when the immune system of the host weakens. Infection with *C. tropicalis* can occur in neutropenic individuals. *Candida* infections have been on the rise since the acquired immunodeficiency syndrome (AIDS) pandemic began. People who have primary immunodeficiencies, which impact the immune system's cell-mediated responses, are also more likely to get *Candida* infections.

Candida species antigens are of two main categories:

1. Cell wall antigens
2. Cytoplasmic antigens

The main antigenic component of the cell wall is mannan. The cell wall contains glucan polymers, which have a lower immunological activity. Antigenic characteristics are exhibited by a number of cytoplasmic products.

PATHOGENESIS

Candida albicans undergoes polymorphism when it switches from a commensal to a pathogenic form in response to environmental changes. During this stage, blastopores undergo a morphological change into hyphae, with pseudohyphae acting as a transitional stage.

Candidalysin, an essential component in the progression of candidiasis, is a toxin that is unique to hyphae. The hyphae of *C. albicans* produce it, and it damages the cells of the host. Candidalysin can weaken the cytoplasmic contents by intercalating with, permeabilizing through, and forming holes in the epithelial membrane. It is the first peptide toxin produced by any human pathogenic fungus to be identified.

Proteins, fibrinogens, and fibronectins are used as adhesions by *Candida. C. albicans* attaches to host cells by the action of adhesins (Als3 and Hwp1), which are mostly produced during hyphae development.

An important mechanism in the promotion of pathogenicity in *Candida* species is the thigmotropism of *C. albicans*. Thigmotropism is the ability of an organism to respond to touch or other physical stimuli. It is also the ability to sense changes in the surface contours and respond to them. Probably, *C. albicans* utilizes this property for tissue invasion. This is also the process that helps it to form biofilms on inanimate surfaces. Thigmotropism is a process that helps bacteria grow biofilms on inanimate surfaces and then spread those biofilms throughout host tissues.

- *Enzymes*: There are three main enzymes produced by *C. albicans*: (1) Hemolysin, (2) phospholipase, and (3) secreted aspartyl protease (SAP). The attachment to host tissue and the rupture of the host cell membrane are both facilitated by hydrolytic enzymes. These enzymes help the pathogen invade blood vessel and mucous membrane surfaces while evading the host immune system.
- *Phenotypic switching*: Morphological changes, such as blastopores becoming pseudohyphae and finally real hyphae, aid in adaptation to different host conditions. Such change allows it to evade immune mechanisms and invade the host tissues.
- *Biofilm formation*: Majority of *C. albicans* infections cause significant morbidity and mortality due to the biofilms similar to that the bacteria form on host surfaces or implants.

CLINICAL FEATURES

Candidiasis or Candidosis

Association of *Candida* with humans could be varied. It could be commensalism or acting as an opportunistic infectious agent or as an allergen. The infection caused by *Candida* species is called candidiasis or candidosis. The clinical manifestations of *Candida* species are given in **Box 20.1**.

Among the fungal infections in the mouth, the most prevalent is candidiasis. Oral *Candida* carriers were originally estimated to be between 35% and 80% of the population. It is believed that >80% of oral fungal isolates contain *C. albicans*, making it the most frequent species in both infected and healthy mouths. *C. glabrata*, *C. dubliniensis*, *C. parapsilosis*, *C. krusei*, and *C. tropicalis* are some of the other *Candida* species found in the mouth.

BOX 20.1 | Clinical classification of candidiasis.

- *Infectious diseases*:
  - *Mucocutaneous manifestations*:
    - Oral: Thrush, stomatitis, glossitis, and cheilitis
    - Alimentary: Esophagitis and gastritis
    - Vulvovaginitis, balanitis, and balanoposthitis
    - Chronic mucocutaneous candidiasis
    - Ocular candidiasis
  - *Cutaneous manifestations*:
    - Intertriginous and generalized
    - Paronychia and onychomycosis
    - Diaper dermatitis
    - Candidal granuloma
  - *Systemic manifestations*:
    - Urinary tract
    - Endocarditis
    - Pulmonary candidiasis
    - Meningitis
    - Candidemia
    - Dissemination
    - Arthritis
    - Osteomyelitis
    - Endophthalmitis
- *Allergic diseases*:
  - Candidids
  - Eczema
  - Asthma
  - Gastritis

The most common predisposing factors for candidal infections are the use of prosthetic replacements, orthodontic appliances, dry mouth (xerostomia), poor oral hygiene, and AIDS. Nutritional deficiencies (iron, folic acid, and vitamin deficiency), endocrinopathy (diabetes, hypothyroidism, hypoparathyroidism) and autoimmune diseases (Sjögren's syndrome, etc.), patients on chemotherapy, and steroids therapy are other factors for the promotion of candidal infections.

Infectious Diseases

Mucocutaneous Candidiasis

Oral Candidiasis

The oral cavity and perioral region are the exclusive domains of primary candidiasis, although systemic conditions might give rise to secondary candidiasis.

When an infection impacts just the mouth and the surrounding areas, it is called primary candidiasis. When the infection is a component of a systemic condition, it is called secondary candidiasis. In its most basic form, there are four candidiasis types: (1) Pseudomembranous, (2) acute erythematous, (3) chronic erythematous, and (4) chronic hyperplastic/nodular.

Pseudomembranous candidiasis: It represents the majority. White plaques or patches appear on the oral mucosa and can be gently scraped off. Typical sites for lesions include the tongue, buccal mucosa, and both the hard and soft palates. Sometimes, it is accompanied with an unpleasant aftertaste.

Acute erythematous or atrophic candidiasis: Painful red lesion on the back of the tongue is a common symptom. Denture stomatitis, prosthetic palatitis, and chronic erythematous or atrophic candidiasis are some of the names for the same condition. The mucosal lesions are red and localized to the locations where the prosthesis is placed.

Chronic hyperplastic candidiasis (Candida leukoplakia): The deep insertion of these white deposits into the oral cavity tissue makes mild scraping ineffective in removing them. Its most prevalent locations are the buccal mucosa and the sides of the tongue.

Angular cheilitis: Redness, erosions, and crusts—sometimes coated with white plaque—are clinical manifestations of an inflammatory illness that affects one or both corners of the lips.

Median rhomboid glossitis: It has no known cause and is frequently linked to secondary *Candida* infection. A nodular or smooth lesion is the clinical manifestation of the alteration that is situated in the center of the tongue.

Gastrointestinal Tract Infections

Esophageal candidiasis: Inflammatory plaques form in the esophagus. They may cause dysphagia, odynophagia, retrosternal burning sensation (acid reflux), epigastric pain, and back discomfort. In human immunodeficiency virus (HIV)-positive persons, esophageal candidiasis is an AIDS-defining condition. Lesions in immunocompromised individuals may progress to stomach producing gastritis. *Small intestine* is sometimes affected. Intestinal infections can be superficial, affecting only the mucosa and submucosa, or deep, affecting the entire intestinal wall and causing tissue damage, perforation, or even distant dissemination. In stool of normal persons, *Candida* may be present in small numbers as commensals. In stool of patients with irritable bowel syndrome (IBS) and inflammatory bowel disease (IBD), *Candida* is found in higher numbers. *Candida* is implicated as one of the probable causative agents of antibiotic-associated diarrhea.

Vulvovaginitis, Balanitis, and Balanoposthitis

- Vulvovaginitis is one of the most common infections caused by *Candida* species. There is itching, burning sensation, and dyspareunia along with white curdy vaginal discharge. As varying percentages of females carry *Candida* in their vagina, interpretation becomes difficult. Local examination shows vulvar erythema and edema. Vulvovaginitis is common in young sexually active females.
- In balanitis and balanoposthitis, there is pruritus, edema, and whitish lesions over glans penis. In some patients, erosions and edema of prepuce may occur. It may lead to phimosis later. As this infection may be transmitted by sexual contact, both the partners should be treated.

Chronic Mucocutaneous Candidiasis (CMC)

CMC is a hereditary immunodeficiency disorder, which is a persistent or recurring infection with *Candida* due to malfunction of T cells. CMC is a collection of illnesses that usually manifest themselves in infancy. It is characterized by recurring and chronic *Candida* infections that can affect the skin, nails, and mucosal surfaces. The chances of systemic spread are minimal. The first symptom is usually oral candidiasis or diaper dermatitis. There are hyperplastic, nodular lesions with white patches and deep crevices. Common symptoms can include nails becoming hyperkeratotic and fragmented with paronychia. Cutaneous lesions are hyperkeratotic, erythematous, and serpiginous plaques. Lips get cracks, and angular cheilitis is seen. Many viral, autoimmune, and endocrine diseases are linked to CMC. Some instances of endocrinopathies include hypoparathyroidism, thyroid abnormalities, and Addison's disease. *Candida* granuloma in CMC is characterized by hyperkeratotic lesions that are disfiguring and well-defined; these lesions can grow to be several centimeters in size and manifest on the scalp, lips, eyelids, or face. Mucosal manifestations of CMC include vulvovaginitis and infections of the oropharynx, larynx, and esophagus.

Infection of Eye

Candida is one of the organisms which may cause keratitis. In a patient with fungemia, it can lead to endogenous endophthalmitis.

Cutaneous Candidiasis

Intertrigo

A typical symptom is inflammation of the skin folds. The axilla, submammary, umbilical, perineum, and under the rings on the hands are typical places that are impacted. People who are overweight or elderly, especially those who have diabetes mellitus, are also more likely to experience intertrigo. Folds between fingers and toes are also the likely sites of affection.

Paronychia and Onychomycosis

Paronychia is inflammation of nail folds of fingers and toes. In onychomycosis, the distal part of nail is affected.

Diaper Dermatitis

Diaper rash is seen in infants after use of diapers which leads to maceration and diaper rash. There are maculopapular lesions with vesicles and satellite pustules. Intertriginous areas of gluteal crease, perineum, and inguinal folds show erythematous rash. Causes are mechanical friction, diaper being soiled with urine and feces, variation in skin pH, and secondary infection with bacteria and *Candida*.

Systemic Candidiasis

Candidemia and Septicemia

It occurs in neonates and adults with immunodeficiencies. Many species may cause this condition, the common ones being *C. albicans*, *C. tropicalis*, *C. krusei*, and *C. parapsilosis*. *C. parapsilosis* is associated with total parenteral nutrition (TPN), while *C. tropicalis* is seen in neutropenic patients. Newly emerging yeasts are *C. auris*, *C. haemulonii*, *C. glabrata*, and *Pichia anomala*.

Disseminated Candidiasis

There may be serious infections of oropharynx and upper gastrointestinal tract. Various predisposing factors are:

- Patients with catheterization
- Broad-spectrum antibiotics for a long duration
- Hematological malignancies
- Transplant recipients
- Severe burns
- Postsurgery
- Hyperalimentation

Urinary Tract Infection

Predisposing factors are:

- Disseminated candidiasis
- Diabetes mellitus
- Pregnancy
- Prolonged use of antibiotics
- Catheterization

Candiduria: The infection or colonization of the kidneys or lower urinary tract might cause this. Indicators of a urinary tract infection include pus cells in urine. The majority of infections is transmitted through bloodborne pathogens. While indwelling drainage devices are prevalent in hospitalized patients, candiduria is rare in otherwise healthy individuals. *Candida* can enter the urine stream through the catheters. The vaginal cavity is a breeding ground for *Candida* species, making women more susceptible to infection.

Endocarditis and Pericarditis

Infection of previously abnormal native valves or prosthetic valves takes place. Pericarditis may be associated with thoracic surgery.

Meningitis

Infection is common in low-birth-weight babies and elderly patients. Meningitis may also follow complicated neurosurgical procedures or ventriculoperitoneal shunts. Chronic meningitis and shunt obstruction may lead to formation of hydrocephalus.

Arthritis

Infection spreads through the hematogenous route or direct inoculation during surgery.

Osteomyelitis

It develops by the hematogenous route. Osteolytic lesions may develop.

Endophthalmitis

It is either manifestation of disseminated *Candida* infection or a rare complication of ocular surgery.

Pancreatitis

Fungal infection in a patient with pancreatitis may turn out to be a severe outcome.

Pulmonary Candidiasis

Pulmonary involvement occurs through systemic infection. Presence of *Candida* in sputum is considered nonpathogenic unless we isolate *Candida* from a lung biopsy sample.

Allergic Diseases

Allergic reaction similar to "id" reaction to dermatophytes may occur in some individuals due to metabolic products. Cutaneous urticaria and eczema are reported.

Candida in AIDS

Patients with AIDS may suffer from a variety of infections due to *Candida*. There may be increased oral carriage, oral candidiasis, esophageal candidiasis, infections of urogenital system vulvovaginitis, balanitis, or hematogenous dissemination. Various oral presentations include thrush, erythema, angular cheilitis, or leucoplakia.

LABORATORY DIAGNOSIS

Specimens will depend on the sites affected. These include swabs collected by rubbing lesions on oral or vaginal mucosa. Sputum, cerebrospinal fluid (CSF), urine, skin and nail scrapings, and tissue biopsies are collected for direct demonstration and culture. Blood for culture can also be submitted. Molecular techniques are available for diagnosis of *Candida*. Serum is submitted for serological tests in some situations.

Microscopy

- Potassium hydroxide (KOH) (10%) slide mount is performed on the specimens collected which depend on the sites of involvement. Specimens including skin or nail scraping and whitish patches from oral mucosa and vagina are collected with sterile swab.
- *Tube KOH*: Biopsy is kept in a tube of KOH overnight and after that wet mount is prepared to see budding yeast cells with or without pseudohyphae.
- Gram staining is performed on suitable specimens for detection of gram-positive yeast cells (4–8 μm), pseudohyphae, and pus cells. Initially, it was thought that presence of pseudohyphae signifies the colonization and tissue invasion. But it should be kept in mind that some *Candida* species do not produce pseudohyphae and may still produce invasive infections.
- Other staining methods used are PAP smear and calcofluor staining method.
- Grocott–Gömöri's methenamine silver (GMS) staining is used to demonstrate fungal element in tissue (black against green background).

Fungal Culture

Sabouraud Dextrose Agar

Specimens are inoculated on two sets of Sabouraud dextrose agar (SDA) slants with antibiotics; one slant is incubated at 37°C while the second slant is incubated at 25°C. Smooth, creamy, and pasty colonies **(Fig. 20.1)** appear in 2–3 days. *C. tropicalis* shows hyphal fringe at the edge of colony. Lactophenol cotton blue (LPCB) mount or Gram staining is performed from the colonies. As the colonies are smooth and pasty, Gram staining is preferred.

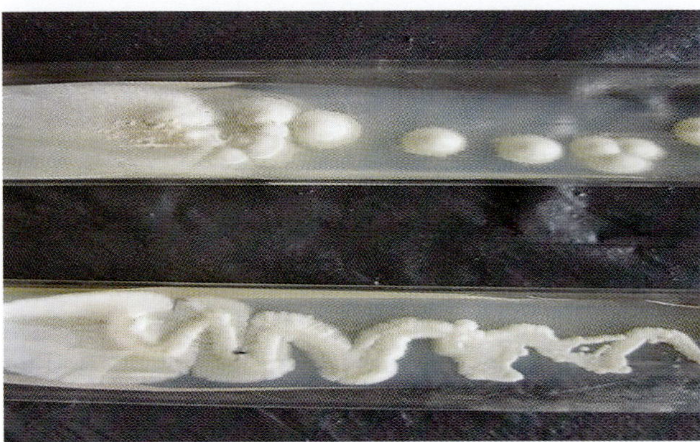

FIG. 20.1: SDA slant showing pasty colonies of *Candida* species. (SDA: Sabouraud dextrose agar)

Candida species grow on blood agar at 37°C after just overnight incubation. Hence, in an unsuspected case, *Candida* may be observed accidentally on blood agar inoculated for bacterial culture.

Brain Heart Infusion Broth for Blood Culture

For diagnosis of candidemia, blood is collected in brain heart infusion broth which is incubated and periodically subcultured on SDA slants. After 48 hours of incubation, before the first subculture, Gram staining is performed from smear prepared from blood culture bottle so that a provisional report for the presence or absence of growth can be given. *Lysis centrifugation test* increases the sensitivity of blood culture. It is a laboratory technique used to detect BSIs caused by fungi, bacteria, or mycobacteria, especially in cases where other blood culture methods have limitations.

Automated Blood Culture Systems

Blood is collected in a blood culture bottle and incubated till a signal is "flagged" or till 5 days. Subculture and smears are prepared from the flagged bottles.

Growth Pattern on Cornmeal Agar

Part of colony is taken from growth on SDA slant and inoculated on cornmeal agar (CMA) by a method known as Dalmau method.

Conventional Diagnosis

Further identification of *Candida* species is done by germ tube test, growth pattern (with special reference to the formation of chlamydoconidia) on CMA, growth on CHROMagar, sugar fermentation tests, and sugar assimilation test. Other biochemical tests which are added are rapid trehalose test, urease test, and formation of surface pellicle in liquid medium.

Germ Tube Test (Reynaud's Braude Phenomena)

- It is used for presumptive identification of *C. albicans* and *C. dubliniensis*. Very small inoculum (to provide light suspension containing approximately 10^5–10^6 cell/mL) is picked up from SDA and emulsified in freshly procured pooled serum in a test tube.
- The suspension is incubated at 37°C. After 2 hours of incubation, a drop of suspension is taken on a grease-free slide and cover slip is placed over the suspension to be observed under low and high power of a microscope.
- If a test is negative after 2 hours, make another preparation after 3 hours from the same suspension which is incubated further. Germ tube formation should not be looked for after 4 hours (hyphae formation may start).
- Along with the test strain, the standard strain of *C. albicans* is tested simultaneously with the same serum as positive control and *C. parapsilosis* as negative control.
- *Germ tube test is a tube-like outgrowth from a conidium or spore; it is the beginning of the hyphae and appears as filaments that are not constricted at their points of beginning* **(Figs. 20.2A to C)**. If filaments with constriction are present, they are pseudohyphae.
- Gram staining may be useful from the suspension which has two advantages. One is that under oil immersion, constriction is easily made out in pseudohyphae and the second is for recordkeeping. The other method to preserve the findings of a germ tube test is addition of formalin. Each batch of serum should be tested with known positive strain as serum may contain inhibitory substances such as ferritin.

Germ tube test has low sensitivity and reproducibility. Some variants of *C. albicans* give this test negative. The test can also be performed on Mueller–Hinton agar. **Table 20.1** shows differences between germ tube and pseudohyphae.

Cornmeal Agar Culture (Dalmau Method)

- The suspected strain is streaked on CMA with Tween 80, and cover slip is placed over the streaking.
- Along with the test strain, the control strain of *C. albicans* is also inoculated.
- The plate is incubated at 25°C for 2–3 days.
- The growth pattern is observed under an inverted microscope. Also, production of chlamydoconidia is observed. If an inverted microscope is not available,

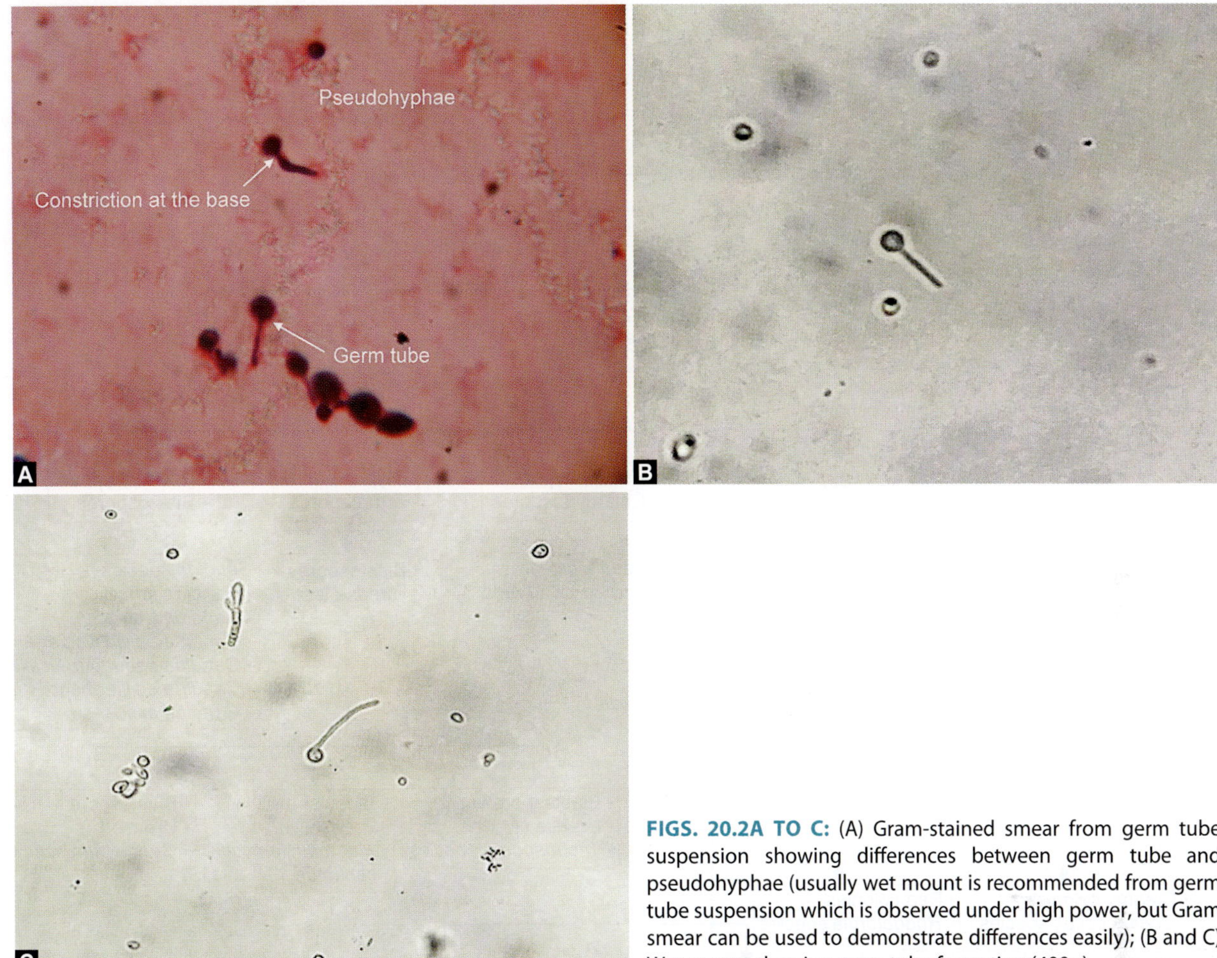

FIGS. 20.2A TO C: (A) Gram-stained smear from germ tube suspension showing differences between germ tube and pseudohyphae (usually wet mount is recommended from germ tube suspension which is observed under high power, but Gram smear can be used to demonstrate differences easily); (B and C) Wet mount showing germ tube formation (400×).

TABLE 20.1: Differences between germ tube and pseudohyphae.

Features	*Germ tube (later forms hyphae)*	*Pseudohyphae*
Growth process	Apical elongation with continuous growth at the tip	Budding with formation of constricted septa
Terminal cell	Elongated and cylindrical	Shorter and more spherical
Cell wall	Uniform and parallel	Constricted at septa, irregular
Septa	Straight and perpendicular, typically complete	Curved, pinched, and often incomplete
Origin of branches	No constriction at the point of branching	Branches arise from constricted areas

one can seal the plate and observe under 10× objective of a light microscope.

- Other different media used for the demonstration of chlamydoconidium are rice starch agar, Staib agar, and tobacco agar.

Flowchart 20.1 shows an algorithm used for the identification of yeast isolated from clinical specimen. Biochemical tests such as sugar fermentation and sugar assimilation which are used for the identification of common *Candida* species are shown in **Tables 20.2 and 20.3**, respectively.

CHROMagar

Colonies of various colors are produced when enzymes from *Candida* species react with a medium that contains diverse chromogenic substrates. Subculturing an isolate colony on this medium and incubating it for 1–2 days comprise the standard procedure. In contrast to the blue colonies produced by *C. tropicalis*, those of *C. albicans* are green in color. One cannot obtain the desired effects if the medium is not from a reputed manufacturer.

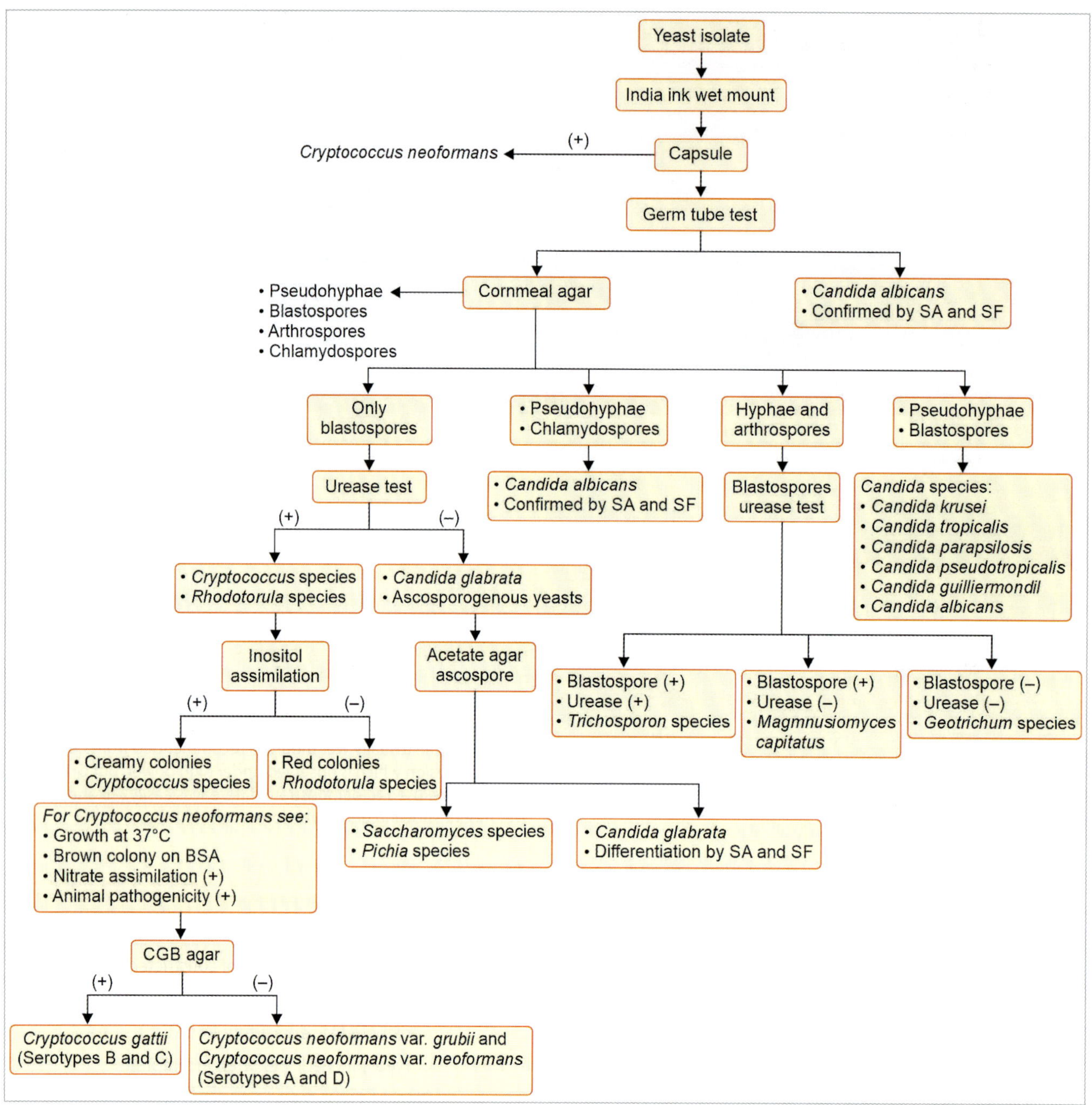

FLOWCHART 20.1: Identification scheme of commonly encountered yeast isolates.
(SA: sugar assimilation; SF: sugar fermentation)

MYCOLOGICAL CHARACTERISTICS

Candida albicans

- *Colony morphology on Sabouraud Dextrose Agar*: The rate of growth is rapid, the colony matures in 3 days. Cream-colored, pasty, smooth colonies are produced on SDA (***see* Fig. 20.1**). Initially after overnight incubation, colonies are small, but after 24–48 hours, the size increases. Sometime, confluent pasty growth may cause confusion as it may closely resemble colonies of *Cryptococcus*; hence, confirmation is done by microscopic examination. Negative stains such as India ink and nigrosine are used to demonstrate capsule. Capsule is absent in *Candida* species. Old colonies may appear wrinkled and show extensions

TABLE 20.2: Fermentation reactions of *Candida* species.

Candida species	*Glu*	*Mal*	*Suc*	*Lac*
Candida albicans	AG	AG	–	–
Candida tropicalis	AG	AG	AG	–
Candida kefyr	AG	AG	AG	–
Candida guilliermondii	AG	–	AG	–
Candida parapsilosis	AG	–	–	–
Candida krusei	AG	–	–	–
Candida glabrata	AG	–	–	–

[A: acid production; G: gas production; Glu: glucose; Lac: lactose; Mal: maltose; Suc: sucrose; –: no reaction)

TABLE 20.3: Assimilation reactions of *Candida* species and growth on TRM.

Candida species	*Glu*	*Mal*	*Suc*	*Lac*	*Cel*	*Gal*	*Tre*	*Raf*	*Mel*	*Xyl*	*Ino*	*Dul*	*TRM*
Candida albicans	+	+	+	+	+	+	+	–	–	+	–	–	PP
Candida tropicalis	+	+	+	–	+	+	+	–	–	+	–	–	M
Candida kefyr	+	–	+	+	+	+	–	+	–	+	–	–	SP
Candida parapsilosis	+	+	+	–	–	+	+	–	–	+	–	–	RP
Candida guilliermondii	+	+	+	–	+	+	+	+	+	+	–	+	PsP
Candida krusei	+	–	–	–	–	–	–	–	–	+	–	–	DP
Candida glabrata	+	–	–	–	–	–	+	–	–	+	–	+	PP

(Cel: cellobiose; Dul: dulcitol; DP: pink and dry; Gal: galactose; Glu: glucose; Ino: inositol; Lac: lactose; M: maroon; Mal: maltose; Mel: melibiose; OP: orange pink; PP: pale pink; PsP: pink and pasty; Raf: raffinose; RP: rose pink; SP: Salmon pink; Suc: sucrose; Tre: trehalose; TRM: tetrazolium reduction medium; Xyl: xylose; +: assimilation positive; - : assimilation negative)

on enriched media as blood agar which are commonly called "feet" which develops at the border of colony.

- *Microscopic morphology*: Yeast cells are round to oval (3.5 × 4–8 µm); pseudohyphae and true hyphae may be present. The germ tube test is positive.
- *Growth pattern on CMA*: Different growth patterns are shown in **Figures 20.3 and 20.4**. Pseudohyphae and (sometimes) real hyphae, along with clusters of spherical blastoconidia (yeast cells) spaced regularly at septa, provide a "spidery" appearance when cultured at 25°C for 72 hours. At the end of hyphae or short lateral branches, the majority of isolates produce terminal thick chlamydoconidia, which are asexual spores with thick walls. Sometimes, these conidia are produced in clusters similar to *C. dubliniensis*. Hence, one cannot rely on these findings. It is observed that in the case of *C. albicans*, chlamydoconidia are produced at the sites where microaerophilic conditions are available. Because microaerophilic conditions are created around the edge of the coverslip placed over CMA, it increases chlamydoconidium production; CMA plates examined under a low-power microscope are likely to show these features. Chlamydoconidium is produced in different areas below the coverslip by *C. dubliniensis*. The location of chlamydoconidia may be terminal or intercalary (within hyphae). When Tween 80 is added to corn meal agar it enhances production of chlamydoconidia. **Figures 20.3 and 20.4** show morphological features of *C. albicans* on

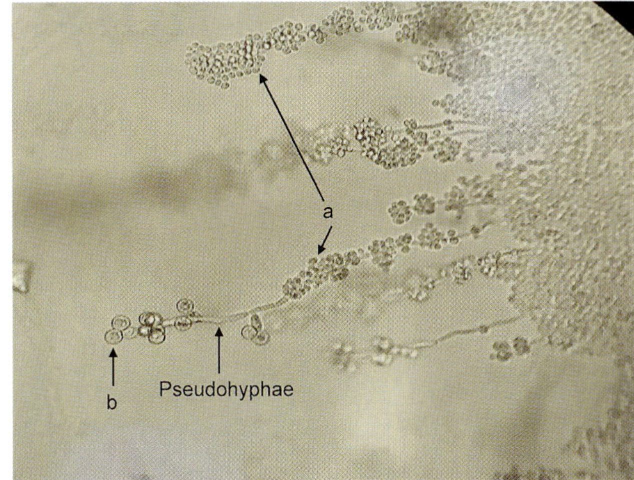

FIG. 20.3: Growth of *Candida albicans* on CMA. (a) Clusters of blastoconidia. (b) Terminal chlamydoconidia (under low power). (CMA: cornmeal agar)

CMA. **Figure 20.5** shows abundant production of chlamydoconidia by *C. dubliniensis* on CMA.

Candida tropicalis

- *Colony morphology*: Rate of growth is rapid, the colony matures in 3 days. Colonies are cream colored, wrinkled near the edge. They may have "mycelial fringe."
- *Microscopic morphology*: Yeast cells are round to oval (3.5–7.0 × 5.5–10.0 µm). The germ tube test is negative.
- CMA (Dalmau plate) at 25°C for 72 hours shows blastoconidia singly or in very small groups all along "long graceful" pseudohyphae **(Fig. 20.6)** (*C. parapsilosis* has short pseudohyphae). A few teardrop-shaped chlamydoconidia may be seen in some isolates only. Their wall is thin as compared to those produced by *C. albicans*.
- *CHROMagar*: Blue-colored colonies are produced.
- *Growth in SABI broth*: *C. tropicalis* produces surface pellicle in SABI broth **(Fig. 20.7)**. This test may be used to differentiate it from *C. parapsilosis*.

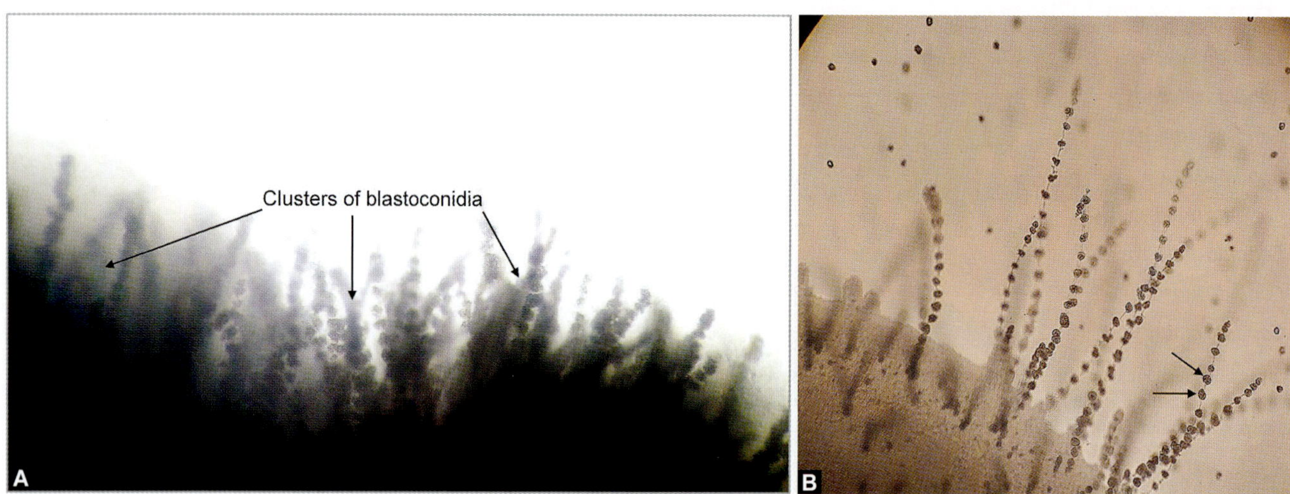

FIGS. 20.4A AND B: One more pattern of *Candida albicans* on CMA (low power). Clusters of blastoconidia at regular intervals giving "spidery appearance".
(CMA: cornmeal agar)

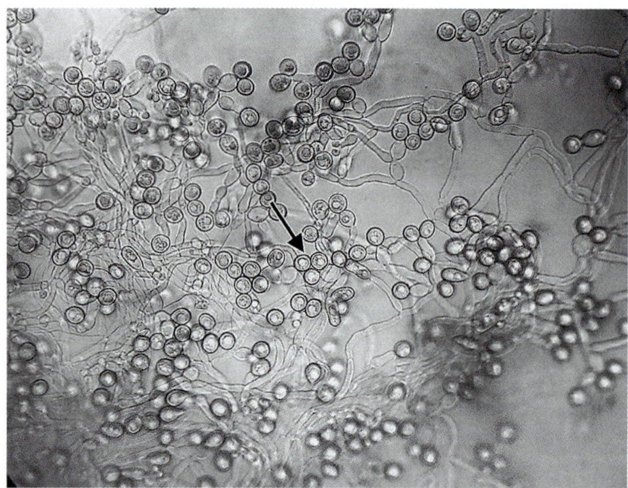

FIG. 20.5: Growth of *Candida dubliniensis* on CMA showing clusters of chlamydoconidia.
(CMA: cornmeal agar)

FIG. 20.6: Growth pattern of *Candida tropicalis* on CMA (100×) low power.
(CMA: cornmeal agar)

Candida parapsilosis

- *Colony morphology on SDA*: Rate of growth is rapid, the colony matures in 3 days.

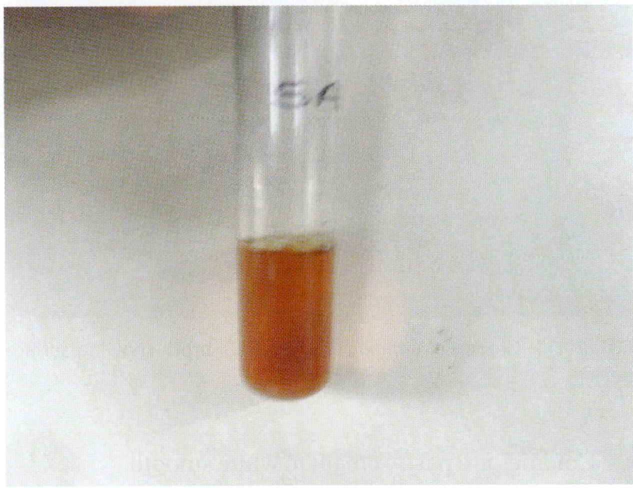

FIG. 20.7: Growth of *Candida tropicalis* in SABI broth.

- Colonies are creamy; sometimes, they show mycelia fringe.
- *Microscopic morphology*: Yeast cells are round to oval, size varying 3–4 × 5–8 μm.
- *CMA*: It shows blastoconidia, single or small clusters along the pseudohyphae. Important characteristics include "sage brush" appearance and some "satellite colonies" away from line of inoculation **(Figs. 20.8A to C)**. Pseudohyphae are relatively short (compared to *C. tropicalis*), crooked or curved, and occasional presence of large hyphal elements called giant cells.

Candida krusei

- *Colony morphology on SDA*: Rate of growth is rapid, and colonies mature in 3 days. Colonies are dry, dull, flat, and creamy to slight tan colored with hyphal fringe.
- *Microscopic morphology*: Yeast cells are oval, size varying 2–6 × 4–10 μm, with single terminal budding.
- *CMA* shows blastoconidia, and pseudohyphae are often present with robust, cells arranged parallel to the main axis. Pseudohyphae with elongated

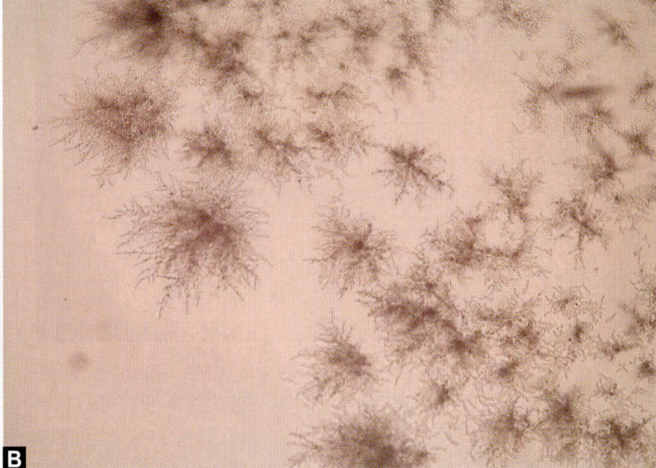

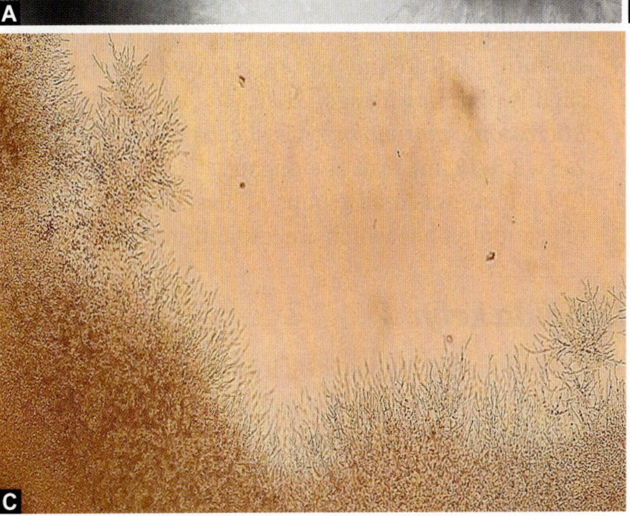

FIGS. 20.8A TO C: Growth of *Candida parapsilosis* on CMA. Note down (A and B) "satellite colonies" and (C) edge of the colony giving "sage brush" appearance.
(CMA: cornmeal agar)

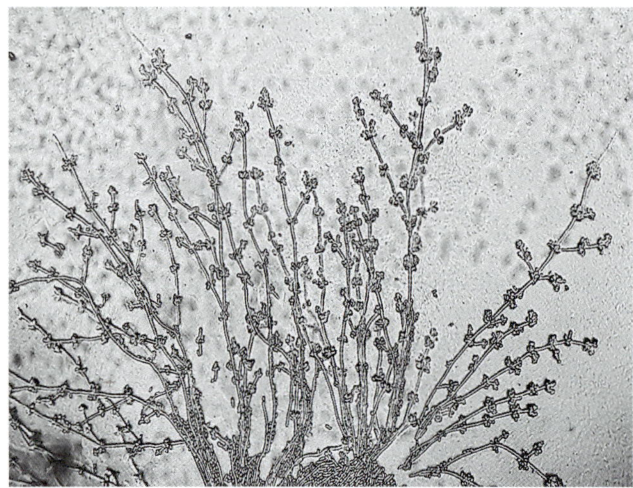

FIG. 20.9: Growth pattern of *Candida krusei* on CMA (low power). (CMA: cornmeal agar)

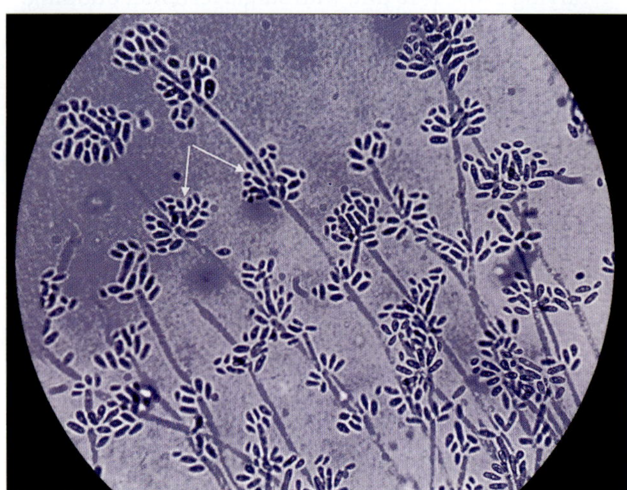

FIG. 20.10: Growth of *Candida krusei* on CMA (high power). Arrangement of pseudohyphae in various directions giving "cross matchsticks" appearance.
(CMA: cornmeal agar)

blastoconidia give "cross matchstick" or (tree)-like appearance **(Figs. 20.9 and 20.10)**. This may be confused with *Blastoschizomyces capitis*. *B. capitis* shows growth in the presence of cycloheximide, assimilates galactose, and shows anneloconidia which are absent in *C. krusei*.

- *Growth in SABI broth*: There is formation of surface pellicle **(Fig. 20.11)** which also extends along the side of tube.

Candida glabrata

- *Colony morphology on SDA*: Rate of growth is rapid; colonies mature in 3–5 days.

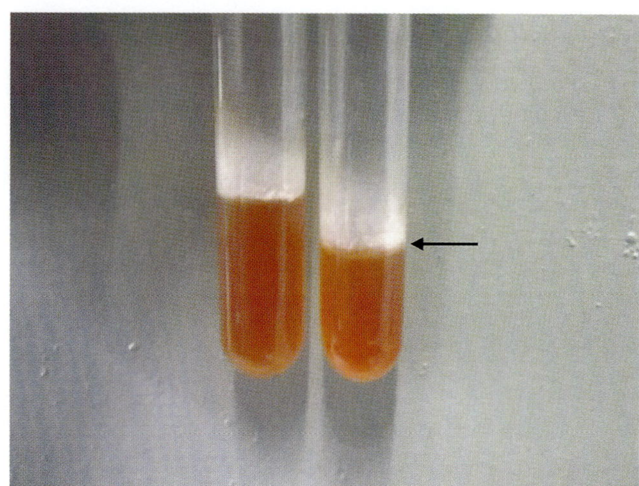

FIG. 20.11: Growth of *Candida krusei* in SABI broth showing surface pellicle.

- Colonies are pastry cream to white smooth.
- *Microscopic morphology*: Yeast cells are small, size varying 2–3 × 3.5–4.5 µm, oval with single terminal budding.
- *CMA*: It shows blastoconidia only, and no pseudohyphae are formed. Short chains of blastoconidia may be formed which may be confused with pseudohyphae. Yeast cells (blastoconidia) on CMA are closely arranged in contrast to that of *Cryptococcus* in which because of capsule produced by each cell, yeast cells show spaces in between. As there are other *Candida* species such as *C. famata* and *C. auris*, one cannot only rely on findings on CMA for identification of *C. glabrata* (*C. glabrata* gives *rapid trehalose* test positive).

Candida guilliermondii

- *Colony morphology on SDA*: Rate of growth is rapid, and colonies mature in 3 days. Colonies are flat, glossy, smooth, and creamy to tan color which may turn slightly pinkish with age.
- *Microscopic morphology*: Yeast cells have size varying 2–5 × 3.3–12 µm, oval or elongate.
- *CMA*: It shows small groups of blastoconidia at septa of pseudohyphae which are few and short.

Candida kefyr

- *Colony morphology on SDA*: It has rapid rate of growth; colonies mature in 3 days and round in shape. Colony is cream-colored smooth.
- *Microscopic morphology*: Round-to-oval yeast cells of size 3–8 × 5–12 µm are present.

- *CMA*: Pseudohyphae with elongate blastoconidia that line up parallel giving "logs in stream appearance."

Candida lypolytica

- *Colony morphology on SDA*: Growth matures in 5 days; the colonies are creamy and smooth.
- *Microscopic morphology*: Round-to-oval yeast cells of size 3–6 × 4–10 µm are produced.
- *CMA*: It shows pseudohyphae and a few true hyphae, bear elongate blastoconidia short-chain forms, and produce a stark, branching appearance. It differs from *C. krusei* by no fermentation of xylose.

Candida dubliniensis

- *Colony morphology on SDA*: It is similar to that of *C. albicans*. Rate of growth is rapid; colonies mature in 3 days.
- *Microscopic morphology*: It is very similar to *C. albicans*.
- *CMA*: It shows pseudohyphae with regular cluster of blastoconidia at regular intervals at septa with large chlamydospores in pairs and clusters, at terminus as well as "intercalary" (within hyphae) **(Fig. 20.5)**. *C. albicans* produces chlamydoconidia on CMA near the edge of the coverslip where microaerophilic conditions are present, while *C. dubliniensis* produces these conidia on all of the area below coverslip as well as edge.
- Differences in colony morphology from *C. albicans* are observed on tobacco agar and Staib agar. *C. dubliniensis* colonies show peripheral fringe and produce large number of *chlamydoconidia.*
- It was first isolated from an HIV patient in Dublin (Ireland), now present worldwide.
- It causes oropharyngeal candidiasis, vaginitis, and BSIs.
- It can rapidly develop resistance to fluconazole.

The differences between *C. albicans* and *C. dubliniensis* are given in **Tables 20.4 and 20.5**.

Candida lusitaniae

Yeast and pseudohyphae are produced, including distinctly curved pseudohyphae, on CMA. It causes infections in patients with hematological malignancies or in stem cell transplant recipients. *Candida lusitaniae* can develop secondary resistance to amphotericin B (AmB).

Candida pelliculosa

Candida pelliculosa (teleomorph—*P. anomala*) is an uncommon cause of neonatal septicemia. *P. anomala* is a free-living yeast found in plants, fruits, and soil and is associated with food and its products, either as a production organism or as a spoilage yeast. The ability to grow in preserved food and feed environments is due to its capacity to grow under low pH, high osmotic pressure, and low oxygen tension. The sexual stage includes the production of hat-shaped ascospores. Budding cells are spherical or elliptical, and pseudohyphae may be present. This organism has potential to cause outbreaks of fungemia in neonatal intensive care unit (NICU).

The *C. haemulonii* complex includes *C. haemulonii sensu stricto, Candida duobushaemulonii, and C. haemulonii var. vulnera.* There is a concern because of the intrinsic antifungal resistance to AmB, azoles, and echinocandins.

Candida pseudohaemulonii has been isolated from BSIs, and molecular studies showed a close phylogenetic relationship with *C. haemulonii* complex. *C. pseudohaemulonii* can be distinguished from this species by the assimilation pattern of esculin, melibiose, L-rhamnose, trehalose, and glycerol.

The clinical manifestations of infections caused by *C. haemulonii* complex members are similar to those observed in the cases caused by *C. albicans* and other nonalbicans *Candida* species.

TABLE 20.4: Differences between *Candida albicans* and *Candida dubliniensis*.

Candida albicans	*Candida dubliniensis*
• Light green or bluish green colonies on CHROMagar	• Dark green color on CHROMagar
• Chlamydospores on appropriate media are arranged singly, occasionally in pairs, and rarely clusters	• Chlamydospores usually plenty, intercalary as well as terminal, and present in pairs or clusters
• Colonies on Staib agar are smooth and shiny	• Rough colony on Staib agar with hyphal fringe
• Assimilation of xylose	• No assimilation of xylose
• *Growth at 45°C*: Present	• *Growth at 45°C*: Absent

TABLE 20.5: Other differences between Candida albicans and Candida dubliniensis.

Characteristics	*Candida albicans*	*Candida dubliniensis*
Biofilm formation	Strong	Less effective
Virulence factors	Adherence, proteases, and filamentous transition	Similar but less pathogenic
Antifungal susceptibility	Susceptible to azoles, echinocandins, and polyenes	Similar but may vary slightly

Fungemia, onychomycosis, peritonitis, leukocytosis, and high fever are features of systemic candidiasis caused by *C. haemulonii sensu stricto*.

Candida duobushaemulonii causes onychomycosis and vulvovaginal candidiasis. *C. haemulonii var. vulnera* causes onychomycosis, lower extremity ulcers, and fungemia.

Candida auris

Candida auris has emerged globally as a multidrug-resistant, healthcare-associated fungal pathogen, presenting challenges in organism identification, antifungal resistance, and high patient mortality. Its ability to colonize the skin and persist in the environment promotes transmission within and between healthcare facilities, a feature unique among *Candida* species. *C. auris*, first identified in East Asia in 2009, has since been isolated on five continents and is notable for its multidrug resistance and treatment challenges. Unlike other *Candida* species, *C. auris* spreads within healthcare settings, contributing to BSIs with high mortality rates (30–60%).

Candida auris was first isolated from the ear canal of a patient in Japan in 2009 and soon after reported in South Korea. Retrospective reviews have shown that the earliest isolates date back to 1996. Since its discovery, *C. auris* has been reported in countries, including India, South Africa, the United States, and the United Kingdom. Clinical isolates have been found in various body fluids and tissues, with BSIs being the most common invasive infection. Most cases occur in patients with significant healthcare exposure and underlying comorbidities.

Risk Factors for Candida auris

BSIs include prolonged intensive care unit (ICU) stays, respiratory illnesses, vascular surgery, and prior antifungal use. Clonal transmission within healthcare facilities is common.

Microbiology and Taxonomy

Candida auris has been phylogenetically linked to the *Clavispora/Candida* clade, closely related to *C. haemulonii* and *C. pseudohaemulonii*. Its genetic sequences, particularly from the 26S D1/D2 and 18S ITS regions, demonstrate this relationship. Studies continue to explore its virulence, antifungal resistance profiles, and potential relatedness across strains.

Virulence Factors

Several studies have investigated the virulence factors of *C. auris*, which include germination, adherence, biofilm formation, and the production of enzymes such as phospholipases and proteinases. While *C. auris* does not form germ tubes, pseudohyphae, or chlamydospores in vitro, it may produce phospholipase and proteinase in a strain-dependent manner. *C. auris* can adhere to plastics and form biofilms, but these capabilities are notably weaker compared to *C. albicans*. Interestingly, some strains of *C. auris* form aggregates that resist disruption in vitro, which contrasts with nonaggregating strains.

Identification in the Clinical Laboratory

Identifying *C. auris* in clinical settings is crucial, especially when isolates are from sterile body sites, as antifungal susceptibility can vary significantly by species.

Phenotypic Characteristics

Candida auris appears as nondescript white-to-cream-colored colonies on SDA and pink to beige on CHROMagar. The yeast forms ovoid to elongated budding cells but does not produce pseudohyphae on CMA or rice Tween 80 agar. It grows well at both 37 and 42°C and assimilates sugars such as N-acetylglucosamine, succinate, and gluconate. These traits distinguish *C. auris* from closely related species such as *C. haemulonii*.

Biochemical Methods

Misidentifications of *C. auris* as other *Candida* species, especially *C. haemulonii*, have been common due to limitations in commercial biochemical testing databases.

Possible misidentifications based on various biochemical methods are as follows:

- *API 20C AUX*: *Candida sake* and *Rhodotorula glutinis*
- *BD Phoenix*: *Candida catenulata*
- *Vitek 2*: *C. duobushaemulonii* and *C. famata*

MALDI-TOF MS

Matrix-assisted laser desorption/ionization-time of flight mass spectrometry (MALDI-TOF MS) is an accurate and rapid method for identifying *C. auris* from pure cultures. However, the current Food and Drug Administration (FDA)-cleared libraries for commercial MALDI-TOF systems, such as the Bruker Biotyper and Vitek MS, do not include *C. auris*.

Molecular Methods

Molecular methods, such as rDNA sequencing of the 28S D1/D2 or ITS 1/2 regions, can accurately identify *C. auris*. Polymerase chain reaction (PCR)-based assays have also been developed. One real-time PCR assay designed by Kordalewska et al. can differentiate *C. auris* from related species such as *C. haemulonii* and *C. lusitaniae.*

Phenotypic Susceptibility

There are no species-specific antifungal susceptibility breakpoints for *C. auris* as of yet. However, *C. auris* isolates typically show high resistance to fluconazole, with minimum inhibitory concentrations (MICs) of ≥16 μg/mL and variable resistance to other azoles, amphotericin, and echinocandins. Posaconazole and isavuconazole have shown the most potency in vitro. However, studies may be skewed by clonal isolates, and false MIC elevations have been reported when using the Vitek 2 susceptibility testing method.

One more effective way to differentiate *C. auris* isolates from other *Candida* species is by growing them at 40–42°C because only *C. auris* can grow at this temperature.

Another form of differentiation is taking advantage of its ability to tolerate high salt concentrations. A culture in broth containing yeast nitrogen base, 10% sodium chloride (NaCl) supplemented with dextrose, dulcitol, or mannitol, can differentiate *C. auris* from *C. haemulonii sensu stricto, C. duobushaemulonii, C. albicans*, and *C. parapsilosis*, which cannot grow under these conditions.

New CHROMagar *Candida* Plus medium showed better performance in the *C. auris* identification, although *C. pseudohaemulonii* resembles *C. auris* in mixed culture colonies; it tends to be much smaller and produces a distinctive blue halo after 72 hours. This makes the misidentification of *C. pseudohaemulonii* with *C. auris* less likely when found in clinical specimens.

RAPID IDENTIFICATION SYSTEMS

API 20C Aux System

API 20C Aux system is a process based on the assimilation of carbohydrates. It entails testing the assimilation of 19 carbohydrates in cupules that are cultured at 30°C for 24–72 hours. Turbidity analysis via computer programs is used for identification. This technique reliably distinguishes between various *Candida* species, including *C. dubliniensis* and *C. albicans.*

API Candida System

API *Candida* system, a 10-tube test, was able to identify five carbohydrates using a battery of acidity and enzymatic assays. Sugar acidification and enzyme activity form the basis of the test's principle. Visual observations of changes in color and morphological features allow for interpretation.

Fluorogenic Membrane Filtration Method

This is more accurate than the CHROMagar method. The enzymatic reaction is detected by passing fluorogenic substrates through a nylon membrane filter. It is helpful for identification of *C. albicans, C. krusei, C. tropicalis*, and *C. glabrata.*

Fungichrom I and Fungi-Fast I Twin Systems

In contrast to the fungi-fast twin system, which has 10 test cupules, the Fungichrom I twin system has 16 test cupules (International Microbio, Parc D'activitésallee D'athenes, France). After being incubated at 30°C for 24–48 hours, the samples are checked for any changes in color.

Vitek

The main concern is that *C. auris* could be incorrectly diagnosed because these tests require distinct fungal colonies and an incubation time of 2–3 days.

MALDI-TOF MS

It is useful for accurate identification of *Candida* species. Even identification of newer species such as *C. auris* is possible.

MOLECULAR METHODS

DNA-based Methods

Various conventional techniques have been utilized for studying the genome of *Candida* species. These include pulsed-field gel electrophoresis (PFGE), restriction enzyme analysis (REA), restriction fragment length polymorphism (RFLP), and amplified fragment length polymorphism (AFLP).

Polymerase chain reaction and its modifications (nested PCR and real-time PCR) that can enhance precise identification and quantification of the *Candida* are available. Microarray is also available now. Nucleic acid sequence-based amplification (NASBA) and peptide nucleic acid-fluorescence in situ hybridization (PNA-FISH) have also been utilized for *Candida.*

Serological Tests for Invasive Candidiasis

- *Antibody*: There are a number of methods for detecting antibodies, including immunodiffusion, immunoprecipitation, immunofluorescence, and slide agglutination.
- *Antigen*: Cell wall components such as cell wall mannoprotein (CWMP), beta-(1,3)-D- glucan is the target and detected by different tests.
- *Candida* mannan and anti-mannan antibody test. This test detects circulating immune complexes (IC) in patients with invasive candidiasis

Candida Enolase Antigen Testing

The major drawback of this method is that beta-D-glucan can be found in other types of fungi, such as *Aspergillus* species and *Pneumocystis jirovecii*, which makes it questionable to use it for diagnosing *Candida* species infections. Still, this test has high negative predictive value that helps to get rid of invasive candidiasis.

- *The Platelia® Candida antigen sandwich EIA* (Bio-Rad Laboratories, Marnes-la-Coquette, France): It can identify *Candida* species mannan using monoclonal antibodies (mAbs). A positive result from the enzyme immunoassay (EIA) is indicated when two separate blood samples show ≥0.5 ng of mannan per milliliter. There will likely be more testing of the test in future, and the inclusion of more specific mAbs might increase the number of species identified.
- *LightCycler® SeptiFast Test* (Roche Diagnostics): From 3 mL of patient blood collected over the course of 6 hours, this test can identify 25 different pathogens in the bloodstream, including five different species of *Candida* (*C. albicans, C. tropicalis, C. glabrata, C. parapsilosis, and C. krusei*) and *Aspergillus fumigatus*.
- *T2 Candida panel* (T2 Biosystems, Lexington, Massachusetts, United States): It is useful for the diagnosis of candidemia and the detection of *C. albicans, C. glabrata, C. parapsilosis, C. tropicalis,* and *C. krusei* in whole blood.

T2 *Candida* is a nonculture-based test. The completely automated T2Dx device is used to collect whole blood samples, which are placed in K2 ethylenediaminetetraacetic acid (EDTA) tubes. It uses a thermostable DNA polymerase and primers for the *Candida* ribosomal DNA operon to amplify the DNA of the lysed *Candida* cells, which were obtained by mechanically beating the cells using beads. The amplicon-induced agglomeration of supermagnetic particles and T2 magnetic resonance (T2MR) measurement are used to detect the amplified *Candida* DNA product.

Each specimen undergoes processing with an internal check to ensure that the results are accurate. The typical turnaround time of the T2 *Candida* panel is <5 hours, and it can detect as few as 1 colony-forming unit (CFU)/mL of whole blood.

Growth in Sabouraud broth: This test is useful for identifying distinct species. After 2 days of incubation at 25°C, *C. tropicalis* in Sabouraud broth generates a thin surface pellicle. On the underside of the tube, *C. krusei* forms broad surface layers. Surface pellicle is not produced by *C. albicans*.

Sugar assimilation pattern: It is a useful and reliable method for the identification of *Candida* species **Figure 20.12** shows the assimilation pattern of tested sugars on yeast nitrogen base agar.

Urease test: *C. krusei* gives this test positive, but it may show strain variation.

Pal's medium (sunflower seed agar) possibly differentiates *C. albicans* from *C. dubliniensis*. Colonies of both species will develop into smooth, creamy-gray colonies after 48–72 hours of development on this medium. On the other hand, a hyphal fringe encircling the colonies is a hallmark of *C. dubliniensis* isolates. Because other *Candida* species (*C. tropicalis, C. parapsilosis,* and *C. krusei*) can also produce a fringe on Pal's agar, it may be prudent to restrict its use to germ tube positive and/or chlamydospore positive isolates.

Whenever any yeast is isolated from clinical specimens, **Flowchart 20.1** is followed.

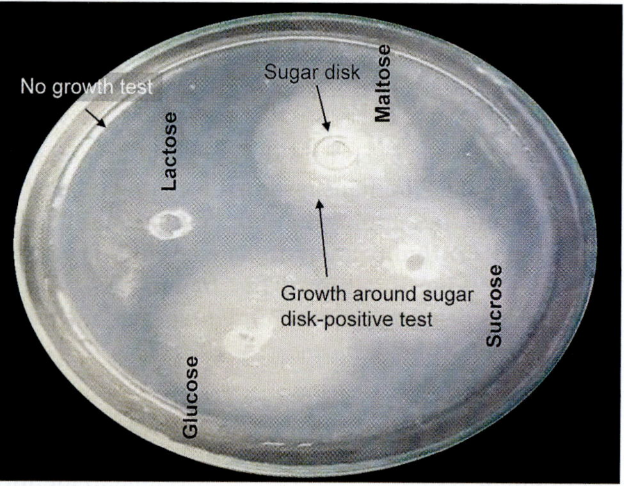

FIG. 20.12: Sugar assimilation test (growth around sugar indicates that sugar is assimilated).

TREATMENT

Candida infections are treated with antifungal medications such as nystatin, clotrimazole, AmB, and miconazole.

Mild or moderate genital *Candida* infections can be treated with antifungal vaginal cream (1, 3, 7 day treatment) or econazole or fluconazole 150 mg orally one-time dose. For recurrent vaginal infections, fluconazole is given on days 1, 4, and 7 and then weekly for 6 months. This treatment can be used for oral thrush. Even oral lozenges act as a substitute form. For oral and mucocutaneous infections, 1% gentian violet is locally applied. Nystatin can be used for resistant mucosal lesions as suspension containing 200,000 units/mL. Systemic candidiasis requires treatment with oral or intravenous (IV) antifungal medications, including caspofungin, fluconazole, and AmB.

For systemic infections:

- AmB—IV is used for 6–10 weeks.
- 5-fluorocytosine can be added to it for disseminated candidiasis.
- Triazoles such as fluconazole, itraconazole, imidazole, and ketoconazole can also be used.

Fluconazole-resistant Species

Disseminated infections are the primary source of fluconazole-resistant species, including *C. tropicalis*, *C. krusei*, and *C. glabrata*. One potential treatment for fluconazole resistance is voriconazole.

CHAPTER

21 Cryptococcosis

INTRODUCTION

Encapsulated yeasts of the genus *Cryptococcus* are the cause of the opportunistic infection known as cryptococcosis, which is present globally. Cryptococcosis can manifest as lung, meningeal, or disseminated infection.

Cryptococcal meningitis became more common during the acquired immunodeficiency syndrome (AIDS) pandemic. It was the second most common opportunistic fungal infection in AIDS patients, after *Candida* species. Additional risk factors for the development of cryptococcosis include immunosuppressive medication, broad-spectrum antibiotics, renal transplantation, and increased steroid use.

HISTORY

A case of a 31-year-old girl with swollen lymphatic glands and a big ulcer across her tibia was reported by Busse and Buschke in 1894. Busse described a yeast form in lesion tissue and called the yeast *Saccharomyces* after culturing it.

Saccharomyces neoformans was the name given to the yeast that Sanfelice isolated from peaches in 1894 with the presumption that the fungus caused tumor. Verse (1914) reported the first case of cryptococcal meningitis in a 29-year-old woman. Benham first used the name *Cryptococcus neoformans* in 1950. Emmons isolated the fungus for the first time from pigeon droppings.

Cryptococcus neoformans has been derived from the Greek words "krypto," which means "hidden," "kokkos," which means "berry," "neo," which means "new," and the Latin word "forma," which means "form."

Serotyping: Based on capsular antigen, *C. neoformans* shows five serotypes: A, B, C, D, and AD. Serotype AD reacts with antisera against serotype A as well as D. It is a hybrid strain of serotypes A and D. Geographic distribution of various serotypes is different as shown in following table **(Table 21.1)**.

TABLE 21.1: Geographical distribution of different serotypes.

Serotypes	*Geographical distribution*
A	Worldwide, including North America, South America, and parts of Asia
B	Predominant in Australia, Southeast Asia, Central Africa, Brazil, Venezuela, and some parts of Europe (e.g., Italy)
C	Common in Southern California, Colombia, and parts of South America
D	Found in Europe (e.g., Denmark, Italy, Switzerland, and France) and parts of North America
AD	Present in various regions globally, including both North and South America

Varieties: Based upon the biochemical and morphological characteristics, three varieties of *Cryptococcus* were earlier classified.

Old classification:

- *C. neoformans* var. *grubii* (serotype A)
- *C. neoformans* var. *gattii* (serotypes B and C) (*C. gattii* has been given separate species status recently)
- *C. neoformans* var. *neoformans* (serotype D)

Non-neoformans cryptococcal species: These were initially considered as nonpathogenic, but human infections occur with them. This group includes *C. albidus*, *C. laurentii*, and few other species. Patients with defective cell-mediated immunity (CMI) may have the infections with *C. laurentii* and *C. albidus*. Catheter-associated fungemia may be caused by these species. They have increased resistance to flucytosine and fluconazole. *C. albidus* is isolated from the skin of healthy people and found in the air. In immunocompromised patients, *C. laurentii* can cause fungemia, oculomycosis, and infrequently diarrhea.

The taxonomy of pathogenic cryptococcal species has evolved due to molecular research, which has replaced more conventional taxonomic categories with more precise molecular and genetic ones. Various genotypes were described.

Medically Important Species

- *Cryptococcus neoformans* species complex:
  - It contains species primarily associated with infections in humans, particularly in immunocompromised individuals [e.g., human immunodeficiency virus (HIV)/AIDS].
  - *Species*:
    - *C. neoformans* (var. *grubii*—genotypes VNI, VNII, and VNB)
    - AD hybrid (VNIII)
    - *Cryptococcus deneoformans* (genotype VNIV)
- *Cryptococcus gattii* species complex:
  - It includes species that can cause infections in both immunocompetent and immunocompromised individuals, often associated with outbreaks.
  - *Species*:
    - *C. gattii* (genotype VGI)
    - *Cryptococcus deuterogattii* (VGII)
    - *Cryptococcus bacillisporus* (VGIII)
    - *Cryptococcus tetragattii* (VGIV)
- *Emerging nonpathogenic Cryptococcus species*: Other environmental species such as *C. albidus* and *C. laurentii* rarely cause infections but may act as opportunistic pathogens in immunocompromised hosts.

Clinical Implications of Classification

- *C. neoformans species complex* is more common globally and typically affects HIV/AIDS patients, causing cryptococcal meningitis.
- *C. gattii species complex* causes more severe disease in immunocompetent hosts and has been implicated in outbreaks in nonendemic regions.
- *Molecular typing* [e.g., multilocus sequence typing (MLST)] is essential for outbreak investigation and understanding pathogenicity differences among genotypes.

> ***You may know this:***
> *Mating types*: The sexual stage of *C. neoformans* is represented by *Filobasidiella neoformans* and *Filobasidiella bacillispora*. "α" and "a" are the two mating types of yeast that exist in laboratory settings. Basidiomycetous teleomorphs are created when they are crossed. The environment and clinical isolates have higher frequencies of the α type.

Of the 37 species of *Cryptococcus* that are commonly found in the environment, only three are usually regarded as pathogens: (1) *C. grubii*, (2) *C. gattii*, and (3) *C. neoformans*.

Newer Classification versus Conventional Classification

The newer *genetic classification* divides *C. neoformans* and *C. gattii* into seven species. As this database is included in the newer diagnostic methods such as matrix-assisted laser desorption/ionization-time of light mass spectroscopy (MALDI-TOF MS) which is not available with many laboratories, some scientists prefer to use conventional classification.

The important differentiating characteristics of three *Cryptococcal* species are given in **Table 21.2**.

EPIDEMIOLOGY

There were isolated cases of cryptococcosis all over the world, but the AIDS pandemic is the most common predisposing factor in the increased incidence of cryptococcal disease. It is the second most common fungal infection in AIDS patients, after candidiasis. The fungus was discovered in pigeon droppings, pigeon nests, and old buildings. Cryptococci thrive in the presence of creatinine at these sites. Pigeons are immune to the disease due to their high body temperature. The fungus was also seen in other avian species such as chickens, parrots, and sparrows, but transmission to human being does not occur. *C. neoformans var. grubii* has been found in avian droppings as well as wood debris from *Cassia grandis* (Pink shower tree) and other trees. The *gattii* variant is associated with flowering of the trees *Eucalyptus canadensis* (river red gum) and *Eucalyptus tereticornis* (forest red gum) which are present in Australia, Brazil, south California, Mexico, Nepal, and India. *C. gattii* is isolated from many places in India. It holds the ability to cause infection in immunocompetent persons. There is a rare report of *C. gattii* causing infections in AIDS patients.

PATHOGENESIS AND VIRULENCE FACTORS

Virulence Factors

- *Capsule*: It is a major virulence factor. It is antiphagocytic. It is made up of glucuronoxylomannan (GXM) and galactoxylomannan (GalXM). GXM is a major capsular polysaccharide. GXM polymer structural differences (which act as antigens) aid in organism serotyping. The capsule has antiphagocytic properties.

TABLE 21.2: Different characteristics of different species.

Features	Cryptococcus gattii	Cryptococcus neoformans var. grubii	Cryptococcus neoformans var. neoformans
Serotypes	B and C	A	D
Teleomorphs	*Filobasidiella neoformans var. bacillispora*	*Filobasidiella neoformans var. neoformans*	*Filobasidiella neoformans var. neoformans*
Prevalence	Tropical and subtropical	Worldwide	Europe
Habitat	Eucalyptus tree	Avian excreta	Avian excreta
Immune status of patient	HIV-negative	HIV-positive	On corticosteroids
Virulence of organism	Low	High	High
Onset of disease	Insidious	Acute	Acute
Fever	+	++	++
Neurological sequelae	++	+	+
Focal CNS lesions	++	+	+
Focal pulmonary lesions	+++	+	+
Cryptococcemia	+	++	++
Skin involvement	Not known	Less frequent	Frequent
Blastospores	Elliptical	Rounded	Rounded
CDBT medium for thymine	Growth with blue-green color	No growth	Growth with orange color
CGB agar	Cobalt blue color	No change	No change
GCP agar	Positive	Negative	Negative
D-proline	Utilized	Not utilized	Not utilized
D-tryptophan	Utilized	Not utilized	Not utilized
Malate assimilation	Positive	Negative	Negative
Mortality	+	++	++
Treatment	Longer with relapse	Shorter	Shorter

(CDBT: creatinine-dextrose-bromothymol blue thymine; CGB: canavanine-glycine-bromothymol blue; CNS: central nervous system; GCP: glycine-cycloheximide-phenol red; HIV: human immunodeficiency virus)

It inhibits dendritic cell (DC) uptake. GXM alters the function of macrophages. GalXM affects cell-mediated immune responses.

- Cell wall mannoproteins, which is the dominant antigen and affects CMI.
- *Melanin*: It is antigenic in nature. Because of its redox properties, it neutralizes free radicals which gives protection to the fungus from intracellular killing in phagocytes. The enzyme phenol oxidase of the organism produces melanin from L-dihydroxyphenylalanine (L-DOPA). These building blocks (L-DOPA) for melanin are available in large quantities in the brain. To a certain degree, it clarifies the brain tropism of *Cryptococcus.*
- *Ability to grow at 37°C*: It is also a virulence factor of *Cryptococcus.*
- *Phenotypic switching*: It is in charge of the organism's survival. The phenotypic switching facilitates the spread of *C. neoformans* and *C. gattii* in the central nervous system (CNS).
- *Cryptococcal phospholipase B1*: It aids in adherence to the lung epithelium, interstitial infection, survival, and replication within macrophages. It also aids in the spread of *Cryptococcus* from the lungs to the blood and lymphatic systems.
- *Urease*: It increases accumulation of immature DCs and induces T helper 2 (Th2) response in mice.
- *Alpha mating type*: It may be a virulence factor as α-matting type represents 90% of clinical and environmental isolates.

PATHOGENESIS

The pathogen *C. neoformans* enters the lungs by inhalation and reaches the alveoli. It can cling to pulmonary epithelial cells (possibly because type II pneumocytes have GXM receptors). *Cryptococcus* inhibits phagocytosis by various virulence factors.

Within macrophages, they escape the phagosome and, after multiplication within the cells, they exit via cell lysis. *Cryptococci* can become trapped in infected macrophages which prevents them from extracellular environment. The interaction of the organisms with alveolar macrophages is a vital step in spreading of organisms in the body.

Cryptococci cross blood–brain barrier by three possible ways as follows:

1. *Transcellular passage through endothelial cells*: Endothelial cells produce microvilli, which pull the cryptococci inside the cells. Coming out through the opposite cell surface, it causes minimal damage to endothelial cells.
2. *Paracellular route between endothelial cells*: Cells retract as a result of the interaction between cryptococci and endothelial cells, and the junction through which organisms pass is loosened.
3. *Trojan horse approach*: Monocytes transport cryptococci through blood vessels.

Transient Colonization or Persistent Colonization

A healthy individual may experience short-lived, asymptomatic carriage of *C. neoformans* after being exposed to environmental fungus, or the illness may be subclinical or self-limiting. It is possible to detect the fungus as a passing sputum sample on occasion. It is possible to isolate *C. neoformans* from sputum multiple times over months or even years in individuals with chronic lung illness who do not have aggressive invasion of the lung parenchyma, provided that the bronchi are colonized asymptomatically for an extended period of time.

CLINICAL FEATURES

Pulmonary Cryptococcosis

In immunocompetent people, pulmonary cryptococcosis symptoms are often modest. Symptoms of pleuritic chest pain, dyspnea, coughing, and fever are signs of pulmonary cryptococcosis in people with AIDS. Pulmonary cavities, pleural effusions, mass infiltrates, hilar lymphadenopathy, and lobar infiltrates are common in people with impaired immune systems. In immunocompromised patients, cryptococcal pneumonia can still cause serious complications even when the CNS is not involved. Serum cryptococcal polysaccharide antigen testing is often negative in the cases of isolated pulmonary cryptococcosis; nevertheless, it can occasionally be positive when there is no evidence of infection at other locations or involvement of the CNS. Regardless of symptoms or serum antigen titer results, a lumbar puncture should be considered to rule out CNS disease in immunocompromised persons if *Cryptococcus* is isolated from the lung or another sterile body region.

In the lung of a patient infected with *Cryptococcus* species, two specialized forms of the fungus have been observed. (1) "Titan cells" are very large (up to 100 μm) forms of *Cryptococcus* seen in patients who develop chronic infection. These forms resist phagocytosis. These cells have thicker cell wall, have huge and tightly composed capsule, and show polyploidy. These can multiply normally to produce normal forms of *Cryptococcus*. (2) "Microcells" are another form of *Cryptococcus* seen in chronic infections. These are not >2 μm in size, with a thick cell wall. It is proposed that such cells play a role in causing CNS infections.

Central Nervous System Disease

Pulmonary cryptococcosis may spread through bloodstream to involve CNS. It produces meningoencephalitis. The signs of meningeal involvement may be present. In severe cases, coma and respiratory failure may occur, and the condition may become fatal. Cranial nerve palsies and hydrocephalus are common. The brain usually has a high number of *Cryptococci*. While most infections spread throughout the body, there are cases where the brain is invaded, leading to the development of solid tumor-like masses in specific areas. The formation of cryptococcoma is seen in immunocompetent individuals, and it is a rare event in AIDS. Intracranial space-occupying lesion (ICSOL) is the hallmark of granuloma. Clinical features include headache, nausea, memory loss, ataxia, seizures, double vision, photophobia, blind spot, and coma. No growth in culture can occur. A culture from a brain biopsy might be necessary to confirm the diagnosis.

Cutaneous Infection

When the fungus spreads from a pulmonary site to another part of the body, the common site is skin next to CNS. Immunocompromised patients are at increased risk. They are common (affecting 5–15% of patients) and often suggest a bad prognosis.

Primary Cutaneous Cryptococcosis

It is due to trauma. Scalp, face, and neck are common sites of infection. The skin lesions may take any form as papule, nodule, abscess, ulcer, granuloma, and cellulitis.

Secondary Cutaneous Cryptococcosis

Hematogenous spread leads to formation of skin lesions in immunocompromised patients. Disease starts with papule, which ulcerates producing thin exudate with a large number of organisms.

Prostatic Infection

The prostate is a common site for cryptococcal infections. Most of the time, there are no symptoms. Urological surgery on the prostate can trigger the reactivation of latent infections.

Ocular Cryptococcosis

Ocular cryptococcosis is rare, although patients with cryptococcal meningitis may experience either (1) sudden blindness from the infection's direct impact on the optic nerve or (2) gradual blindness over a period of weeks or months due to increased intracranial pressure.

Osseous Cryptococcosis

About 10–15% of patients will experience bone lesions. There may be osteolytic lesions. Affected areas may include the pelvis, bony protrusions, cranial bones, ribs, and spine.

Visceral Cryptococcosis

By way of hematogenous transmission, infections might manifest in any organ or tissue. Typically discovered only at autopsies, this is a very grave finding despite how uncommon it is.

Observations of Clinical Forms of Infection with *Cryptococcus gattii*

Pulmonary cryptococcosis and meningoencephalitis can be caused by *C. gattii* infections in otherwise healthy individuals. Their immunological condition permits patients to mount a greater immune response, which in turn improves their prognosis. Patients often experience hydrocephalus, papilledema, and elevated cryptococcal antigen titers, in addition to cerebral mass lesions. Multiple enhancing lesions on CT scans indicate meningoencephalitis in some cases.

DIFFERENTIAL DIAGNOSIS

Infections can sometimes resemble the symptoms of cancers of the respiratory system or CNS. A pulmonary infection should be differentiated from tuberculosis, sarcoidosis, candidiasis, histoplasmosis, or coccidioidomycosis and nocardiosis. Since both cryptococcal meningitis and tuberculous meningitis can appear similar, it is important to distinguish between the two.

LABORATORY DIAGNOSIS

Direct Examination

India Ink or 10% Nigrosin

Microscopical analysis of cerebrospinal fluid (CSF) prepared with India ink for the detection of encapsulated yeasts is the gold standard for diagnosing cryptococcal meningitis. This is a negative staining technique. Instead of India ink, Nigrosin 10% can be used. **Figure 21.1** shows cryptococcal capsule in negative stain. Centrifuged samples are preferable for analysis. *Cryptococcus* is a globular-shaped, capsulated yeast cell with variation in size (from 5 to 20 µm in diameter). Budding with narrow-based, single bud per yeast cell may be seen. The capsule is clearly delineated against a dark background. It has been observed that in cases of non-AIDS-related cryptococcal meningitis, the sensitivity of India ink staining of CSF ranges from 30 to 50%, but in cases of AIDS-related illness, it can reach up to 80%. Red blood cells (RBCs), lymphocytes, and pus cells may create confusion while observing wet mount.

- *Modified India ink (India ink with 2% chromium mercury)*: Both the outside and inside of a structure are more clearly shown in this mount.
- *Calcofluor staining*: It increases the chances of detection of the organisms.
- *Gram staining*: *Cryptococcus* is gram-positive yeast.

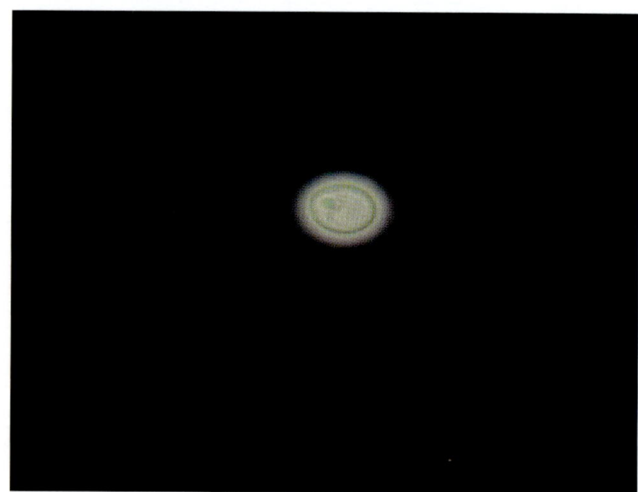

FIG. 21.1: India ink preparation showing a capsulated yeast cell of *Cryptococcus* (400×).

- *Analysis of CSF findings*: Proteins are increased, sugar is reduced, and 10–100 lymphocytes/mm^3 are seen.
- *Other staining methods*: Giemsa **(Fig. 21.2)**, periodic acid-Schiff (PAS), and Grocott-Gömöri's methenamine silver (GMS) stains are used for lymph node aspirate and other specimens.
- *Mayer's mucicarmine stain*: It stains the capsule rose colored.
- *Most specific stain is Alcian-blue* for capsule demonstration.
- *Masson-Fontana stain* detects melanin of the organism; hence, it is used for identification of capsule-deficient strain.
- *Capsule enhancement*: It can be done by growing the organism in 1% peptone or inoculation in a susceptible animal such as mouse.

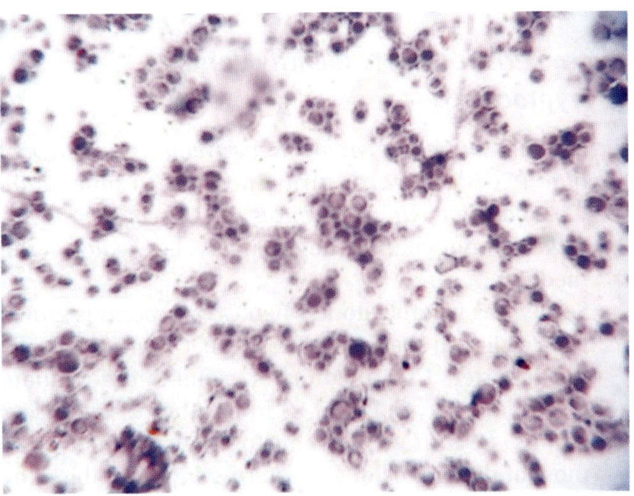

FIG. 21.2: Yeast cells of *Cryptococcus neoformans* (Giemsa stain).

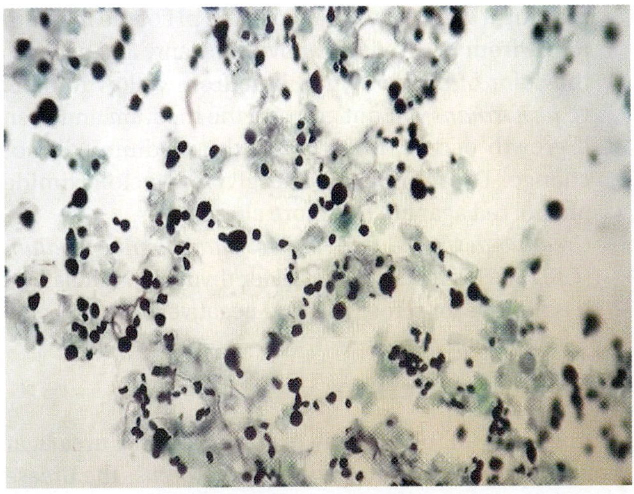

FIG. 21.3: Yeast cells of *Cryptococcus neoformans* (GMS stain) (1,000×).
(GMS: Grocott-Gömöri's methenamine silver)

Histopathology

The polysaccharide capsule is stained red when using Mayer's mucicarmine to stain tissue specimens. Because the capsule has ruptured after fixation, a clear zone surrounds the cryptococci in this stain. When looking for organisms in tissues that lack a capsule, the Masson-Fontana stain can be helpful. **Figure 21.3** shows black yeasts in GMS staining performed on section of lung.

Culture

List of Media

These include Sabouraud dextrose agar (SDA) slants without Actidione (which inhibits *Cryptococcus*), blood agar, chocolate agar, brain heart infusion (BHI) agar, cysteine-heart hemoglobin agar, birdseed agar (Staib's agar), Pal's sunflower seed agar, and tobacco agar. The media are incubated at 25 and 37°C in biochemical oxygen demand (BOD) incubators.

Chocolate agar with 5–10% CO_2 enhances capsule production.

Colonies appear in 48 hours. Culture media can be stored at ambient temperature for 2–4 weeks. Colonies are mucoid, buff to cream colored on SDA slants as shown in **Figure 21.4**.

Circular, capsulated budding yeast, with a diameter ranging from 5 to 20 µm, with prominent capsule are seen in smears prepared from colonies. At 37°C, more cells become elongated. *C. gattii* also generates cells that are oval-to-lemon shaped and measure 3–5 × 3–7 µm in diameter. As the incubation period lengthens, the colonies of the fungus change color from orange-tan to brown.

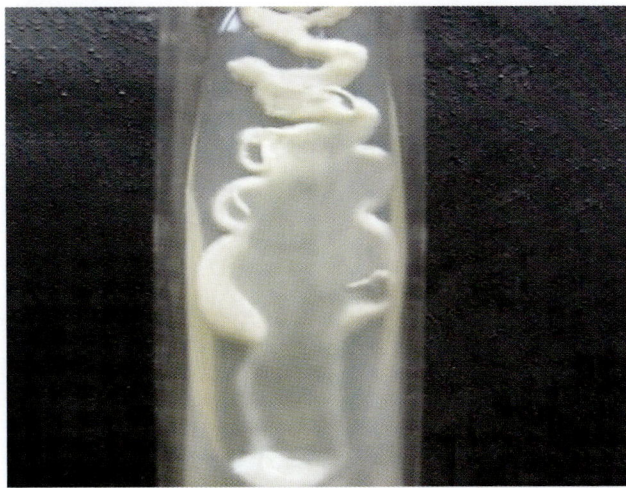

FIG. 21.4: SDA slant showing mucoid growth of *Cryptococcus neoformans*.
(SDA: Sabouraud dextrose agar)

Melanin Production

The "brown colony" effect is a way to identify *C. neoformans*. For demonstration of brown effect, "birdseed" agar (Staib's agar), Pal's sunflower seed agar, or tobacco agar is used **(Fig. 21.5)**. A loopful of the colony grown on SDA is inoculated on these media. Then these media are incubated at 30°C. After 2 or 3 days, colonies of *C. neoformans* grown on Staib's agar, as well as on Pal's sunflower seed agar, will turn a deep tan to brown hue. The principle of the test is to look for an enzyme phenol oxidase (laccase), by *Cryptococcus* species. Caffeic acid is the substrate for the enzyme. End result is the formation of melanin.

The test is performed on birdseed agar. A colony of *Cryptococcus* is streaked on "birdseed" agar. Birdseed is also known as niger seed or *Guizotia abyssinica*. The extract of the seeds contains caffeic acid.

Staib's agar is a selective niger seed agar that contains antibiotics. It should be used for primary isolation of *Cryptococcus* from specimens likely to be contaminated by gram-negative bacilli.

After 2 or 3 days, colonies of *C. neoformans* grow on birdseed agar showing tan to brown colored colonies due to production of melanin. Pal's sunflower seed agar also serves the same purpose.

The enzyme responsible for colony browning, phenol oxidase (laccase), is inhibited by glucose; hence, it is important to keep the glucose concentration in the medium below 0.1%. Melanin production can also be achieved using mustard seed agar and tobacco agar. Thus, the "brown colony" effect is a way to identify *C. neoformans*.

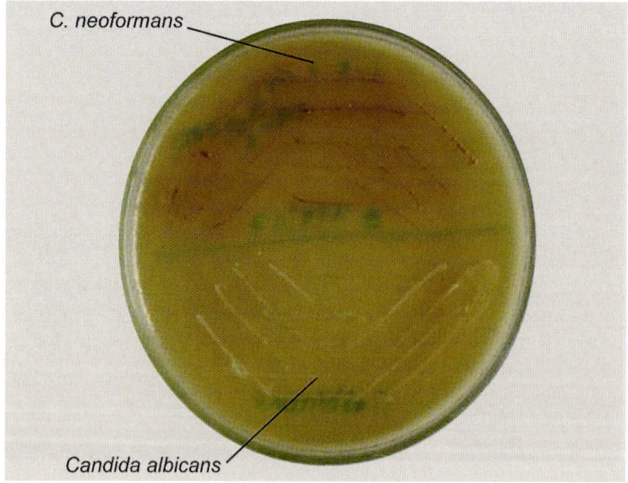

FIG. 21.5: Birdseed agar showing brownish growth of *Cryptococcus neoformans*.

Caffeic Acid Test Disks

Filter paper disks impregnated with caffeic acid when smeared heavily by the colonies will turn brown after incubation at 37°C for 30 minutes to 4 hours if the reaction is affirmative.

Biochemical Tests for Identification of Cryptococcus

Sugar assimilation test, Christensen's urea test, rapid urease test, and inositol and nitrate assimilation tests are used for identification at the genus level. Every cryptococcal strain assimilates inositol and nitrate, nonfermentative, and urease-positive. Also, all species of *Cryptococcus* produce brown effect. *C. neoformans* can be detected in as little as 15 minutes with the rapid urease test.

Characteristic Used to Identify Variants of Cryptococcus

- *Medium containing canavanine–glycine–bromothymol blue (CGB)*: *C. gattii* turns medium to blue while *C. neoformans var. neoformans* and *C. neoformans var. grubii* do not change the original yellow color of the medium.
  Serotyping is rarely done when *Cryptococcus* is grown from a clinical specimen. Therefore, *C. gattii* is usually not reported. CGB medium is useful to differentiate *C. gattii* (serotype B and C) from other *Cryptococcus* strains. *C. gattii* is resistant to L-canavanine, while most of the strains of *C. neoformans* are inhibited by this agent. Glycine in the medium is the only source of carbon in this medium. *C. gattii* can utilize glycine but *C. neoformans* cannot. Therefore, when *C. gattii* is growing it will lead to change in the pH of the medium to rise from 5.8 to a level above neutrality and changes the color of bromothymol blue from yellow to blue. *C. neoformans* will not grow on the medium and even if growth occurs, the color of the medium will not change. D-proline agar and glycine cycloheximide phenol red agar are two more alternatives.
- *Creatine-dextrose-bromothymol blue-thymine medium (CBDT)*: This medium is used for thymine assimilation. It is positive for serotype D and negative for serotype A.

Urease Production

Putting a loopful of a colony on Christensen's urea agar is one way to identify the genus *Cryptococcus*. The urease produced by the pathogenic species of this genus splits urea, which releases ammonia, which increases the pH.

As a result, the agar's color changes from pale yellow to pink or magenta, often within hours, as a result of the pH-related alteration. *C. neoformans* can be detected in as little as 15 minutes with the fast urease test. Rapid urease test is done by using urea broth heavily inoculated by the colonies. Results are available within 4 hours.

Carbohydrate Assimilation

The API 20C kit can identify the assimilation profile. Nonpathogenic *Cryptococcus* species, such as *C. albidus*, *C. laurentii*, *C. luteolus*, *C. terreus*, and *C. uniguttulatus*, can occasionally be isolated from clinical specimens taken from nonsterile areas. Identifying these species can help rule out *C. neoformans* and *C. gattii*. Brown colony effect on birdseed agar is not produced by any of these species. The API 20C panel does not include all of the necessary assimilation or other tests to distinguish between *Cryptococcus* species. It is possible for phenol oxidase-positive *Trichosporon* species to be mistakenly scored as *C. neoformans* when using the API 20C. Under the microscope, the structure on cornmeal agar can differentiate these two.

Serological Tests

Detection of cryptococcal polysaccharide capsular antigen (CrAg) can be done by latex agglutination (LA) tests, lateral flow assay (LFA), and enzyme-linked immunosorbent assay (ELISA) test.

Crypto-LA test: Serum, CSF, and blood aliquots can all be submitted to the test. This test is utilized for both quantitative and qualitative purposes, and it helps with diagnosis and prognosis evaluations. Urine has a low titer compared to CSF, which has a medium one. It is possible to connect CSF titers with mortality. *Disseminated Trichosporonosis* or rheumatoid arthritis might lead to false-positive results. To prevent false-positive results, pronase should be added to the serum before testing. It is possible to overcome the reasons of false negatives, which arise from a prozone effect at very high antigen titers, by diluting the sample. Possible causes of false-negative results in LA tests include an inadequate specimen storage procedure, a low fungal load (as seen in chronic low-grade meningitis or early stages of illness), and the test itself. An important titer value is 1:8.

Eiken LA test: It is used to detect antigen in serum. It is a more sensitive and specific test than the crypto-LA test. The test is useful in the diagnosis of pulmonary infection.

Lateral flow assay: The test is very simple to perform; hence, it is a popular point-of-care test having sensitivity and specificity similar to the agglutination test.

Antibody tests: Though these tests are not reliable for the diagnosis due to cross-reaction, they have prognostic values. Indirect immunofluorescence (IF), complement fixation test (CFT), and agglutination test are available.

Restriction fragment length polymorphisms (RFLP), pyrolysis-mass spectrometry, and polymerase chain reaction (PCR) are used as the typing tests.

Animal pathogenicity test: The Swiss Albino mice is used for this test. The routes of inoculation are intraperitoneal, intracerebral, or intracerebellar. The animal dies in about 7–10 days, and if the animal survives, autopsy is done after 2 weeks. The yeast cells can be demonstrated from various body fluids and organs.

Culture conditions favoring capsule enhancement are:

Diluted Sabouraud medium: To do this, *Cryptococci* are incubated in a Sabouraud broth solution that is diluted 1/10 with water. Using a diluent such as phosphate buffered saline (PBS), 3-(N-Morpholino)-propanesulfonic acid (MOPS), or 4-(2-hydroxyethyl)-1-piperazineethanesulfonic acid (HEPES) buffer at a concentration of 0.05 M and a pH of 7.3 significantly enhances these results. The diluted Sabouraud's medium either broth or agar can be incubated at either 30 or 37°C. Capsule development can be induced by incubating *Cryptococci* on an agar medium that contains 10% fetal bovine serum in PBS at 37°C.

- *CO_2*: Incubation of the yeast in RPMI 1640 (Roswell Park Memorial Institute) medium in a CO_2 incubator enhances capsule formation.
- *Limited iron medium*: Depleting iron in a chemically defined medium provides a stimulus for inducing capsule formation.

TREATMENT

Treatment is initiated with amphotericin B (liposomal formulation at 3–4 mg/kg/day), or the lipid complex at 5 mg/kg or conventional amphotericin B at 0.7 mg/kg/day. Any one of these can be used along with flucytosine 25 mg/kg every 6 hours (100 mg/kg/day) for at least 2 weeks and until improvement. Patients who respond to amphotericin B may be switched to fluconazole, 400–800 mg/day, for 8–10 weeks. Final therapy is suppressive phase with fluconazole 200 mg once daily.

CHAPTER

22 *Pneumocystis jirovecii*

INTRODUCTION

Pneumocystis jirovecii pneumonia (PJP) is a fungal infection that mostly strikes the immunocompromised patients, presents as atypical pneumonia, and can be fatal in its severe form. Initial *P. jirovecii* infections are associated with a 10–20% mortality risk in acquired immunodeficiency syndrome (AIDS) patients, and PJP is one of the AIDS-defining illnesses. The reservoir of an infection is human beings, and the mode of infection is inhalation. The lungs are primarily involved; spread outside of the lungs is rare. The use of cytotoxic cancer treatment, treatment for collagen-vascular disorders, stem cell transplant recipients, or organ transplant patients acts as predisposing factors along with AIDS.

HISTORY

Pneumocystis carinii was first described by Carlos Chagas in 1909. He was using experimental animals to study human infections of *Trypanosoma cruzi*. He observed sickle and rounded forms, which he identified as male and female *Trypanosoma* stages. Antonio Carini was conducting research on *Trypanosoma lewisi* lung infection in rats. He forwarded the slide to the Pasteur Institute. In 1912, Dr and Mrs Delanoë examined the slides and identified the organism as a distinct species of protozoan parasite named *P. carinii* (in the honor of Antonio Carini). Pneumonia epidemics were documented in the overcrowded and undernourished European orphanages after the World War II.

The etiology of interstitial plasma cell pneumonia was determined to be *Pneumocystis* by Otto Jirovec along with Joseph Vanek (1951). In 1976, Jakob Frenkel suggested that the name *P. carinii* be used for rat-infecting species and *P. jirovecii* for human-infecting species. Molecular genetic analysis connected this creature to fungi instead of protozoa.

Initially, this organism was thought to be protozoa, which is related to *Microsporidia*. The following characteristics pointed to it being protozoa:

- There was no growth in fungal culture media; growth required tissue cultures or cell lines.
- There was an absence of ergosterol in cytoplasmic membrane. Hence, it is resistant to antifungal drugs that inhibit ergosterol synthesis.
- It is sensitive to antiprotozoan agents, such as pentamidine and trimethoprim-sulfamethoxazole (TMP-SMZ).

It is classified as fungus based on the following criteria:

- It stains with fungal stain Grocott–Gömöri's methenamine silver (GMS) in the same way as other fungi.
- It contains chitin at all stages of its lifecycle. Many enzymes, such as chitinase, attack the cell wall of *Pneumocystis* in the same way they attack fungi.
- Synthesis of proteins *Pneumocystis* elongation factor 3 and thymidylate synthase are similar to ascomycetic fungi.
- Cyst wall ultrastructure resembles fungi.
- Studies using r-RNA show that it is a fungus.

TAXONOMY

At this time, it is thought of as belonging to the Pneumocystidales order of Pneumocystidomycetes, the genus *Pneumocystis*, and the Ascomycota subphylum Taphrinomycotina.

EPIDEMIOLOGY

Pneumocystis jirovecii is ubiquitous. The mammalian lung seems to be its sole habitat. As far as science is aware, there is no independent living organism. It is still unknown where *P. jirovecii* can be found. It is conceivable for healthy persons to have transient colonization. Infants infected with *Pneumocystis* for the first time, people with chronic lung illness, and the elderly are at risk of becoming silent reservoirs. It is typical for *Pneumocystis* to colonize the airways of people with chronic obstructive pulmonary disease (COPD).

One could argue that *P. jirovecii* is a part of the human microbiome, as even healthy individuals undergo temporary colonization. Transmission through the air can cause asymptomatic carriage of *P. jirovecii* to begin in hosts with impaired immune systems.

The initial cases of *Pneumocystis* pneumonia were documented in the 1970s in individuals suffering from hypogammaglobulinemia, congenital immunodeficiencies, hematological malignancies or individuals who had been administered corticosteroids or cytotoxic drugs for lymphoproliferative diseases. Once known as *P. carinii* pneumonia (PCP), PJP was officially recognized as the first opportunistic infection that defined AIDS in 1981 by the Centers for Disease Control and Prevention (CDC), United States. Prior to the AIDS crisis, less than 100 cases of PCP in humans had been reported.

Cases increased dramatically in the decades after the 1982 start of the AIDS epidemic. After reaching 20,000 cases in 1991, the suggestion to provide chemoprophylaxis against PCP to all HIV-positive individuals with a CD4 cell count < 200 cells/μL caused the incidence of PCP to decline. Once more, following the introduction of extensive highly active antiretroviral therapy (HAART) targeting the HIV virus in 1995, there was a precipitous fall. Although the number of PCP cases has decreased significantly, this type of pneumonia is still the leading cause of death among untreated HIV-positive individuals.

Other conditions, apart from low CD4 count due to HIV, predisposing to PCP are:

- Cytotoxic therapy and steroid therapy in hematological malignancies such as lymphoma, leukemia, and Hodgkin's disease
- Iatrogenic-induced immunosuppression
- Congenital immunodeficiency
- Cushing's syndrome
- Protein-calorie malnutrition

LIFECYCLE

Due to historic reasons, the lifecycle of pneumocystis is still described using parasitic terminologies.

It occurs in the lungs. There are both asexual and sexual cycles. Asexual division takes place by tropic forms (*trophozoites*) and sexual cycles produce cysts with eight intracystic bodies (also known as *sporozoites*) within. The lifecycle is divided into three stages: (1) *Trophozoite* (vegetative), (2) *cyst*, and (3) *sporozoite*. *Precyst (sporocyst)* is an intermediate stage between the trophozoite and cyst stages.

The zygote is formed after the first mating. Then sporogenesis begins. The zygotic nucleus first goes through meiosis and then through mitosis. Precysts and then cysts are formed. After some time, excystation takes place and sporozoites come out of cyst. Sporozoites get converted into trophozoites. Excystation of some of the trophozoites takes place, cysts are formed, and also eight intracystic bodies (sporozoites) are produced. By the asexual cycle, trophic forms multiply by binary fission.

- *Trophozoites*: These are pleomorphic and ellipsoid in shape when examined under a light microscope in unfixed preparations, but can appear ameboid after fixation and analysis under an electron microscope. Their size ranges from 2 to 5 μm. They are haploid and mononuclear, with a single mitochondrion. They appear in groups. They are plentiful in the foamy substance that fills the alveoli. These forms are thin and flexible and covered with filopodia, which they use to attach to epithelial cells (type I pneumocytes).
  Asexual reproduction: Trophozoites divide by binary fission.
  Sexual reproduction:
  - *Precyst (sporocyst)*: It is a stage of the sexual cycle that leads to the formation of cysts.
  - *Cysts*: They are large, 4–6 μm in size, oval, thick wall with eight sporozoites (also known as *intracystic bodies*). When sporozoites are released from cysts, empty cysts are produced which are known as navicular bodies. They appear black in GMS stain and reddish purple in Toluidine Blue O stain.
  - *Sporozoites*: They are oval or peach in shape and 1–2 μm in size. The basophilic cytoplasm and reddish-purple nucleus are visible in Giemsa stain.

The mature cyst wall ruptures, releasing the eight sporozoites, which are then converted to trophozoites. The empty cysts are visible as navicular bodies, which are black when stained with GMS and reddish purple when stained with Toluidine Blue O.

PATHOGENESIS AND PATHOLOGY

Lungs are the most common site of infection for *P. jirovecii* in susceptible people. To change from its smaller trophic to larger cystic form, pneumocystis fungus adheres to alveolar epithelial cells (type I pneumocytes). The inflammatory reaction of the host causes considerable lung injury and decreased gas exchange, leading to hypoxia and possibly respiratory failure.

Although most cases of *Pneumocystis* involve the alveoli, few cases of disseminated infection can occur in people with very weak immune systems. Patients undergoing nonsystemic or second-line prophylaxis may see extrapulmonary symptoms such as hepatosplenomegaly and lesions on the skin, eyes, ears, or thyroid. In advanced diffuse pneumocystis, all the lung lobes are affected.

Foamy eosinophilic honeycombed exudate and thickening of the alveolar interstitial spaces are the two main characteristics revealed by hematoxylin and eosin (H&E) in histopathology. Hyperplasia and hypertrophy of type II pneumocytes, interstitial edema, infiltration of mononuclear cells, and moderate fibrosis are the causes of the interstitial thickening. More harm is done by inflammation in the lungs than by the fungus itself. In order to stimulate polymorphonuclear neutrophil (PMN) cells to invade the site of inflammation, macrophages engulf *P. jirovecii* and secrete interleukin-8 (IL-8). PMNs cause lung damage by releasing free radicals, cationic proteins, and proteinases. Impaired oxygenation is caused more by the input of PMN than by the load of *P. jirovecii*. Lung tissue is directly damaged by $CD8^+$ T-lymphocytes, leading to increased inflammation. The alveolar lumens are filled with *P. jirovecii* as the $CD4^+$ T-lymphocyte count drops below 200 cells/μL.

Adult respiratory distress syndrome (ARDS) like presentation: Severe instances may lead to the development of a hyaline membrane and interstitial fibrosis accompanied by swelling. Lung compliance, total lung capacity, and vital capacity alterations, an increased alveolar–arterial [alveolar partial pressure of oxygen (PAO_2)–arterial partial pressure of oxygen (PaO_2)] oxygen gradient, and diminished diffusing capacity all lead to decreased oxygenation. ARDS is comparable to this picture of widespread lung injury.

Lung stiffness and difficulty breathing are symptoms of PCP, which are caused by a decrease in the production of surfactant phospholipids. These lipids ordinarily serve to lower alveolar surface tension. The last stage can mirror other restrictive lung illnesses in its progression toward severe interstitial fibrosis and contiguous cyst-like airspaces, which give the lung a "honeycomb" or "sponge-like appearance."

Granulomatous lesions and cavitary disease are two further reactions that the organism may occasionally initiate.

CLINICAL PRESENTATION

- There is no pathognomonic combination of symptoms.
- Increasingly coughing that does not resolve itself over a few weeks or months. Symptoms such as shortness of breath, fever, and nonproductive cough are common.
- Chest discomfort gets worse over a period of days or weeks.

  In moderate situations, HIV-positive patients may have a normal pulmonary examination at rest, but when they exert themselves, they will experience tachypnea, tachycardia, and diffuse dry ("cellophane") rales. Oxygen deprivation can be minor [$PaO_2 \geq 70$ mm Hg in ambient air or an alveolar–arterial O_2 difference (A-a) $DO_2 < 35$ mm Hg] or substantial. A late symptom of severe hypoxia is cyanosis.
- Pleural effusion, intrathoracic adenopathy, and cavitation are rare complications.
- Pneumothorax, asymmetric disease, nodules, blebs, cysts, and localization to the higher lobes are all examples of unusual presentations.
- *Extrapulmonary pneumocystosis*: Patients with advanced HIV infection who are using aerosolized pentamidine alone or who are not getting prophylaxis are at risk of developing extrapulmonary pneumocystitis. Most often, the organs that are implicated include the kidneys, thyroid, spleen, liver, bone marrow, gastrointestinal tract, and eyes. From unanticipated results to autopsies to fast spread across many systems, the clinical picture can be rather varied.

RADIOGRAPHY

In PCP, the hallmark high-resolution computerized tomography (HRCT) finding is bilateral, symmetrical ground-glass appearance, most commonly seen in the perihilar region. The "crazy paving" pattern can be caused by alveolitis and involvement of the interlobular septum.

IMMUNITY

Microbial Factors

Two main categories of *P. jirovecii* antigens have been established. One is the multifunctional major surface glycoprotein (MSG) molecule. The trophic forms of *P. jirovecii* are able to attach themselves firmly to type I pneumocytes because MSG binds to alveolar extracellular matrix (ECM) proteins. The mannose residues in MSG trigger phagocytosis and inflammation when they attach to the mannose receptors found on alveolar macrophages. As an additional indicator of infection, another antigen complex consists of a 35–45 kDa glycoprotein.

Host Factors

Alveolar macrophages: They engulf attached *P. jirovecii* via several pattern recognition receptors (PRRs), acting as the lung's initial line of defense. After being engulfed by phagosomes, *P. jirovecii* undergoes degradation through lysosome fusion. Lung epithelial cells and macrophages release reactive oxygen species (ROS), cytokines, and chemokines that promote inflammation [e.g., tumor necrosis factor-alpha (TNF-α) and IL-8]. Lymphocyte-derived products, especially interferon gamma (IFN-γ), are essential for activation of alveolar macrophages. Macrophages lose some of their ability to phagocytose *P. jirovecii* when they become infected with HIV. This happens as there is reduction in the expression of surface mannose receptors. The death of alveolar macrophages during an infection is caused in part by apoptosis.

CD4+ T-lymphocytes: Their action on PCP involves bringing in effector cells like macrophages and activating them to eliminate *Pneumocystis*. An HIV-positive person becomes susceptible to *P. jirovecii* when CD4+ T-lymphocyte count drops to <200 cells/μL.

Polymorphonuclear neutrophils and CD8+ T-lymphocytes: The presence of elevated CD8+ T-lymphocytes and PMN lung inflammation are hallmarks of severe PCP. PMNs cause damage to alveolar and capillary epithelial cells by releasing ROS and proteinases.

When it comes to protecting the host from *P. jirovecii*, B lymphocytes play a crucial role. Antibody opsonization enhances alveolar macrophage phagocytosis and killing. It is possible that PCP is caused by reduced local antibody production.

Pneumocystis jirovecii: Alteration of Pulmonary Surfactants

There are a number of ECM proteins that *P. jirovecii* can attach to, including vitronectin, fibronectin and collectin 3, surfactant proteins A and D (SP-A and SP-D). *P. jirovecii* is able to connect to alveolar macrophages more effectively when its primary surface glycoprotein, MSG, binds to SP-A and SP-D.

Surface tension increases significantly, and hypoxemic respiratory failure occurs in PCP patients due to surfactant downregulation caused by *P. jirovecii* infection.

Immune reconstitution inflammatory syndrome (IRIS): If a patient's immune system recovers at the same time that they stop taking systemic steroids or are undergoing cancer treatment, or if their CD4$^+$ T-lymphocytes recover rapidly following antiretroviral medication, then the patient will experience IRIS. Since nonsevere PCP is present in patients with PCP-related IRIS, the degree of immunological recovery determines the severity.

LABORATORY DIAGNOSIS

- *Pulmonary function tests*: Vital capacity, total lung capacity, and carbon monoxide diffusion capacity in one breath are all reduced. Gallium scans are more accurate.
- *Method considered gold standard*: Staining bronchoalveolar lavage (BAL) fluid with immunofluorescent and colorimetric techniques (specificity 95% and sensitivity 95%).
- Noninvasive test for β-(1 → 3)-D-glucan in serum/BAL is also quite sensitive. Negative test can rule out PCP.
- It is recommended to first induce sputum in AIDS patients, and if that fails, to move on to BAL. The use of BAL in bronchoscopy allows for the successful acquisition of microscopic evidence of *P. jirovecii.* The sensitivity and specificity of cytocentrifuge smears of BAL fluid are 81–90% and 90–100%, respectively, when stained or on using immunofluorescence. Only in extreme cases should an open lung biopsy be considered.
- *GMS, Toluidine O, Gram–Wiegert staining*: These stains make it easy to identify cysts by staining their walls (cystic stage). There are clusters visible in the smear **(Fig. 22.1)**. The most sensitive and user-friendly technique is Gram–Wigert staining.
- *Wright Giemsa or its variant—Giemsa-like rapid stain (Diff-Quick, polychrome methylene blue staining)*: These are easy and rapid to perform. The drawback is that they are not selective stain for internal contents of cyst nuclei of developmental stages and trophic forms.

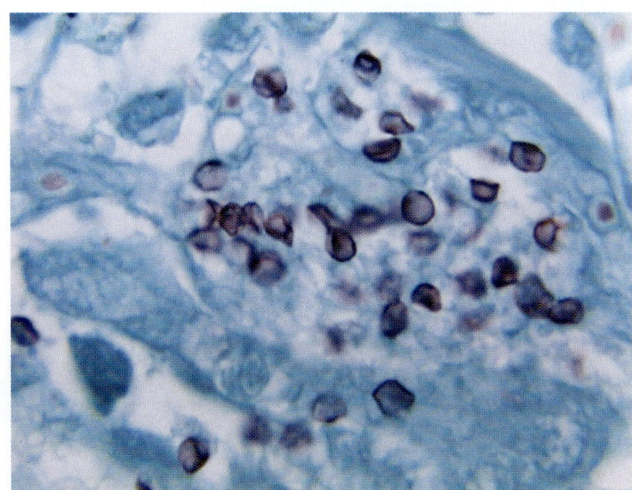

FIG. 22.1: GMS-stained smear showing cysts (1,000×). (GMS: Grocott–Gömöri's methenamine silver)
Source: Public Health Image Library CDC.

- *Phase contrast microscope* with vital dyes provides rapid diagnosis.
- *Tinctorial stain such as May-Grünwald and Papanicolaou* (PAP) smear stain intracystic sporozoites as well as trophozoites.
- *Giemsa*: It stains trophozoites as deep blue. It does not stain cyst wall **(Fig. 22.2)**.
- *Immunofluorescence* with monoclonal antibodies to both cyst and trophozoite is developed but false-negative results may occur.
- *H&E stain*: It demonstrates typical granular, foamy, and honeycombed material in alveoli **(Fig. 22.3)**.
- *Giemsa stain* shows reddish nucleus and blue cytoplasm.
- *GMS* shows black-colored organisms **(Fig. 22.1)**.
- *Calcofluor stain* is easy to perform and is a rapid method. The direct fluorescent antibody (DFA) method (Merifluor Pneumocystis and Meridian Bioscience of Cincinnati, OH) uses monoclonal antibody staining, which has a few benefits: It can detect both trophic forms and cysts, which might be morphologically confounded with *P. jirovecii,* and it can exclude *Candida* that could be mistaken for *P. jirovecii.*
- *Fungitell® Test for β-(1 → 3)-D-glucan*: Measurement of β-(1 → 3)-D-glucan levels in the serum, plasma, or BAL fluid may be useful in the diagnosis of PCP. Its levels >31 pg/mL in serum is a useful marker for the diagnosis of PCP. Because it is noninvasive, the Fungitell test may be useful as a rapid presumptive screen, before confirmatory microbiologic tests are done.
- *DNA probe*: It is used to detect the organism in BAL sample.
- *Nested polymerase chain reaction (PCR)*: It has 80% sensitivity.
- *Real-time PCR*: It is a rapid, sensitive, and specific method.

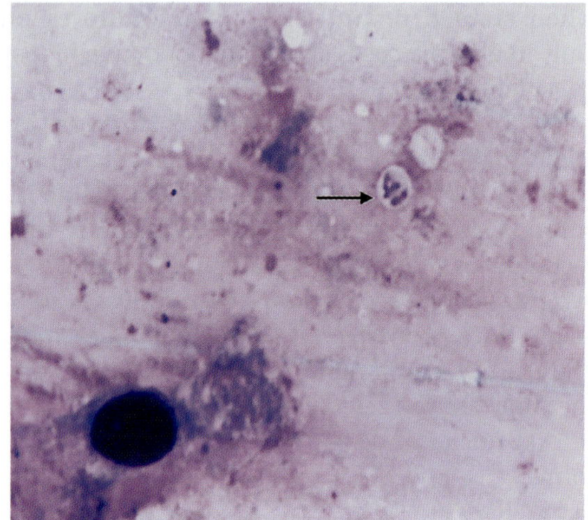

FIG. 22.2: Giemsa stain showing the fungus (1,000×).
Source: Public Health Image Library CDC.

In Vitro Cultivation

Efforts have been made to find in vitro procedures that can speed up the creation of pathogenic organisms. When cultivating *Pneumocystis*, it was a common practice to employ specific cell lines, such as Mv1 from mink, human embryonic lung (HEL) from human lung fibroblasts, and A 549 from human lung cancer.

Utilizing a three-dimensional air-liquid interface culture system established by the CuFi-8 respiratory epithelial cell line, the initial triumph was attained in 2014. Direct cultivation and propagation of *P. jirovecii* from BAL samples is achieved using this method.

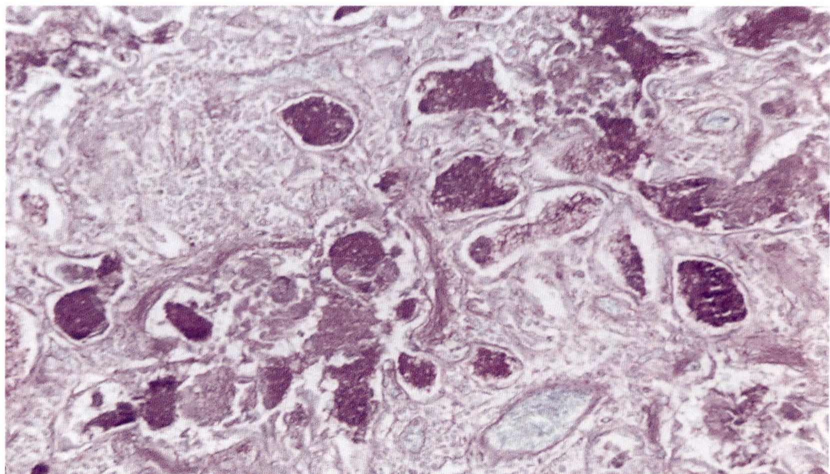

FIG. 22.3: Lung biopsy stained with H&E—alveolar spaces filled with exudate containing fungus (400×).
(H&E: hematoxylin and eosin)
Source: Public Health Image Library CDC.

TREATMENT AND PROPHYLAXIS

- As there is no ergosterol in the cytoplasm of the organism, it is resistant to commonly used antifungal drugs. A combination of TMP and SMZ (or SMX) is the drug of choice for treatment as well as prophylaxis. It is given orally, and the doses are TMP as 15–20 mg/kg/day and SMZ 75–100 mg/kg/day.
- The second line of drug is pentamidine isethionate [4 mg/kg/day, intravenous (IV) for 3 weeks]. It is suitable for patients who cannot tolerate TMP-SMZ.
- Dapsone is another alternative drug.
- Atovaquone in the dose of 750 mg orally thrice a day for 3 weeks is given to mild-to-moderate cases. It has few adverse effects and is suitable in patients with glucose-6-phosphate dehydrogenase (G-6-PD) deficiency who do not tolerate other drugs.
- Primary prophylaxis is given to those patients who never had PCP (1) if their CD4 count is <200/mm^3 or (2) if they develop oral thrush or (3) unexplained fever > 100°F for >2 weeks.
- Secondary prophylaxis is given to HIV-seropositive patients who have already had an episode of PCP.

The standard guidelines for prophylaxis are as follows:

- Preventative PCP treatment is necessary for patients with a CD4 count < 200/mm^3 or for higher-count patients who experience esophageal candidiasis or an unexplained fever > 100°F for longer than 2 weeks. Patients with CD4 counts < 200/mm^3 are advised to take a lifelong prophylactic.
- Prophylaxis should be administered to all individuals who have experienced a prior episode of PCP. This medication can be given to patients unless they have a known sensitivity to TMP-SMZ. Other treatment plans should be considered in the event that TMP-SMZ is well-tolerated.

[There is some incidence reported showing point mutations in its dihydropteroate synthase (*DHPS*) gene. Combination of TMP-SMZ and caspofungin which shows synergistic activity may be tried in future.]

CHAPTER

23 Microsporidiosis

INTRODUCTION

Microsporidiosis is an opportunistic fungal infection caused by *Microsporidia* species which are obligatory intracellular organisms. In humans, they are opportunistic organisms affecting patients with underlying immunodeficiency such as acquired immunodeficiency syndrome (AIDS). The genus was previously placed in kingdom Protozoa but has now been shifted to kingdom Fungi. The most common species which cause human infections are *Enterocytozoon bieneusi* and *Encephalitozoon intestinalis*. The fungus produces diarrhea with weight loss or may cause infections of other sites, including disseminated infections. The disease, microsporidiosis, is one of the emerging fungal infections.

HISTORY

Gluge, in 1838, recorded the first report of microsporidia existence in fish. In 1857, *Nosema bombycis* was found by Professor Carl Wilhelm von Nägeli, the first microsporidia. The severe sickness caused by *N. bombycis* was called pebrine that affected silkworms. It almost wiped out the silk industry in Germany, Italy, and France in Europe. It is well known that Louis Pasteur's research saved the silk industry in Europe.

Microsporidia were a mystery for a long time; scientists could not agree on what they were. Some suggested that they were yeast like organisms whereas others suggested that they were creatures related to fungi, creatures, protozoa, cancer cells, or broken red blood cells. Balbiani, in 1882, suggested the separate taxon microsporidia for it. The molecular phylogenetic analysis disproved the earlier theory that microsporidia are a primitive protozoon. In 2008, microsporidia were grouped as a basal branch or a sister group of fungi.

It is now known that microsporidia are obligate intracellular fungi. Microsporidia have been known to cause sickness in a wide range of hosts, including insects such as honeybees and silkworms, and vertebrates, including fish, cattle, rabbits, rats, dogs, and primates.

In the year 1959, the first human case was described from a Japanese child. In 2001, Sehgal et al. reported the first case of intestinal microsporidiosis in India. In 2003, Sharma et al. reported the first case of ocular illness.

MYCOLOGY

Although microsporidia were formerly thought of as simple protozoa, they are now known to belong to the kingdom Fungi. Chitin and trehalose, a shared life cycle, and a shared arrangement of DNA all make them look like fungi. Microsporidia are widely distributed in nature, with 170 genera and almost 1,300 species of which 15 have been reported from human diseases. The pathogenic species are listed in **Table 23.1**, but *E. bieneusi* and *E. intestinalis* are the most common human pathogenic species.

The spores of the fungus have a thick three-layered wall, and they can survive chlorine concentrations present in drinking water. The polar filaments or polar tubes can invade the host. The mode of transmission is exactly not known, but ingestion, inhalation, and inoculation are the most suspected modes of transmission.

Microsporidia have well-defined nuclei and plasma membrane, but they lack organelles seen in eukaryotes.

MORPHOLOGY (FIG. 23.1)

The infective and extremely hardy spore form can survive in nature. In living organisms, it takes on an oval shape with dimensions of 0.5 μm in width and 1–1.5 μm in length. It has a three-layered cell wall. The three layers are (1) proteinaceous exospore, (2) chitinous endospore, and (3) plasma membrane. Exospore is electron-dense and endospore is electron-lucent. The organelles found

TABLE 23.1: Various species of microsporidia.

Species	Synonyms	Common name	Known infections	Host specificity
Anncaliia algerae	*Nosema, Brachiola*	–	Various, including in immunocompromised hosts	Human and other mammals
Anncaliia connori	*Nosema*	–	Rare, in immunocompromised hosts	Human and other mammals
Anncaliia vesicularum	*Brachiola*	–	Rare, in immunocompromised hosts	Human and other mammals
Encephalitozoon cuniculi	–	–	Systemic infections, especially in immunocompromised individuals	Human and rabbits
Encephalitozoon hellem	–	–	Conjunctivitis, keratitis, and systemic infections	Human and other mammals
Encephalitozoon intestinalis	–	–	Diarrhea and systemic infections in immunocompromised individuals	Human and other mammals
Encephalitozoon (undetermined)	–	–	Various, poorly characterized	–
Endoreticulatus	–	–	Rare, in immunocompromised hosts	Human and other mammals
Enterocytozoon bieneusi	–	–	Diarrhea and systemic infections	Human and other mammals
Microsporidium ceylonensis	–	–	Rare, in immunocompromised hosts	Human and other mammals
Microsporidium africanum	–	–	Rare, in immunocompromised hosts	Human and other mammals
Nosema ocularum	–	–	Ocular infections	Human and other mammals

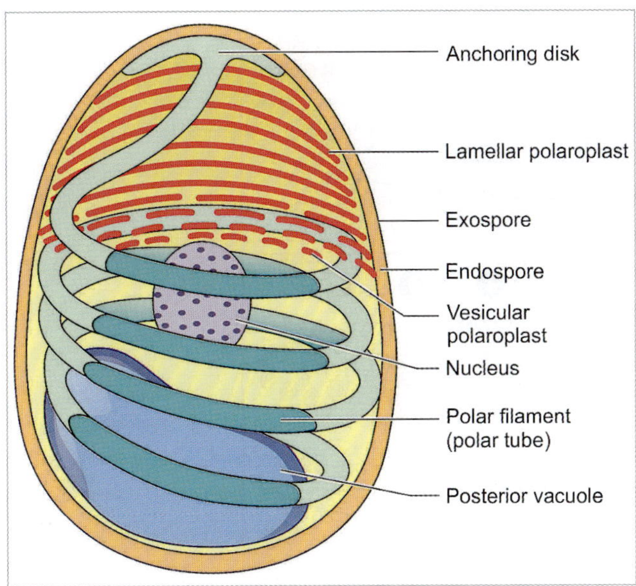

FIG. 23.1: Morphology of microsporidian spore.

in cytoplasm are nucleus, ribosomes, anchoring plate, polaroplast—lamellar and tubular, coiled polar tube (six coils), polar sac, and a posterior vacuole.

Anchoring plate, polaroplast—lamellar and tubular, and coiled polar tube (six coils) make up the extrusion mechanism of the spore. These structures are diagnostic for microscopic appearance. The infectious material, sporoplasm (cell membranes), is injected into the host cell by means of a tubular extrusion mechanism that resembles a spring. Inside the host, the fungus utilizes host cell machinery for energy and multiplies in host cytoplasm.

Human microsporidia can infect several organ systems; immunocompromised individuals, such as those living with human immunodeficiency virus (HIV)/AIDS, often experience recurrent diarrhea as a symptom. Additional clinical signs include encephalitis, keratitis, sinusitis, myositis, and systemic disease.

Infections in humans have been linked to microsporidia belonging to several genera and species, such as *Nosema, Enterocytozoon, Encephalitozoon, Pleistophora, Trachipleistophora, Brachiola, Anncaliia, Tubulinosema, Endoreticulatus*, and *Microsporidium*. Some kinds of microsporidium are zoonotic, which means they can infect animals as well as people. The spore of a microsporidian has an unusual form. Infectious spores are produced by microsporidia during their life cycle. These spores are the only part of the life cycle that can survive outside of the host cell because of their resistance to environmental influences.

LIFE CYCLE AND PATHOGENESIS (FIG. 23.2)

Humans contract the disease most commonly through eating contaminated spores, but it can also spread through inhalation and indirect skin contact.

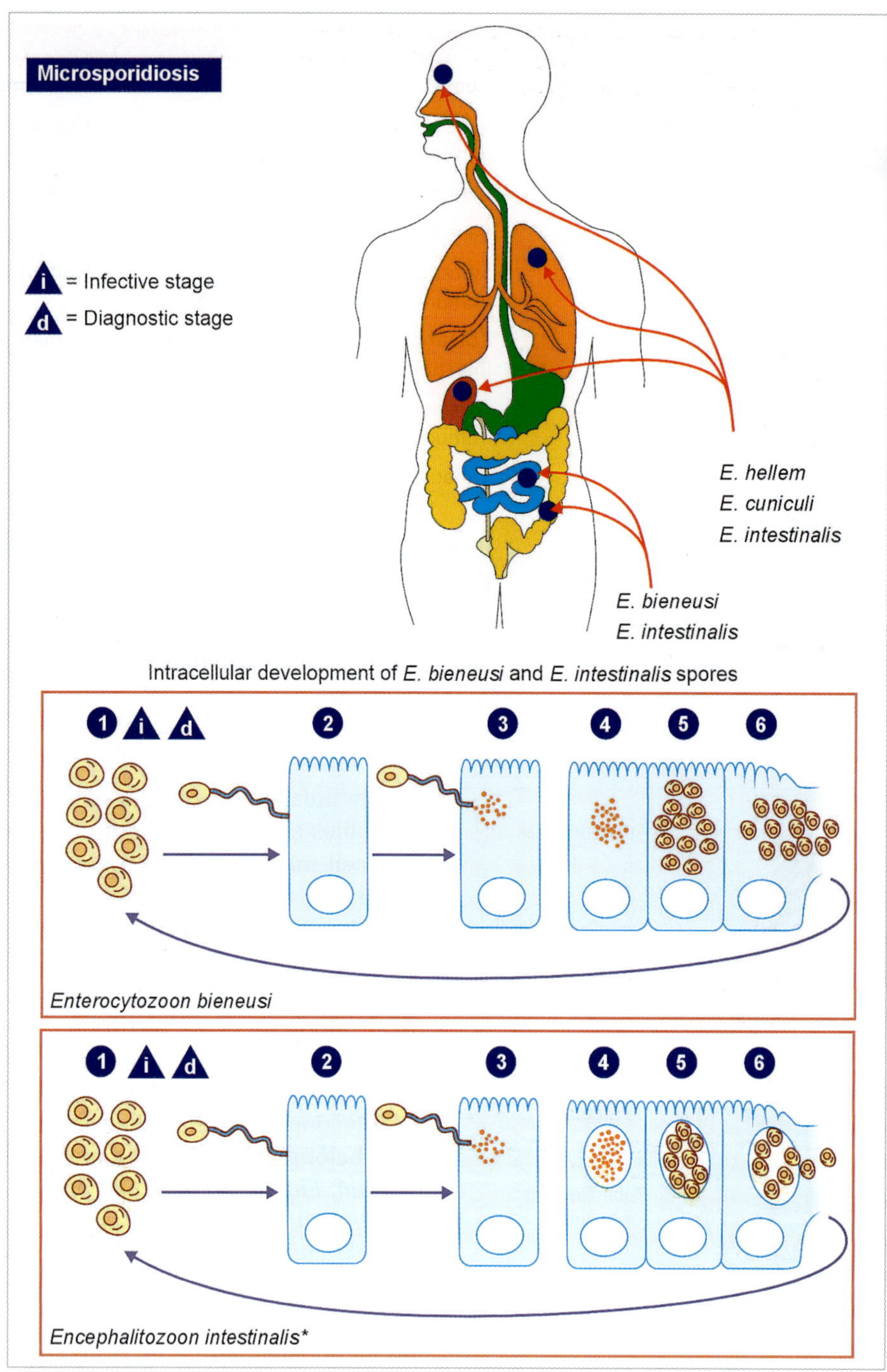

*Development inside parasitophorous vacuole also occurs in *E. hellem* and *E. cuniculi*.

FIG. 23.2: Life cycle.

Extrusion of Sporoplasm

The infectious spore material, known as sporoplasm, is introduced into the host cell, the enterocyte, through injection. For injecting the sporoplasm, the polar tube extends from the spore as a long, flexible cylindrical structure. This process is aided by polar sacs, polaroplasts, elevated pH, and calcium ions. The first is to puncture the plasma membrane of the host cell; the second is to enlarge the host cell's plasma membrane to encase the growing sporoplasm.

Asexual Cycle

Within the host cells, the sporoplasm divides into many meronts. There are several ways to multiply: Binary fission, schizogony, or plasmotomy. Plasmotomy involves dividing the cytoplasm without considering the nuclei in order to produce progeny with numerous nuclei. Meronts are free-floating, round-to-elongated structures in the host cell's cytoplasm or vacuole.

Sporogony

Meronts mature into sporonts. They are enclosed by a double-layered cyst wall and either directly change into sporoblasts or become multinucleated to create sporangial plasma before transforming into sporoblasts. Sporoblasts go through sporogony and become spores. Spore can be released by lysis of the host cell. Some of these microsporidia that infect humans have been successfully cultivated in various cell lines. *Vittaforma corneae*, a human microsporidium, was one of the first microsporidia to be successfully cultivated in humans. It was grown using a variety of cell lines, including SIRC cells, MDCK cells, and rabbit embryo fibroblasts.

EPIDEMIOLOGY

Human infections caused by microsporidia have been recorded on every continent with the exception of Antarctica. Surface water is a common habitat for microsporidia. Other water sources, such as groundwater, tertiary sewage effluent, hospital effluent, and municipal drinking water, may harbor microsporidia that can cause illness in humans. Before the AIDS pandemic, human infections with microsporidia were rare. However, seroprevalence rates recorded for microsporidiosis in humans varied from 0 to 42% before the AIDS era, and this data was primarily derived from serology. Human microsporidial infections increased in number as the AIDS epidemic progressed. The prevalence of gastrointestinal microsporidiosis in HIV-positive persons varied between 2 and 70%, depending on the study population and diagnostic methods used.

Risk Factors for Microsporidiosis

- *Immunosuppression*: Individuals with a low CD4 T-lymphocyte count (below 50–100 cells/mm^3) are highly susceptible to microsporidial infections.
- *Transplantation*: Those who have received a transplant of the kidney, liver, heart–lung, or pancreas are at risk of infection from donor-infected tissues.
- *Corticosteroid use*: Patients using corticosteroids, including prednisone, have had chronic bilateral keratoconjunctivitis as a result of *Encephalitozoon* species.
- *Consumption of untreated water*: Particularly for those who travel frequently or live in areas with inadequate water cleanliness, it increases the likelihood of contracting a microsporidial infection.
- *Contact lens use*: Contact lenses increase the risk of eye infections when not cleaned and hygienically maintained properly.
- *Water exposure*: Things such as soil, hot springs, and untreated water supplies fall into this category. Any water-based leisure activity in areas where microsporidia are prevalent has the potential for infection.
- *Travel*: The chance of contracting microsporidiosis increases when one travels to areas where the disease is common.

Modes of Transmission

- *Zoonotic transmission*: Direct evidence of zoonotic transmission has been recorded in situations where people became ill after coming into contact with diseased animals.
- *Waterborne transmission*: Waterborne infection is a common pathway for microsporidial infection. Ingestion of polluted water or consumption of food cooked with contaminated water might result in illness. Microsporidial spores can also be detected in sewage discharge, providing a concern if effective water treatment is not implemented.
- *Foodborne transmission*: Consumption of raw or undercooked meat, along with unwashed produce, has been associated with microsporidial illnesses.
- *Horizontal transmission*: Oral transmission has also been recognized as a possible route for horizontal transfer, such as through oral–anal contact during sexual activity.
- *Vertical transmission*: Several animal species have reported vertical transmission, but no humans have been found to do so yet.
- *Inoculation and eye exposure*: In some cases, microsporidial spores can be introduced into the body through inoculation into open wounds or through exposure to the eye.

Host–Parasite Interactions in Microsporidia

Polar Tube and Invasion Mechanism

A unique structure called the polar tube is utilized by microsporidia in their invasion method. This structure allows the parasite's nucleus and sporoplasm to transfer from the spore to the host cell.

Spore Wall Proteins and Host Cell Interaction

- It is thought that spore wall proteins (SWPs), particularly those found in the exospore, have a function in invasion by attaching to host cells or initiating signaling.
- Various SWPs have been discovered, including but not limited to SWP1, SWP2, SWP3, and SWP4.
- Post-translational glycosylation modifies certain SWPs; this modification may play a role in spore adhesion to mucin or host cells as they travel through the gastrointestinal (GI) system.

Polar Tube Proteins and Host Cell Interaction

Microsporidia include six polar tube proteins, numbered PTP1 through PTP6, some of which interact with host cells.

Sporoplasm Proteins and Host Cell Interaction

As the spore invades, it uses the polar tube to release its sporoplasm into the host cell. It has been demonstrated that a sporoplasm surface protein 1 (SSP1) binds to the host cell surface at the location of the polar tube contact.

Microsporidia acquire energy through interactions with voltage-dependent anion channels (VDACs) in host cells, which in turn interact with SSP1.

Nutrient Acquisition

The host cell provides microsporidia with nutrients, such as ATP. Energy acquisition by microsporidian meronts is dependent on their interaction with host mitochondria.

IMMUNITY

It is possible to produce antibodies that target microsporidia by recognizing their polar tube and spore wall. People with impaired cell-mediated immunity, such as those living with HIV/AIDS, are at an increased risk of contracting microsporidiosis. Chronic infection with high antibody titers and ongoing inflammation can be a consequence of microsporidial infections in specific cases. Research has shown that in order to completely eradicate microsporidial infections, gamma interferon (IFN-γ) is essential. Infection is more likely to occur in CD8+ cell-deficient mice, and CD8+ T cells help reduce tissue burden.

CLINICAL FEATURES

Factors such as the host's immune status, the particular microsporidian species involved, and the mode of transmission can cause infections in humans to differ greatly. Some of the symptoms that can occur in a patient with human microsporidiosis are listed as follows:

- *Intestinal microsporidiosis: chronic diarrhea*: *E. bieneusi* and *E. intestinalis* induce microsporidiosis, and one of the most prevalent clinical signs is chronic diarrhea. People with impaired immune systems, such as those living with HIV/AIDS, frequently exhibit this symptom.
- *Myositis*: Microsporidia can cause muscle inflammation (myositis) in some cases. For example, *Anncaliia algerae* has been associated with myositis in humans.
- *Kidney and urogenital infection*: Microsporidial infections can affect the kidneys and urogenital tract, leading to conditions such as nephritis and urogenital infections.
- *Cholangitis*: Some microsporidial species, such as *E. bieneusi*, can cause inflammation of the bile ducts (cholangitis). This condition may lead to symptoms such as jaundice and abdominal pain.
- *Ascites*: Ascites, the accumulation of fluid in the abdominal cavity, can occur as a result of microsporidial infections.
- *Sinusitis*: Infections involving the sinuses, such as sinusitis, have been reported in cases of microsporidiosis.
- *Hepatitis*: Microsporidia can cause inflammation of the liver (hepatitis), which may lead to symptoms such as jaundice and abdominal discomfort.
- *Keratoconjunctivitis*: Microsporidial infections can affect the eyes, leading to conditions such as keratoconjunctivitis. This may manifest as eye pain, redness, and vision problems. Use of contact lens may act as a predisposing factor.
- *Disseminated infection*: In severe cases, microsporidial infections can become disseminated, spreading throughout the body. Pneumonitis, sinusitis, nephritis, cystitis, hepatitis, peritonitis, infection of brain, and skin lesions may occur as a part of disseminated disease.
- *Asymptomatic infection*: Not all individuals infected with microsporidia develop noticeable symptoms. Some may carry the infection without experiencing clinical manifestations, especially if they have a healthy immune system.

Enterocytozoon bieneusi

In most of the AIDS patients, chronic diarrhea cases are caused by *E. bieneusi*, making it the most common microsporidium causing human sickness. Prolonged diarrhea, loss of appetite, and low body weight without fever can be symptoms of an infection with *E. bieneusi*. Fatigue and wasting syndrome are common outcomes of malabsorption. Sclerosing cholangitis, which occurs when it invades the biliary system's epithelium, is another possible outcome.

Encephalitozoon (Encephalitozoon Species*)*

Encephalitozoon cuniculi, Encephalitozoon hellem, and *E. intestinalis* are among many species of *Encephalitozoon* that infect mammals and can spread to many organs.

Encephalitozoonidae infections can lead to a variety of symptoms and conditions, including but not limited to sinusitis, bronchiolitis, nephritis, keratitis, peritonitis, hepatitis, gastroenteritis, cerebritis, cystitis, urethritis, prostatitis, nodular skin lesions, and systemic infection. Immunocompromised individuals, such as those with HIV/AIDS, organ transplant recipients, or who are using immunomodulatory drugs, are at an increased risk of contracting these diseases. An infection known as interstitial nephritis can manifest in AIDS patients who have contracted an *Encephalitozoon* species.

Anncaliia Species

- Many species of the *Anncaliia* genus have been found in people, including *A. algerae, Anncaliia connori*, and *Anncaliia vesicularum*.
- *A. algerae* infection has been linked to keratitis, infection of the vocal cord, severe myositis, and skin abscesses.
- Myositis and disseminated infection can also be caused by *A. vesicularum* and *A. connori*.

Vittaforma corneae

- *V. corneae* can cause keratoconjunctivitis in both healthy individuals and HIV-infected patients.
- Outbreaks have been associated with exposure to soil.
- This pathogen can also cause enteritis, and dissemination has been observed in immunocompromised hosts.

LABORATORY DIAGNOSIS

Feces, biopsies of the small intestine, sputum, urine, corneal smears, small intestine content, body fluids, duodenal aspirate, bronchoalveolar lavage (BAL), cerebrospinal fluid (CSF), and biopsies of organs are among the samples taken. The confocal microscopy is proved to be very useful.

Light Microscopy

The most common way to diagnose gastrointestinal microsporidiosis is by analyzing stool samples for the presence of spores. It is usual for disseminated microsporidial infections to involve the kidneys, which means that urine specimens should also be obtained in case of spore shedding in urine.

Chromotrope 2R technique: The spores and their surrounding wall have a pinkish-red color with a central belt-like line. It takes approximately 90 minutes and is a laborious process.

Quick-hot Gram-chromotrope staining: It takes only 10 minutes. Spores stain dark violet, with belt-like strips.

Modified trichrome stain (MTS): Microsporidia appear as red refractile structures against a blue background. Various modifications are Weber green MTS, Ryan blue MTS, and Kokosin hot method of MTS.

Modified acid-fast staining: 1% acid alcohol is used as a decolorizing solution. Spores are acid-fast and appear red.

Fluorescent microscope: Fungi-Fluor and Uvitex 2B can be used for detection in stool and urine samples.

Culture

Being obligate intracellular organism, it cannot grow on any bacterial or fungal culture media. Various cell lines used for cultivation are monkey kidney, rabbit kidney cells (Vero, RK13), human fibroblast cell culture (MRC-5), and MDCK cell line. It is useful for antigen preparation and drug susceptibility testing.

Serologic Tests

Antibody Detection

- Antibodies to *E. cuniculi* are detected by indirect immunofluorescence assay (titer—1:16).
- Microagglutination test (titer above 1:160).
- *Enzyme-linked immunosorbent assay (ELISA) and Western blot*: They are used to detect antibodies against the C1 Hsp70 protein of *E. cuniculi* and *E. intestinalis* but they have less specificity.

Antigen Detection

Direct immunofluorescence (DIF) is used for antigen detection.

Molecular Biology-based Techniques

- Molecular techniques, such as polymerase chain reaction (PCR), have become important for diagnosing microsporidial infections.
- PCR-based tests using various genetic markers, including small subunit ribosomal ribonucleic acid (SSU rRNA), large subunit rRNA (LSU rRNA), and intergenic spacer regions, can detect different microsporidian species in clinical samples.
- Nucleic acids are isolated from clinical specimens, and PCR can detect microsporidia with high sensitivity (detecting as low as 100–1,000 spores/mL).
- Real-time PCR has been found to be three times more likely to detect microsporidia compared to traditional microscopy.
- In situ hybridization with rRNA probes can also identify microsporidia at the species level but is less commonly used due to lower sensitivity and complexity.

TREATMENT

The treatment of microsporidiosis depends on the specific microsporidian species causing the infection and the patient's immune status. Some key points regarding the therapy of microsporidiosis are as follows:

- *Immune reconstitution*: Improving immune function by combination antiretroviral treatment (cART) is critical in immunocompromised persons, particularly those with advanced AIDS and very low CD4+ cell counts. This immune reconstitution can result in symptom relief and microsporidia eradication. Immune reconstitution inflammatory syndrome (IRIS) is uncommon in microsporidiosis.
- *Dehydration and malnutrition management*: Severe dehydration, malnutrition, and wasting syndrome should be managed with fluid support and nutritional supplementation.
- *Antimotility agents*: Diarrhea can be controlled using antimotility agents as needed.
- Specific treatments for microsporidial species are as follows:
    - *E. bieneusi*: There is currently no highly effective commercial therapy for this species. Fumagillin has shown effectiveness in clinical trials and is available through expanded access programs. Alternatives include nitazoxanide and albendazole, but their efficacy may be limited, especially in patients with low CD4 counts.
    - *Encephalitozoonidae (systemic infections—E. cuniculi, E. hellem, and E. intestinalis)*: Albendazole is the treatment of choice, given at 400 mg twice daily.
    - *Encephalitozoonidae keratoconjunctivitis*: Topical fumagillin solution can be used, along with albendazole if systemic infection is present.

Although there is no hard and fast rule on how long microsporidiosis treatments should last, it is recommended that patients continue taking their medication for at least 4 weeks. It should be considered to continue therapy if immunosuppression remains (for instance, a CD4 count below 200 cells/μL).

Other Medications

Several other medications have been reported as treatments for microsporidiosis, including atovaquone, furazolidone, itraconazole, nitazoxanide, thalidomide, and more. However, the efficacy of these treatments may vary, and they are generally used in specific cases or when other options are unavailable.

Potential New Therapies

Various potential new therapeutic approaches for microsporidiosis are being explored, including synthetic polyamines, calmodulin inhibitors, calcium antagonists, chitin synthesis inhibitors, topoisomerase IV inhibitors, and others. These approaches aim to target specific aspects of microsporidia biology and metabolism.

CHAPTER

24 *Talaromyces marneffei (Penicillium marneffei)*

INTRODUCTION

Talaromyces marneffei (Penicillium marneffei) is a thermally dimorphic fungus that is endemic to Southeast Asia, and the disease is seen in immunocompromised patients such as human immunodeficiency virus (HIV)-infected persons. Talaromycosis is an acquired immunodeficiency syndrome (AIDS)-defining illness. Other people at risk include those undergoing immunosuppressive treatment for stem cell or solid organ transplant. In host cells, it occurs in yeast-like forms, and in the environment (as well as a media at 25°C), it occurs in a filamentous form. It is the only dimorphic fungus in the genus *Penicillium* or *Talaromyces.* The mold releases a brick-red pigment into the growing media, which is easily identifiable. Such a type of pigment may also be produced by other *Penicillium* species, but they are not dimorphic. The inhalation of conidia is the mode of infection. Inhaling the conidia causes them to transform into fission yeast once they enter the host's tissues. People living in or visiting Southeast Asia and the surrounding areas are the most common carriers of disseminated talaromycosis.

HISTORY

The fungus was first isolated by Capponi et al. in 1956 from bamboo rats. In the first known instance of *P. marneffei* human infection, *G. Segretain* got a needle prick that contained *P. marneffei* spores. Lymphangitis and a small nodule appeared at the infection site 9 days after the injury. He named the fungus species *marneffei* in honor of Hubert Marneffe, the then director of the Pasteur Institute (Indo-China). In 1973, the first human case of spontaneous infection was documented by DiSalvo et al. in a Southeast Asian patient with Hodgkin lymphoma.

Prior to the publication of the first case of penicilliosis infection in an AIDS patient by Piehl et al. in the year 1988, there were less than 40 cases recorded in Southeast Asia, but penicilliosis infections increased with the HIV pandemic.

MYCOLOGY

The genus *Penicillium* has just one species of dimorphic fungus, *P. marneffei* (now *T. marneffei*). Yeast-like forms are present in the host and media incubated at 37°C, while filamentous (mold) forms are present in the environment as well as media incubated at 25°C.

The yeast-like form divides in two by fission rather than budding. Hence, a transverse septum is formed at the time of fission. Inside the cells of the reticuloendothelial system, round or oval cells measuring 3–4 µm, comparable to *Histoplasma,* are seen. The extracellular forms consist of yeast cells and a few longer, curved forms (8–13 µm) that resemble sausages, forms not seen in *Histoplasma.*

Under conditions of 25–30°C, its colony matures in about 3 days. Cycloheximide inhibits its growth; hence, Sabouraud dextrose agar (SDA) with cycloheximide is not used for primary isolation. At 25°C, colonies of *P. marneffei* will have a greenish-yellow hue with a noticeable red diffusible pigment, as seen in **Figure 24.1**. Red diffusible pigment formation is severely inhibited at temperatures between 35 and 37°C. Hyaline septate hyphae and fruiting structures composed of branching metulae and phialides that produce chains of spherical conidia producing a brush-like appearance are characteristic of this mold's similarity to other *Penicillium* species.

Some other species of *Penicillium* that can infect humans are *Penicillium citrinum, Penicillium cretaceum, Penicillium dupontii, Penicillium glaucum, Penicillium purpurogenum,* and *Penicillium decumbens.*

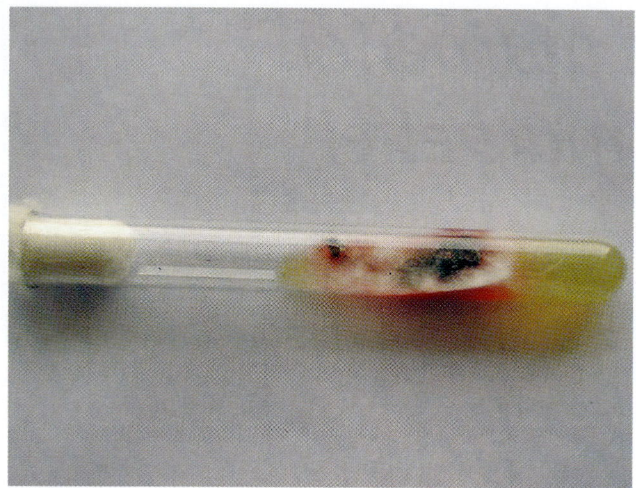

FIG. 24.1: SDA slant with growth of *T. marneffei*.
(SDA: Sabouraud dextrose agar)

Species such as *P. purpurogenum*, *Penicillium atroroseus*, *Penicillium minioluteum*, and *Penicillium albobiverticillius* may also produce pigment that is similar to *T. marneffei*, although they are not dimorphic. Moreover, these are not pathogenic to humans.

TAXONOMY

This fungus is a member of the order Eurotiales, family Trichocomaceae, class Plectomycetes, phylum Ascomycota.

EPIDEMIOLOGY

The disease is endemic in Southeast Asia. Thailand, Southwest China (including Hong Kong), parts of Malaysia, northeast India (especially Manipur state along the Myanmar border), Taiwan, and Vietnam are places with higher prevalence of the disease. A growing number of cases of talaromycosis have been reported in recent years among travelers to and from endemic locations. The ecological niche of the fungus is unclear. Some species of rats (bamboo rats) are infected with fungus, but its role in the transmission of the disease is unclear.

Inhalation of conidia from the environment and subsequent dispersion to different parts of the body during immunosuppression are possible airborne modes of transmission. One possible explanation for *P. marneffei*'s inability to thrive in nonsterile soil is that it cannot compete effectively with other soil bacteria.

The Centers for Disease Control and Prevention (CDC) recommends the use of a Biosafety Level-2 (BSL2) cabinet while handling culture and suspected specimens.

Incidence

In Southeast Asia, talaromycosis is seen as an opportunistic infection that defines AIDS. The rate of its spread is proportional to the rate of AIDS in the area. Among AIDS patients in northern Thailand, it ranks third among opportunistic illnesses. People living with HIV/AIDS or other immunocompromised conditions who reside in or visit endemic areas of Southeast Asia are at risk of developing talaromycosis.

Risk Factors

Individuals who are particularly at risk for developing penicilliosis include:

- *People with AIDS*: Those living with AIDS whose CD4+ T-lymphocyte count falls below 200 cells/μL are highly susceptible to penicilliosis.
- *HIV-negative immunocompromised patients*: Patients with collagen vascular illnesses and those undergoing immunosuppressive or cytotoxic treatment for hematologic malignancies.
- *Travel or residence in endemic areas*: If a febrile immunocompromised patient has a history of visiting or living in Southeast Asia and displays pertinent clinical symptoms such as umbilicated skin lesions, talaromycosis should be examined as a possible diagnosis.

Transmission

Airborne conidia are the main mode for the transmission of talaromycosis. The exact ecological niche of *P. marneffei* is not known. It is associated with bamboo rats and their burrows in regions where it is endemic. Crucially, it is not believed that humans can contract the fungus directly from bamboo rats.

On the contrary, rat burrows are likely to be the source of aerosolized soil conidia.

IMMUNOLOGY AND PATHOGENICITY

Host Factors

The host's defense against the fungus is in the form of pulmonary alveolar macrophages and circulating monocytes. When exposed to *T. marneffei* conidia, circulating monocytes experience an oxidative burst, resulting in superoxide generation. Thus, cell-mediated immunity (CMI) is important in defense against the fungus. The deficiency of CD4+ cells contributes to severity of the disease as cytokines produced by CD4+ cells stimulate CMI responses.

Microbial Factors

- *Morphogenesis*: *T. marneffei* is the only *Talaromyces* species that shows temperature-sensitive dimorphism which plays an important role in its pathogenesis.
- *Pathophysiology*: *T. marneffei* enters through the inhalation of conidia into the lungs. From there, the disease progresses systematically, affecting the mononuclear phagocytic system.

PATHOLOGY

Pulmonary-disseminated talaromycosis has its origins in the lungs and has the potential to spread to other organs through the bloodstream. In the lung, it can cause purulent or granulomatous lesions with central necrosis. Symptoms that patients may encounter include elevated body temperature, cough, decreased appetite, swollen lymph nodes, and the appearance of new skin lesions. This condition progresses gradually over several weeks before seeking medical attention. Other clinical signs include fungemia (fungus in the blood), anemia, generalized lymph node enlargement, and liver and spleen enlargement. These symptoms can resemble those of histoplasmosis, another fungal infection prevalent in the same geographic area.

Skin lesions: In over 85% of patients, there is skin involvement. The forehead, upper limbs, and belly are common sites for these lesions, which manifest as papules with necrotic centers or maculopapular. These lesions can take the appearance of umbilicated papules like those of molluscum contagiosum. It is important to remember that cryptococcosis and histoplasmosis, two other fungal illnesses, can cause very similar skin lesions.

Osseous involvement: Bones such as the ribs, long bones, skull, vertebrae, scapula, and temporomandibular region might be affected by multiple lytic lesions.

Multiorgan dissemination: The fungus has the ability to impact several organs such as the tonsils, skin, kidneys, liver, gut, meninges, pericardium, and adrenals, suggesting that in extreme instances, it might spread far.

Relapsing penicilliosis: Roughly half of all patients will experience relapses if maintenance treatment is not administered or if their CD4+ T cells do not completely recover.

LABORATORY DIAGNOSIS

Direct Examination

Clinical specimens such as skin lesions, sputum, bone marrow aspirates, peripheral blood smears, cerebrospinal fluid (CSF), bronchoalveolar lavage (BAL), and urine are collected. Bone marrow aspirates and peripheral blood smears are most helpful. Smears from liquid specimens can be stained by Giemsa stain. Impression smears can be prepared from biopsies and stained by Giemsa, Grocott-Gömöri's methenamine silver (GMS), and periodic acid-Schiff (PAS) stains.

Histopathology

- Skin lesion tissue sections and swollen lymph nodes, kidney, and liver fine-needle aspirate samples can be histologically examined for the presence of tiny yeasts.
- Unlike other fungal diseases such as *Histoplasma capsulatum and Cryptococcus neoformans*, *T. marneffei* is easily identifiable by its characteristic transverse septa in its yeasts. The septum is best seen in GMS stain, as shown in **Figure 24.2**. Special stains like GMS and PAS are essential for observing *T. marneffei* in tissue sections. Macrophages harboring fission yeast cells may be one of the findings. *T. marneffei* does not stain well with hematoxylin and eosin (H&E).

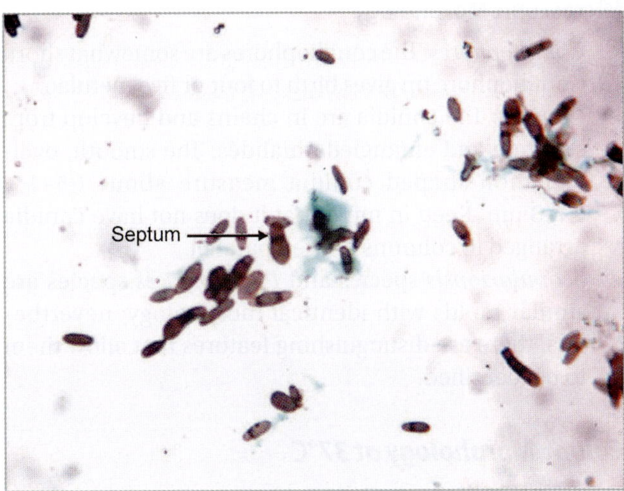

FIG. 24.2: GMS-stained smear showing yeast cells of *T. marneffei* (1,000×).
(GMS: Grocott–Gömöri's methenamine silver)

Culture

Blood cultures; bone marrow; and clinical samples such as skin biopsy, aspirates, and biopsy specimens all have a high rate of recovery in culture.

Colony Morphology (Mold Form) at 25°C

Figure 24.1 shows the colony characteristics of the fungus. Flat, downy, or woolly yellow-orange, gray-green mold colony develops on SDA without cycloheximide with antibacterial agents at 25°C has a white border. The reverse shows a bright red diffusible pigment. It grows rapidly within 2 days.

It should be remembered that not all strains of *T. marneffei* produce characteristic red pigment. Similarly, allred pigment producers are not *T. marneffei*. *Penicillium rubrum*, *P. purpurogenum*, *P. citrinum*, and *Penicillium janthinellum* also produce red pigment. *Paecilomyces* colony may have similar features. To differentiate *T. marneffei* from all these fungi, mold-to-yeast conversion and vice versa must be performed.

Mold-to-yeast (M-Y) Conversion

The enriched media such as Brain Heart Infusion Agar (BHIA), cottonseed agar, and Pine's medium along with SDA (without actidione) are used for demonstration of mold-to-yeast conversion. Many subcultures are required to show the conversion to yeast cells fully; otherwise, yeast forms would be mixed with hyphae.

The exoantigen test may be useful to confirm the dimorphic nature of the isolate.

Microscopic Morphology

- *Conidiophores*: The conidiophores are somewhat short. Conidiophore tip gives birth to four or five metulae.
- *Conidia*: The conidia are in chains and develop from separate and entangled phialides. The smooth, oval- to lemon-shaped conidia measure about 1.5–4 × 0.7–3 µm. Keep in mind that it does not have conidia arranged in columns or even parallel.
- *Scopulariopsis* species and *Paecilomyces* species are similar molds with identical morphology; nevertheless, there are distinguishing features that allow them to be identified.

Colony Morphology at 37°C

Fission Yeast Form

Cultures

The fission yeast does not produce red pigment and the colony has a smooth, beige, cerebriform appearance when cultured on blood agar at 37°C.

Microscopic Morphology

Fission yeast: At a temperature of 37°C, *T. marneffei* can transform into yeast by growing on blood agar or a semisynthetic medium that contains certain nitrogen sources. Yeast cells can be round or long, measuring between 3 and 8 µm in length. They divide by fission instead of budding, and they have a transverse septum, as shown in **Figure 24.1**. Prior to separation, cross walls are created. Yeast in vitro (in culture) looks very much like yeast in vivo (within the host). Yeast forms may resemble arthroconidia. The septum of yeast cells is best demonstrated by GMS staining.

A newer technique, matrix-assisted laser desorption/ionization time-of-flight (MALDI-TOF), is used for the identification of the isolate.

Serological Tests

Indirect enzyme immunoassay (EIA) is used for the detection of antibodies. The recombinant *T. marneffei* mannoprotein (Mp1) is used as an antigen in this EIA. Indirect immunofluorescence (IDIF) test and immunoblot assay are also applied for antibody detection.

Patients with *T. marneffei* shed antigens in their blood and urine. Various methods for detecting antigens have been created. There is an EIA using a double layer of antibodies, one targeting carbohydrate epitopes and the other rabbit polyclonal capture antibodies. The sensitivity and specificity of this approach were found to be satisfactory. This is an additional EIA that uses monoclonal antibodies (mAbs) against particular proteins in the yeast culture supernatant. The specificity of this approach was excellent, while its sensitivity was moderate.

Enzyme immunoassay built to detect galactomannan antigenemia—a diagnostic tool for *Aspergillus* infections—has the potential to cross-react with serum from AIDS patients who have talaromycosis. It is useful for monitoring antifungal therapy.

The detection of antigenuria was accomplished by the use of an antigen-capture sandwich EIA. Antibodies were generated in rabbits that had been immunized with whole dead fission yeast forms of *T. marneffei*.

Other antigen detection tests are latex agglutination (LA) and immunodiffusion.

A Western blot test using anti-Mp1p antibodies is useful for the detection of antigen in culture filtrates of *T. marneffei*.

A mAb against galactomannan of *Aspergillus fumigatus* can be applied for the detection of the fungus in formalin-fixed tissue.

Enzyme-linked immunosorbent assay (ELISA) antibody against 4D1 of *T. marneffei* is used for antigen detection with the advantage that it does not cross-react with other fungi.

Genetic Identification

Genomic analysis is possible with molecular techniques such as DNA sequencing. The internal transcribed spacer 2 (ITS2) region of rRNA genes can be specifically targeted by universal fungal primers, allowing for specific detection. This area can be sequenced to identify *T. marneffei* with greater precision.

Exoantigen Test

The identification of culture was achieved through the development of a particular exoantigen test that utilized the immunodiffusion (ID) technique. The reference antigen used was the concentrated culture filtrate obtained from standard strain *T. marneffei* 6-week-old, 25°C shaking cultures. For cultures with unusual colony morphology or that were hard to convert, an identification test using rabbit antiglobulin produced against this antigen could positively identify *T. marneffei*. A positive reaction is indicated by the presence of two to four distinct precipitin lines. The exoantigen test is useful for distinguishing *T. marneffei* from other species. When doing an identification test, it is possible to distinguish between these two closely related species by using anti-*T. marneffei* antiglobulin adsorbed with *Penicillium primulinum* antigens.

An enzyme-linked immunosorbent assay (ELISA)-based antibody test was developed with a recombinant *T. marneffei* mannoprotein (Mp1p) for the serodiagnosis of *T. marneffei* infection. Evaluation of the test revealed high specificity (100%) and approximately 80% sensitivity in HIV-seropositive patients infected with *P. marneffei*. Another ELISA-based technique for mannoprotein Mp1p detection in patient samples also made use of the anti-Mp1p antibody.

TREATMENT

For individuals with severe penicilliosis or multiorgan dissemination, amphotericin B (AmB) monotherapy is the recommended primary therapy. AmB is known to be effective in treating these severe cases. Itraconazole (ITC) is commonly used for maintenance therapy.

In case of mild-to-moderate penicilliosis, ITC is used as the primary therapy.

Amphotericin B is given at a dose of 0.6 mg/kg daily for 2 weeks, followed by oral ITC (400 mg/day) for the subsequent 10 weeks.

For individuals living with AIDS who have recovered and maintained a CD4+ T-lymphocyte count of ≥100 cells/μL, secondary prophylaxis with antifungal therapy may be indicated to prevent relapses.

It is important to note that antifungal therapy is essential for individuals with talaromycosis, as the disease can be fatal if left untreated, especially in persons living with AIDS and those with severe forms of infection. The choice of therapy may depend on the severity of the disease, individual patient factors, and response to treatment.

Itraconazole is the antifungal medication of choice for treating and preventing relapses of primary penicilliosis.

CHAPTER

25 Aspergillosis

INTRODUCTION

The opportunistic invasive mycosis known as aspergillosis is caused by fungi belonging to the genus *Aspergillus*. There are various clinical forms caused by *Aspergillus*. These include invasive aspergillosis, pulmonary aspergillosis, tracheobronchitis, extrapulmonary dissemination, allergic bronchopulmonary aspergillosis, keratitis, otomycosis, and mycotoxin intoxication. Aspergillosis is the second most common opportunistic fungal infection after candidiasis. These fungi are ubiquitous, present on decaying organic matter.

Though there are many species in the genus (at least 150), *Aspergillus fumigatus, Aspergillus flavus, Aspergillus terreus, Aspergillus glaucus, Aspergillus nidulans,* and *Aspergillus niger* are the most common pathogenic species.

The saprophytic fungus *Aspergillus* is found in abundance in organic compost piles, leaf litter, moldy hay, and other decomposing plant materials. While the majority of species break down intricate plant polymers, others are able to utilize human tissues, old parchment, or even feces as substrates. Using *A. nidulans*, researchers have examined metabolic processes and cell cycle dynamics. Various species pose a threat to human and animal health by contaminating wheat and other crops with toxic chemicals.

HISTORY

Aspergillus infections were first recorded in the eighteenth century. Italian scientist Micheli (1729) was the pioneer in attempting the scientific research on fungi which led to the identification of *Aspergillus*. He noticed the presence of a head (or vesicle) with radiating spores from the head which was similar to aspergillum (*Aspergillum* is a brush or perforated globe used by priests to sprinkle holy water during a part of the ceremony called the "asperges"). It was in 1809 when Link first described *A. flavus*.

Virchow documented four cases of pulmonary and bronchial aspergillosis in 1856. Some other early examples of aspergillosis were summarized by Renon in 1897, Cawley in 1947, and Hinson et al. in 1952.

The first major monograph on the genus was published in 1926 by Tom and Church. By 1965, the previous system of classifying *Aspergillus* had been determined to be outdated, and a new system that included 151 species organized into 18 groups had been established.

Modern Advances

- Further research employing DNA hybridization and thin-layer chromatography improved species taxonomy.
- Continuous updates and improvements in classification methods continue to refine our understanding of *Aspergillus* species.

MYCOLOGY

Almost 90% of infections are associated with three common species which are *A. fumigatus, A. flavus*, and *A. niger*. Other pathogenic species include *A. terreus, A. nidulans, A. glaucus, A. versicolor, A. clavatus,* and *A. oryzae*. One type of specialized hypha called *conidiophore* arises from *foot cell* present on vegetative hypha. The conidiophore develops into a *vesicle* or *head* by enlarging at its tip. The *phialides* are arranged on a vesicle that forms conidia. In a *uniseriate arrangement*, they come straight out of the vesicle. In a *biseriate* design, *metulae* first attach to the vesicle and then *phialides* attach to the metulae.

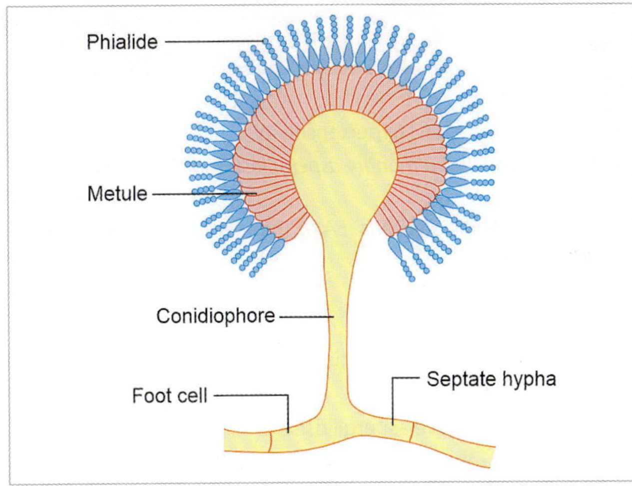

FIG. 25.1: Different parts of aspergillus.

Metulae attach to the vesicle. Along the phialide, the conidia arrange themselves in a chain, with the basipetal pattern with youngest at the base. The phialides encase the entire vesicle in certain species, but in others, they encase only a fraction of it. Refer **Figure 25.1** to see different parts of *Aspergilus.*

CLASSIFICATION

Taxonomically, most of the *Aspergillus* species are classified under the phylum Deuteromycota. Some species multiply by asexual as well as by sexual method (sexual spores-ascospores) and are included in the order Eurotiales of family Trichocomaceae in class Plectomycetes of phylum Ascomycota.

IMMUNITY AND PATHOGENESIS

The innate immunity is important in defense against aspergillosis. The cells which give protection are macrophages and neutrophils.

Spore inhalation is the mode of infection. Conidia are picked up by phagocytes in the lungs of an immunocompetent host. Immune response is mediated by neutrophils, macrophages, and pulmonary epithelial cells. At body temperature, the conidia germinate into hyphae. When alveolar macrophages are activated by chemicals originating from the fungal cell wall, such as β-1,3-glucan (BDG), phagocytes begin to accumulate. To keep an infection under control, cytokines are released, which attract neutrophils. These cells then kill the invading hyphae by generating reactive oxygen derivatives. If any of these steps is hampered, the infection can spread.

Angioinvasion by *Aspergillus* is well known; thrombosis in blood vessels leads to tissue destruction and facilitates the spread of the infection to other parts of the body.

When *Aspergillus* colonizes an existing cavity in people with preexisting lung disease, a large collection of fungal hyphae, fibrin, and other debris can form a mass—an aspergilloma. In allergic bronchopulmonary aspergillosis (ABPA), instead of the usual immune response, there are type I or type III hypersensitivity responses. Immune hyperactivity is experienced by certain people with asthma and cystic fibrosis, which can trigger ABPA. The absence of angioinvasion and the limitation of hyphae to an existing lung are distinguishing features of chronic pulmonary aspergillosis (CPA) and aspergilloma (no angioinvasion), two forms of pulmonary aspergillosis. People with sarcoidosis or chronic obstructive pulmonary disease (COPD) often have these. These are associated with structural lung disease that already exists as well as mild immunological abnormalities. Invasive pulmonary aspergillosis (IPA) or COPD without angioinvasion can develop as the dosage of immunosuppressant medication increases, e.g., with corticosteroid treatment for COPD.

Virulence Factors of *Aspergillus*

The fungus is more harmful because its conidia are smaller and germinate at a faster rate. Their diameter is 2–3 μm. Opportunistic pathogens thrive in environments with temperatures over 37°C, where they can develop rapidly.

The conidia of *A. fumigatus* adhere to one another using surface proteins and residues of sialic acid. The hyphal wall contains BDG. Dectin 1 is its binding site on host macrophages and neutrophils. Hydrophobic proteins form a rod-shaped outer coat of *A. fumigatus* conidia that prevents phagocytosis.

One of the harmful compounds secreted by *Aspergillus* is *gliotoxin*, which inhibits the immune system's cell function. It reduces ciliary motility on epithelial cells and triggers cell death in macrophages and T lymphocytes. *A. fumigatus* is a *verruculogen*, meaning it weakens the epithelium's defenses against invasion. The *proteases* it produces either accelerate colonization of the lung matrix or break down soluble host proteins. *A. fumigatus* strains that cause disease produce a protein called *elastase*, which attaches itself specifically to the elastin found in lung tissue. *Aspartyl proteinase* is produced by growing hyphae and can break down elastin, collagen, and fibronectin.

EPIDEMIOLOGY

Aspergillus species are found all over the world. They are saprophytic fungi that actively degrade organic materials. Aspergilli thrive on a variety of substrates, including hay, grain, decomposing plants, cloth, leather, fabrics, cheeses, and preserved foods. *A. fumigatus*, a blue-green mold, grows and sporulates on food items kept at room temperature or even in the fridge at temperatures lower than room temperature. *A. flavus* is harmful to all living beings. Tree nuts, cottonseed, peanuts, rice, and maize are all infested. Among the toxins and carcinogens produced by *A. flavus* is aflatoxin.

A. terreus possesses an innate resistance to amphotericin. In hospitals, spores of *Aspergillus* may be detected.

There should not be more than 500–700 conidia per cubic meter in hospital air. The fungus possesses the ability to cause nosocomial outbreaks.

The Centers for Disease Control and Prevention (CDC) recommends the following measures such as directed room airflow: Certain examples of directed room airflow include high-efficiency particulate air (HEPA) filtration of incoming air, a high air change rate per hour (12), and a positive air pressure in the patient room relative to the corridor.

Fungal spores can be found in a variety of places, including condensation in HVAC systems, ductwork filters and insulation, behind vapor barriers in buildings, and any source of moisture (leaks, vapor barriers) that encourages mold growth.

Possible sources also include showerheads, shower stalls, and tanks that store cold water. There have been aspergillosis epidemics caused by construction works in healthcare facilities.

CLINICAL FEATURES

Infected spores of *Aspergillus* typically reach the lower respiratory system through inhalation. Sinuses, the gastrointestinal (GI) tract, or even the skin (via intravenous catheters, lengthy skin contact with sticky tapes, or burns) can be entry points for IPA. Various clinical forms of aspergillosis are shown in **Box 25.1**.

Patients receiving lung transplants, those living with human immunodeficiency virus/acquired immunodeficiency syndrome (HIV/AIDS), and cancer patients undergoing chemotherapy are at an increased risk for the infection. When the absolute neutrophil count is below 500 cells/mm^3, neutropenia becomes the most important risk factor. Factors that increase the likelihood of infection after hematopoietic stem cell transplant (HSCT) include a number of immune system abnormalities, an extended period of neutropenia before the transplant, the use of numerous antirejections or anti-graft-versus-host disease (GVHD) medications, parenteral nutrition, antibiotic usage, and an extended length of hospital stay.

BOX 25.1 Clinical forms with pathogenesis mechanisms.

Allergic forms:
- *Asthma:* It is a type I hypersensitivity
- *Allergic bronchopulmonary aspergillosis (ABPA):* It is type I and type III
- *Extrinsic allergic alveolitis (EAA):* There is type III only or with type I or IV

Noninvasive colonization:
- Aspergilloma
- Nonpulmonary, local infection

Invasive aspergillosis:
- Pulmonary invasive aspergillosis
- Chronic necrotizing pulmonary aspergillosis
- Disseminated aspergillosis

The diseases produced by *Aspergillus* are:
- Pulmonary disease
- Central nervous system (CNS) aspergillosis
- Peripheral nervous system (PNS) aspergillosis
- *Aspergillus* endocarditis
- Cutaneous aspergillosis
- Miscellaneous infections

Pulmonary Diseases

The pulmonary disease is broadly divided into four categories:
1. Allergic aspergillosis
2. Aspergilloma
3. Invasive aspergillosis
4. Chronic necrotizing pulmonary aspergillosis (CNPA)

Allergic Aspergillosis

Atopy in patients, when exposed to the spores, manifest as bronchial asthma. The damage is produced due to type I hypersensitivity reactions. There is progressive lung damage which results in decreased lung function. Another type of allergic presentation is in the form of ABPA in which type III hypersensitivity responses cause the majority of damage. The patients present with breathlessness, fever, and cough. Repeated attacks cause lung damage. The growing fungus and mucus may block the airways, and the material may be coughed out. There may be the presence of hyphae in coughed material when there is obstruction to the airways. The patients may develop hypoxia. The areas of collapse may be seen in chest X-ray.

Aspergilloma

The preexisting cavity in the lungs caused by pulmonary tuberculosis gets colonized with the fungus which is surrounded by fibrous tissue. The fungal ball is mostly solitary. Its size may be as large as approximately 8–10 cm. The chest X-ray shows mobile opacity in the cavity with crest of air in the upper margin producing air crescent or "Monod's sign." After turning the patient from supine to prone, the fungus ball's location changes, which is an interesting and variable sign. Less frequently, patients may develop coughing, shortness of breath, or fever.

Invasive Aspergillosis

The fungus grows in lung tissue. It may spread to other organs. On rare occasions, the aspergilloma could enlarge. Most people with aspergilloma do not even know they have it. Although most people experience mild hemoptysis; in rare cases, particularly in patients with underlying tuberculosis, severe and even fatal hemoptysis can occur. Fungal endotoxins and mechanical stimulation of exposed vasculature within the cavity from the fungus ball's movement are potential causes of the bleed. This type of pulmonary aspergillosis is associated with high morbidity. The predisposing factors for invasive aspergillosis are:

- Neutropenic patients (especially with hematopoietic malignancy)
- Advanced AIDS
- Children with chronic granulomatous disease
- Transplant recipients
- Patients on steroids
- Long-term administration of antibiotics

Chronic Necrotizing Pulmonary Aspergillosis

It is commonly seen in patients with COPD, bronchiectasis, pneumoconiosis, and other conditions which cause local defenses to alter. During the pathogenesis, a new cavity may be formed in the lungs. The radiological findings are variable, either areas of consolidation or cavity formation.

Aspergillus Endocarditis

Both natural and prosthetic valves are susceptible to the development of endocarditis. Large fungal vegetations develop on the valves. The risk factors for *Aspergillus* endocarditis include immunosuppression, injectable drug use, antibiotic therapy, and concomitant bacterial endocarditis. Emboli can get dislodged from the vegetation, travel through the bloodstream, and get deposited in the CNS, producing a stroke. Pericarditis and myocarditis may also occur.

Cutaneous Aspergillosis

Both neonatal percutaneous infections and contaminated bandages applied to burn victims can lead to primary cutaneous infections. A secondary cutaneous infection may develop in immunocompromised people as a result of hematogenous spread.

Central Nervous System Aspergillosis

The CNS is involved as a result of hematogenous dispersion from the main focus, which is either the respiratory system or the GI tract. The majority of individuals is immunocompromised, and infection is frequently a postmortem diagnosis. *A. fumigatus, A. flavus, A. terreus,* and *A. versicolor* are the causative species. Brain abscess (intracranial mass, single or multiple), meningitis, ventriculitis, epidural abscess, intracranial aneurysms, or rhinocerebral form leading to meningitis are the many manifestations of aspergillosis of the brain.

Peripheral Nervous System Aspergillosis

Aspergillus species may colonize or invade the nose and paranasal sinuses. The most common species are *A. flavus* and *A. fumigatus*. Similar to mucormycosis, it may have the following presentations: Allergic sinusitis and noninvasive, invasive, or fulminant type. There may be facial mass, ptosis, periorbital cellulitis, or orbital cellulitis. Further spread from orbit to brain may occur by fungi penetrating through the cranium bones.

Other Infections

These include keratitis, endophthalmitis, otomycosis, mastoiditis, osteomyelitis, and rarely onychomycosis.

RADIODIAGNOSIS

To identify the lesion and its precise location, imaging techniques, including MRI and CT scans, are utilized. Invasive aspergillosis is diagnosed using a CT scan.

DIFFERENTIAL DIAGNOSIS

The lesions of invasive aspergillosis should be differentiated from deep mycotic infections. Many *Aspergillus* presentations are also similar to those of mucormycosis. Granulomatous lesions may resemble neoplasms.

LABORATORY DIAGNOSIS

The diagnostic tests are summarized in **Table 25.1**. Conventional methods for the diagnosis include microscopy and culture. As the fungus is saprophytic, it exists everywhere in the environment; repeated isolation of the fungus is required to prove its pathogenic role.

Direct Examination

Aspirates, sputum, bronchoalveolar lavage (BAL), transbronchial biopsy, and other biopsy materials are all examples of direct examination specimens. Hyaline septate hyphae with acute angle branching will be revealed by the 10% potassium hydroxide (KOH) mount. The ideal hyphal diameter ranges from 3 to 6 µm, and they should have the characteristic narrow angle (45°C) and "dichotomous" branching. In dichotomous branching, the terminal tip of a hypha bifurcates into two rather than producing side branches. The branches may appear like fingers making "V" sign. The hyaline, septate hyphae can be seen with other fungi causing hyalohypomycosis such as *Fusarium* species or *Scedosporium* species. Hence, culture is essential.

Tube KOH is performed for a biopsy specimen that is left overnight because the biopsy material is not easily softened. To enhance the sensitivity of direct microscopy, fluorescent microscopy (direct immunofluorescence) or calcofluor white preparations are performed. Hyphae can be stained with hematoxylin and eosin (H&E) **(Fig. 25.2)**. The staining of cells of the hyphae and the surrounding tissue is quite similar. An experienced person can notice the *Aspergillus* hyphae in the tissue stained with H&E. Some distorted hyphae may be confused with nonseptate hyphae. However, it should be kept in mind that mixed infections of *Aspergillus* with mucormycosis are known to occur, especially in cases of paranasal sinusitis.

The fungal-specific stains Grocott–Gomori methenamine silver (GMS) and periodic acid-Schiff (PAS) are preferred. While GMS stain may be more sensitive, PAS stain can identify inflammation and tissue structure.

When stained with GMS or PAS, the hyphae seem to be 3–6 µm wide, densely septate, and dichotomously branched at acute angles.

Septate hyphae along with a head or vesicle of *Aspergillus* may be seen in a sputum sample if the fungus gets free space in aspergilloma. When *Aspergillus* species invade blood vessels, it causes the formation of mycotic thrombi, which can be found in tissues. The fungus

TABLE 25.1: Diagnostic tests for clinical types of aspergillosis.

Disease	*Microscopy*	*Culture*	*Serology*	*Skin test*
Allergic bronchopulmonary aspergillosis (ABPA)	Positive	Positive	Moderate (type I and III hypersensitivity)	Strongly positive
Aspergilloma	Positive	Strongly positive	Often positive (depending on the case)	Not typically used
Invasive aspergillosis	Positive	Positive	Weakly positive	Variable

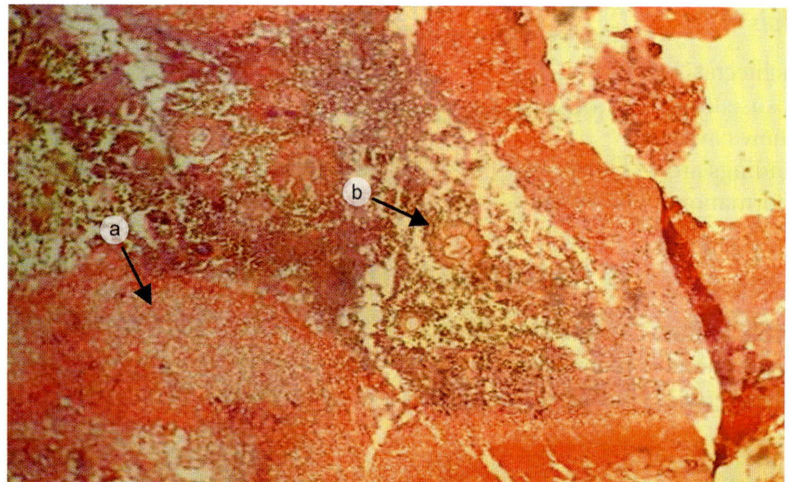

FIG. 25.2: Biopsy from nasal mucosa stained with H&E with hyphae (a) and head of *Aspergillus* (b) (400×). (H&E: hematoxylin and eosin)

grows in radial or parallel arrays in tissues when the host immune system is weak, as in an immunocompromised host invasive aspergillosis. As in the *Mucorales*, the hyphae can twist and bulge into strange shapes. In terms of noninvasiveness and the development of dichotomous, acute angle branching, some hyaline mold hyphae (such as *Fusarium* species and *Pseudallescheria/ Scedosporium* species) may resemble aspergilli.

When *Aspergillus* species are isolated from body fluids or secretions, it is important to note the following:

- Because aspergilli are so ubiquitous in nature, cultures taken from body fluids such as sputum, urine, stool, or wounds do not tell us much. Repeated isolation and correlation with histopathological findings and signs and symptoms are necessary.
- It is more important to use cultures from BAL fluid or transbronchial brush biopsy.
- *Biopsy sites that are typically sterile*: These cultures are very important and should be reported right away.
- *Blood cultures for Aspergillus*: It is unclear what role *Aspergillus* fungemia plays in the clinical manifestations of invasive aspergillosis.

Culture

For culture, Sabouraud dextrose agar (SDA) slants without cycloheximide are employed, and they are incubated at 25 and 37°C. In the first week, the cultures are inspected daily for the existence of growth and then twice a week for the next 4 weeks. To see sporulation, Czapek–Dox Agar and Malt extract agar are utilized. *Aspergillus* species grow quickly. Tease mounts or lactophenol cotton blue (LPCB) mounts created from slide culture are used to record morphological results.

Keep an eye out for the characteristic shape of *Aspergillus* species. *Penicillium* lacks vesicles, which distinguishes it from *Aspergillus,* which has a vesicle or head. The thick-walled, sterile Hulle cells are produced as terminal or intercalary cells. On SDA, homothallic *Aspergillus* species (such as *A. nidulans*) can produce Cleistothecia. In that species, Hulle cells can be found near the cleistothecia. The exoantigen tests can be used for the identification of species.

Aspergillus fumigatus

It may thrive and produce spores at temperatures as high as 48°C and as low as 20°C.

Colony morphology: On SDA-Emmons agar, the usual isolates form rapidly expanding colonies that range in color from blue-green to gray-turquoise (*smoky green*) as shown in **Figure 25.3** with the opposite side being either white or uncolored. A velvety and fuzzy texture characterizes the colony. The whitish area at the colony's periphery represents the mycelial growth zone.

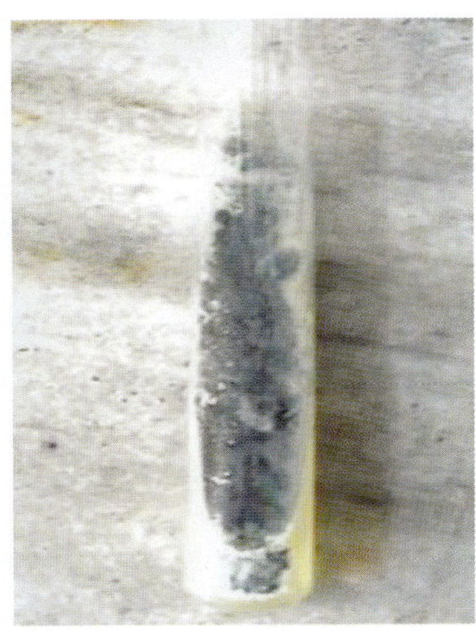

FIG. 25.3: Smoky green colored colony of *Aspergillus fumigatus* on SDA slant.
(SDA: Sabouraud Dextrose Agar)

A hyaline, smooth-walled, *short* (as compared to that of *A. flavus*) conidiophore is present. The phialides of this species run parallel to the axis of the conidiophore and fill the upper part of the vesicle; the species is *uniseriate.* These features are shown in **Figures 25.4A and B**. The conidia are gray, green, or blue-green.

Aspergillus flavus

The colonies have a velvety texture and a parrot green coloration **(Fig. 25.5)** and golden to brown on the reverse. The conidiophore is long and rough-walled. Phialides extend in all directions and cover nearly the whole surface of the vesicle as shown in **Figure 25.6**. It may be uniseriate or biseriate. The conidia are yellow to green.

Aspergillus terreus

A velvety cinnamon-brown, rarely a brilliant orange-brown, is the color of a colony. The back of the colony is a light golden color. The vesicle is biseriate, and its phialides are columnar and located on its upper portion as shown in **Figure 25.7**. There is a second kind of "accessory conidia" called aleuroconidia. These tiny aleuroconidia attach themselves to the hyphae that are submerged in agar material using short pedicels.

Aspergillus glaucus

The colony is green with yellow areas, sometimes brown. The reverse is yellow to maroon. The species is uniseriate. Phialides are loosely arranged. Ascus may be seen **(Fig. 25.8)**.

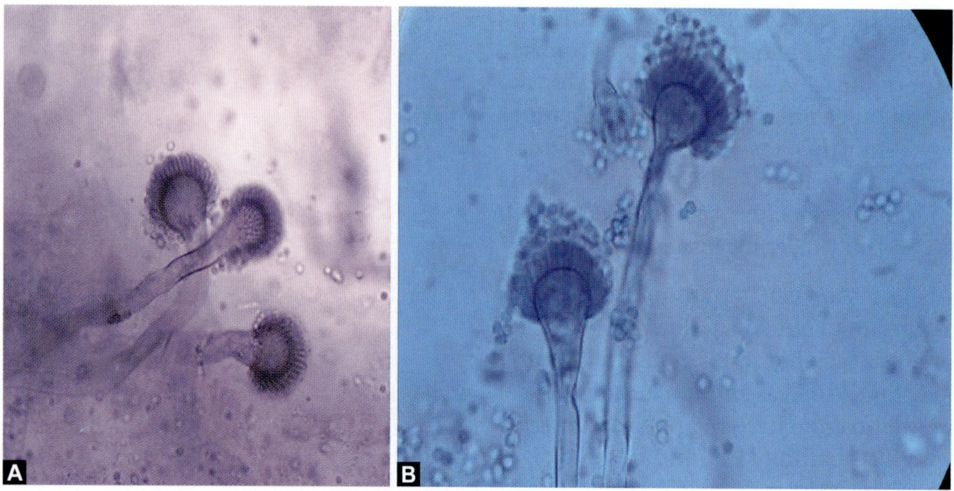

FIGS. 25.4A AND B: LPCB mounts of *Aspergillus fumigatus* (400×).
(LPCB: lactophenol cotton blue)

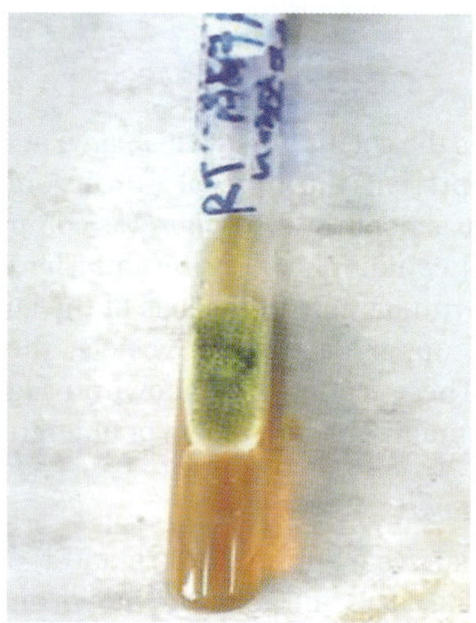

FIG. 25.5: SDA slant with growth of *Aspergillus flavus*.
(SDA: Sabouraud Dextrose Agar)

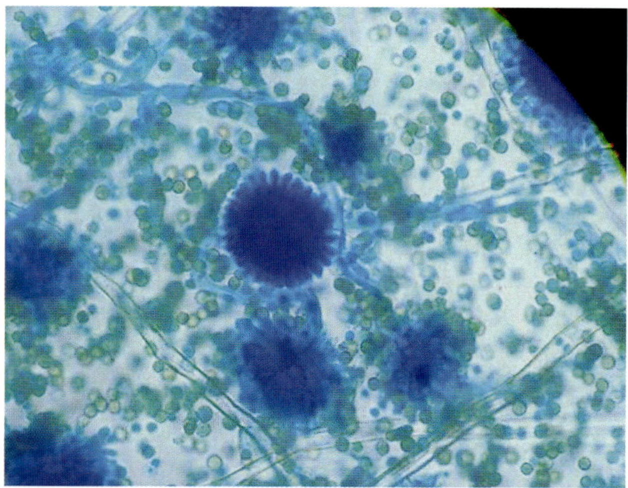

FIG. 25.6: LPCB mount of *Aspergillus flavus* (400×).
(LPCB: lactophenol cotton blue)

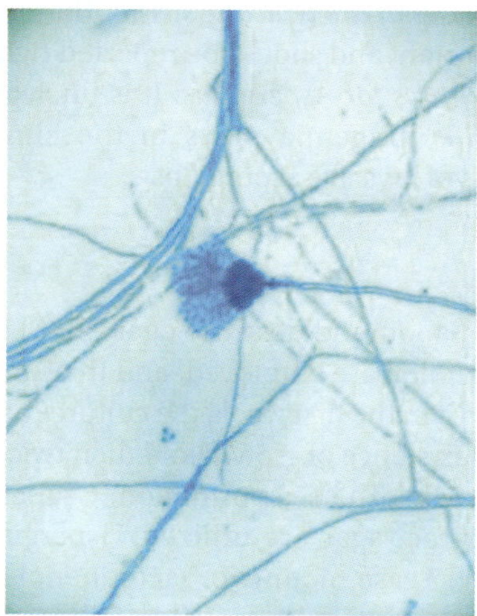

FIG. 25.7: LPCB mount of *Aspergillus terreus* (400×).
(LPCB: lactophenol cotton blue)

Aspergillus nidulans

Colonies are green with dark red brown. The reverse is olive to gray to brown. Cleistothecium contains reddish-brown ascospores surrounded by Hulle cells as shown in **Figure 25.8**.

Aspergillus niger

Colonies are black due to black conidia and the reverse white to yellow. Phialides are biseriate, arranged all over the surface of the vesicle.

Serological Tests

Detection of antibodies: Aspergilloma patients with precipitating immunoglobulin G (IgG) antibodies are quite numerous. The levels of total serum IgE, specific IgE, and IgG are higher in ABPA. One commercially available test

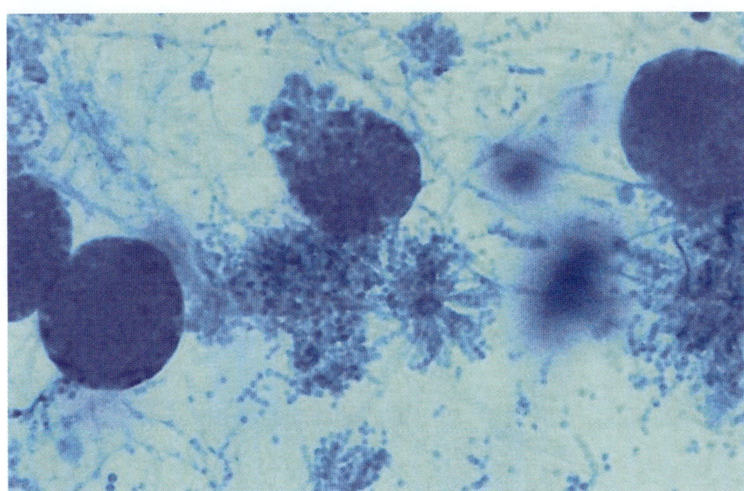

FIG. 25.8: LPCB mount of *Aspergillus glacus* (400×). (LPCB: lactophenol cotton blue)

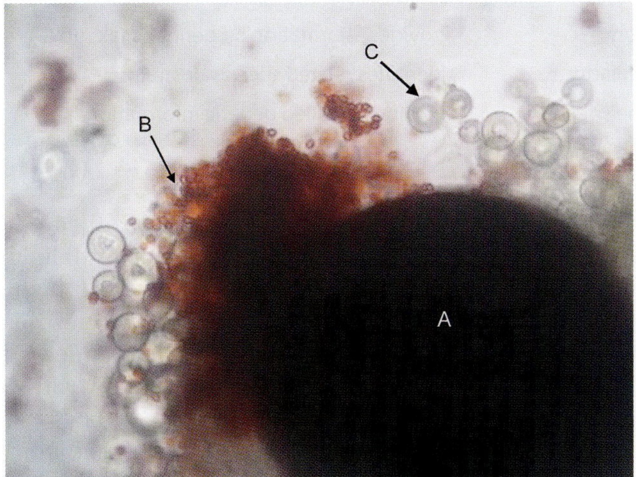

FIG. 25.9: (A) Ascus, (B) ascospores, and (C) Hulle cells of *Aspergillus nidulans*.

is antibody detection by immunodiffusion. Specifically, the antigen is a culture filtrate, cell wall, or cytoplasmic extract of *A. fumigatus*. Another test to detect antibodies is enzyme-linked immunosorbent assay (ELISA).

Antigen detection: Methods make use of ELISA, latex agglutination (LA), and immunoblot. The soluble antigen may be detected in serum, urine, or other body fluids. A Western Blot test is developed for antigen detection in cerebrospinal fluid (CSF).

Illness activity is associated with galactomannan (GM) production, and GM concentration may serve as a predictor of illness outcome. Negative outcomes are predicted by GM concentrations that remain despite antifungal therapy.

Serum GM can be detected in cases of invasive aspergillosis using the Platelia® *Aspergillus* EIA antigenemia test (Bio-Rad Laboratories, Inc.). False-positive results may occur in colonization of the intestine, cyclophosphamide cross-reaction, and dietary GM adsorption from a damaged gut. A false-positive GM test at an achievable serum level is produced by certain batches of the antibiotic combination piperacillin–tazobactam.

One new antigen test for diagnosing: It uses a *lateral flow device* format to detect an extracellular glycoprotein antigen that the fungus only produces when it is actively growing. It is specific for *Aspergillus* species. The test was tagged before GM or BDG in an immunoassay. The innovative test targets a variety of *A. fumigatus* antigens, including Cf2 on the surface of the growing fungus, antigens associated with the cell wall, proteinases, and gliotoxin and its derivatives.

G-test: To find out if there is any circulating β-(1,3)-D-glucan, the G-test is used. Detecting invasive mycosis, the test is incredibly sensitive (–20 pg/mL). But its lack of specificity limits its utility; this glucan is present in the cell walls of the vast majority of fungi, including *Aspergillus, Candida*, and *Pneumocystis.*

Detection of D-mannitol: It was tried in experimental animals by using gas liquid chromatography which is being assessed for the diagnosis of invasive aspergillosis.

Molecular Methods

Genotypic methods are analysis of genomic DNA, mitochondrial DNA, ribosomal DNA, restriction fragment length polymorphism (RFLP), detection of G + C values, and polymerase chain reaction (PCR)-based amplification.

Polymerase chain reaction is now part of standard diagnostic procedures using commercial kits that use serum, plasma, or BAL as its bases. Some have speculated

TABLE 25.2: Typing methods for *Aspergillus* species.

Marker category	***Description***	***Examples/Details***
A. *Phenotyping*		
Morphotyping	Identification based on colony and conidial morphology	*Aspergillus fumigatus* (brush-like conidia)
Biotyping	Classification based on metabolic and biochemical profiles	Nutrient utilization patterns
Chemotyping	Identification based on metabolic by-products	Aflatoxins produced by *Aspergillus flavus*
Secondary metabolites	Analysis of by-products produced by fungi	Aflatoxins, ochratoxins
Isoenzyme pattern	Differentiation based on enzyme activity profiles	Variations in enzyme patterns among species
Protein profiles	Identification based on protein expression	SDS-PAGE patterns
Ubiquinone typing	Analysis of ubiquinone content in the fungal cells	Variations in ubiquinone profiles
B. Genotyping		
Restriction fragment length polymorphism (RFLP)	Differentiation based on DNA fragment lengths after restriction enzyme digestion	Identifies genetic variation
PCR-based amplification	Amplification of specific DNA regions for identification	Useful for species-specific identification
G + C values	Determination of DNA base composition	Provides information on genetic makeup
DNA complementarity	Measurement of the degree of DNA similarity	Identifies related species or strains
RNA sequence	Analysis of RNA sequences to determine species	Provides detailed genetic information

(SDS-PAGE: sodium dodecyl sulfate–polyacrylamide gel electrophoresis)

that its sensitivity could approach 96% when combined with GM detection results in BAL. As anticipated, the PCR has an extremely high specificity—as high as 100% in certain experiments. The ability to use probes against resistance-associated mutations for the identification of azole resistance is an additional benefit of PCR.

Point-of-care tests: The lateral flow devices are available. They detect GM, or extracellular glycoprotein. Both precision and sensitivity are above 70%.

Various typing methods used for *Aspergillus* species are given in **Table 25.2**.

TREATMENT

Voriconazole is the drug of choice. Liposomal amphotericin B (AmB) can be given as primary therapy if voriconazole is not tolerated or contraindicated. Alternative agents for salvage therapy include AmB lipid complex, the echinocandins (caspofungin, micafungin, or anidulafungin), posaconazole, or itraconazole. Combination therapy is usually not recommended; it is given for those with failure of primary therapy with a single agent.

Some clinical isolates of *Aspergillus terreus and Aspergillus flavus* may show antifungal resistance. Very seldom have reports been made of *A. fumigatus* isolates that had a decreased sensitivity to azoles. The amphotericin B (AmB) susceptibility of less common species such as *Aspergillus glaucus, Aspergillus lentulus, Aspergillus nidulans, Aspergillus ustus*, and *Aspergillus versicolor* may be reduced. Voriconazole may be preferable to AmB due to its greater penetration into the central nervous system.

CHAPTER

26 Mucormycosis

INTRODUCTION

Fungi causing mucormycosis are saprophytic fungi with hyphae that are broad, ribbon-like, hyaline, aseptate, or sparsely septate. These fungi are "angioinvasive," meaning they invade and obstruct small- and medium-sized blood vessels, especially arteries. Necrosis of the surrounding area and embolism are common. "Mucormycosis" is an umbrella term for diseases caused by fungi in the family *Zygomycota*, which includes two orders: (1) *Mucorales* and (2) *Entomophthorales*.

TAXONOMY

Phylum *Glomeromycota* is divided into two subphyla: (1) *Mucoromycotina* and (2) *Entomophthoromycotina*. *Mucoromycotina* fungi word cause *Mucormycosis*, while *Entomophthoromycotina* fungi cause—a type of subcutaneous mycosis. The previous name for the group of fungi causing mucormycosis was zygomycosis.

MYCOLOGY

The basic morphological unit of fungi causing mucormycosis is described in the subsequent paragraphs. The various parts of fungi are shown in **Figures 26.1A and B**.

Hyaline hyphae that are broad and mostly aseptate (or sparsely septate) form the vegetative mycelium of all *Mucorales* species.

The stolon is the part of the hypha that joins two clusters of rhizoids together as a part of the vegetative mycelium. It grows laterally, thus expanding the colony. Broad and upright atop the vegetative mycelium is the sporangiophore—a type of hypha that bears sporangia. Both branching and unbranched sporangiophores are possible depending upon the genus. Sporangiospores are produced within sac-like structures called sporangia,

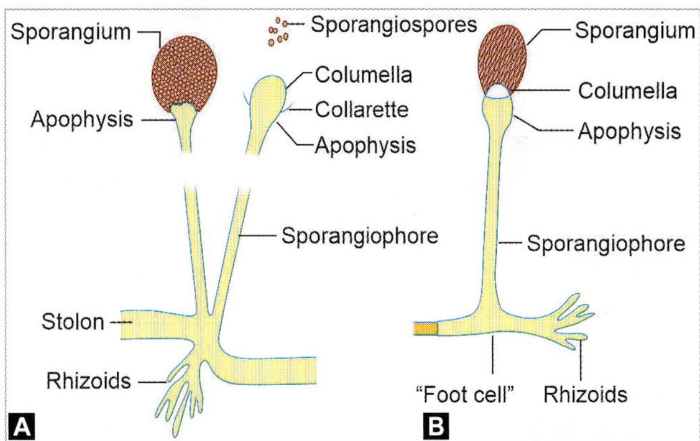

FIGS. 26.1A AND B: Basic morphological features of fungi causing mucormycosis.

which are situated at the tip of the sporangiophore. Rhizoids usually originate from the stolon and resemble roots. But the position of rhizoids may vary. Some species easily show zygospores **(Fig. 26.2)** in the laboratory media.

Initially, these fungi may be classified on the basis of sporangium producers or sporangiole producers or merosporangiole producers as shown in **Table 26.1**.

- *Sporangium producers*: Sporangia are defined as sack-like structures that contain many asexual sporangiospores that would be passively released, e.g., *Rhizopus, Rhizomucor, Mucor, Absidia, Mortierella, Apophysomyces*, and *Saksenaea*.
- *Sporangiole producers*: Sporangiola (plural of sporangiole) are single-celled or few-celled asexual structures that grow on stalks borne from inflated vesicles. They can be found on vesicles that arise at the tips of branched or unbranched sporangiophores. Each sporangiole emerges from the vesicle on a stalk known as a sterigma.
- *Merosporangium producers*: Fungi in this group are distinguished by the production of spores within

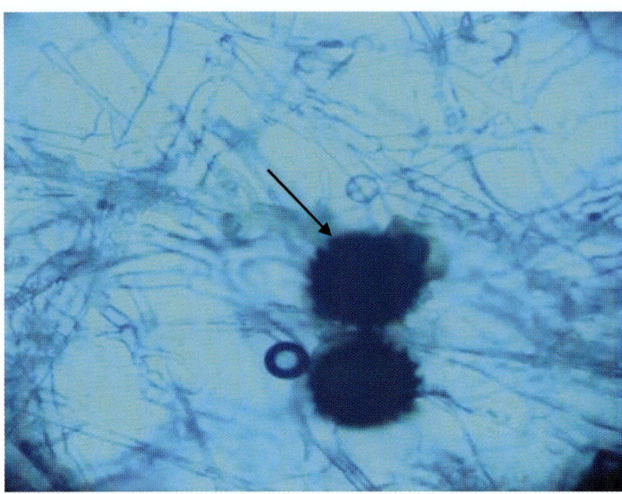

FIG. 26.2: LPCB mount showing ornamental zygospores (400×). (LPCB: lactophenol cotton blue)

TABLE 26.1 List of fungi causing mucormycosis and their classification.

Sporangium producers	*Sporangiole producers*	*Merosporangiole producers*
• *Rhizopus* • *Rhizomucor* • *Mucor* • *Lichtheimia* (earlier *Absidia*) • *Mortierella* • *Apophysomyces* • *Saksenaea*	• *Cunninghamella bertholletiae* • *Cokeromyces recurvatus*	*Syncephalastrum racemosum*

a tubular bag known as a merosporangium. These merosporangia are borne on the terminal swelling of sporangiophore. A single spore column is generated.

Further identifying and differentiating characteristics are summarized in **Tables 26.2A and B**.

Differentiating features of nonglobose sporangia-producing fungi are given in **Table 26.3**.

These fungi are saprophytic and distributed all over the world. They are known as "bread molds." They have low virulence.

ROLE OF IRON IN MUCORMYCOSIS

- Free iron is required by *Mucorales* for their growth. In humans, most of the iron is bound to proteins. Patients with diabetic ketoacidosis may be at a higher risk of these illnesses because iron bound to proteins is released.
- Macrophage phagocytic activity and neutrophil oxidative burst are both inhibited by the low pH that occurs in ketoacidosis.

TABLE 26.2A: Differentiation of sporangium-producing *Mucorales* based on the presence or absence of rhizoids, their position, branched or unbranched sporangiophores, and shapes of sporangia.

Organism	*Sporangium morphology*	*Apophysis and columella morphology*
Rhizopus	Globose; variation in size with species and variety	Together are globose; apophysis is small and may be inconspicuous
Mucor	Globose; 15–80 µm wide; deliquescent	Columella present, but no apophysis; collars may also be present
Rhizomucor pusillus	Globose with smooth, opaque walls; usually 40–60 µm, may be up to 80 µm	Pyriform, subglobose, to spherical; 20–45 µm wide
Mortierella wolfii	Globose and small (15–50 µm); often fails to sporulate	Little or no columella; large collarette left after deliquescence
Absidia corymbifera	May be globose, but more often pyriform, 20–80 µm in diameter	• *Apophysis*: Flask shaped • *Columella*: Dome shaped, occupying about 50% of sporangium

- Role of deferoxamine: *Mucorales* get additional iron from deferoxamine that is used as a chelating agent for patients with iron overload. Deferoxamine is also used in some cases of chronic renal disease on dialysis.

MODES OF TRANSMISSION

The main way that these fungi spread disease is believed to be by the *inhalation* of spores that can be found in the environment. Excavation, construction, or contaminated air conditioning filters have been associated with several outbreaks of rhinocerebral or pulmonary zygomycosis. The other mode of infection is *percutaneous* infection. Trauma acts as the predisposing factor. Tattoos, injection sites, and catheter insertion sites are all potential entry points for zygomycotic infections. Infections in the context of natural disasters or healthcare-associated mucormycosis epidemics have been documented. Infected materials include hospital construction material, bandages, and laundry. Rarely, infection may occur by ingestion.

IMMUNITY

Cell-mediated immunity, particularly polymorphs and macrophages, plays an important role in protection.

TABLE 26.2B: Further identification of *Mucorales*.

Fungus	Sporangium morphology	Rhizoids	Sporangiophore morphology	Zygospores
Rhizopus	Round to oval, often 4–6 µm wide (may be larger); ridged	Abundant, often well-developed	Predominantly unbranched; position is above rhizoidal tufts	Present
Mucor	Smooth walled; oval to round; mostly 3–5 µm, some larger	Absent	Predominantly branched	Present; chlamydoconidia may be present
Rhizomucor pusillus	Smooth walled, globose to broadly ellipsoidal; 3–5 µm	Primitive and rare	Extensively and irregularly branched; more typically monopodial; occur between rhizoidal tufts	Present with warts on surface; red, brown, or black; 45–70 µm wide
Mortierella wolfii	Cylindrical or kidney shaped, 6–10 by 3–5 µm	Primitive	Tall, 450 µm long, arising from stolon; branched, in whorls; occur between rhizoidal tufts	Zygospores not seen; chlamydoconidia may be seen

TABLE 26.3: Differentiating features of the nonglobose sporangium-producing *Mucorales*.

Fungus	Colony	Sporangium	Apophysis and columella	Sporangiospores
Absidia corymbifera	Floccose; first white, turning brown to greenish brown with age	*Pyriform*, 20–80 µm in diameter	• *Apophysis*: Flask shaped • *Columella*: Dome shaped, occupying about 50% of the sporangium	Round to oval, 2–3 by 3–5 µm
Apophysomyces elegans	Floccose, rapidly growing colonies; pale gray to yellowish, turning brown at 37°C	*Pyriform*, 20–58 µm in diameter	• *Apophysis*: Prominent bell or "champagne glass" shaped • *Columella*: Dome shaped, 18–28 µm	Oval and light brown, 5.4–8.0 by 4.0–5.7 µm
Saksenaea vasiformis	Floccose; white colonies	*Flask-shaped* sporangium 20–50 by 15–45 µm; apical end has a gelatinous plug which dissolves	• *Apophysis*: Flask shaped • *Columella*: Dome shaped, 11–15 µm	Oval, 1.4–1.2 by 2.8–4.2 µm

Macrophages prevent infection through phagocytosis. The susceptibility to mucormycosis infection increases in individuals whose monocytes, macrophages, and neutrophils are impaired, such as in diabetics. Patients with diabetic ketoacidosis may be at a higher risk of these illnesses because iron bound to proteins is released. Both macrophage phagocytic activity and neutrophil oxidative burst inhibition are hindered by the low pH that characterizes ketoacidosis.

PATHOGENESIS AND PATHOLOGY

Similar to *Aspergillus*, mucorales are "angioinvasive," preferring blood arteries. Fungi cause thrombosis, hemorrhage, and infarction when they attack the elastic lamina of arteries, both big and small. The fungus has an affinity for the elastic lamina. An essential virulence component unique to the pathogenesis of *Mucorales* is the high-affinity iron permease (FTR1), which enables the pathogen to survive in iron-poor settings. The spore coat (CotH) protein is present on the surfaces of *Mucorales* spores. Fungal virulence factors also include calcineurin (CaN), serine and aspartate proteases (SAPs), and the alkaline *Rhizopus* protease enzyme (Arp).

CLINICAL FEATURES

In most cases of mucormycosis, there is some underlying predisposing factor, but cases have also been reported from normal individuals. The predisposing factors are listed in **Box 26.1**. The mucormycosis was reported in high numbers in coronavirus disease 2019 (COVID-19) patients. The newer species of mucormycosis cause emerging infections.

Rhinocerebral Mucormycosis

It is a severe infection with high mortality. It is the most common infection caused by mucormycosis. Most of the patients have diabetes mellitus, hyperglycemia, and

BOX 26.1 Predisposing factors for the development of mucormycosis.

- Hematological malignancy
- Leukemia
- Lymphoma
- Multiple myeloma
- Neutropenia
- Antineoplastic chemotherapy
- Corticosteroid therapy
- Antirejection therapy
- Diabetes mellitus (types I and II) with or without diabetic ketoacidosis
- Solid organ transplantation
- Bone marrow and peripheral blood stem cell transplantation
- Deferoxamine therapy
- Burns
- Trauma
- Malnutrition in children
- Intravenous drug use

ketoacidosis. The other immunocompromising condition is leukemia. The infection spreads from the nasal mucosa to the paranasal sinuses through the turbinate bone and then involves the orbit and brain. The massive invasion of blood vessels causes infarction. There may be cavernous sinus thrombosis. The onset is acute and all the consequences occur within a short period, usually within a week.

To begin, the patient exhibits fungal sinusitis symptoms such as facial pain, nasal discharge, epistaxis, headache, black eschar on the palate, periorbital cellulitis, ophthalmoplegia, proptosis, ptosis, orbital pain, diplopia, and sudden loss of vision. Through the cribriform plate, the infection spreads from the nose to the brain. In rhino-orbito-cerebral mucormycosis, the infection spreads from paranasal sinuses through orbital apex to brain.

Blood vessels are involved, resulting in vasculitis and cavernous venous thrombosis. The fifth and seventh cranial nerves may be damaged. Spread can also occur to the lungs, skin (necrotizing fasciitis and ulcer over the face), and other organs on occasion. The radiological findings are very typical, revealing the bony destruction and the extent of spread (**Fig. 26.17** depicts radiological image of fungal rhinosinusitis that may evolve rapidly to involve orbit and even brain). Many patients may recall having had teeth extracted in the past. Although other pathogens can cause the disease, *Rhizopus* and *Rhizomucor* are the most common.

Cutaneous Mucormycosis

Both immunocompetent and immunocompromised persons can develop cutaneous mucormycosis. Any number of deeper tissues, including the bones, muscles, and tendons in the area, can get infected. In the context of disseminated infection, it occurs less frequently. Lesions start with painful redness and swelling and then develop into necrosis and, in many cases, necrotizing fasciitis over the course of a few days. "Hairy pus" lesions can develop cotton-like growths. Among trauma patients, cutaneous mucormycosis can be caused by burns, decubitus ulcers, or gangrenous cellulitis. Contaminated dressings pose a risk of infection. Primary cutaneous infections caused by *Saksenaea* and *Apophysomyces* are becoming more common. Although cutaneous mucormycosis has a good prognosis, some patients die as a result of its rapid spread.

Pulmonary Mucormycosis

Infection takes place through the inhalation of sporangiospores. Due to the destruction of blood vessels, there is damage to lung parenchyma. The clinical features are chest pain and dyspnea with or without hemoptysis. The CT scan shows a reverse halo sign. Rarely, the fungal colonizes in a preformed cavity and presents as fungus ball.

Gastrointestinal Mucormycosis

It is believed to be caused by ingestion of spores through contaminated foods such as fermented milk, porridge, herbal products, and even alcohol. Potentially implicated parts of the gastrointestinal (GI) tract include the stomach (gastric ulceration) and the intestines (intestinal involvement, bowel perforation, etc.). Gastric bleeding is the initial symptom experienced by a large number of people. The risk of stomach infection following surgery is low. Some of the symptoms include melena, hematemesis, abdominal discomfort, and diarrhea. According to the autopsy results, this clinical type is more prevalent than initially believed. When diagnosing a condition, an endoscopic examination is useful.

Renal Mucormycosis

Patients with an immunodeficiency syndrome or a history of intravenous drug use are also at a higher risk of developing renal mucormycosis. In a fungal infection of the bloodstream, hematogenous seeding occurs, leading to this condition. Flank pain, fever, and hematuria are common symptoms. Pyelonephritis may develop in patients with impaired immune systems. Multiple abscesses with collection of perinephric pus and renal infarctions are also possible. Using CT or MRI, the true level of involvement can be ascertained. For diagnosis, a kidney biopsy sample is needed.

Disseminated Mucormycosis

Disseminated mucormycosis is more common in patients with serious immunocompromised diseases. There is a 96% documented fatality rate for this presentation, even with adequate therapy. A person's lungs, kidneys, intestines, heart, and brain could all get infected. The infectious agent spreads hematogenously after entering the body through lungs or wounds. Pneumonia, brain abscess, subarachnoid hemorrhage, GI bleeding, hepatitis, acute myocardial infarction, endophthalmitis, and prosthetic valve endocarditis are all possible presentations. *Saksenaea* and *Apophysomyces* are the most common etiological agents; others include *Rhizopus* species, *Mucor* species, *Cunninghamella bertholletiae*, *Apophysomyces* species, and *Lichtheimia*, but rare pathogens such as *Cokeromyces recurvatus* may also exist.

RADIODIAGNOSIS

Computed tomography and MRI are helpful in diagnosing most of the cases, especially the rhino-orbito-cerebral mucoromycetes. These techniques detect soft-tissue involvement as well as spread of infection.

DIFFERENTIAL DIAGNOSIS

Bacterial infections such as orbital cellulitis, rhino-cerebral aspergillosis, and infection due to *Pseudallescheria boydii* are a few conditions which give a similar presentation. Pulmonary involvement is difficult to differentiate from bacterial pneumonia. Few cases of Oomycetes are confused with cutaneous mucormycosis in which histopathological findings will settle the diagnosis.

LABORATORY DIAGNOSIS

Direct Examination

Rapid dissemination of the disease makes prompt preliminary reporting based on microscopic results critical. The diagnostic process involves the collection of various samples, such as nasal scrapings, biopsies or exudates, hard palate lesions, sputum, bronchoalveolar lavage (BAL) fluid, burns, or other wounds.

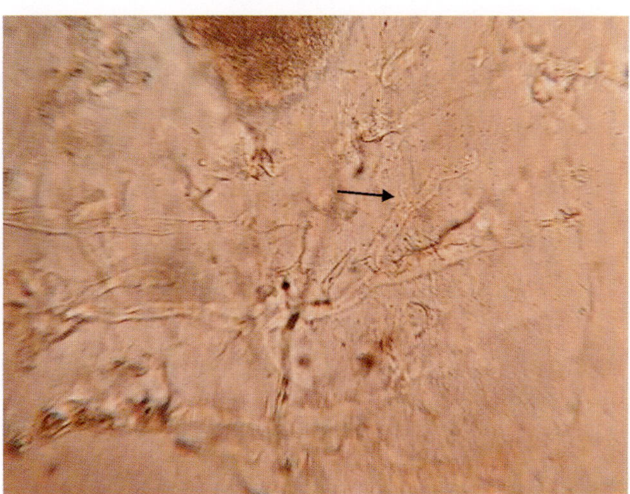

FIG. 26.3: KOH mount showing broad aseptate hyphae with wide-angle division (400×).
(KOH: potassium hydroxide)

Potassium Hydroxide Mount

The hyphae in these specimens are "ribbon like," with branches that branch at irregular intervals and are either nonseptate (coenocytic) or sparsely septate as shown in **Figure 26.3**.

After preparing the specimens with potassium hydroxide (KOH), fluorescent brighteners such as calcofluor can be used for direct observation.

The hyphae often lose their staining and take on either a gram-positive or a gram-negative appearance when Gram staining is applied **(Fig. 26.4)**.

Histopathology

In contrast to periodic acid-Schiff (PAS) staining, hematoxylin and eosin (H&E) staining makes fungal components readily apparent **(Fig. 26.5)**. The hyphae may be seen well with Grocott-Gömöri's methenamine silver (GMS) **(Fig. 26.6)**, making it the most helpful stain for these fungi. In tissue, large hyaline nonseptate hyphae having a diameter of 5–15 µm and branching at wide angles can be observed. Hyphae often droop, making them look like little *ribbons*. Typically, short hyphal components close to or even inside blood arteries might be seen. It should be kept in mind that hyphae may occur wrinkled, *collapsed*, or *bizarrely shaped* ("varicose"). Hyphae cross-sections might be mistaken for yeast cells. *Mucorales* often have branching that is both random and at right angles, as opposed to the acute-angle branching

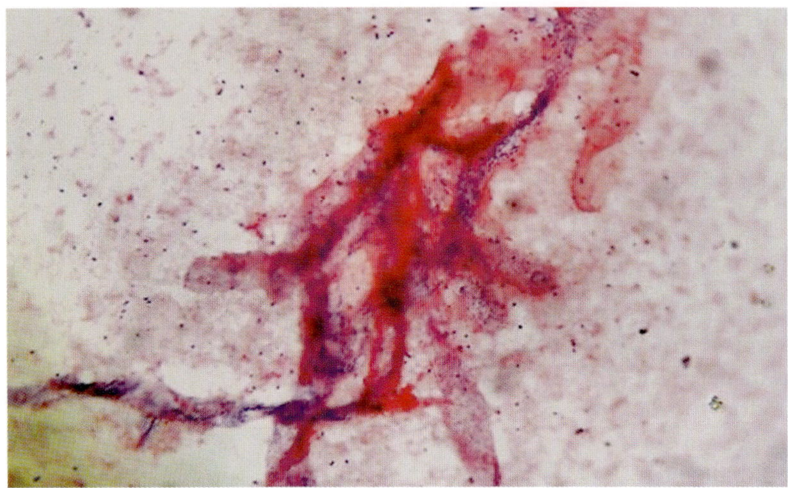

FIG. 26.4: Gram-stained smear showing broad gram variable, aseptate hyphae with "ribbon"-like appearance (1,000×).

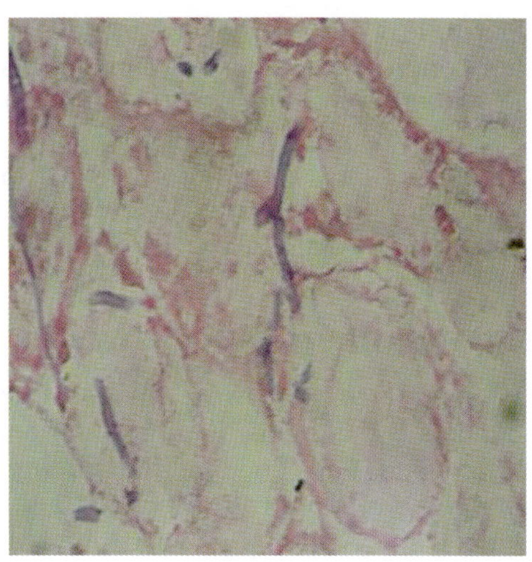

FIG. 26.5: H&E-stained biopsy with aseptate hyphae (400×).
(H&E: hematoxylin and eosin)

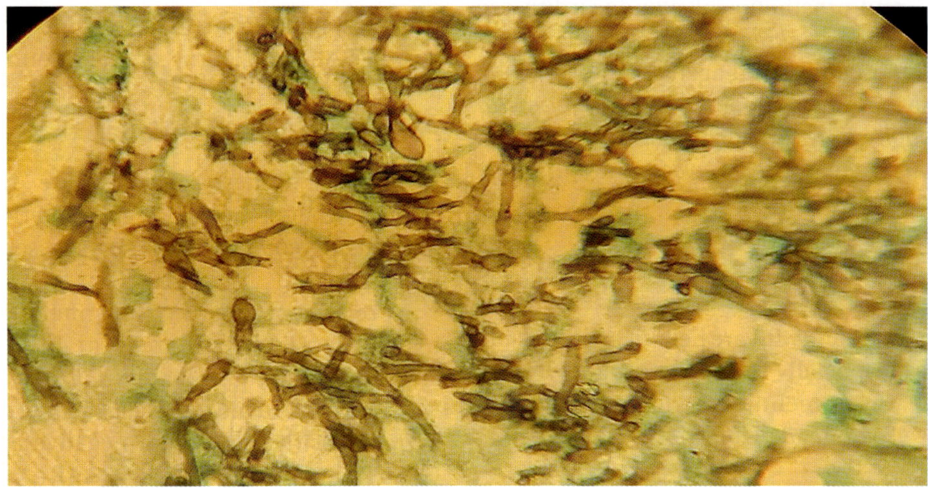

FIG. 26.6: Biopsy stained with GMS stain showing black, broad hyphae of mucormycosis (400×).
(GMS: Grocott–Gömöri's methenamine silver)

of Aspergilli. An infarct is linked to a neutrophilic reaction. Tissues infected with *C. recurvatus* or *Mucor circinelloides* will exhibit yeast-like characteristics.

Culture

The aseptate hyphae are fragile. They may be disrupted and their viability lost during the preparation of biopsy tissue for culture using tissue grinders. Crushing of tissue is avoided. If the material is not minced, it is immediately inoculated into culture media. Specimens from both sterile and nonsterile sites are used as culture materials. In light of the fact that these fungi are prevalent laboratory contaminants, it is important to exercise caution when interpreting isolates obtained from nonsterile sources, such as sputum, nasal sinus aspirates or scrapings, hard palate lesions, burns, or other wounds. The repeated isolation and correlation of microscopy with culture and clinical features are very essential.

Due to their susceptibility to cycloheximide, the preferred medium is modified Sabouraud dextrose agar (SDA) with antibiotics but no cycloheximide. It is possible for certain species of *Mucorales* to thrive in temperate environments. Thus, to facilitate species differentiation, it is optimal to culture samples at temperatures of 25, 35, 40, and 45°C. Different terms are used while describing colonies such as "lid lifters," "cotton candy," or floccose growth as shown in **Figure 26.7**. "Pin molds" are the unassisted eye's perception of sporangiophores with sporing heads.

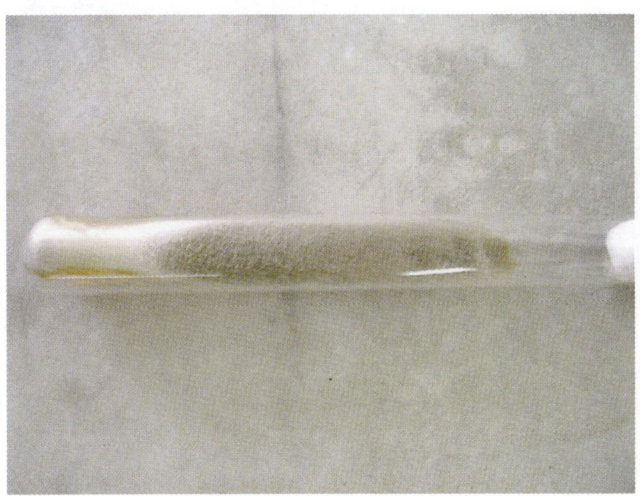

FIG. 26.7: SDA slant with fluffy growth (cotton candy) filling the whole tube of *Rhizopus* species.
(SDA: Sabouraud Dextrose Agar)

Failure to Grow

Mucorales are notorious for failing to grow from histopathologically confirmed biopsy specimens in many cases. Because tissue grinding may kill their sparsely septate fragile hyphae (cytoplasm leaks out), processing may influence poor recovery of *Mucorales* from both autopsy and biopsy specimens. The simplest option is to mince the tissue. To stimulate fungal growth, minced tissue slices can be placed directly on culture medium. Despite *Mucorales* invasion of blood vessels, blood cultures are rarely positive. Nonetheless, these molds can be recovered from blood cultures, which should not be overlooked.

Failure to Sporulate

Majority of *Mucorales* species are sporulating on common media such as SDA, cornmeal agar (CMA), or potato dextrose agar (PDA); however, there are a few outliers. Only sterile hyphae can be produced by *Apophysomyces elegans* and *Saksenaea vasiformis* under standard culture conditions. An improved alternative would be Czepek Dox agar. To encourage sporulation, start cultures on agar with cornmeal, sucrose, and yeast extract or tap water and then move them to a 1% agar block submerged in water. Grass and hay can be added to 1% saline agar in the Padhye and Aiello method to produce sporulation.

Rhizopus

The most common species causing infection is *Rhizopus arrhizus (Rhizopus oryzae)*. Colonies are white to light gray initially which become darker with maturation of sporangia. The position of rhizoids is just below the points from where sporangiophores arise (nodal). The sporangiophores are brown, erect, single or in groups, unbranched. Sporangia are globose, hyaline at the start, and become gray, dark brown, or black when mature.

Sporangiospores have longitudinal striations. The findings of the lactophenol cotton blue (LPCB) mount of *Rhizopus* is shown in **Figures 26.8A to C**. *R. arrhizus* has larger sporangiospores, while *Rhizopus microsporus* has small sporangiospores and sporangia. Taxonomically, the group *R. microsporus* is created to include all the species of *Rhizopus*. One emerging species is *Rhizopus homothallicus* which shows ornamental (surface projections are present) zygospores.

Rhizomucor pusillus

Colonies are initially white, then become gray and dark afterward. **Figure 26.9** shows the LPCB mount of *Rhizomucor* species. Sporangiophores are branched. Rhizoids are poorly formed which are internodal; they are formed in between and not at the points from where sporangiophores arise. Sporangia are brown and spherical. Sporangiospores have smooth walls and are globose to ellipsoidal. There is no apophysis. The temperature growth range is wider (20–60°C).

Rhizomucor pusillus can assimilate sucrose but has no thiamine dependence. It is significantly more sensitive to the statin drug lovastatin than *R. miehei*. *R. miehei* cannot assimilate sucrose but has a partial thiamine growth requirement.

Lichtheimia Species (Absidia)

Colonies that are white at first turn gray after prolonged incubation. *Lichtheimia corymbifera* can grow at temperatures ranging from 24 to 52°C.

Cycloheximide inhibits growth. The microscopic features are shown in **Figure 26.10**. It has internodal rhizoids. The stolon (the space between the rhizoids) is where the sporangiophores emerge. A prominent septum is present on the sporangiophore. Their species name comes from the fact that they are either hyaline or light gray in color and have simple branching or are arranged in whorls or clusters called corymbs. The sporangium is pyriform or pear shaped. The apophysis has a unique conical or funnel shape. Its diameter ranges from 100 to 150 μm. Columella can be either hemispherical or short ovoidal in shape. Sporangiospores are 2–3 × 3–4 μm in size and have a round to ellipsoid form. Zygospores are round (50–80 μm), brownish with rough walls. Two species, *L. corymbifera* and *Lichtheimia ramosa*, are known to infect humans.

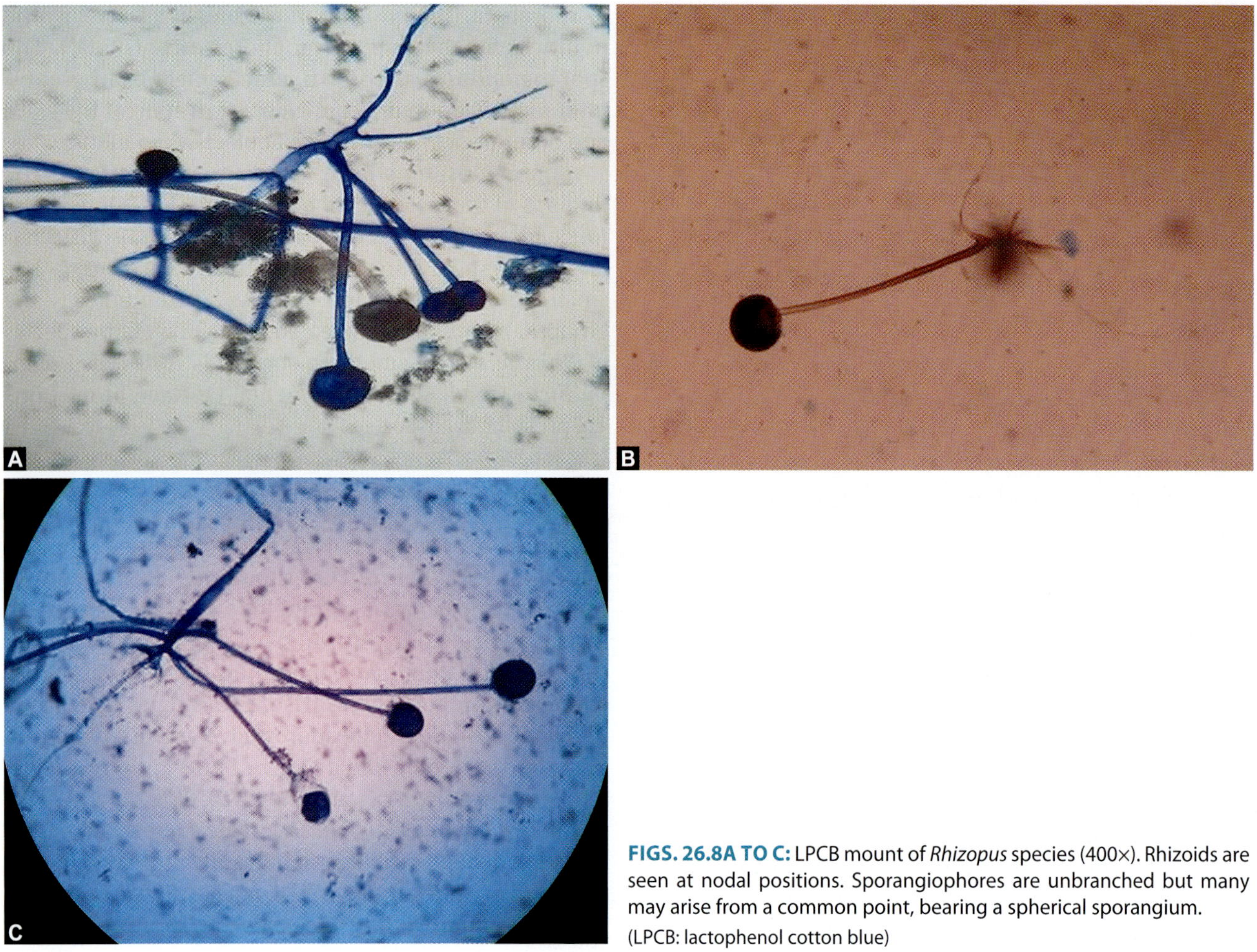

FIGS. 26.8A TO C: LPCB mount of *Rhizopus* species (400×). Rhizoids are seen at nodal positions. Sporangiophores are unbranched but many may arise from a common point, bearing a spherical sporangium.
(LPCB: lactophenol cotton blue)

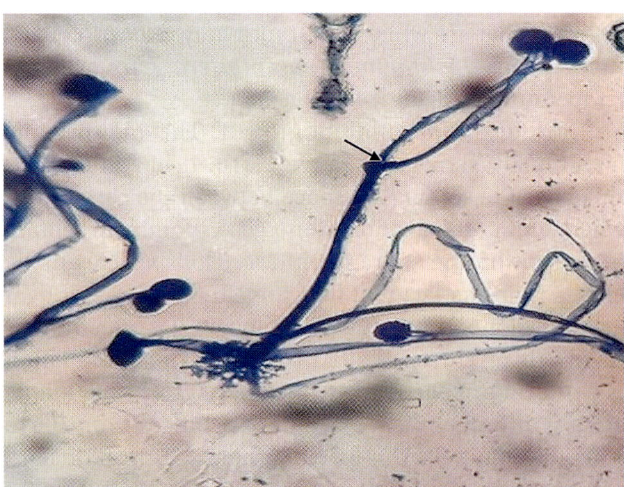

FIG. 26.9: LPCB mount of *Rhizomucor* species showing branched sporangiophore (400×).
(LPCB: lactophenol cotton blue)

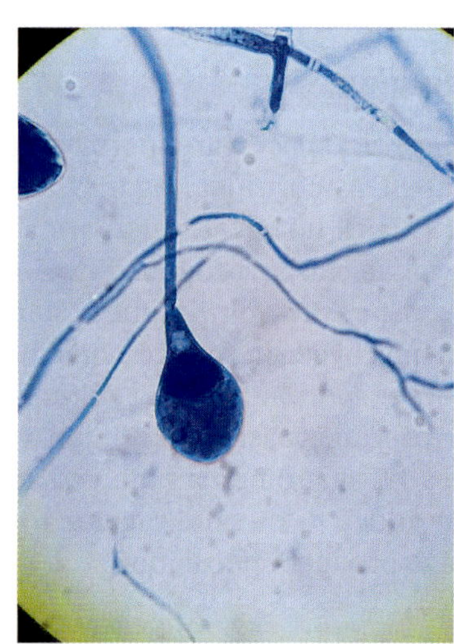

FIG. 26.10: LPCB mount of *Absidia*.
(LPCB: lactophenol cotton blue)

Mucor Species

Figures 26.11A and B show the characteristics of *Mucor* species. Globose, smooth sporangiophores are seen. The sporangiophores are branched. No rhizoids are found. There is no apophysis. A zygospore's suspensors are not appendaged. Rare mucormycosis agents include *M. circinelloides* and *Mucor ramosissimus*. *M. circinelloides* produces colonies that are pale gray-yellowish and turn brown at 37°C as they grow slowly at temperatures below 39°C. As a rule, the sporangiophores of *M. circinelloides* are sympodially branching. Sporangiophores are deliquescent, meaning they liquefy, and they bear sporangia that are spherical and 25–80 µm in diameter.

Apophysomyces elegans

The white colony turns buff with age. *A. elegans* is resistant to cycloheximide and can survive in environments as hot as 43°C. Since *A. elegans* does not easily sporulate on typical mycologic media, one must employ specific growth conditions that are low in nutrients and subject the organism to high incubation temperatures. A 1% agar block in water will promote sporulation in 3 weeks when incubated at 25°C. It is possible that sporulation can be facilitated under these conditions (37°C and 10–12 days incubation) by adding 1% agar with a small amount of yeast extract.

Unbranched sporangiophores develop from the tips of stolon-like hyphae in *A. elegans*.

Underneath the prominent apophyses are robust, grayish-brown sporangiophores.

The shape of an *apophysis* can range from bell shape or even *champagne glass*. Cells in the *foot* can develop into sporangiophores. A tuft of rhizoids is produced by the foot cell. The morphology of the sporangia is pyriform. A columella with a dome form is present. In contrast to *Absidia,* the sporangiophore displays a *brown thickening* just below the apophysis. *A. elegans, Apophysomyces trapeziformis, Apophysomyces ossiformis, Apophysomyces variabilis* (the most common in India), and *Apophysomyces mexicanus* are the five species that are currently significant. There is no zygospore formation in this species.

Saksenaea vasiformis complex

White colonies **(Fig. 26.12)** could be tricky to sporulate. Long-necked, vase shaped (or flask shaped) sporangia are seen as shown in **Figure 26.13**. Rhizoids with dark pigmentation are visible. After dissolving the gelatinous

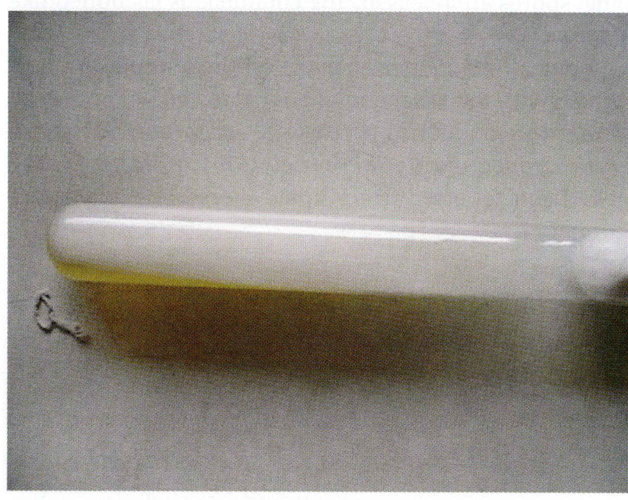

FIG. 26.12: Fluffy growth of *Saksenaea vasiformis* on SDA slant. (SDA: Sabouraud dextrose agar)

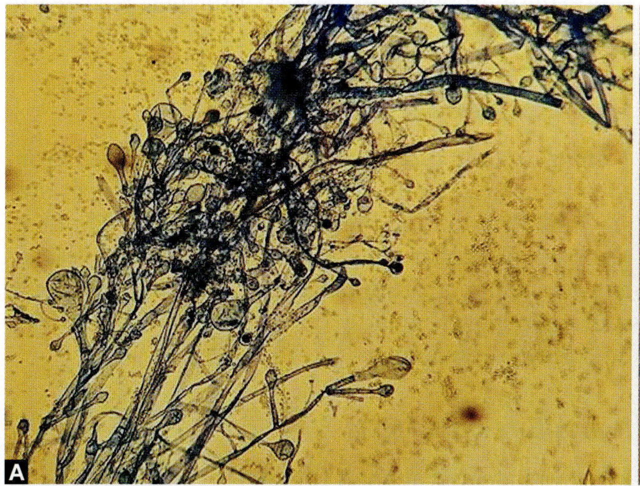

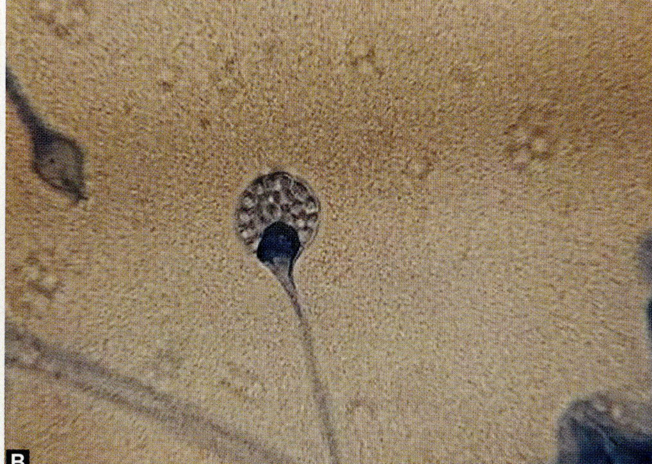

FIGS. 26.11A AND B: LPCB mounts of *Mucor* species (400×). (LPCB: lactophenol cotton blue)

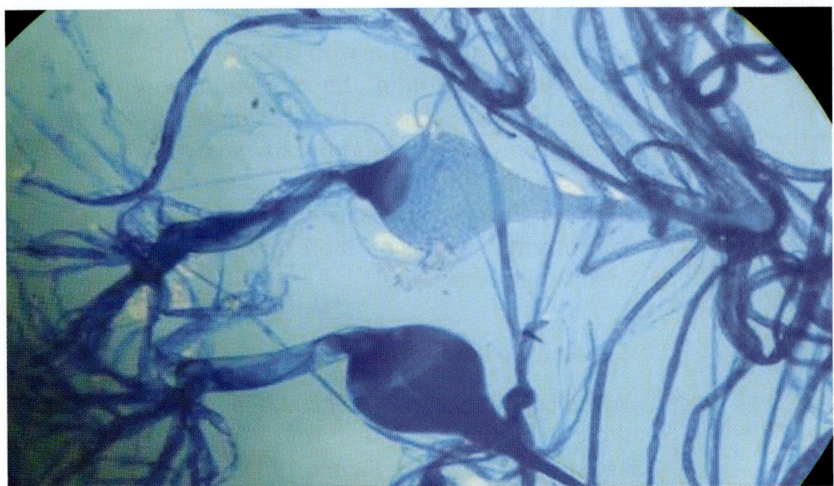

FIG. 26.13: LPCB mount of *Saksenaea* species (400×).
(LPCB: lactophenol cotton blue)

plug, spores are released. The columella is fashioned like a dome.

Four different species make up the complex *S. vasiformis*. With the exception of *Saksenaea oblongispora*, all of the aforementioned species—*S. vasiformis, Saksenaea erythrospora,* and *Saksenaea loutrophoriformis*—have been reported from India. There is no zygospore formation.

Syncephalastrum racemosum

Aerial mycelium is white initially and later turns gray against a white background. There are chains of spores formed in tubular sporangia called *merosporangis* as shown in **Figure 26.14**.

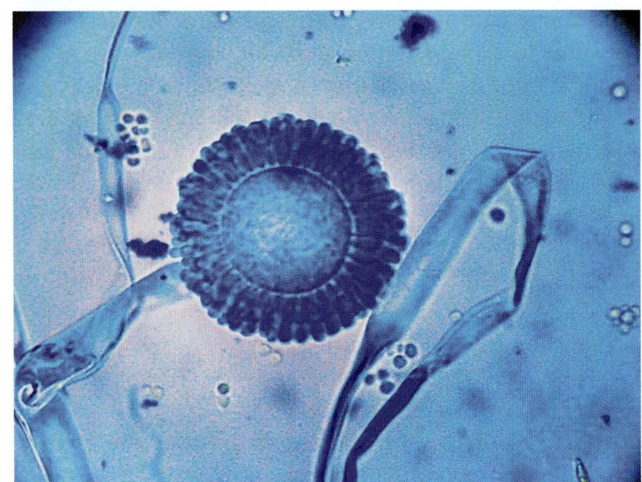

FIG. 26.14: LPCB mount of *Syncephalastrum* (400×).
(LPCB: lactophenol cotton blue)

Cunninghamella bertholletiae

The colony is gray in color. The sporangiophores are erect with a whorl of short branches at the apical region, each holding a swollen vesicle. Each sporangiole has one spore. Sporangioles are pear shaped to oval, and they are distributed all over the vesicle and attached with denticles as shown in **Figures 26.15A and B**.

Cokeromyces recurvatus

About 10 days of incubation at 30°C, broad sporangiophores with terminal vesicles are formed with elongated curved stalks or pedicles **(Fig. 26.16)**. Sporangia are globose. Short sporangiophores terminate at the apex into a single vesicle that bears several curved to twisted pedicles. Sporangia are formed at the tip of each pedicle.

Zygospores are usually seen. On brain heart infusion (BHI) agar at 37°C, yeast-like pasty colonies develop in 2 days, with large thick-walled spores with multiple buds. Due to the morphology of the yeast form there is chance of misdiagnosing it as *P. brasiliensis*.

Thamnostylum Species

Thamnostylum lucknowense was first isolated from soil in Lucknow, India. Colonies are fast-growing; they are initially white and later turn brownish. Whorls of recurved, pedicellate sporangiola are formed on vesicles on sporangiophores. Sporangiola have 8–16 oval, smooth sporangiospores. It is a rare cause of rhino-orbital mucormycosis in humans.

Nonculture-based tests

Improved identification of culture specimens is possible with matrix-assisted laser desorption ionization—time

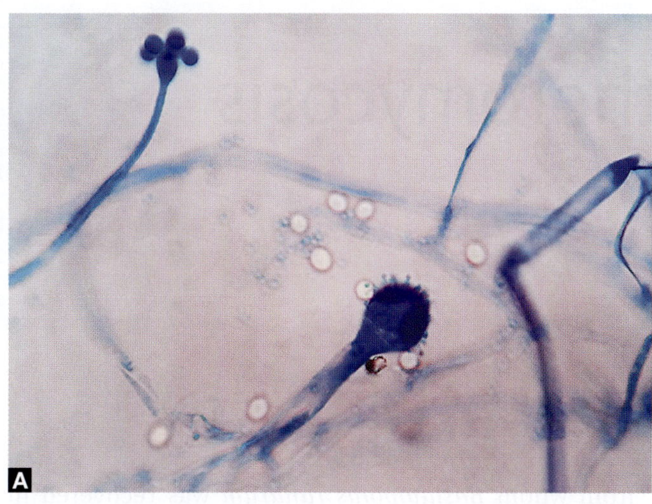

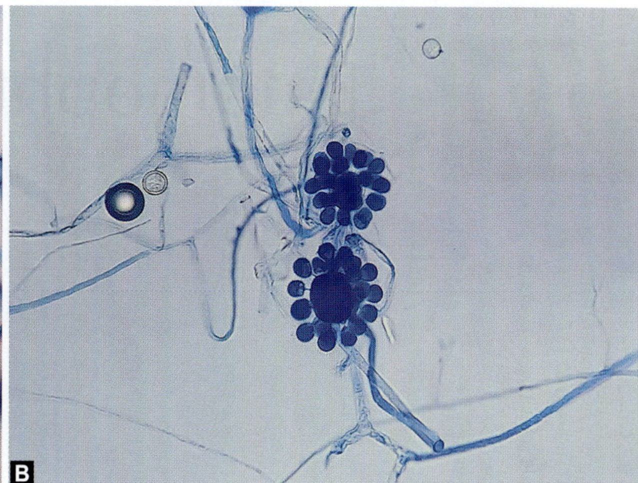

FIGS. 26.15A AND B: LPCB mount of *Cunninghemella* species (400×). (LPCB: lactophenol cotton blue)

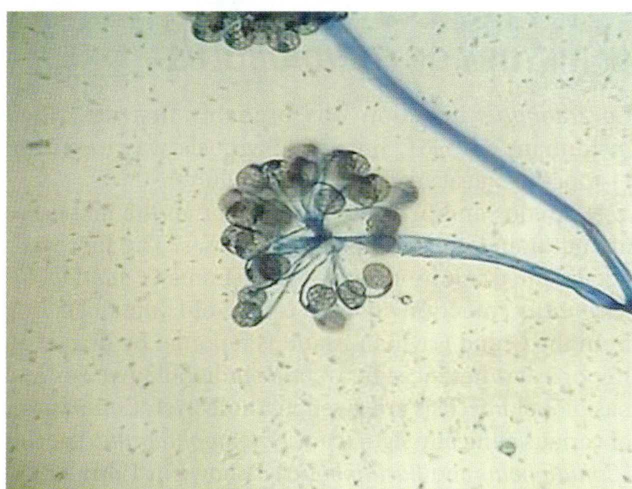

FIG. 26.16: *Cokeromyces* species.

of flight (MALDI-TOF) mass spectrometry. The capacity of molecular technologies, such as polymerase chain reaction (PCR)-based approaches, to enhance detection in tissues and frequently assist in species-level identification through targets like the internal transcribed spacer (ITS) or 18S ribosomal RNA, has led to their increased use.

Currently, there are enzyme-linked immunosorbent assay (ELISA) assays that target serum *Rhizomucor pusillus* and *R. arrhizus* antibodies, as well as Western immunoblotting that targets cytoplasm, hyphae walls, and septate for the diagnosis of mucormycosis. *Mucorales*-specific interferon (IFN)-producing T lymphocytes have recently been tested using ELISA (ELISpot) or immunocytofluorimetric assays.

Immunohistochemistry with newly commercialized monoclonal antibodies against *R. arrhizus* is another option for diagnosing mucormycosis (sensitivity 100%, specificity 100% for mucormycosis), which can be helpful in cases where cultures come back negative.

TREATMENT

The following approaches are used in the treatment of mucormycosis:

- Rapid correction of the underlying condition
- Surgical debridement
- Antifungal treatment
- Adjunctive therapy as hyperbaric oxygen

The drugs useful against mucormycosis are amphotericin B, posaconazole, and isavuconazole. Other azoles are useful against mucormycosis. Cytokines such as interferon γ and granulocyte-macrophage-stimulating factors (GM-CSFs) are adjunctively used to treat mucormycosis in neutropenic patients.

CHAPTER

27 Entomophthoromycosis

INTRODUCTION

In the context of the family Entomophthorales of fungi, "Entomophthoromycosis" describes long-lasting infections that start under the skin. The word entomophthoromycosis is derived from two Greek words "entomon,"which means "insect", and phthora that means "destroyer". Genera *Conidiobolus* and *Basidiobolus* are pathogenic to people. In people with healthy immune systems, the infection stays under the skin and in the subcutaneous tissues. Persistent fibrosis and scarring can lead to a worsening of deformity, lymphatic blockage, further disfigurement, and a loss of function at the site of infection.

HISTORY OF *BASIDIOBOLUS*

The first report of Entomophthorales human infection came from Indonesia in a boy with subcutaneous swelling from whom *Basidiobolus ranarum* was recovered in pure culture. Those authors mentioned that in 1925, Van Overeem, also in Indonesia, described a lesion in a horse and *B. ranarum* was recovered.

HISTORY OF *CONIDIOBOLUS*

Conidiobolus infection was probably first described in humans in 1961, but the diagnosis was based on histopathological analysis without culture.

Emmons and Bridges (1961) reported the first cases of conidiobolomycosis in Texan horses. The first well-documented culture-positive case of human *Conidiobolus coronatus* infection in an 11-year-old Jamaican boy from the Grand Cayman Island is reported by Bras et al. Important differences between conidiobolomycosis and basidiobolomycosis are given in **Table 27.1**. Comparison of various clinically significant *Entomophthorales* species (*Conidiobolus* and *Basidiobolus*) is shown in **Table 27.2**.

TABLE 27.1: Differences between conidiobolomycosis and basidiobolomycosis.

Features	***Conidiobolomycosis***	***Basidiobolomycosis***
Anatomical sites	Face, nasal area	Trunk, thigh, buttocks
Lesions	Firmly attached to the underlying tissue	Not firmly attached to the underlying tissue
Age	Primarily adults	Primarily children
Visceral involvement	Not usually seen	Gastrointestinal involvement
Causative agents	*Conidiobolus coronatus*, *Conidiobolus incongruus*, *Conidiobolus lamprauges*	*Basidiobolus ranarum*
Colony morphology	Flat, waxy colonies that become powdery with a short aerial mycelium; petri dish lid covered with conidia ejected from older cultures; colonies white, buff, tan, or brown	Flat, furrowed colonies with a waxy texture; yellowish to gray
Morphology of conidia	Conidia are round to pyriform, with prominent papillae on the wall giving rise to secondary conidia	Primary asexual spores are globose, forcibly discharged, phototropic, and produced singly at the tip of the conidiophore

Continued

Continued

Features	*Conidiobolomycosis*	*Basidiobolomycosis*
Sexual spores	Rarely produced but within the larger of the two gametangia	Zygospores have two closely appressed beak-like appendages
Microscopic features	• Conidia often have a distinct papilla and are usually found in clusters • Aerial hyphae are less pronounced	Conidia are typically more isolated, with a pronounced beak-like structure in sexual spores
Histopathological findings	Histology may show granulomatous inflammation with necrosis and conidia within the tissue	Histology reveals a more diffuse, granulomatous inflammation with abundant necrotic tissue and zygospores
Treatment	Antifungal medications such as itraconazole or ketoconazole; surgical debridement may be necessary in severe cases	Antifungal medications, such as itraconazole or ketoconazole; surgical intervention may be required for extensive cases
Diagnosis	Clinical presentation, microscopy of tissue samples, and culture	Clinical presentation, microscopy, and culture
Epidemiology	Found predominantly in tropical and subtropical regions	More common in tropical and subtropical areas, often in agricultural or rural settings

TABLE 27.2: Comparison of various clinically significant *Entomophthorales* species (*Conidiobolus* and *Basidiobolus*).

	Conidiobolus lamprauges	*Conidiobolus coronatus*	*Conidiobolus incongruus*	*Basidiobolus ranarum*
Sexual conidia (zygospores)	Size 12–18 μm and 15-40 μm, with a single large globule	Not produced	Larger in size with numerous globules	With beak-like appendages
Asexual conidia	Globose to obovoid, 15–22 μm	Globose, 25–45 μm	Globose, 16–34 μm	Globose
Secondary conidia	Present	Present	Present	Absent
Villose conidia	Absent	Present	Absent	–
Multireplicative conidia	Absent	Present	Present in a few strains	–

MYCOLOGY

In case of agents of mucormycosis, the spores are released passively after rupture of the sporangium wall, while in case of *Entomophthorales*, the spores are forcefully ejected. The fungi are seen in soil, decaying vegetation, gastrointestinal tract (GIT) of amphibians, and insects (insect pathogens). Based on the etiological agents, the diseases are named conidiobolomycosis (caused by the genus *Conidiobolus*) and basidiobolomycosis (caused by *Basidiobolus*).

TAXONOMY

Among the first groups of Zygomycota were the *Entomophthorales* and *Mucorales*. The genera *Basidiobolus* and *Conidiobolus* made up the order *Entomophthorales*. It was necessary to reclassify *Mucorales* and *Entomophthorales* because of their distinct evolutionary histories. Zygomycota is no longer a taxonomic group. *Basidiobolomycetes*, *Neozygitomycetes*, and *Entomophthoramycetes* are now all considered to be members of a single subphylum, the *Entomophthoramycota*. *Conidiobolus* species is an example of an Entomophthoramycete, whereas *Basidiobolus* species is an example of a Basidiobolomycete.

HABITAT AND GEOGRAPHICAL DISTRIBUTION

Many species of *Basidiobolus* are both saprobic and parasitic. Insects, woodlice, decaying plants, and the excrement of reptiles and amphibians contain these conidia. In addition to humans and horses, the species can also be found in dogs, bats, and other mammals.

All over the tropics and subtropics, from South America to India, Pakistan, Uganda, Kenya, the Ivory Coast, Myanmar, and Ghana, *Basidiobolus* species is found. Additionally, reports have come in from the southeast United States, including Arizona, and England.

Conidiobolus is a saprobic and invasive fungus. All the beaches in India, the East Coast of the United States, and the United Kingdom contain *Conidiobolus*, as well as soil and decomposing plant matter. Extremely high humidity is ideal for *Conidiobolus* spore development. This means that tropical regions tend to have the highest number of cases. Sheep, horses, and insects are all hosts for this particular kind of parasite. The excrement of amphibians, such as lizards and frogs, also contains conidia.

SPECIES OF MEDICAL IMPORTANCE

The important species of *Conidiobolus* are *C. coronatus*, *Conidiobolus incongruus*, and *Conidiobolus lamprauges*.

Various species of *Basidiobolus* are *B. ranarum*, *Basidiobolus haptosporus*, and *Basidiobolus meristosporus*. Molecular taxonomy and restriction enzyme analysis have shown that *B. ranarum* is synonymous with *B. haptosporus* and *B. meristosporus*. Only *Basidiobolus ranarum* has ever been associated with human illness among the *Basidiobolus* species.

There are two species of *Conidiobolus* that can cause illness in humans: (1) *C. coronatus* and (2) *Conidiobolus incongruous*. The former is responsible for most human infections. The sheep and horses are the primary hosts of the *C. lamprauges*. It has been documented as a source of infection in patients with impaired immune systems.

MODE OF TRANSMISSION OF *BASIDIOBOLUS*

- Insect bites or low-level trauma followed by injections with proper aseptic cleaning of the injection site are two possible entry points for the fungus into human hosts. These organisms are carried on the surface of insects and mites.
- Another possibility is that amphibians ingest these infected insects and then pass the fungus on through their excrement, which might contaminate even small wounds. Contaminated soil and plants can spread disease.

MODE OF TRANSMISSION OF *CONIDIOBOLUS*

The primary route of infection is believed to be the inhalation of fungal spores present in the air. These spores can colonize the nasal passages or paranasal sinuses, leading to chronic rhinosinusitis.

LIFE CYCLE

Entomophthorales produce multinucleated sticky conidia that are forcefully ejected. Conidia germinate and develop a germ tube that allows them to enter potential hosts when they settle on them. If the expelled conidia land somewhere other than the intended host, secondary small conidia can form.

PATHOLOGY OF *CONIDIOBOLUS* AND *BASIDIOBOLUS*

The infection affects the subcutaneous tissue. Penetration of adjacent anatomical sites is rare. When hematoxylin and eosin (H&E) is used to stain tissues, those that are infected show signs of inflammation and extensive fibrosis. The reaction includes the presence of many eosinophils and the formation of a red envelope surrounding the invading hyphae. The term for this is the Splendore-Höeppli effect (S–P). Deposited here are antigen–antibody complexes. Infected tissues of both entomophthoralean and mucoralean (usually, we prefer terms such as *Entomophthorales* and *Mucorales*) fungi have broad hyphae. However, eosinophils and the S–P phenomenon, which are absent in mucoralean fungus, become crucial in differentiating these two pathogen types.

The hyphae are 8–12 µm broad, sparsely septate, and unbranched, forming either short filaments in the shape of ribbons or tiny rings (hyphae that have been cross-sectioned). The severity of the inflammation is proportional to the disease's progression. It is possible to see neutrophils and eosinophils surrounding the hyphae in severe cases. In chronic cases, histiocytes, lymphocytes, and sometimes giant cells are seen, with a small number of eosinophils.

Angioinvasion is *not* a feature of Entomophthorales.

Differential diagnosis of rhinoentomophthoramycosis: Atypical mycobacterial cutaneous infections, squamous cell carcinoma, chromoblastomycosis, sporotrichosis, paracoccidioidomycosis, blastomycosis, coccidioidomycosis, pythiosis, rhinosporidiosis, tuberculosis of the mucosa, and nocardiosis are to be considered as differential diagnosis.

CLINICAL FEATURES

Conidiobolomycosis

The inferior nasal turbinate is the site of infection. The infection gradually spreads to the paranasal sinuses and then, usually, the skin around the nose, glabella, cheekbones, and upper lip on both sides. Symptoms include a stuffy nose, a runny nose, and persistent sinusitis. Swelling of the face, which may spread to the upper lip and cheek, may appear gradually; it is firm and painless. It is possible to feel the swelling through the skin. Tumor-like swellings that grow over time and cause significant deformities. Lesions are accompanied by reddening of the skin. A mass resembling the swelling develops, which can be easily extracted from deeper tissues. A "doughnut-lifting sign" describes this appearance. It does not affect bones. Swelling of the hard and soft palates, which occurs within the mouth, can spread to the larynx and throat, leading to difficulties in swallowing and other symptoms.

Differential Diagnosis of Conidiobolomycosis

The condition should be differentiated from soft-tissue tumors. Histopathological examination of the tissues shows the presence of aseptate hyphae.

Basidiobolomycosis

Subcutaneous Basidiobolomycosis

In contrast to *Conidiobolus*, the subcutaneous tissue of the lower limb is affected. The infection takes place through small abrasions of the skin following a thorn prick or through insect bite. The trunk, upper arm, shoulder, and axilla are all impacted by the *B. ranarum* infection that persists under the skin. More susceptible to the disease are children residing in tropical and subtropical regions. Males are more affected than females. A subcutaneous nodule develops into a solid, woody mass as the lesion advances. A firm, discrete, and painless mass under the skin is what it looks like. An enlarged, infected limb might grow to be two or three times its typical size. The "bathing trunks" area—buttocks and thighs—are the most common sites, although it can also spread to the subcutaneous tissues nearby. It is possible for smaller lesions to form as satellites, with well-defined borders. It could be painful to deal with large lesions. While swelling of regional lymph nodes is possible, bone involvement is often minimal. It is quite rare for an underlying condition to be present.

Gastrointestinal Basidiobolomycosis

It has an impact on children and grown-ups alike. For intestinal basidiobolomycosis, the most common symptoms are as follows: (1) Mucous and bloody diarrhea, (2) epigastric discomfort, (3) low fever that comes and goes, (4) bleeding inside the intestines, (5) vomiting, and (6) the growth of tumor-like masses in the tissues of the stomach and intestines. The presence of intestinal ulcers and nodular masses is similar to Crohn's disease. It has also been reported that the invading hyphae spread to the pancreas, liver, and lymph nodes. There have also been reports of unusual cases of systemic illness affecting the muscles, maxillary sinus, and mouth in addition to the lungs. Elephantiasis, mycetoma, and sporotrichosis are the diseases that need to be distinguished from basidiobolomycosis.

Differential Diagnosis of Basidiobolomycosis

Elephantiasis, mycetoma, sporotrichosis, and infection of atypical mycobacteria should be ruled out. The gastrointestinal lesions should be differentiated from Crohn's disease and malignancy.

LABORATORY DIAGNOSIS OF BASIDIOBOLOMYCOSIS

The gold standard for laboratory diagnosis is still culture of tissue. The hyphae of certain species of *Conidiobolus* and *Basidiobolus*, however, are susceptible to damage when the tissue is homogenized. Acute and chronic inflammatory infiltration is observed in the biopsy along with ribbon-shaped hyphae that are wide, thin-walled, sparsely septate. Use of a fluorescence microscope to examine wet mount preparations improves the sensitivity of diagnosis compared to H&E staining, which is low.

Media such as Sabouraud dextrose agar (SDA), potato dextrose agar (PDA), and cornmeal agar (CMA) are utilized for specimen inoculation in culture. At 30°C, colonies expand at a moderate pace, whereas at 37°C, growth is slow. A glabrous or waxy colony ranging in color from gray to beige is the early morphology of *Basidiobolus* species. **Figures 27.1A and B** show colonies of *Basidiobolus* on SDA slant and SDA plate. Aerial hyphae cover this colony as it gets radially furrowed with time. The SDA slant is white on the back.

The hyphae are aseptate or sparsely septate. As a result of producing ballistoconidia, satellite colonies are formed. The sporangiophores cover the inside of the tube and plate with spores because they forcefully release the terminal sporangiospore.

The primary asexual spores that are produced at the tip of the conidiophore are globose which are forcibly released. The secondary conidia are produced which are clavate with a wide base and adhesive tip. They are not discharged. Sporangiospores may produce meristospores by cleavage. Intercalary zygospores are produced with a smooth wall and a *beak-like appendage* which is the remain of copulatory tubules. **Figures 27.2A and B** show zygospores with beak-like appendages.

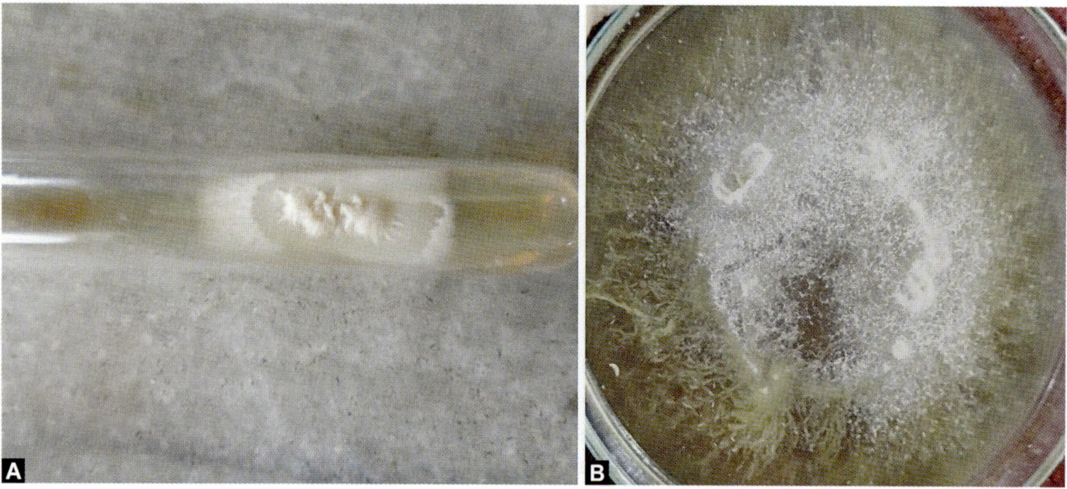

FIGS. 27.1A AND B: (A) Colony of *Basidiobolus* on SDA slant; (B) Growth of *Basidiobolus* on SDA plate.
(SDA: Sabouraud dextrose agar)

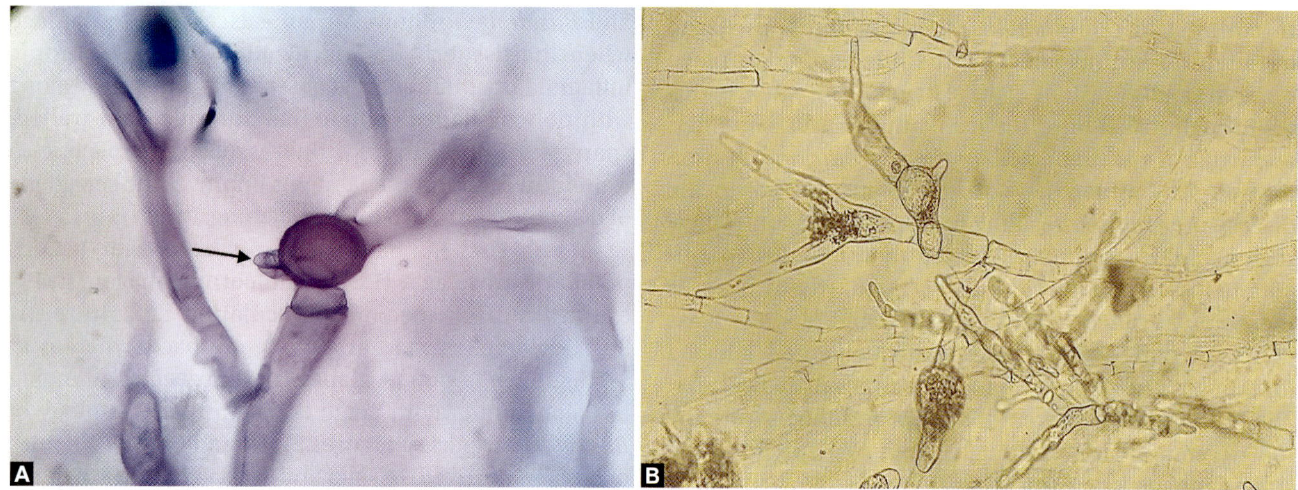

FIGS. 27.2A AND B: LPCB mount and wet mount (zygospore with beak-like projection).
(LPCB: lactophenol cotton blue)

LABORATORY DIAGNOSIS OF CONIDIOBOLOMYCOSIS

For specimen inoculation, SDA, PDA, and CMA are the media that are utilized.

A set is kept at 37°C, while the other is kept at 25°C. *Conidiobolus* species develops sporadic white aerial hyphae and quickly grows into glabrous, flat, beige-to-brown colonies on conventional medium at 37°C for 3–5 days. The colonies later have white reverses. The colonies' centers become powdery. Sporangiospores, released by short, nonbranching sporangiophores, cover the inside of the culture tube or the lid of the plate.

Lactophenol cotton blue (LPCB) mount: In addition to the sporangiola, the sporangiospores of *Conidiobolus* have a clearly visible *papilla*. The spores can have *villi*, which look like little hairs. These structures are shown in **Figures 27.3A and B**. It is named *C. coronatus* because of the villous corona that surrounds the spore. Additionally, papilloconidia can be observed as elongated cells with a terminal knob.

Sexual spore production is useful for the speciation of the genus *Conidiobolus*. The most common species *C. coronatus* does not produce zygospores. At first, the colonies of *C. incongruus* look similar, but as time goes on, they dry out. At 37°C, growth is optimal, whereas at 25°C, it is almost nonexistent.

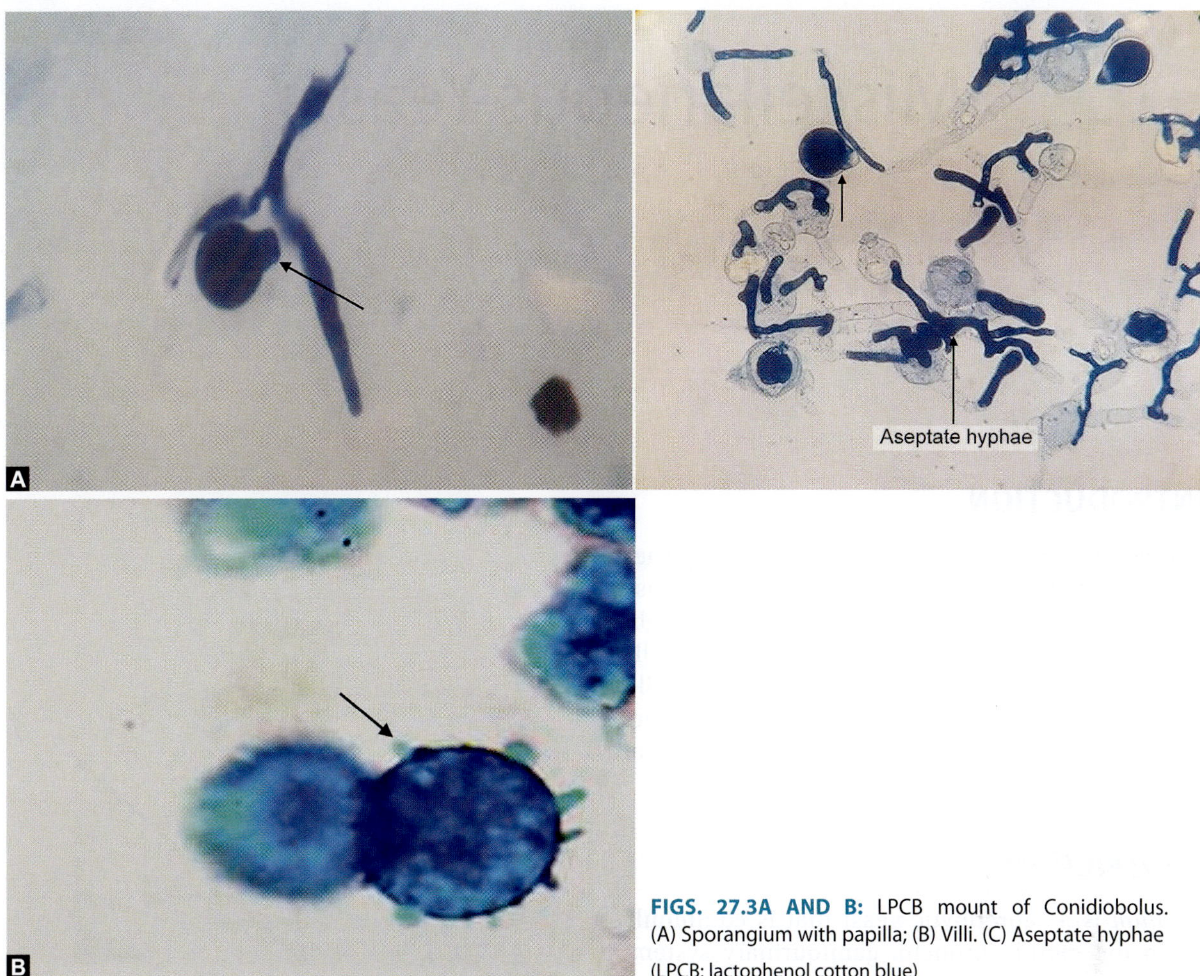

FIGS. 27.3A AND B: LPCB mount of Conidiobolus. (A) Sporangium with papilla; (B) Villi. (C) Aseptate hyphae (LPCB: lactophenol cotton blue)

TREATMENT OF CONIDIOBOLOMYCOSIS AND BASIDIOBOLOMYCOSIS

Saturated solution of potassium iodide (SSKI) is administered orally at a dosage of 20 mg/kg/day, with a daily maximum dose of 2 g/kg. Even after the lesions have disappeared, the medication should be taken for another month. When treating a rhinosinusitis infection, a combination of surgical debridement, SSKI and itraconazole works well. Hyperbaric oxygen is potentially helpful in facilitating recovery. In some cases of conidiobolomycosis, surgical intervention may be necessary.

CHAPTER

28 Miscellaneous Yeasts

INTRODUCTION

Some yeasts *Cryptococcus* species and *Candida* species are already covered. In this chapter we consider those yeasts that might be saprobes or commensals and might produce infections in humans. Infections occur usually in immunocompromised host. Almost all cause mild infections but some could be serious. Their characters are described in the chapter. Some have industrial importance.

GEOTRICHUM

Geotrichum is a saprophytic yeast that is commonly found in the mouth, bronchi, genitourinary system, and gastrointestinal tract (GIT). *Geotrichum candidum* is a single species in the genus. *Geotrichum* contains fast-growing colonies and hyphae that are frequently dichotomously branched at the colony boundary. In immunocompromised people, the genus can cause skin, oral, lung, and GIT infections. *Geotrichum* forms white-to-cream colonies that are smooth or hairy at 25°C. At 37°C, development is exceedingly sluggish and resembles mold growth.

Microscopically, arthroconidia are found **(Fig. 28.1)**. These are distinguished from *Trichosporon* by the lack of blastoconidia and a negative urease test. Arthroconidia generate hyphae from one corner, giving them a "hockey-stick" look. Nystatin, gentian violet, and amphotericin B are the medications utilized in the therapy.

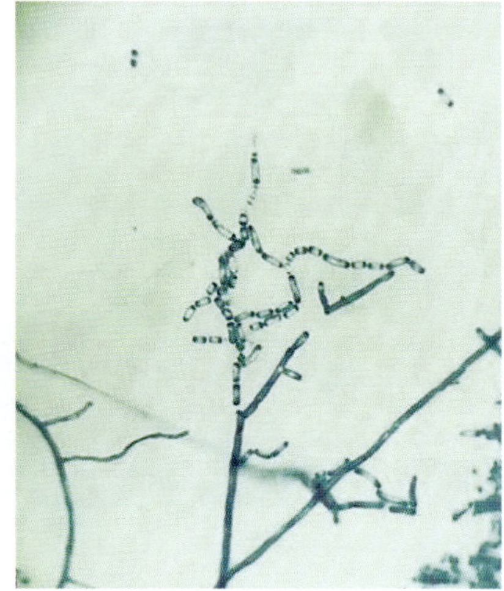

FIG. 28.1: LPCB mount of *Geotrichum* (400×). (LPCB: lactophenol cotton blue)

MAGNUSIOMYCES CAPITATUS

This fungus was previously known as *Geotrichum capitatum* or *Blastoschizomyces capitatus*. It may be found in the environment and has been isolated from diverse places such as the oral mucosa, skin, and respiratory tract. It can infrequently produce widespread illness in immunocompromised people, particularly neutropenic ones. Direct microscopy reveals hyphae. The colonies on Sabouraud dextrose agar (SDA) are glabrous and range in color from white to yellow. The presence of annelloconidia at the tip of the conidiophore distinguishes it from other yeasts **(Figs. 28.2 and 28.3)**. It lacks urease, develops in SDA with cycloheximide, and exclusively assimilates glucose and galactose. Amphotericin B and flucytosine are used in the therapy.

RHODOTORULA

Rhodotorula species are named after the carotenoid pigments that give their colonies their characteristic pink, coral, orange, or red hues. Some species of *Rhodotorula* are significant for medicine, such as *Rhodotorula glutinis*, *Rhodotorula mucilaginosa* (formerly *Rhodotorula rubra*),

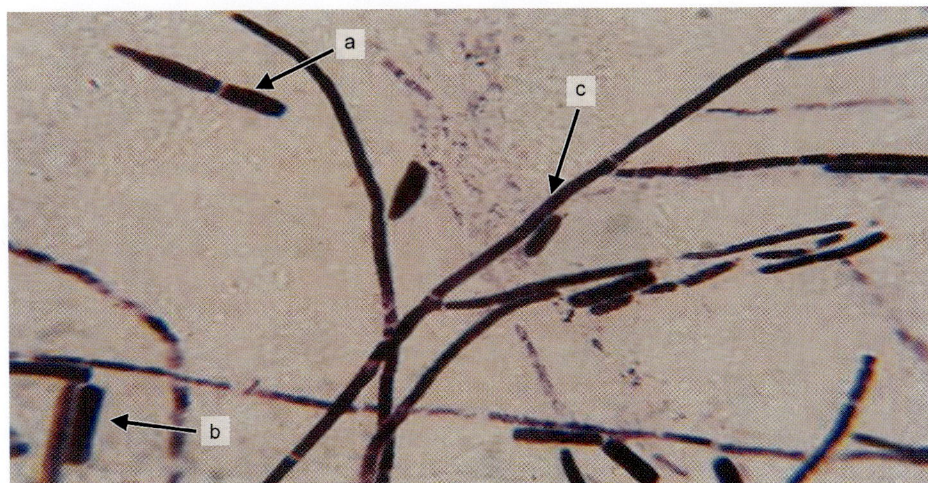

FIG. 28.2: LPCB mount of *Magnusiomyces capitatus*. (a) Annelloconidia; (b) Arthroconidia; (c) True hyphae (×1,000).
(LPCB: lactophenol cotton blue)

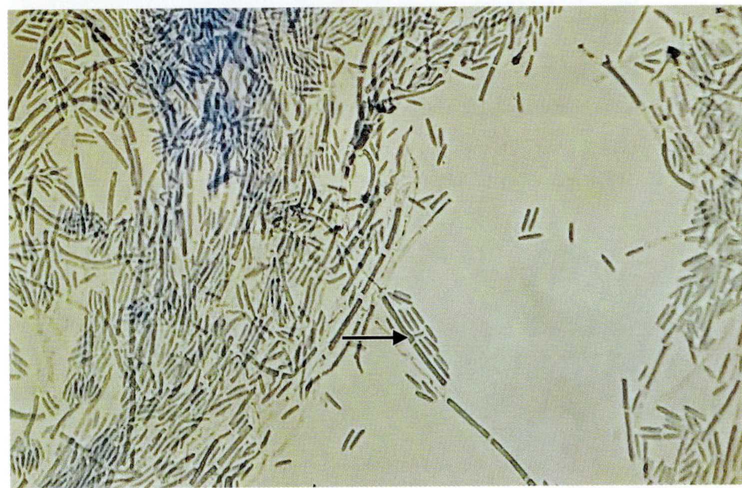

FIG. 28.3: *Magnusiomyces capitatus* under high power showing annelloconidia.

and *Rhodotorula minuta*. Yeast like these are seen in soil, in the air, and even on the surfaces of leaves. Milk and cheese may contain *Rhodotorula* species. These microbes, dwell in the oral cavity, on the skin, in the nails, and in the mucous membranes of gut and respiratory tract. They can be isolated from feces. It may cause skin infections, keratitis, fungemia, CNS infections. Risk factors are immunocompromised state, chronic liver and kidney disease, indwelling central venous catheter. It may cause peritonitis in patients on peritoneal dialysis. Monopolar ellipsoid budding yeast *R. mucilaginosa* produces a little amount of pseudohyphae. The budding yeast *R. glutinis* is ellipsoid in shape and has many polarities; it also makes primitive pseudohyphae. Budding yeast *R. minuta* is ellipsoid-shaped and monopolar; it does not generate pseudohyphae. Colonies on SDA produce orange pigment, as shown in **Figure 28.4**.

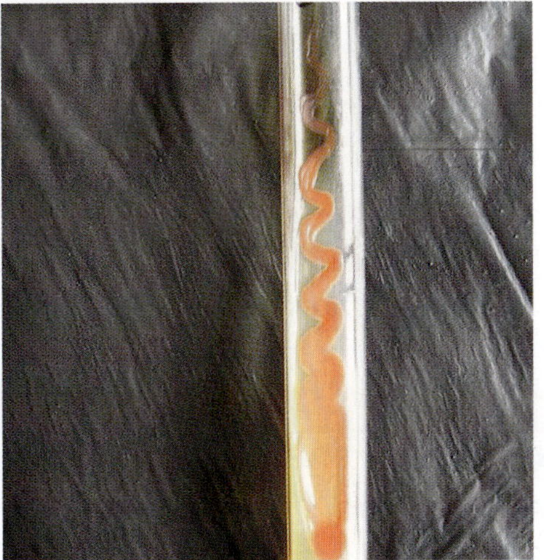

FIG. 28.4: Growth of *Rhodotorula* on SDA.
(SDA: Sabouraud dextrose agar)

TRICHOSPORON

Trichosporon is a saprophytic yeast that may colonize the skin, GIT, and respiratory tract and has been found in feces, sputum, blood, and central venous catheters. As a result, when it is isolated from clinical specimens, it should be reported with caution. *Trichosporon* species include *Trichosporon asahii*, *Trichosporon ovoides*, *Trichosporon mucoides*, *Trichosporon inkin*, *Trichosporon asteroids*, *Trichosporon cutaneum*, *Trichosporon loubieri*, and *Trichosporon pullulans*. Trichosporon infections are both superficial and systemic. "White piedra" is caused by *T. inkin*, *T. ovoides*, and *T. mucoides*. Onychomycosis can be caused by *Trichosporon*. Endocarditis, pneumonia, brain abscess, osteomyelitis, and otomycosis are the systemic illnesses caused. One of the reasons of false-positive latex agglutination tests for *Cryptococcus* is the cell wall antigen of *Trichosporon*. SDA colonies are yeast-like, cream-colored, and wrinkled with furrows. True hyphae, arthroconidia, and blastoconidia are seen when smear is prepared from cornmeal agar (CMA). The findings can be confirmed by lactophenol cotton blue (LPCB) preparation **(Fig. 28.5)**. The Gram-stained smear may show an arthroconidium with two blastoconidia attached at one end giving "rabbit ear" appearance, as shown in **Figures 28.6A and B**. Speciation can be done by Vitek or sugar assimilation tests **(Table 28.1)**.

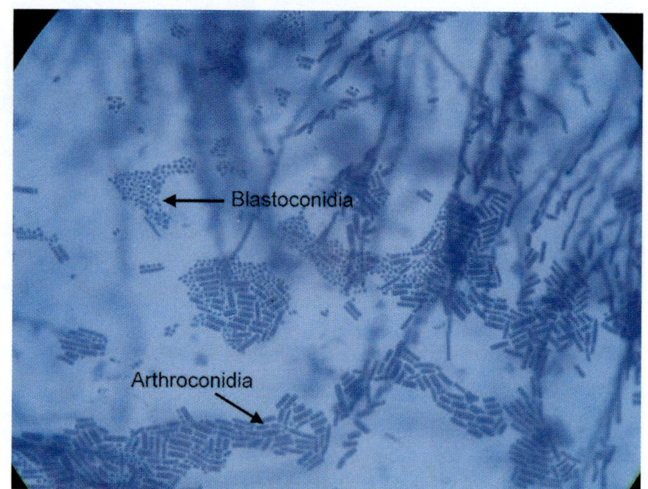

FIG. 28.5: LPCB mount of *Trichosporon* (400×).
(LPCB: lactophenol cotton blue)

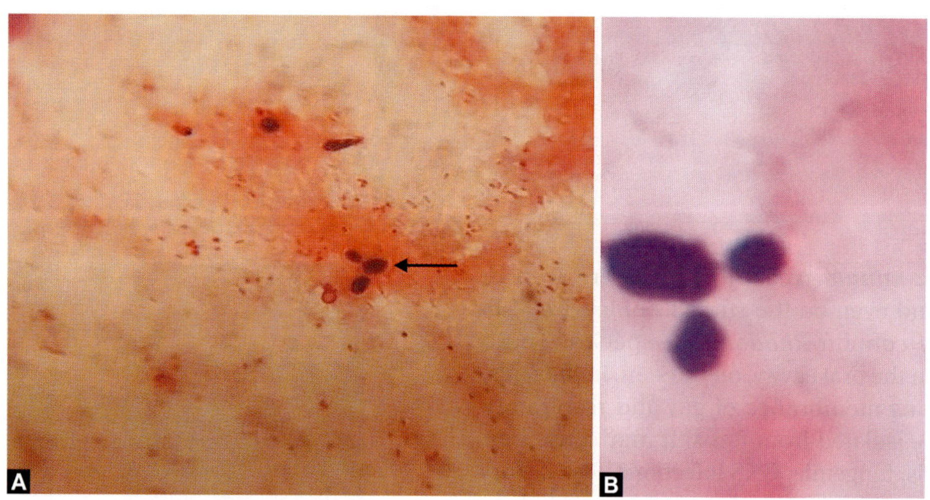

FIGS. 28.6A AND B: Gram-stained smear of *Trichosporon* showing "rabbit ear" appearance (1,000×).

TABLE 28.1: Assimilation patterns of clinically significant *Trichosporon* species.

Trichosporon species	*Growth at 37°C*	*L-rham*	*Mel*	*Raff*	*Rib*	*Xyl*	*L-arab*	*Gala*	*Sorb*	*Ino*
Trichosporon asahii	+	+	–	–	v	v	+	–	–	–
Trichosporon cutaneum	–	+	+	+	+	+	+	–	+	+
Trichosporon inkin	+	–	–	–	–	–	–	–	–	+
Trichosporon mucoides	+	+	+	+	+	+	+	+	+	+
Trichosporon ovoides	+	+	–	v	–	v	–	–	–	–

Differences between Geotrichum, *Magnusiomyces*, and *Trichosporon* are given in **Table 28.2**.

SACCHAROMYCES

Saccharomyces cerevisiae is sometimes known as "baker's yeast" or "brewer's yeast." Yeast is utilized in fermentation and as an adjuvant in protein supplements. The budding yeasts are circular to oval in shape, with rudimentary pseudohyphae on occasion. **(Fig. 28.7)**. The yeast has been found in instances of oral thrush, vulvovaginitis, and fungemia, as well as the human respiratory system, GIT, and genitourinary tract.

TABLE 28.2: Comparative features of *Trichosporon, Magnusiomyces capitatus*, and *Geotrichum* species.

Species	*Blastoconidia*	*Annelloconidia*	*Urease*
Trichosporon	+	–	+
Magnusiomyces capitatus	+	+	–
Geotrichum	–	–	–

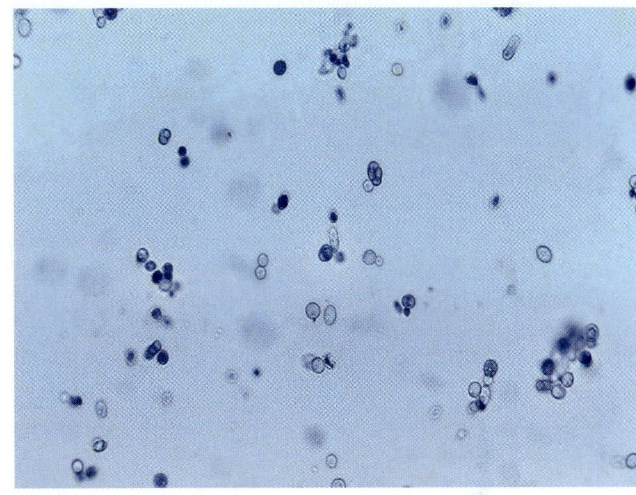

FIG. 28.7: Yeast cells of *Saccharomyces* (×400).

SECTION

6

Miscellaneous Mycoses

Section Outline

CHAPTER

29 Ocular Infections

INTRODUCTION

Though bacterial infections of different components of eye, fungal infections are also on rise. There are many predisposing factors of which most common is trauma. Both molds and yeasts may cause infections of eye.

MYCOTIC KERATITIS OR FUNGAL KERATITIS

A serious eye emergency, mycotic or fungal keratitis (FK) can infect the cornea and cause blindness if left untreated. Infectious agents of FK include yeasts and filamentous fungi. Both geographical location and occupational exposure play a role in the etiology and predisposing risk factors.

Different regions have different rates of FK; the lowest rates are in Europe, while the highest rates are in Asia and Africa. *Aspergillus* and *Fusarium* species are the most often found fungi that cause FK globally. The most frequently isolated yeast is *Candida* species.

The incidence of FK is on the rise because of:

- Increased use of topical antibiotics after minor trauma or abrasion
- Increased availability and use of topical steroids
- Increased prevalence of diabetes mellitus across the regions
- Improved culture and microbiology services in these countries, meaning that underdiagnosed cases are now being reported
- Widespread use of contact lenses

RISK FACTORS

- Agricultural laborers, who are often younger men, are more likely to suffer from FK due to the prevalence of trauma in this population. Comorbidities affecting both the eyes and the body, such as diabetes and ocular surface disease, are more common risk factors in the elderly.
- *Injury*: This is especially the case when injuries involving vegetative matter or injuries sustained during farming are involved. Direct inoculation with fungal conidia can occur after an injury with plant materials.
- The intensity of FK may be associated with diabetes. The ocular surface microenvironment can be changed by hyperglycemia, which includes changes in enzyme activity and commensal organisms. As a result, fungal adhesion, proliferation, and corneal penetration become simpler.
- Traditional eye medicines: These are not exactly sterile, but they contain plant material—usually herbs or dried leaves—and could be a way to infect the cornea with microbes, especially for fungal illnesses.
- Glucocorticoids, which are topical steroids, have been associated with immunological dysregulation and an increased risk of invasive fungal infection in individuals.
- Conditions that have already damaged the eye's surface: These include disorders of the inflammatory ocular surface, corneal exposure, dry eye, blepharitis, chronic epithelial defects, and other abnormalities of the ocular surface.
- Optical contact lenses: The likelihood of FK occurrence is conditional on the lens type, replacement frequency, and cleaning method. The composition of the solution for contact lenses is also important. People all across the globe who wear soft contact lenses and have used a certain kind of tainted contact lens solution have been sickened with *Fusarium* keratitis.
- Prior ocular procedures: Potential risk factors for developing *glaucoma* include cataract surgery, laser refractive surgery or corneal transplantation, intravitreal injections for retinal illness, and the

frequent use of corticosteroid periocular injections to treat diabetic macular edema.

CAUSATIVE AGENTS

The list of fungi responsible for FK is given in **Table 29.1**. Filamentous fungi are the most common pathogens which include *Aspergillus* and *Fusarium* species. The infections of dematiaceous fungi are also rising.

PATHOGENESIS

The fungi cannot pass through an intact corneal epithelium. Trauma allows fungi to enter the corneal stroma. Mycotoxins, fungal cellular components, and fungal enzymes like elastase aid in the deeper penetration of the fungus.

Coagulation necrosis and keratocyte loss are present. Collagenous fibers also develop edema. The membrane of Descemet may be breached by hyphae. In about 50% of cases of FK, hypopyon develops. Hypopyon is a collection of white blood cells (WBCs) in the anterior chamber in response to infections of cornea. It is usually sterile. When a hypopyon forms, neutrophil exudate is present.

CLINICAL FEATURES

Ocular pain, redness, lacrimation, discharge, diminished vision, gritty sensation, and photophobia are common symptoms that patients present with.

TABLE 29.1: Common agents of keratomycosis.

Category	*Agents*
Hyaline hyphomycetes	• *Aspergillus* species (*Aspergillus flavus* and *Aspergillus fumigatus*) • *Fusarium* species (*Fusarium solani* and *Fusarium oxysporum*) • *Acremonium* species • *Paecilomyces* species • *Purpureocillium lilacinum* • *Penicillium* species • *Scedosporium apiospermum*
Phaeoid hyphomycetes	• *Curvularia* species • *Bipolaris* species • *Alternaria* species • *Exserohilum* species • *Fonsecaea pedrosoi* • *Aureobasidium pullulans* • *Colletotrichum dematium*
Yeast-like fungi	*Candida* species (*Candida albicans, Candida tropicalis*, and *Candida krusei*)

Keratitis and ulcer are evident during an eye examination. Severe ulcerative lesions are usually accompanied by an anterior chamber reaction or hypopyon.

Torch-light examination reveals lid edema, blepharospasm, and matted eyelashes. The conjunctiva is congested. The most common feature of FK is a grayish-white corneal infiltrate with diffuse borders or irregular, feathered margins. The size, depth, and extent of corneal infiltrate can be judged by a slit lamp. When an ulcer forms, it has raised edges and firm slough. Elongated lines of fungal hyphae beyond the central part of the ulcer and feathery satellite stromal lesions are seen. Other features such as endothelial plaque, thinning, descemetocele, and perforation can also be seen if present. The satellite lesions that surround the central wound are referred to as "ring abscesses." An "immunological ring" that may form locally in the corneal stroma surrounding the infection may be seen in some cases.

In *Candida* keratitis and ulcer, the corneal infiltrate is yellowish white. *Candida* keratitis usually follows ocular surface diseases; compared to history of trauma in cases of ulcer due to filamentous fungi. Bacterial keratitis is comparable to *Candida albicans*-induced keratitis, except that the progression of corneal ulcer is gradual.

Dematiaceous FK is a persistent low-grade keratitis with little structural damage.

Stromal keratitis, which can be more localized, is distinguished by small ulcerations and a collar button structure.

Fusarium keratitis is distinguished by the absence of ring infiltrate and raised lesions. In *Aspergillus flavus* keratitis, the feathery border and ring infiltrates are apparent.

DIFFERENTIAL DIAGNOSIS

History taking is equally important to reach a diagnosis, similar to physical examination. Keratitis and ulcers caused by bacteria, *Acanthamoeba*, herpes simplex, and atypical mycobacteria have to be differentiated. Some are "sterile corneal ulcers." It is many a time difficult to differentiate FK from bacterial keratitis. In bacterial keratitis, a complaint of foreign body sensation with every blink, prominent necrotic areas, and purulence are noted. In case of *Acanthamoeba,* there is usually a history of contact lens wearing, and photosensitivity is disproportionate to the ulcer. In case of FK, there is a history of trauma, especially with vegetable matter; there are dense stromal infiltrate, early formation of hypopyon, and satellite lesions. In herpetic keratitis, there is photophobia, but pain or foreign-body sensation is NOT a complaint. A "sterile" ulcer is usually peripheral, <1 mm in size, with clear stroma and no inflammation.

LABORATORY DIAGNOSIS

The involvement of fungi can be suspected by using a confocal microscope. The fluorescein dye may be used to visualize the ulcer.

Specimen

Corneal scrapping is obtained by an experienced ophthalmologist by scraping the cornea with a no. 15 Bard–Parkar surgical blade from the base and margins of ulcers, using 4% xylocaine as a local anesthetic agent. A platinum spatula may be used to get the material.

Microscopy

Wet preparations with 10% potassium hydroxide (KOH) and calcofluor white are observed under low power and high power for the presence of fungal elements. A fluorescence microscope is required to observe slides stained with calcofluor white. A Gram-stained smear will demonstrate gram-positive fungal elements, yeasts with either pseudohyphae or hyphae, depending upon the etiological agent. Special stains as periodic acid-Schiff (PAS) and Grocott–Gömöri's methenamine silver (GMS) can be performed on biopsy.

Culture

Corneal scapings are inoculated on Sabouraud dextrose agar (SDA) and blood agar plates by making "C"- or "S"-shaped inoculation to differentiate growth over the inoculum from growth on other parts of the plate which may be due to contamination. Two slants of SDA without actidione are inoculated and incubated at 25 and 37°C.

Media are observed daily in the first week and thereafter twice a week for the presence of growth. We have to wait for at least 4 weeks before reporting it as sterile.

The isolate is identified by gross examination of colonies and microscopically by performing lactophenol cotton blue (LPCB) mounts. Slide cultures can be performed on cornmeal agar or potato dextrose agar to enhance sporulation. The description of fungi is given in individual chapters.

Newer Technique

Newer techniques include polymerase chain reaction (PCR) and matrix-assisted laser desorption ionization-time of flight mass spectrometry (MALDI-TOF MS) (on direct specimen for corneal ulcer). Noninvasive techniques such as in vivo confocal microscopy (IVCM) and anterior segment optical coherence tomography (AS-OCT) are also available. IVCM can reveal branching white lines in the infiltration area when the lesion is caused by filamentous fungi. Ophthalmic B-scan ultrasonography is useful in the follow-up of cases suspected to be progressing to endophthalmitis.

TREATMENT

Various agents used for treating FK are given in **Table 29.2**. A topical agent is useful for treatment, and oral fluconazole can be added for filamentous fungi. Extensive debridement is successful, particularly in case of infections caused by dematiaceous fungi. Therapeutic penetrating keratoplasty or lamellar keratoplasty is done for refractory cases.

ENDOPHTHALMITIS

Introduction

Inflammation of the vitreous or aqueous fluids and other intraocular tissues can cause blindness in rare cases of endophthalmitis. Fungal endophthalmitis occurs when fungus invades the eye, either internally by hematogenous spread or externally through puncture wounds and surgeries. The etiological agents are listed in **Table 29.3**.

Exogenous Endophthalmitis

The infectious microbes found in the outside world or on the surface of the eye are the culprits behind

TABLE 29.2: Treatment of mycotic keratitis.

Fungal type	*First choice*	*Second choice*
Filamentous fungi	• Natamycin 5% ointment • *Alternative*: Amphotericin B 0.5% drops + flucytosine • *Adjunctive*: Itraconazole 1% cream + 200–400 mg PO • *Supportive*: Silver sulfadiazine cream 1%	• Amphotericin B 0.5% drops + flucytosine • Silver sulfadiazine cream1%
Yeast-like fungi	Amphotericin B 0.15% drops + flucytosine (1% drops + 150 mg/kg PO)	• Fluconazole (0.5% drops + 200 mg PO) • Miconazole 1% drops

TABLE 29.3: Etiological agents of endophthalmitis.

Category	*Fungal agents*	*Common features*
Exogenous endophthalmitis	*Candida species:* • *Candida glabrata* • *Candida tropicalis* • *Candida parapsilosis* *Others:* • *Paecilomyces* species • *Fusarium* species • Acremonium species • *Curvularia lunata*	• Typically associated with trauma or surgery • Common in postoperative infections. Fungal elements are introduced directly into the eye
Endogenous endophthalmitis	*Candida albicans:* • *Aspergillus flavus* • *Aspergillus fumigatus* *Others:* • *Histoplasma capsulatum* • *Coccidioides* species • *Blastomyces dermatitidis* • *Cryptococcus neoformans* • *Sporothrix schenckii* • *Fusarium* species	• Results from systemic infection with dissemination to the eye • Common in immunocompromised individuals • Fungal elements spread through the hematogenous route

exogenous endophthalmitis. There are three distinct forms of exogenous fungal endophthalmitis: (1) Postoperative, (2) posttraumatic, and (3) FK-derived. Compared to endogenous infection, these occur more frequently. Despite how uncommon it is, postoperative endophthalmitis is most commonly associated with fungi, specifically species of *Aspergillus* and *Candida*. For posttraumatic endophthalmitis, bacteria are the most common culprits, whereas *Aspergillus* is the most common fungus. Concomitant spread of FK is the rarest cause of fungal endophthalmitis.

Possible causes of exogenous endophthalmitis include FK, penetrating trauma, and intraocular surgery. The pathophysiology of external fungal endophthalmitis typically originates in the aqueous humor.

Fungal causes of acute-onset postoperative endophthalmitis are uncommon.

Several factors can increase the likelihood of FK-induced endophthalmitis, including the use of contact lenses, damage caused by organic debris, and laser-assisted in situ keratomileusis (LASIK).

Endogenous Endophthalmitis

Of all cases of endophthalmitis, only 5–15% are caused by internal factors. A compromised blood-ocular barrier is the usual mechanism for its hematogenous dissemination. Fungemia occurs most commonly in immunocompromised individuals or those who utilize intravenous drugs for endogenous endophthalmitis. Fungi are the most typical culprits when it comes to endogenous endophthalmitis.

Established risk factors for endogenous fungal endophthalmitis include:

- Human immunodeficiency virus (HIV) and other immunosuppressive diseases
- Underlying malignancy
- Broad-spectrum antibiotic therapy
- Corticosteroid therapy and other immunosuppressive therapies
- Gastrointestinal (GI) trauma or surgery
- Intravenous hyperalimentation
- Indwelling intravenous catheters
- Intravenous drug abuse
- Neutropenia
- Diabetes mellitus
- Renal insufficiency
- Recent hospitalization
- Organ transplant
- Hemodialysis
- Pregnancy, abortion, and postpartum state
- Lung disease (specific to *Aspergillus*)

Clinical Features of Endogenous Endophthalmitis

Subacute decreased vision, ocular discomfort, photophobia, and a red, irritated eye are some of the clinical signs and symptoms of endogenous fungal endophthalmitis. Eyelid swelling, congestion in the conjunctiva and around the cornea, inflammation in the anterior chamber (with or without a hypopyon), redness absent, and haze or exudates from the vitreous will all be found during a physical examination. Nonspecific fundus findings include intraretinal hemorrhages, infarcts in the nerve fiber layer, Roth spots, and cotton-wool spots. The ability to see the fundus may be impaired due to inflammation within the eye. In most cases, the presence of vitreous haze and creamy white lesions at the level of the choroid and retina can be used to identify *Candida* chorioretinitis. Lesions in the early stages lie flat on the choroid and show little to no vitritis. They have the potential to invade the vitreous and retina if not treated, as they can cross the blood–retina barrier. There is a higher risk of tractional detachment and retinal traction when the lesions are quite elevated, have extensive vitritis, and eventually heal with scarring. The lesions are usually many and affect both sides of the body in about 65% of instances. Vitreous abscesses are another hallmark of *Candida* endophthalmitis. In cases of *Aspergillus* endophthalmitis, the posterior pole is affected by larger, more severe, and more hemorrhagic chorioretinal lesions that are yellow-white in color. In most cases, *Aspergillus* invades the choroidal and retinal arteries, leading to ischemic infarctions and full-thickness retinal necrosis.

Exogenous Endophthalmitis

Puffball lesions in the vitreous cavity are the outward signs of this condition. The symptoms of fungal endophthalmitis, which can occur after surgery or trauma, usually manifest a few weeks or months after exposure. Vision problems, inexplicable pain, swelling of the eyelids or cornea, inflammation of the anterior chamber, hypopyon, vitritis, or open purulence are some of the symptoms that patients report. There may be clumps instead of a diffuse appearance to the inflammation within the eye. FK is most commonly caused by mold infections, which can manifest as fuzzy or feathery-edged infiltrates or satellite lesions on the cornea.

DIAGNOSIS

Ultrasound B-scan

Ophthalmologists can use the nonspecific information it gives to guide their surgical planning, such as the extent to which the infection has spread, where the infection is concentrated, and whether or not there is retinal detachment or abscesses.

Microscopy and Culture

When patients exhibit symptoms that are compatible with fungal endophthalmitis but blood cultures come back negative, cultures of intraocular fluids can help confirm the diagnosis. One limitation of vitreous cultures is their low sensitivity. Fine-needle aspiration and diagnostic vitrectomy are two methods for obtaining vitreous samples; the latter is associated with a better diagnostic yield, particularly when done early. Although the yield for cultures is significantly lower for aqueous samples collected by fine-needle aspiration, it is still possible.

Any instance of endogenous endophthalmitis warrants a full systemic infection workup, including blood cultures. Endogenous fungal endophthalmitis cannot be ruled out only because blood cultures come out negative. Positive blood cultures are obtained in only 50–75% of patients with endogenous *Candida* endophthalmitis. An ophthalmologist should be consulted immediately for all patients who have been diagnosed with systemic fungemia in order to conduct a thorough evaluation of the eyes. If the results come back negative, one will need to retake the test 2 weeks later.

Polymerase Chain Reaction

The ability to detect culture negative cases makes PCR a preferred method to provide faster results with higher sensitivity and specificity. Anterior chamber paracentesis is a less invasive alternative to vitreous aspiration and biopsy for detecting fungal DNA in aqueous samples using PCR.

Beta-D-glucan

Measuring levels of intraocular fluid beta-D-glucan may be a significant finding.

FUNGAL INFECTIONS OF OCULAR ADNEXA—FUNGAL DACRYOCYSTITIS

Fungal dacryocystitis accounts for 5% of all acquired dacryocystitis cases. It is common in females.

Etiological agents

- *Acremonium*
- *Candida*

- *Paecilomyces*
- *Rhizopus*
- *Aspergillus*
- *Dermatophytes*

Clinical Features

Clinical features include pain, erythema, induration, heaviness, and tenderness at medial canthus. Eyelids may become edematous. There may be rupture of lacrimal sac. Canaliculitis presents with mucopurulent discharge and unilateral conjunctivitis. If there is swelling of the lacrimal sac, aspiration is performed to relieve discomfort. Oral treatment is necessary.

Eyelid infection: May be caused by *Sporothrix, Blastomyces dermatitidis,* and *Paracoccidioides brasiliensis.*

Eyelashes may be infected by *Candida, Malassezia,* and *Microsporum canis.*

CHAPTER

30 Otomycosis

INTRODUCTION

Otitis externa is an infection of the external ear canal, i.e., the external auditory canal (EAC). Most cases of otitis externa are due to bacteria. When fungi are the causative agents, the condition is known as otomycosis. Otomycosis, often known as a fungal ear infection, is a superficial fungal infection. It happens when some fungal species, such as molds (like *Aspergillus*) and yeasts (like *Candida*), multiply and invade the skin lining of the ear canal. Itching, ear discharge, feeling of ear canal obstruction, pain, and reduced hearing are common symptoms of this illness. Otomycosis can occur as an acute, subacute, or chronic condition.

ANATOMY OF THE EXTERNAL AUDITORY CANAL

- The external auditory canal (EAC) is also known as external acoustic meatus.
- It is a tubular structure (2–2.5 cm in length) extending from the auricle—the protruding part of the outer ear to the ear drum, i.e., the tympanic membrane.
- The inner lining comprises skin extending from the outer surface of the eardrum to the auricle.

Intact skin acts as a barrier, housing modified sweat glands producing cerumen (ear wax) with antimicrobial properties. It also discourages insects to enter.

MICROBIAL ECOLOGY OF THE HEALTHY EXTERNAL AUDITORY CANAL

Healthy EAC skin hosts various microbial species, including *Staphylococcus* species, *Corynebacterium* species, *Bacillus* species, *Streptococcus* species, and gram-negative bacilli (*Pseudomonas aeruginosa* and *Escherichia coli*). Some fungi, mainly *Aspergillus* and *Candida* species, can also be seen. Normally, these microbes live in a benign, saprophytic state. Impaired host defensive mechanisms, particularly nonspecific, may allow them to become pathogenic.

The etiological agents of otomycosis are listed in **Table 30.1**.

EPIDEMIOLOGY

- *Climatic influence*: Tropical and subtropical areas with lengthy summers and rainy seasons are otomycosis hotspots because these climate conditions are ideal for fungal development.
- *Host-related factors*: Several factors can contribute to otitis externa, including the EAC's anatomy, local ear canal trauma, hearing aids, immunocompromised status, previous antibacterial treatment resulting in secondary fungal infection, and autoinoculation in patients with untreated dermatomycosis.
- *Disruption of the EAC microbiota*: Chemical usage, such as soaps, shampoos, antiseptics, and excessive antibacterial ear drops, alters the EAC microbiota, promoting fungal overgrowth.
- *Clothing habits*: Wearing head coverings or traditional clothes, such as turbans or veils, is connected with an increased risk of otomycosis, particularly in certain locations.
- *Swimming and sauna*: Frequent swimming, sauna usage, and spa treatments elevate the risk of infection.
- *Underlying health conditions*: Diseases such as diabetes, immunosuppression, prolonged systemic antibiotic use, retroviral infections, malignancies, otologic procedures, and prematurity are predisposing factors for otomycosis.
- *Global prevalence*: South America, Central America, Africa, and Asia are all home to yeast and mold species that can cause otomycosis.
- *Seasonal variation*: Some seasonal variations are suggested.

TABLE 30.1: Etiological agents of otomycosis.

Agent type	*Common agents*	*Less common agents*	*Emerging concerns*
Molds	*Aspergillus niger* complex and *Aspergillus tubingensis*	*Aspergillus flavus* complex, *Aspergillus terreus, Aspergillus fumigatus, Aspergillus versicolor,* and *Aspergillus luchuensis*	*Aspergillus sydowii*—detected in immunocompromised cases
Yeasts	*Candida albicans*	*Candida parapsilosis, Candida lusitaniae, Candida guilliermondii, Candida auris, Candida tropicalis, Candida krusei,* and *Candida glabrata*	
Uncommon fungi	*Cryptococcus species, Rhodotorula species, Geotrichum candidum, and Trichophyton mentagrophytes*		
Other mold genera		*Penicillium, Scopulariopsis, Chrysosporium, Fusarium, Alternaria, Paecilomyces, Aureobasidium* species, *Acremonium* species, and certain *Mucorales* group species	*Saksenaea vasiformis* and *Scedosporium apiospermum*—rare cases

Gender and Age Distribution

There are conflicting findings about gender prevalence, with some research indicating a higher frequency in men. The age range of 25–45 years is most typically afflicted, while frequency increases with age.

Disrupting the equilibrium between bacterial and fungal growth, particularly if nonspecific and specific bodily defense mechanisms are disturbed, might transform these germs from saprophytes into pathogens.

CLINICAL FEATURES

Inflammatory Characteristics of External Auditory Canal Condition

Inflammatory Manifestations

- It affects the skin and subcutaneous tissues, with severe instances extending to the eardrum and auricle.
- It exhibits a mild-to-severe spectrum, manifesting as localized/diffuse, acute/chronic, and infectious/noninfectious etiologies.
- It is predominantly caused by bacteria (up to 90%), commonly by *P. aeruginosa* and *Staphylococcus aureus*. Fungi contribute the rest.
- Otomycosis typically begins asymptomatically but may lead to recurrent infections, occasionally extending to the middle ear.
- In severe instances, it may spread to surrounding tissues, and rarely, to deeper structures, more prevalent in immunocompromised individuals.
- *Varied pathogenic behavior*: *Aspergillus* rarely damages tissues; *Candida* initiates with exudation, progressing to granulomatous inflammation.
- It presents with symptoms such as itching, otorrhea, ear canal blockage sensation, pain, headache, tinnitus, EAC edema, redness, epithelial desquamation, and impaired hearing.

Noninflammatory Factors Influencing External Auditory Canal Condition

Contributing Causes

Contact/allergic dermatitis or systemic diseases (e.g., seborrheic dermatitis, psoriasis), potentially leading to secondary bacterial or fungal infections.

DIAGNOSIS

Clinical Assessment and Examination

Diagnosis primarily relies on patient history, clinical presentation, and otoscopic examination of the ear canal and eardrum.

Sample Collection Swabbing Technique

- Use sterile cotton or rayon-tipped swabs to collect samples.
- Gently swab the affected areas of the EAC.
- Ensure thorough contact with the site of infection without causing discomfort or injury to the patient.

- For deeper infections or discharge, reach the affected area to gather appropriate material.

Scraping Technique

Use a sterile curette or spatula to scrape the surface of the affected area. Perform scraping carefully to collect tissue debris, cerumen, or discharge from the external ear canal. Avoid excessive pressure to prevent causing injury or bleeding in the sampled region.

Microscopic Examination

Methodology: Wet mount microscopy involves native or potassium hydroxide (KOH)/lactophenol preparations for direct examination of patient samples.

Culture

- *Media selection*: Employ selective media tailored for specific microbes. For yeasts, use Sabouraud agar with dextrose/maltose and antibacterial agents; for molds, use media with a higher carbohydrate concentration and antibacterial agents but without actidione.
- *Culture conditions*: Optimal conditions for yeast are 48–72 hours at 37°C in an aerobic atmosphere and for molds 7–14 days at 26–28°C in an aerobic atmosphere. Some molds require specific temperatures for growth.
- *Serial examinations*: Slants are observed daily in the first week and thereafter twice a week.
- *Species differentiation*: Utilize biochemical assays, assimilation tests, or automated systems (e.g., VITEK®) for yeast species identification and antifungal susceptibility testing.

Advanced Techniques and Future Directions

- *Nonculture methods*: Ongoing research explores techniques such as matrix-assisted laser desorption ionization–time of flight mass spectrometry (MALDI-TOF-MS), molecular analyses, and machine learning to expedite diagnosis and improve accuracy.
- *Machine learning in microscopy*: Artificial intelligence (AI) models applied to microscopic images (otoendoscopy and histological) offer potential for automated diagnosis with high accuracy rates, especially in identifying specific fungal genera.

TREATMENT GUIDELINES

Treatment guidelines are given in **Table 30.2**.

TABLE 30.2: Treatment guidelines for otomycosis.

Treatment options	*Characteristics*
Clotrimazole (topical imidazole)	• Considered a first-line topical treatment for uncomplicated otomycosis in many international guidelines • May exhibit varying effectiveness against *Aspergillus*-related otomycosis
Nystatin	Used as a local treatment in some regions; however, its efficacy against *Aspergillus* species remains debatable
Miconazole, bifonazole, and isoconazole	Show varied effectiveness against different yeast and mold species, potentially useful against *Aspergillus* species according to some studies
Lanoconazole and luliconazole	Show potential effectiveness against *Aspergillus* species, but their use in otomycosis treatment needs further evaluation
Terbinafine and naftifine	Recommended in certain regions for otomycosis; however, constant laboratory monitoring is advised
Systemic antifungals	• Reserved for severe cases or when local therapies fail • Triazole antifungals (e.g., fluconazole and itraconazole) are suggested, especially in complicated cases with mastoiditis or meningitis due to their broader spectrum
Advantages of ointments	• Preferred over liquid formulations due to their longer residence on the skin's surface; they are considered safer for use in cases of perforated eardrums • Liquid formulations may be used by soaking cotton wool or gauze pads
Additional considerations	• Antiseptics, acidifying agents, and anti-infective agents with corticosteroids may not have significantly increased efficacy compared to antifungal drugs in otomycosis treatment • Extensive ear canal debridement is recommended

CHAPTER

31 Hyalohyphomycosis

INTRODUCTION

Hyalohyphomycosis is a term used to describe infections caused by a diverse group of fungi that produce *hyaline (nonpigmented) hyphae* in tissues. These infections are opportunistic in nature and are seen predominantly in immunocompromised individuals. The fungi involved in hyalohyphomycosis belong to several genera and species within the class *Hyphomycetes*, but they all share the characteristic of producing filamentous, septate hyphae without melanin or dark pigmentation.

CAUSATIVE AGENTS

Hyalohyphomycosis is caused by a variety of hyaline fungi, including:

- *Acremonium*
- *Fusarium*
- *Paecilomyces*
- *Penicillium*
- *Scopulariopsis*
- *Scedosporium apiospermum*
- *Aspergillus* (nonmelanized species)

MORPHOLOGY

- Infections are characterized by the presence of *hyaline, septate hyphae* in tissue.
- These fungi are distinguishable from dematiaceous fungi, which cause *pheohyphomycosis* and produce darkly pigmented hyphae.

EPIDEMIOLOGY

- Hyalohyphomycosis is globally distributed, with fungi found in soil, decaying vegetation, and water.
- Infections are usually opportunistic and occur in individuals with:
    - Neutropenia
    - Organ transplants
    - Prolonged corticosteroid use
    - Cancer or other immunosuppressive conditions

CLINICAL MANIFESTATIONS

- *Localized infections:* Keratitis, cutaneous or subcutaneous lesions, sinusitis, and onychomycosis
- *Invasive infections:* Disseminated disease involving lungs, brain, heart, or other organs, especially in severely immunosuppressed individuals
- *Nosocomial infections*: Infections associated with hospital environments, often related to contaminated medical devices such as catheters

DIAGNOSIS

- *Direct microscopy:* Visualization of hyaline, septate hyphae in tissue samples.
- *Culture:* Growth of the causative fungi on standard fungal media.
- *Histopathology:* Detection of hyphae in tissues using special stains such as periodic acid-Schiff (PAS) or Grocott–Gömöri's methenamine silver (GMS).

TREATMENT

- *Antifungal therapy:*
    - Specific antifungal agents depend on the fungal species involved. Common treatments include:
        - Voriconazole
        - Amphotericin B
        - Posaconazole
        - Itraconazole
    - Resistance is variable, particularly in *Fusarium* and *Scedosporium* species.
- *Surgical intervention:* In some cases, surgical debridement of infected tissue is necessary, especially in localized infections.

- *Immune restoration:* Optimizing the immune status of the patient is crucial for successful treatment.

The types of arrangements of conidia help to identify some important species. *Scedosporium, Lomentospora,* and *Pseudoallescheria boydii* have conidia arranged singly along the conidiophore. *Acremonium* species show conidia in clusters at the tip, while *Aspergillus, Penicillium, Paecilomyces,* and *Scopulariopsis* show conidia arranged in chains.

SCEDOSPORIUM SPECIES

There are two important species of *Scedosporium*: *Scedosporium prolificans* and *Scedosporium apiospermum*; the latter has the teleomorph *P. boydii.* Molecular phylogenetic investigations were applied in detail in 2005. They kept two primary "species": (1) *S. prolificans* and (2) *S. apiospermum*, which includes the teleomorph *P. boydii.*

The genus *Scedosporium* includes the following species: *Scedosporium angustum, Scedosporium aurantiacum, S. apiospermum, Scedosporium boydii, Scedosporium cereisporum, Scedosporium dehoogii, Scedosporium desertorum, Scedosporium ellipsoideum, Scedosporium fusoideum,* and *Scedosporium minutispora.*

Scedosporium angustum, S. apiospermum, S. boydii, S. ellipsoideum, and *S. fusoideum* are considered a species complex. *S. apiospermum, S. boydii,* and *S. dehoogii* show extensive genetic diversity that suggests the presence of cryptic species; that is, *S. prolificans* was considered only distantly related to *Scedosporium* and was reclassified as *"Lomentospora prolificans,"* and the genus *Lomentospora* was reinstated for this species.

Infections caused by S. apiospermum are:

- Sinusitis (fungal ball)
- Endophthalmitis
- Pneumonia
- Central nervous system (CNS) infections
- Cutaneous infections
- Bones, joint infections
- Mycetoma
- Otitis externa
- Mycotic keratitis
- Disseminated disease is more common in immunocompromised patients with involvement of the lungs, brain, skin, and heart.
- In patients with cystic fibrosis (CF), these fungi may get colonized subsequently leading to invasive disease.

Histopathology

The hyphae of *Scedosporium* species look similar to those of other hyaline molds, such as *Aspergillus, Fusarium,* and *Paecilomyces* species, and are thus difficult to distinguish. Hyphae may branch at acute angles, lack pigmentation, and be septate. Some experts believe that *Scedosporium* and *L. prolificans* are strongly indicated by their unevenness and the fact that their branches span two parallel hyphae to form an H-shaped pattern. It should be mentioned that *L. prolificans* often has melanized hyphae. Slices stained with GMS reveal lemon-shaped conidia borne at the hyphae's either terminal end or lateral side. Conidia with a purple hue or those that are located within blood vessels are also visible inside tissues. Thrombosis occurs frequently in blood vessel walls.

Inflammation is characterized by granulomas, hyphae inside the vasculature, and the presence of multinucleate giant cells. A gray-black color and cycloheximide susceptibility are two characteristics that set *L. prolificans* apart from other *Scedosporium* species.

Lomentospora prolificans

- *Colony*: Downy to cottony texture, reverse-dark brown or gray, almost black.
- Conidiogenous cells are flask-shaped with basal swelling, solitary or branched conidiophores, conidia—globose to subglobose, and thick-walled 3 × 5 µm as shown in **Figure 31.1**.

Scedosporium apiospermum

- It does not grow at 40°C
- *Colony:* White gray, becoming darker gray or brown, reverse is dark brown or gray, almost black
- *Conidiogenous cells*: Cylindrical solitary or branched conidiophores, conidia—globose to subglobose, and thick-walled 5–7 × 4–6 µm **(Figs. 31.2 and 31.3)**.

Enzyme activity, carbohydrate consumption patterns, and growth at 40 and 45°C are some of the phenotypic identification methods. While tests can help with species identification, they are unable to differentiate between *S. apiospermum* complex species. For quick and affordable identification of *Scedosporium* species or *L. prolificans*, matrix-assisted laser desorption ionization-time of flight mass spectrometry (MALDI-TOF MS) is used.

Direct Detection in Clinical Specimens by Molecular Methods

Methods such as species-specific multiplex polymerase chain reaction (PCR) using real-time PCR or oligonucleotide arrays are examples of this type of method, similar to broad-range PCR and DNA sequencing. Clinical specimens are tested and identified for the presence of *Scedosporium* and *Lomentospora* species.

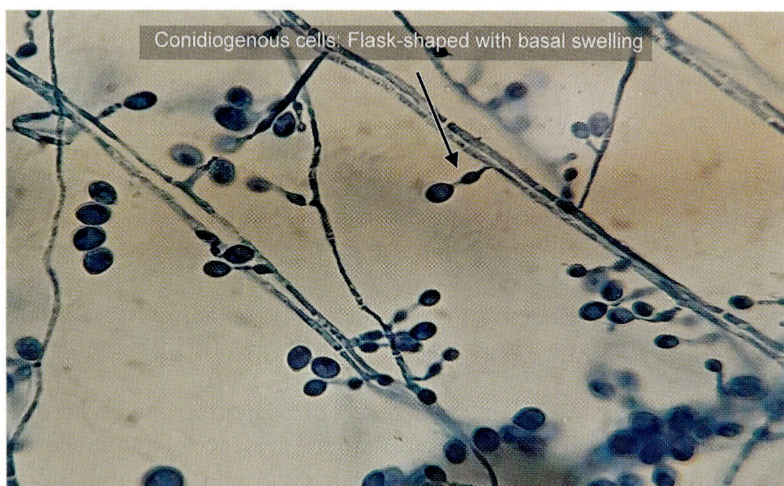

FIG. 31.1: LPCB mount of *Lomentospora* under oil immersion (1,000×).
(LPCB: lactophenol cotton blue)

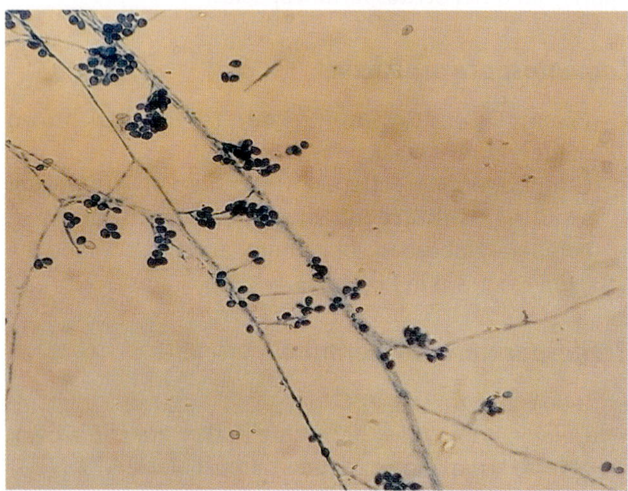

FIG. 31.2: LPCB mount of *Lomentospora* (400×).
(LPCB: lactophenol cotton blue)

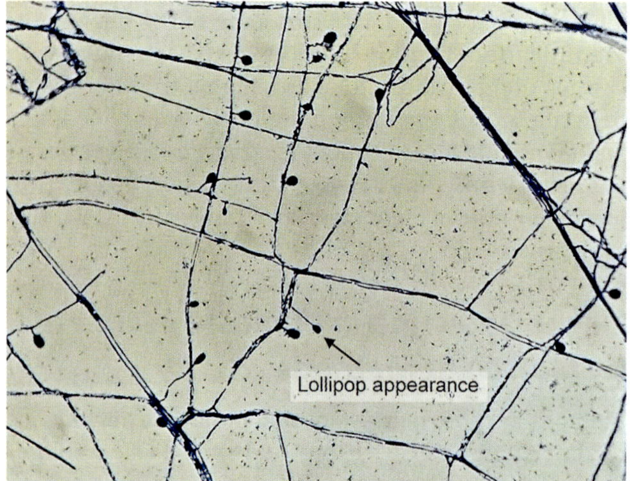

FIG. 31.3: LPCB mount *Scedosporium apiospermum* (400×).
(LPCB: lactophenol cotton blue)

FUSARIUM

The most common species of *Fusarium* that infect humans are *Fusarium solani, Fusarium oxysporum, Fusarium verticillioides* (*Fusarium moniliforme*), and *Fusarium chlamydosporum*. Species complexes have replaced many previously recognized species; one such example is the *F. solani* species complex (FSSC). There are some associations between specific disease and fungal species. For instance, keratitis in sugarcane workers is caused by *F. sacchari*, but pneumonia is caused by *F. verticillioides*. Several species of *Fusarium* are known to cause illness in humans, animals, and plants. Mycotoxicosis and invasive sickness are two human diseases that can be caused by *Fusarium* species. When it comes to individuals with hematologic malignancies or stem cell transplants, invasive mold mycosis caused by *Fusarium* species is second only to *Aspergillus* species. The majority of the cases of *Fusarium* mycosis occur in patients with a neutropenic condition.

Clinical Features

Cutaneous Infections

Erythema and subcutaneous nodules surround the skin lesions. It is one of the pathogens responsible for dermatomycosis and onychomycosis. *Fusarium* species induce macerated interdigital infection, which is particularly common in tropical areas and can be mistaken for dermatophytosis. It can also induce fasciitis.

Skin Lesions from Hematogenous Dissemination

Patients being treated for hematologic malignancies who get a positive blood culture for *Fusarium* species have painful skin sores. The skin rash contains huge red or gray annular lesions (1–2 cm diameter), which are extremely characteristic "target" lesions. The extremities and trunk are the most commonly afflicted areas. Central ulceration develops in the lesions.

Superinfection of Burns and Diabetic Ulcers

Species of *Fusarium* can infect immunocompromised hosts, including those with diabetic ulcers or severe burns. It has the potential to invade deeper tissues and spread to healthy skin.

Disseminated Fusarium Mycosis

Inhalation of conidia, ingestion, cutaneous damage, or a chronic nail infection are all potential entry points for the illness. One can observe the following kinds of presentations:

- Unresponsive fever to antibiotics, particularly in leukemia patients or those undergoing stem cell transplantation.
- Nasal polyposis
- A paronychia may develop around infected toenails, and cellulitis may manifest at skin breakdown sites or surrounding skin lesions.
- Symptoms similar to invasive pulmonary aspergillosis, including pleuritic chest discomfort, coughing up blood, and hemoptysis.
- Infection spreading outside the lungs to the brain and spinal cord.
- Disseminated *Fusarium* mycosis differs from invasive aspergillosis in that *Fusarium* causes skin lesions and yield positive blood cultures. Most commonly, *F. solani, F. oxysporum*, and *F. verticillioides* are implicated.

Keratitis

Injury with plant debris is the mode of infection. Fungal keratitis is becoming more common as soft contact lenses are more widely used. Either preexisting ocular problems or inadequate care and disinfection are to be blamed. The rapid initiation of intensive treatment is necessary in cases with fungal keratitis, which constitutes a medical emergency. In just a few short weeks, an infection with *F. solani* can cause complete blindness in the affected eye.

Endophthalmitis

It may also be caused by *Fusarium.*

Peritonitis

Patients undergoing continuous ambulatory peritoneal dialysis (CAPD) for chronic renal failure run the risk of contracting a *Fusarium* infection.

Toxicosis

Fumonisins, trichothecenes, and zearalenones are all compounds that might cause a variety of symptoms (these are covered in Chapter—Mycotoxicosis).

Sabouraud dextrose agar (SDA) plate without chlorhexidine is seeded with corneal specimens that have "C-"-shaped streaks on it to differentiate between the infectious strain and accidental contamination. Some forms of *Fusarium* are fuzzy or cottony and grow rapidly. Brown, pink, purple, white, and yellow are some of the surface colors. The reverse side could be a shade of blue, brown, red, or violet.

The presence and shape of microconidia, the number and location of chlamydospores, the number and shape of septations inside macroconidia, the shape of their foot cells, and the presence of sporodochia and sclerotia are all morphologic characteristics as shown in **Figures 31.4 to 31.6**. The presence of multicellular, spindle-shaped macroconidia is an important feature of *Fusarium* species.

Fusarium solani

Colony morphology: Quickly adapting to new environments, it has a cottony white-cream obverse and a cream reverse.

Microscopic Morphology

Macroconidia: The phialides support a profusion of macroconidia with three to five septa that are thick-walled and have a sickle shape. Sporodochium is formed when macroconidia cluster together.

Microconidia: Microconidia that range in size from one to three cells, with an oval to kidney form, and are produced on long phialides (*F. oxysporum* has short phialides). It is possible that chlamydospores are plentiful and present.

Fusarium oxysporum

The aerial mycelia have a purple tint, the surface is cottony, and the underside might be anything from colorless to dark purple; the growth rate is fast.

When compared to *F. solani*, phialides are shorter. Macroconidia have thin walls and foot-shaped basal cell.

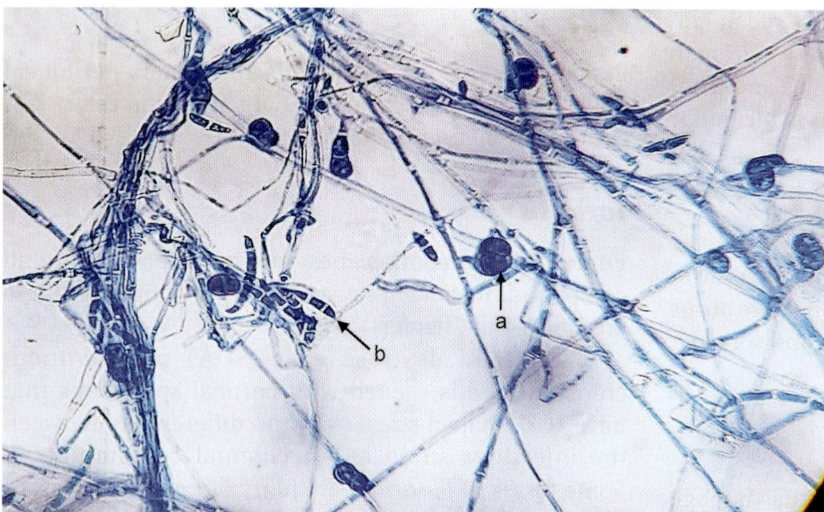

FIG. 31.4: LPCB mount showing (a) chlamydoconidium; and (b) macroconidium

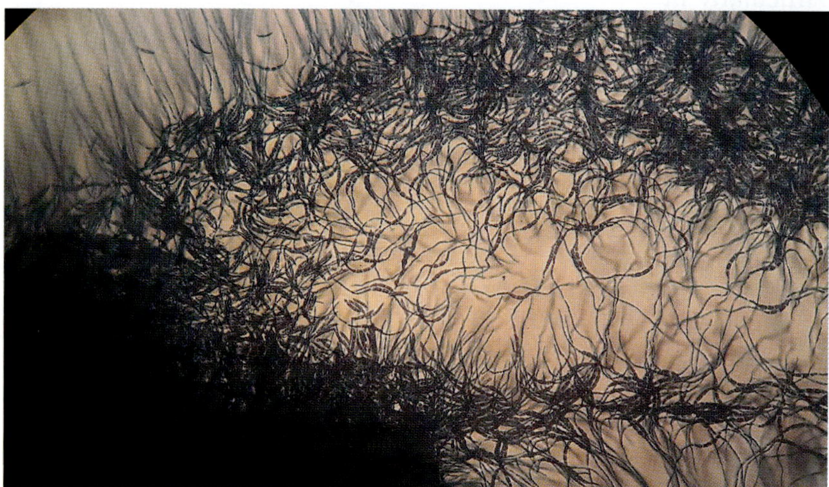

FIG. 31.5: Sporodochium shown by some *Fusarium* species.

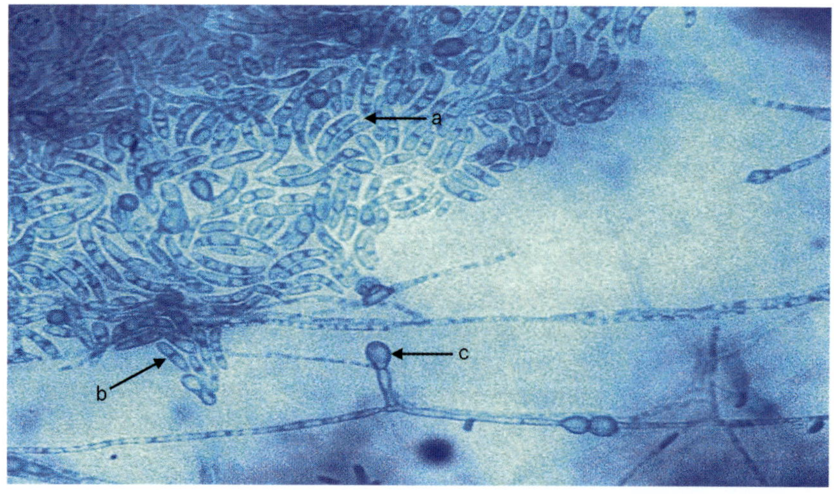

FIG. 31.6: LPCB mount of *Fusarium oxysporum* showing (a) macroconidia, (b) microconidia, and (c) chlamydoconidia (400×).

(LPCB: lactophenol cotton blue)

The colony has tan or orange color. There is presence of paired chlamydoconidia.

Slender phialides that produce clusters of ovoid unicellular conidia are the finding in case of *Acremonium*. Acremonium is to be differentiated from *Colletotrichum* and *Cylindrocarpon*. In *Colletotrichum*, the macroconidia have the form of beans. Also, septae are present. *Cylindrocarpon* has oblong conidia and chlamydoconidia without foot cell.

Treatment

The success in maximum patients is seen with liposomal Amphotericin B, and voriconazole with terbinafine therapy is given in cases of disseminated infections.

PAECILOMYCES

A hyaline hyphomycete, *Paecilomyces* present worldwide. It may ruin crops, food, and paper, and it can be retrieved from the ground and the air. The fungus is clinically relevant because of its potential resistance to sterilization methods, frequent contamination of medicinal lotions and creams, and colonization of clinical items such as catheters and plastic implants.

However, *Paecilomyces* species can infect immunocompromised individuals and are seen to infect hosts with healthy immune systems. *Paecilomyces lilacinus* and *Paecilomyces variotii* are the two most pathogenic species. *P. lilacinus* is renamed as *Purpureocillium lilacinum.*

Disease

Fungi often enter the body by airborne particles, indwelling catheters, or through the skin. In rare cases, *P. lilacinus*-contaminated fluids have led to infections of the skin or ocular tissues.

Keratitis

The two most common clinical entities are endophthalmitis and keratitis. Infections involving intraocular lenses, nonsurgical injuries involving foreign bodies, ophthalmic surgery, the use of contact lenses, and the use of topical or systemic corticosteroids act as the most common risk factors. There were a few cases where no known risk factors were identified.

Cutaneous and Subcutaneous Infections

Skin eruptions such as erythematous macules, papules, vesicles, or nodules with a necrotic core are among the many possible clinical manifestations of these illnesses. Additional instances of infections affecting soft tissues, such as cellulitis, have also been documented.

Other Infections

Other infections include onychomycosis, vaginitis, pleural effusion, sinusitis, osteomyelitis, disseminated infection, and fungemia. Indwelling central venous catheters act as a predisposing factor for fungemia.

Laboratory Diagnosis

It is important to distinguish the fungus from the species of *Penicillium*. Phialides in *Paecilomyces* are clustered, flask-shaped, tapering at the end, and typically divergent. The conidiophore's axis is the point at which phialides bend. Conidia are seen in chains **(Figs. 31.7 to 31.9)**.

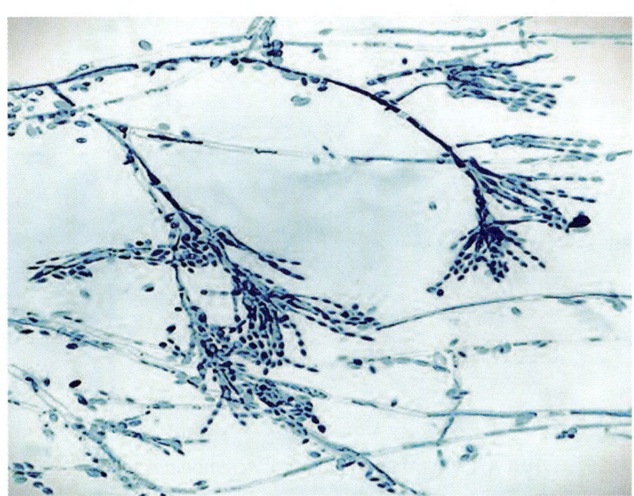

FIG. 31.7: LPCB mount of *Paecilomyces* (400×).
(LPCB: lactophenol cotton blue)

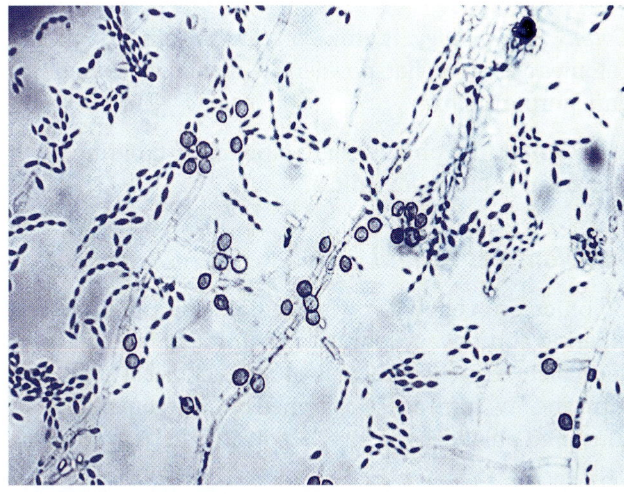

FIG. 31.8: *Paecilomyces* species showing chains of conidia (400×).

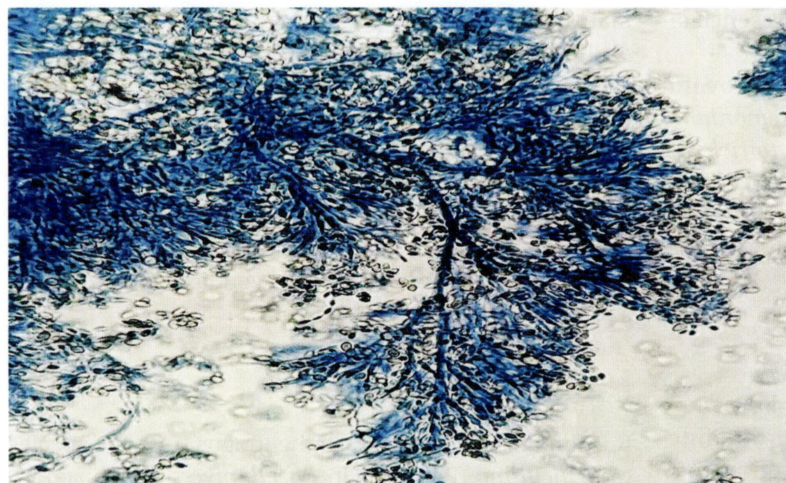

FIG. 31.9: LPCB mount of *Paecilomyces* (Medusa head appearance) (400×).
(LPCB: lactophenol cotton blue)

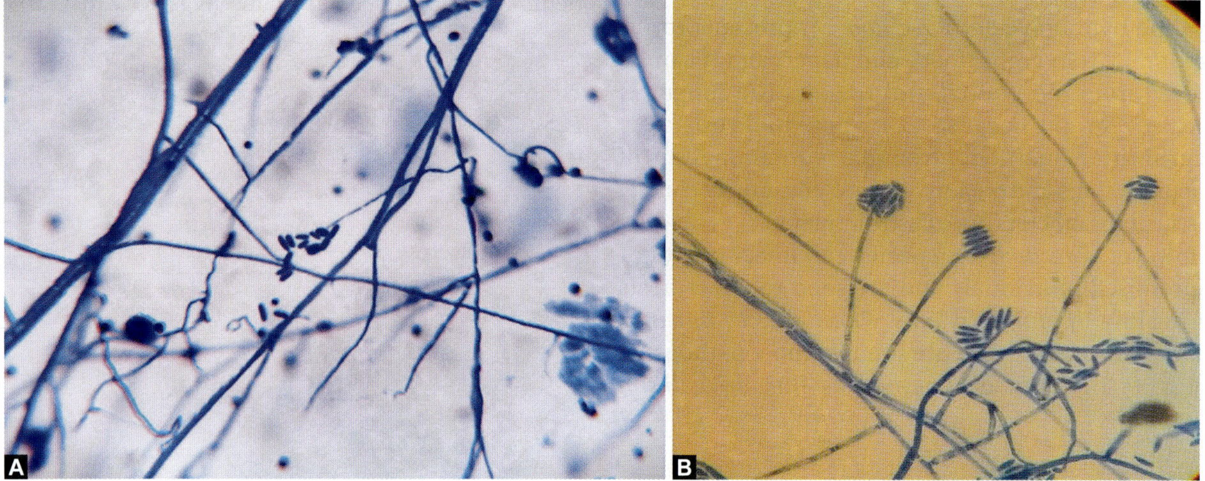

FIGS. 31.10A AND B: (A) LPCB mount of *Acremonium* species (400×); (B) LPCB mount of *Acremonium* (400×).
(LPCB: lactophenol cotton blue)

Paecilomyces lilacinum

Colony morphology: It grows on SDA within 3 days. The colonies are white, flat, powdery, with mauve (sometimes dark purple) color.

Microscopy: The phialides are elongated, tapering, with elongated or ellipsoid conidia.

Paecilomyces variotii

Colonies are yellow-brown in color. The phialides are tapering abruptly, cylindrical or ellipsoidal, and occur in verticillate branches. There is a long cylindrical neck. "M" form and "W" form are seen formed by divergent phialides. Clustered phialides can give "Medusa head" appearance.

ACREMONIUM SPECIES

This saprophytic fungus is found in rotting plants, food, and soil. Colonies begin flat and gradually become fluffy, velvety, glabrous, yellowish, or pinkish. Conidiophores are not present. Conidiogenous cells are upright and taper toward the tip. Conidia are one-celled that are cylindrical to-globose in shape and appear as *balls* at the tip of conidiogenous cells **(Figs. 31.10A and B)**. The fungus was originally known as *Cephalosporium,* then *Acremonium kiliense*, and finally *Sarocladium kiliense.* Mycetoma, keratitis, onychomycosis, endophthalmitis, arthritis, osteomyelitis, endocarditis, pneumonia, and subcutaneous infection are all caused by this fungus.

SCOPULARIOPSIS

These are found in dirt, decaying plants, and animal waste. *Scopulariopsis brevicaulis* and *Scopulariopsis brumpti* are the most prevalent species that cause human infection. In leukemic individuals, *S. brevicaulis* produces onychomycosis, cutaneous infection, and pneumonia. The colonies are white and powdery and have a brownish or cream-colored back. The conidiophore is shorter, and the conidia in chains are huge (49 µm), thick-walled, and *rough.* In acquired immunodeficiency syndrome (AIDS) patients, *S. brumpti* has been linked to hypersensitivity pneumonitis, onychomycoses, and pulmonary infection. It features branching conidiophores and *smooth*-walled conidia **(Figs. 31.11A and B)**.

CHRYSOSPORIUM

Chrysosporium is a genus of saprophytic, filamentous fungi found primarily in soil, animal remains, and keratinized materials such as hair, feathers, and nails. These fungi are hyaline molds, meaning they lack pigmentation in their hyphae. While generally regarded as nonpathogenic, some species are opportunistic pathogens.

Medical Importance

Although most *Chrysosporium* species are saprobes, a few have been associated with opportunistic infections in humans and animals, particularly in immunocompromised individuals. These include:

Human infections (rare):

- Cutaneous or subcutaneous lesions
- Pulmonary infections
- Disseminated infections, especially in immunosuppressed individuals
- Often confused with *Blastomyces* or other dimorphic fungi due to overlapping features

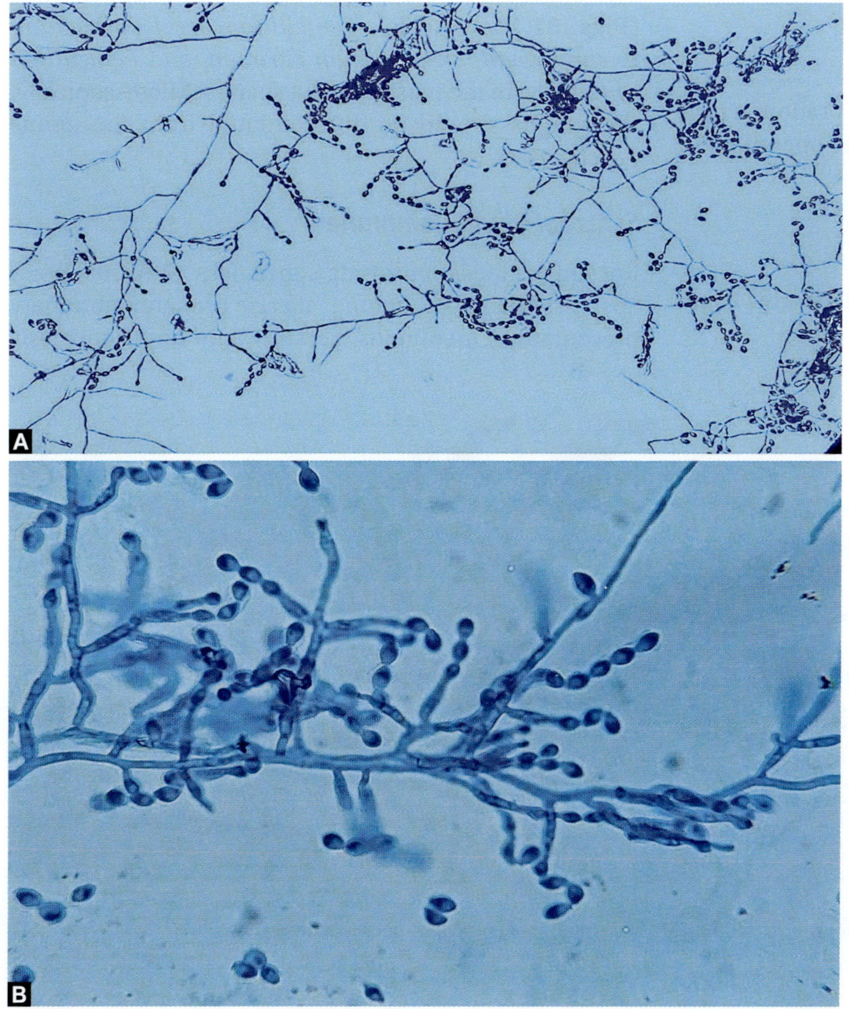

FIGS. 31.11A AND B: (A) LPCB mount of *Scopulariopsis* species (400×). (B) LPCB mount of *Scopulariopsis* under oil immersion (1,000×).
(LPCB: lactophenol cotton blue)

Differentiation from Related Fungi

- *Chrysosporium* may resemble *dimorphic fungi* such as *Blastomyces dermatitidis* and *Histoplasma capsulatum* in culture, but it lacks the thermally dimorphic characteristics of these pathogenic fungi.
- *Chrysosporium* does not grow at human body temperature (37°C) in most cases, unlike its pathogenic relatives.

Treatment

- Treatment is rarely required for saprophytic *Chrysosporium* contamination.
- *For rare pathogenic cases*:
    - *Topical or systemic antifungals* such as itraconazole or amphotericin B may be used.
    - Immune reconstitution in immunocompromised patients is essential for better outcomes.

Key Species

- *Chrysosporium keratinophilum*
- *Chrysosporium tropicum*
- *Chrysosporium queenslandicum*

These species are keratinophilic and predominantly environmental but may occasionally cause opportunistic infections.

Beauveria species

Beauveria bassiana is a pathogen on silkworm. It has been isolated from lungs.

Trichoderma Species

These fungi are soil-borne, also found in wood. The fungus is isolated from skin, lungs, and oral mucosa. Infections are mainly seen in immunocompromised cases.

The colonies are white, turning green. Reverse is pale yellow. The tips of conidiophores are phialides at wide angles. Conidia are present in clumps at the tips of phialides.

Penicillium Species

It is one of the most common laboratory contaminants. *Penicillium chrysogenum (Penicillium notatum)* and *Penicillium griseofulvin* are the antibiotic-producing species. Allergic illness, keratitis, otomycosis, onychomycoses, and deep infections such as endophthalmitis, endocarditis, peritonitis, pericarditis, esophagitis, and mycotoxicosis can all be caused by the *Penicillium* species. The colonies are powdery, blue-green, with white, red, and brown reverse growth. Conidiophores can be unbranched or branched, with secondary branches termed metulae bearing round, smooth, or rough conidia. The entire structure has a "paint brush" appearance **(Figs. 31.12A and B)**. *Penicillium brevicompactum, P. chrysogenum, Penicillium citrinum,* and *Penicillium commune* are the most frequent species. Microscopically, the fungus should be differentiated from the genus *Paecilomyces.*

Schizophyllum Commune

Rot fungus feeds on rotting substances. Sinusitis, brain abscess, fungal ball in lung, allergic bronchopulmonary presentation, meningitis, keratitis, and onychomycosis

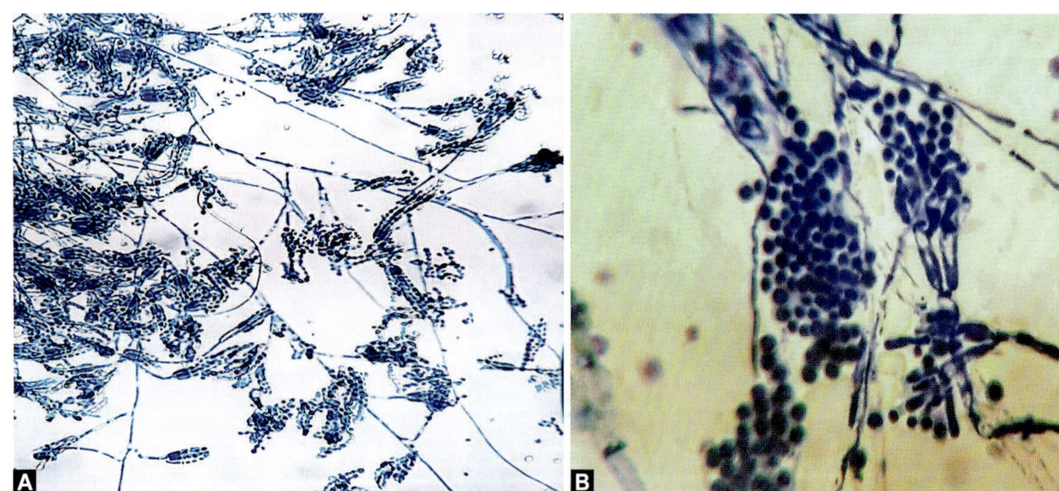

FIGS. 31.12A AND B: (A) LPCB mount of *Penicillium* species (400×). (B) LPCB mount of *Penicillium* species under 1,000×.
(LPCB: lactophenol cotton blue)

are all caused by this fungus. It belongs to the phylum Basidiomycota and has both binucleate (dikaryotic) and monokaryotic stages. The binucleate stage has hyphae with *"clamp connections"* and *spicules.* The clamp connection is hook-like outgrowth from hyphae which forms a bridge between two parts. There is basidiocarp (mushroom) production. Fruiting bodies are uncommon in monokaryotic stages with septate hyphae. The organism resembles a loose Chinese fan or undulating waves of tightly packed corals. What we call "gillies" or "split gills" might be any shade of pale white or creamy yellow. Its thin, thick, spongy crown has a diameter of around 1–4 cm. The "gills" on the underside of the cap of a split-gill mushroom are named after their unusual longitudinally divided structure. The colonies on 2% malt extract agar are spreading, fuzzy, and a pale shade of grayish-brown to white. They are also producing fruiting bodies that can be seen under a microscope quite quickly. Some isolates may not produce fruiting bodies for as long as 12 weeks. Sessile fruit bodies resemble kidneys and have several lobes, as well as split gills on the underside. "Clamp connections" characterize the wide, hyaline hyphae. The four basidiospores are carried by the basidia on the upright sterigmata.

Findings of cycloheximide sensitivity and a bleach-like odor are noteworthy because the monokaryotic stage does not have fruiting structures.

Hormographiella Species

It is rarely involved in human disease, although cases of endocarditis, endophthalmitis, and lung infection in neutropenic patients have been reported. On microscopic examination, other structures are absent and only arthroconidia are seen. It has a prominent conidiophore that is broader than the conidiogenous hypha.

CHAPTER

32

Adiaspiromycosis and Emergomycosis

INTRODUCTION

The fungal disease that causes granulomatous pulmonary disease in animals and occasionally in humans is known as *adiaspiromycosis.* It is caused by *Emmonsia* species and has peculiar forms known as "adiaspores" in tissues. Emergomycosis is a systemic fungal infection that manifests as a cutaneous and widespread illness in immunocompromised persons caused by dimorphic fungi from the genus *Emergomyces.* Following a taxonomic review, several of the most significant species of the genus *Emmonsia* are now classified among the fungi that cause emergomycosis.

ADIASPIROMYCOSIS

The two clinically significant species causing human infections are (1) *Emmonsia crescens* and (2) *Emmonsia parva.*

Rats and other rodents are common animals infected though more than 96 animal species have been reported to harbor *E. crescens*. Human adiaspiromycosis was initially reported from the Americas, Israel, and Europe. Those who work with soil, in plant nurseries, or in the construction, demolition, or restoration of historic buildings are more likely to be exposed to the fungus. It is believed that inhalation of soil-borne conidia is the primary route of transmission.

HISTORY

The first report (1942) came from a rodent suffering from a pulmonary disease. Chester et al. demonstrated spherule-like structures with asexual spores in the lungs of the infected rodent and labeled the fungus as *Haplosporangium parvum,* thinking it as an agent of mucormycosis. *H. parvum* was given the new genus name *Emmonsia* by Ciferri and Montemartini as a tribute to the eminent mycologist Chester Wilson Emmons. Human infection was first documented from France by Doby-Dubois in the year 1964.

The name of the disease *adiaspiromycosis* (a-not or without + dia-through + speirein-to scatter or disperse) was suggested by Emmons and Jellison for a lung infection in which no dissemination or multiplication of inhaled spores occurred. The term *adiaconidium (adiaspore)* is derived from the typical conidia of a fungus with a unique property of progressive enlargement of its size without multiplication.

MYCOLOGY

Two species, *E. parva* and *E. crescens,* cause the disease. The adiospores (adiaconidia) produced by *E. crescens* are large (50–700 μm), while those of *E. parva* are small (20–70 μm). The wall of adiaconidia of *E. crescens* is quite thick (20–70 μm) as compared to that of *E. parva. E. crescens* is multinucleate. The species *E. crescens* shows adiaconidia when grown at 37°C, while *E. parva* shows a mycelial form at 37°C.The growth of *E. crescens* is inhibited by the addition of actidione (cycloheximide). The species of the genus *Emmonsia* are considered dimorphic as they can be converted from a mycelial form to adiaconidia. The differences between the two imported species are given in **Table 32.1**.

TAXONOMY

The causative agents of adiaspiromycosis belong to the family Moniliiaceae, class *Hypomycetes* in phylum deuteromycetes.

EPIDEMIOLOGY

Rodents may serve as one of the zoonotic reservoirs of the fungus; however, the disease is rare in humans. Infection

TABLE 32.1: Differences between two *Emmonsia crescens* and *Emmonsia parva*.

Characteristics	*Emmonsia crescens*	*Emmonsia parva*
Adiaconidia (adiaspores)	Produced	Produced
Size of adiaconidia	50–500 µm (maximum 700 µm)	10–25 µm (maximum 40 µm)
Growth at 37°C	Adiaconidia	Mycelial
Growth at 40°C	Inhibited	Adiaconidia
Cycloheximide	Reduced growth	No inhibition

in humans occur by inhalation of conidia of the fungus present in dust. The asexual conidia after entering lungs get converted to adiaconidia which may increase in size and damage lung tissue. Dissemination may occur rarely in immunocompromised hosts. The majority of human infections are caused by *E. crescens.* The disease is so uncommon that only 70 cases are reported all over the world, including India. The species of *E. parva* is restricted to the southwestern USA, Eastern Europe, Kenya and Australia, while *E. crescens* is seen worldwide with few exceptions as Africa and Australia. An outbreak of conjunctivitis is reported from Brazil.

PATHOGENESIS

Conidia enter during inhalation and expand in size without replication in alveoli. The response looks like a granuloma without necrosis or caseation which is made up of epithelial cells, macrophages, lymphocytes, plasma cells, a few neutrophils, and fibrous tissue. The Splendore-Hoeppli phenomenon exists. Conidia that have collapsed seem crescent and are most likely nonviable. The granuloma in the alveoli may get calcified.

CLINICAL FEATURES

The majority of instances of adiaspiromycosis is asymptomatic, and they are restricted to the lungs. The fungal elements may cause mechanical damage. Chest radiographs can reveal pulmonary infection or can be discovered incidentally in surgical lung specimens or autopsy material. The severity is determined by host variables as well as the amount of conidia in the infected material.

Solitary Adiaspiromycosis

This form is a self-limiting pulmonary infection, mostly asymptomatic, diagnosed by chance during histopathological findings.

Localized Disease

Infection is limited to the original site of infection and a solitary pulmonary nodule.

Disseminated Disease

This is a diffuse granulomatous disease which may cause compression of airways. The clinical features are fever, cough, dyspnea, fatigue, and night sweats. The other organs involved may include skin, peritoneum, and bones (osteomyelitis). Only severe cases may present with respiratory failure.

Radiodiagnosis

The X-ray findings of nodules may be easily confused with tuberculosis. There may be bilateral reticulonodular infiltrations.

Differential Diagnosis

It is important to differentiate this disease from coccidioidomycosis and rhinosporidiosis based on the presence of spherules. *C. immitis* spherules are smaller in size (30–60 µm) with trilaminar walls that are 2 µm thick and contain endospores in size from 2 to 5 µm. Rhinosporidium has sporangia with a diameter of 200–300 µm and contains thousands of endospores inside. Adiaconidia do not have endospores, hence appear empty.

LABORATORY DIAGNOSIS

The specimens collected are fine-needle aspiration and biopsy tissue. The sputum and bronchoalveolar lavage (BAL) examinations usually yield poor results even in severe cases. The stains used for histopathological examination are hematoxylin and eosin (H&E), periodic acid-Schiff (PAS), Grocott-Gömöri's methenamine silver (GMS), and Gridley fungal stains.

Histopathological observations include the presence of thick-walled adiaconidia **(Fig. 32.1)** with a trilaminar wall that are round to oval in shape and 50–500 µm in size. The GMS and PAS stains indicate a trilaminar wall, but the H&E stain reveals two layers: (1) An exterior eosinophilic layer and (2) an interior hyaline layer.

Emmonsia crescens has adiaconidia that are 5–10 times bigger than *E. parva.* Histopathologic sections may reveal some types of rings that are empty and contain eosinophilic granules but do not contain endospores. All three processes—fixation, embedment, and sectioning—are likely to be blamed for the missing structures of the ring. Actually, at temperatures below 37°C, the multinucleate, dormant adiaspores of *E. crescens* can germinate and cause hyphal development **(Fig. 32.2)**.

Epithelioid and giant cell granulomas surround each adiaspore within its thick and fibrous capsule. The adiaconidia appear as empty bodies, but small eosinophilic globules may be seen attached to the inner surface of the wall.

Fungal Culture

Sabouraud dextrose agar (SDA) slants without cycloheximide are used for culture. The other medium used is brain heart infusion (BHI) blood agar. The colonies are glabrous or velvety with a pale brown center, and the reverse is cream to pale brown.

Colony Morphology

There are two distinct colony morphologies that can be seen: (1) One is characterized by a rough, powdery growth with pale orange to gray-orange aerial mycelium covering a reddish-ray surface with an irregular margin and a reddish-brown reverse and (2) the other is characterized by a yellowish-white to orange-white colony with a dense woolly center and a broad, smooth margin.

In its most basic form, the mold can be described as having identical hyaline, septate hyphae, each with a terminal conidium (aleurioconidium) **(Fig. 32.2)** and short conidiophores. A single conidium can develop on any of one to three spine-like pegs that protrude from the inflated apex of the conidiophore. Conidia can be subglobose, ovoid, or pyriform, and they range in size from 2.5 to 3.5 µm. The wall's surface is either perfectly smooth or slightly roughened. At 37°C, *E. crescens* produces adiaspores, which can reach a size of 70 µm in diameter (though they may reach a diameter of 700 µm in vivo) **(Fig. 32.1)**.

Sporulation of the fungus is increased on potato dextrose agar (PDA). For differentiation, growth pattern is observed when grown at 40°C. The conidia and hyphae of *E. parva* undergo degeneration, but uninucleate adiaconidia are produced that increase in size. The

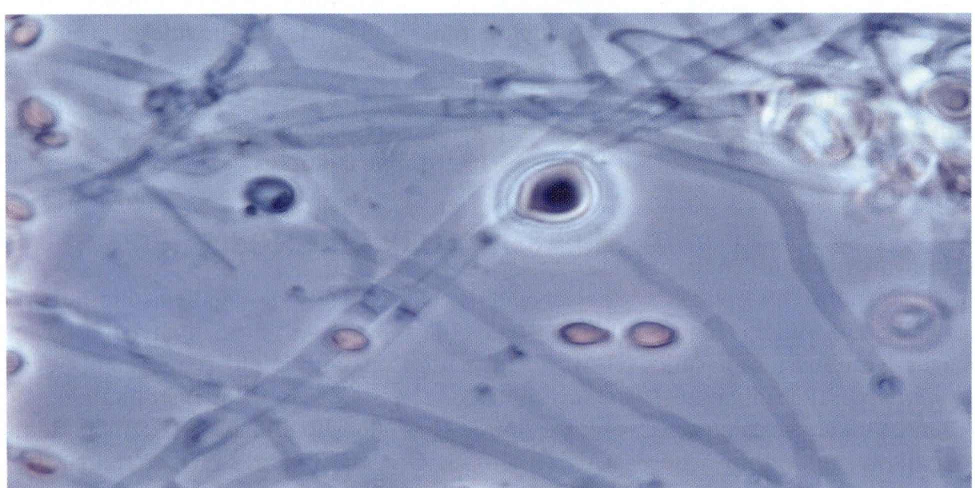

FIG. 32.1: LPCB mount showing adiaconidia (400×).
(LPCB: lactophenol cotton blue)
Source: Public Health Image Library CDC.

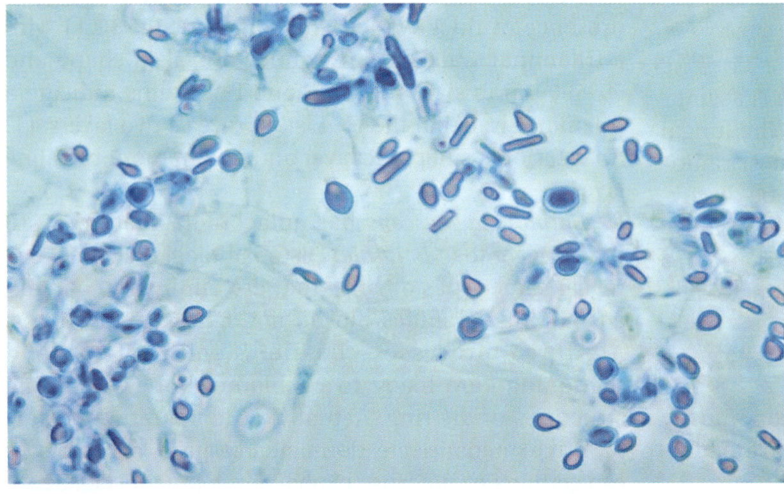

FIG. 32.2: LPCB mount of *Emmonsia* species (400×).
(LPCB: lactophenol cotton blue)
Source: Public Health Image Library CDC.

E. crescens isolates grow better on phytone yeast extract agar. The colonies appear at 37°C and not at 40°C. Thick-walled multinucleate adiaconidia are produced by *E. crescens*. The urease test is positive.

The exoantigen may show nonspecific precipitation lines with other fungi. Polymerase chain reaction (*PCR*) has a possible use for adiaspiromycosis diagnosis. *No serological tests* for the detection of antigen or antibodies are available.

Treatment

The role of antifungal drugs is definitely not known. Itraconazole may be given 200 mg/day.

EMERGOMYCOSIS

Introduction

This clinical condition is caused by a novel dimorphic fungus of the genus *Emergomyces*. It has been associated with cutaneous and disseminated infection, especially in immunocompromised individuals. The disease is known as emergomycosis.

Several new species of fungi that are phylogenetically and morphologically related to *Ajellomycetaceae* emerged during the 1970s. Five fungi that resemble *Emmonsia* were placed into the new genus *Emergomyces* in 2017 as a result of a taxonomic revision. Deadly disseminated mycosis outbreaks are reported in North America, Europe, Africa, and Asia.

Emergomyces pasteurianus, Emergomyces africanus, Emergomyces canadensis, Emergomyces orientalis, and *Emergomyces europaeus* are the five separate species included in the genus. *E. pasteurianus* shows morphological similarity to *Emmonsia* but in host tissues and on media incubated at 37°C, it shows yeast-like cells instead of adiaconidia.

Asia, Africa, Europe, and North America are the four continents from which emergomycosis has been documented so far. The following is a list of places where each species is found:

- *E. pasteurianus*: Asia (including India), Europe, France, Spain, Netherlands, Uganda, and South Africa
- *E. africanus*: South Africa, Zimbabwe, and Lesotho
- *E. canadensis*: Canada and the United States
- *E. orientalis*: China
- *E. europaeus*: Germany

The most extensive burden of the disease has been observed among human immunodeficiency virus (HIV)-infected patients of South Africa.

Virulence Factors and Pathogenesis

Inhalation of soil-borne conidia is the mode of infection with *Emergomyces* species. Inside the host, yeast-like cells form that can spread outside the lungs.

The pathogenesis of emergomycosis remains mostly unknown. Both *E. pasteurianus* and *E. africanus* have the virulence genes that are seen in other members of the family Ajellomycetaceae. Possible environmental interactions between eukaryotic organisms may help maintain pathogenic potential in mammals.

Clinical Features

Like yeast, these fungi can reproduce and spread outside of the lungs. Patients with impaired immune systems, such as those with acquired immunodeficiency syndrome (AIDS), are the only known hosts of disseminated infection. Immunosuppressive drug use, hemophilia, solid organ transplantation, and neutropenia are other underlying risk factors.

Cutaneous Emergomycosis

It is the most common clinical presentation of the disease in which various types of skin lesions such as plaques, papules with or without crusts, and ulcers are seen. The lesions heal with scarring.

Disseminated Emergomycosis

The cervix, lymph nodes, skin, lungs, liver, spleen, and bone marrow are all parts of the body that *Emergomyces* can infect. The morphologies of cutaneous lesions can vary among individuals.

Signs of pulmonary involvement include consolidations, reticulonodular infiltrates (both localized and diffuse), lobar atelectasis, effusions, and hilar lymphadenopathy.

Differential Diagnosis

The condition should be differentiated from histoplasmosis, cryptococcosis, sporotrichosis, and blastomycosis. The skin lesions resemble those of varicella, scrofuloderma, papular HIV eruption, secondary syphilis, pyoderma gangrenosum, guttate psoriasis, drug reactions, Kaposi sarcoma, and guttate syphilis.

If a chest radiograph shows pulmonary lesions, tuberculosis could be the diagnosis. Yeasts resemble *Blastomyces dermatitidis* or *Histoplasma capsulatum*, depending upon the species.

Laboratory Diagnosis

Diagnostic procedures include histopathology analysis, fungal culture, and molecular testing. Blood, skin, lymph node aspirate, induced sputum, bone marrow, lymph node tissue, and trephine biopsy are among the specimens that are taken.

Direct Examination

Yeast cells with narrow-based budding are seen in various preparations such as potassium hydroxide (KOH), calcofluor white (CFW), H&E, PAS, and GMS.

Histopathology

Using hematoxylin-eosin, PAS, and GMS stains, intracellular yeasts with surrounding inflammatory response in the affected tissue can be visualized. A skin biopsy finding includes the presence of chronic granulomatous and/or suppurative dermal infiltrates of histiocytes, multinucleated giant cells, plasma cells, and intracytoplasmic, narrow-based budding yeasts ranging in size from 2 to 5 µm.

Fungal Culture

The standard media for primary cultures include SDA, malt extract agar (MEA), and PDA. Initially smooth and glabrous, colonies turn powdery, somewhat elevated, and wrinkled after 2 weeks. They can range in color from yellowish white to brown. The reverse side is a buffish-ochre hue. A slender conidiophore grows at an angle from a from thin, hyaline hypha. Occasionally, you will see short secondary conidiophores adorned with "florets" of individual, single-celled, subspherical conidia, and the conidiophores themselves are somewhat inflated at the tip. In order to convert mold to yeast, a colony is subcultured on BHI agar, which contains 5% sheep blood. The colony is then kept at 35°C. Colonies emerge from incubation 2–3 weeks later, appearing cerebriform, pasty, and ranging in color from yellowish white to tan. Yeast cells with a narrow base and a small oval shape can be seen in a Gram-stained colony smear.

Polymerase chain reaction is the method of choice for identification of the isolate.

Treatment

It is questionable if antifungal drugs play a role. Some promising outcomes have been observed with ketoconazole, thiabendazole, and itraconazole.

CHAPTER

33 Allergic Fungal Diseases

INTRODUCTION

Fungi can induce allergies in various parts of the body such as respiratory system, conjunctiva (allergic conjunctivitis), and skin (atopic dermatitis, id reaction). These are grouped in an entity called allergic fungal diseases (AFD). The various clinical conditions of AFD could be manifestations of hypersensitivity type I, III, or IV.

Fungi associated with AFD include a variety of species, with some of the most common ones being the following:

- *Aspergillus fumigatus*: This is one of the most prevalent fungi associated with AFD, including allergic bronchopulmonary aspergillosis (ABPA) and severe asthma with fungal sensitization (SAFS).
- *Alternaria alternata*: *Alternaria* species are frequently implicated in fungal sensitization and AFD, particularly in milder cases.
- *Cladosporium herbarum*: Similar to *Alternaria*, *Cladosporium* is often found in the environment and can lead to fungal sensitization and AFD in susceptible individuals.
- *Penicillium species*: Some *Penicillium* species, such as *Penicillium chrysogenum*, have been associated with AFD, especially in cases of severe asthma.
- *Candida species*: *Candida* can cause AFD, including bronchitis, especially in individuals with underlying respiratory conditions.
- *Malassezia species*: *Malassezia* is typically a skin commensal but can cause skin-related AFD, such as atopic dermatitis.
- *Trichophyton species*: *Trichophyton* is known for causing dermatophyte infections but can also contribute to AFD when inhaled.
- *Rhizopus species*: Although less common, some species of *Rhizopus* have been associated with AFD, particularly in individuals with compromised immune systems.
- *Epicoccum nigrum*: This fungus can trigger AFD in some cases and is occasionally included in diagnostic testing panels.
- *Fusarium species*: *Fusarium* is known to cause infections and can be associated with AFD, particularly in severe cases.

A variety of terminology exists to classify allergic and respiratory conditions attributable to fungal exposure:

A. Allergic fungal airway disease (AFAD)
B. Extrinsic allergic alveolitis (EAA)/hypersensitivity pneumonitis (HP)
C. ABPA/allergic bronchopulmonary mycoses (ABPM)
D. SAFS

The terms given as B, C, and D above are types of AFAD. In addition, allergic rhinitis, allergic sinusitis, and asthma are also other allergic conditions related to the respiratory tract.

There are certain associations between a few organisms, sources, and specific allergic syndromes. Farmer's lung is caused by *Faenia rectivirgula* contaminating stored hay. Bagassosis occurs due to sugarcane containing *Thermoactinomyces sacchari*. Maple bark stripper's disease is caused by *Cryptostroma corticale. Alternaria* species present in wood pulp is responsible for wood pulp worker's disease. The list of organisms causing allergic diseases is given in **Table 33.1**.

ALTERNATIVE TERMINOLOGY FOR FUNGAL-DRIVEN AIRWAY DISEASES

In recent years, alternative terminology has emerged to describe fungal-related airway diseases.

"Airway mycoses" highlights the immunological and physiological significance of fungi growing in the airways, emphasizing their role as pathogens rather than harmless colonizers. "Fungal asthma" is proposed as an umbrella term covering SAFS, ABPA/M, and fungal bronchitis, primarily in pediatric populations. "Fungal bronchitis" is characterized by cough, mucoid sputum, and airway dysfunction, responding well to antifungal treatment, especially in individuals with AFAD. Only thermotolerant fungi cause AFAD. The fungi that can grow at body temperature are called "thermotolerant fungi." High levels of IgE to thermotolerant fungi and signs of fungal-related lung injury are the hallmarks of AFAD. However, the concept of fungal infection causing bronchitis remains somewhat contentious, though positive cultures for certain fungi may serve as biomarkers for antifungal therapy response.

Classification of hypersensitivity pneumonitis according to occupation or antigen exposure yields several variants. For instance, there is farmer's lung, gerbil-keeper's lung, and woodworker's lung. Proteins derived from birds and animals constitute a significant source of antigens in causing diseases such as bird fancier's lung, furrier's lung, and animal handler's lung, among others. Pigeons are the principal source of avian allergen in HP, along with parakeets, parrots, doves, chickens, and turkeys. Maple bark stripper's disease, bagassosis, byssinosis, and lycoperdonosis are some other examples of HP/EAA.

Metal working fluid (this is a fluid used as a lubricant or coolant for machines; aerosols produced may be inhaled and act as allergens) or humidifier water, sauna bath water contaminated with bacteria, proteins from avian blooms, or chemicals such as isocyanates are other sources of allergens to those working in industries. Persons exposed to such situations may get EAA.

Though antigens differ in each condition, the basic pathophysiology is the same. The concepts of laboratory diagnosis, prognosis, prevention, and treatment also remain the same. Hence, these are discussed in only farmer's lung.

TABLE 33.1: Causative agents of allergic diseases.

Category	Agent
Fungal agents—hyaline hyphomycetes	*Aspergillus fumigatus*
	Aspergillus flavus
	Aspergillus niger
	Penicillium simplicissimum
	Penicillium rubrum
Bacterial agents—actinomycetes	*Faenia rectivirgula* (formerly *Micropolyspora faeni*)
	Thermoactinomyces candidus (formerly *Micromonospora candidus*)
	Thermoactinomyces vulgaris (formerly *Micromonospora vulgaris*)

Farmer's Lung

Farmer's lung disease (FLD) is a type of *HP*. The main cause of FLD is inhalation of biological dust, which can be found in straw, moldy hay, or other agricultural goods. This happens frequently while storing straw, grain, or other agricultural items in places with a lot of humidity.

In the seventeenth century, the disease was initially recognized by the Italian researcher Bernardino Ramazzini. He found that farmers and breeders were more likely to have the disease because they were constantly breathing in organic dust. (Organic dust contains molds, pollen, bacteria, pesticides, feed and bedding particles, hairs of animals, feathers and droppings of birds, fertilizers, and methane). Now it is known that these can act as sensitizing agents. Campbell in 1932 first described farmer's lung as a separate clinical entity from Britain in 1932.

Causative agents of farmer's lung are shown in **Table 33.2**. Most cases of farmer's lung are caused by thermophilic actinomycetes such as *Saccharopolyspora rectivirgula* (earlier *Micropolyspora faeni* or *Faenia rectivirgula*) and *Thermoactinomyces vulgaris*, as well as fungi such as *Aspergillus* species. Other causes include *Penicillium simplicissimum* and *Penicillium rubrum*. But causes differ substantially from one part of the world to another.

Pathophysiology

Farmer's lung develops most commonly in persons exposed to moldy hay. The hay, straw, or grains get the growth of bacteria and fungi if stored in damp conditions. In dry weather, when such material is handled, the bacteria and fungi get aerosolized easily. This is especially true when the activity is in a poorly ventilated building/room/godown. When breathed in, allergens irritate the airways and the areas between them. To start, type III hypersensitivity develops after inhaling an allergen. This is a localized type III hypersensitivity.

TABLE 33.2: Causative agents of farmer's lung.

Bacteria	• *Thermoactinomyces candidus* • *Thermoactinomyces vulgaris* • *Faenia rectivirgula*
Fungi	• *Aspergillus fumigatus* • *Aspergillus flavus* • *Aspergillus niger* • *Penicillium rubrum* • *Penicillium simplicissimum*

The development of granulomas happens as the disease advances. Upon continuous acute exposure, serum immunoglobulin G (IgG) antibodies specific to the inhaled antigen can be found at quite high titers. Chronic and ongoing hypersensitivity reactions (type IV) to antigens mediated by T cells cause fibrosis.

Clinical Features

There is a slow start. Both the extent of exposure and the illness's severity influence the clinical presentation.

Typically, the disease entity is described as acute, subacute, and chronic.

Acute form: Patient presents with dry cough, difficulty breathing, fever, myalgia, and joint pains. It is easy to mistake the acute symptoms for a viral infection.

Subacute form: It has an insidious onset. The patient has mild fever, cough, shortness of breath, and myalgia.

Chronic form: It is a prolonged process of low-grade fever, weakness, loss of appetite, loss of weight, chronic cough, shortness of breath, and night sweats.

To aid in the diagnosis of this ailment, a thorough history should be collected, including details such as geographical areas, occupation, systematic risk exposure, and the duration of symptoms.

Diagnosis

Lymphocytosis is an important finding in the diagnosis of FLD. High-resolution computed tomography (HRCT) scans further help in the diagnosis. The most noticeable characteristics include mosaic patterning, air trapping, centrilobular nodules, and diffuse ground-glass opacities. Septal thickening, ground-glass opacities, fibrosis, bronchiectasis (usually affecting the higher lobes more heavily), and symptoms of pulmonary hypertension are chronic manifestations. Smokers are at an increased risk for developing emphysema.

Additional methods include sputum cultures, antigen detection, and enzyme-linked immunosorbent assay (ELISA) examination of serum antibodies.

Due to the fact that antibodies (IgG) can remain in the body for up to 10 years after farming has stopped, detecting them is useless since it just shows past exposure. Additionally, antibodies can exist in some people even in the absence of overt symptoms.

Many patients with hypersensitivity pneumonitis/farmer's lung have decreased diffusing capacity of the lung for carbon monoxide (DLCO) and forced mid-expiratory flow (FEF 25–75%). Bronchoalveolar lavage (BAL) results can be helpful in certain situations. An increased number of lymphocytes, moderate neutrophils, few eosinophils, and macrophages in BAL fluid indicate interstitial inflammation that is a hallmark of FLD. The CD4/CD8 ratio is low in BAL fluid.

In order to diagnose fibrotic diffuse interstitial lung disorders, transbronchial lung cryobiopsy (TBLC) is used. The last diagnostic option is a surgical lung biopsy.

Differential Diagnosis

Differential diagnoses include COPD, pulmonary fibrosis, organic dust toxic syndrome (a disease that affects smokers), and viral infections.

Complications: Patients requiring ventilatory assistance and vasopressors may exhibit symptoms of respiratory failure and shock.

Treatment

The primary measure should be to stay away from potential environmental hazards. In the short term, steroids may alleviate symptoms but they have no effect on long-term functional outcomes. Patients' conditions have improved while using mycophenolate, although more research is required to confirm this.

Vaccinations, oxygen supplements, diuretics, and noninvasive ventilation may be necessary in cases of chronic illness. As a last resort, a lung transplant could be considered. We must prioritize preventive actions. In addition to alleviating symptoms, the powered dust respirator helmet has improved functionality. Since symptoms still affect 63% of patients even after 5 years following an acute episode, strict primary preventative measures are necessary. The early detection of farmer's lung is crucial for determining the prognosis. Research has indicated that 8% of individuals experience worsening symptoms following acute bouts. The stated mortality rate is 1%. Eight years following diagnosis was the average lifetime.

EXTRINSIC ALLERGIC ALVEOLITIS

The immunologically mediated disease known EAA or HP develops when a person becomes hypersensitive to certain antigenic organic material that they inhale repeatedly. This material can come from a variety of sources, including spoiled hay or wood bark, metal working fluid or humidifier water contaminated with bacteria, proteins from avian blooms, or chemicals such as isocyanates.

ALLERGIC BRONCHOPULMONARY ASPERGILLOSIS

About 2.5% of the world's population is exposed to ABPA. The highest estimate for the prevalence of ABPA aggravating asthma in the Indian community is approximately 5%.

Pathogenesis

Causative fungi are various species of *Aspergillus*. The conidia are small enough to fit into airways, measuring only 2–3.5 μm. Even while many people with asthma are exposed to spores, it does not mean that they all develop the disease. In persons who develop ABPA, the immune responses fail to eliminate the spores, leading to aberrant Th2 immune responses and spore persistence; several deficiencies in innate and adaptive immunity have been discovered. In people with a family history of the condition, spores can transform into hyphae. The outer coat of germinating conidia is lost, revealing several fungal proteins such as D-glucan and galactomannan.

Typically, phagocytes are able to identify these fungal proteins and eliminate some of the fungus. As a result of fungal growth-induced exocytosis of several proteins, a Th1 CD4+ T-cell response is induced, which helps macrophages and neutrophils eliminate the fungi. Meanwhile, interleukin (IL)-4, IL-5, IL-13, CCL17, IL-9, and other substances are secreted by ABPA's immunological response, which is mostly Th2 CD4+ T cells. Inflammation, brought on by the Th2 response, manifests itself in mast cell degranulation and a massive infusion of eosinophils and neutrophils. Both total IgE and IgA, as well as *Aspergillus*-specific IgA, are produced. There are a number of symptoms associated with ABPA, including mucus clogging and eosinophilic pneumonia. Bronchitis, pulmonary fibrosis, and COPD are all inflammation-related conditions.

Pathology

- Thick mucus plugs in dilated bronchi are a common pathological sign, which is known as bronchiectasis.
- Airway secretions demonstrate inflammatory cells, mucin, Curschmann's spirals, and Charcot–Leyden crystals, which are indicative of eosinophilic inflammation.
- Fungal organisms inhabit a limited number of spaces.
- In patients with ABPA, inflammatory cells such as eosinophils and neutrophils invade the airways.
- Within the lung parenchyma, eosinophils predominate in a mixed chronic inflammatory response.
- In addition to organizing pneumonia and bronchocentric granulomatosis, bronchiolitis obliterans can occur.

Clinical Features

- In addition to poorly managed asthma, persons without a history of bronchial asthma may very rarely get ABPA.
- On rare occasions, ABPA is identified by systematic screening of asthmatic patients, even when the patient does not exhibit any symptoms.
- Symptoms include leukopenia, mild fever, decreased appetite, and generalized aches and pains.
- A brownish mucus plug is expected to be expelled.
- Those who have had bronchiectasis for a long time are more likely to experience clubbing (66%).
- It is unusual to hear coarse crackles during auscultation, yet polyphonic wheezing is prevalent.
- Characteristics of respiratory failure and pulmonary hypertension can be detected during a physical examination.
- It is important to distinguish between other pulmonary disorders when localized auscultatory abnormalities develop during ABPA exacerbations.

Immunological Investigations

- Currently, the gold standard for screening asthmatic patients for ABPA is an elevated level of *A. fumigatus*-specific IgE in serum.
- *Test for Aspergillus on the skin*: A skin prick or intradermal injection reaction to *A. fumigatus* antigen tests the immediate type I hypersensitivity to *Aspergillus*. It gives comparable results to having high IgE antibodies against *A. fumigatus*. The sensitivity of this test is around 88–94%. However, the potential for anaphylaxis, incompetence of the technical personnel doing the test, and the absence of antigen standardization are some drawbacks of skin testing. Consequently, it is not advised to conduct skin testing nowadays.
- When diagnosing and monitoring patients with ABPA, measuring blood total IgE is a helpful test. When screening for ABPA in asthmatic patients, serum total IgE (cutoff 500 IU/mL) has a strong sensitivity (96%) but a poor specificity (24%).
- *Immunoglobulin G specific to A. fumigatus*: When compared to the previously employed immunodiffusion test, the sensitivity of the commercially available enzyme immunoassay is over 90%.
- *Eosinophil count in peripheral blood*: A peripheral blood eosinophil count of >1,000 cells/μL is traditionally considered as a key criterion for the diagnosis

of ABPA; however, a count of >500 cells/μL is considered to be the acceptable cutoff in many studies.

- *Cultures of sputum*: Because *A. fumigatus* fungi are so common, a positive culture of the sputum provides support for the diagnosis of ABPA but cannot prove it.
- *Tests for pulmonary function*: These are crucial for determining the lung disease severity level. When the diffusion capacity is reduced, these tests typically reveal an obstructive problem.
- A commonly used yet less sensitive and specific diagnostic test for diagnosing invasive pulmonary aspergillosis is the detection of galactomannan in serum or BAL fluid.
- Overexpression of thymus and activation-regulated chemokine (TARC, CCL17) has been studied in ABPA patients because of the predominance of the Th2 immune response.

Algorithm for the diagnosis of ABPA:

- *Measurement of A. fumigatus-specific IgE*: If levels exceed 0.35 kUA/L, proceed to measure total serum IgE.
- *Assessment of total serum IgE*: If total IgE exceeds 500 IU/mL, additional investigations are warranted, including—
  - Thin-section CT scan of the chest
  - *A. fumigatus*-specific IgG
  - Peripheral blood eosinophil count
- *Classification based on imaging*:
  - *ABPA-S*: ABPA without bronchiectasis on CT
  - *ABPA-B*: ABPA with bronchiectasis
  - *ABPA-HAM*: ABPA with high-attenuation mucus
- *Follow-up recommendations*: Annual measurement of total serum IgE is recommended in patients with elevated *A. fumigatus*-specific IgE, as approximately 40% of allergic sensitized (AS) patients may develop ABPA.

MAPLE BARK STRIPPER'S DISEASE

Maple bark stripper's disease is due to the inhalation of conidia of *Cryptostroma corticale*, and the disease is common in people working with the maple bark tree. The clinical features are cough, dyspnea, fever, night sweats, and substernal pain. There may be the formation of granulomas with small conidia within phagocytic cells.

BAGASSOSIS

Bagassosis is due to thermophilic actinomycetes present in dust from bagasse which is from sugarcane. In addition to spores, the bagasse contains fiber, silica, and quartz. Manifestations are similar to farmer's lung.

LYCOPERDONOSIS

Lycoperdonosis is due to the conidia of *Lycoperdon* species, commonly known as puff balls. The disease is similar to allergic lung disease.

BYSSINOSIS

Byssinosis is also called dusty cotton disease which is due to a fungus present in dust from the cotton-producing plant.

ALLERGIC RHINITIS

There is evidence linking allergic rhinitis to exposure to wet environments or fungi. Longitudinal studies indicate that adult-onset asthma is more likely to develop in individuals with pre-existing allergic rhinitis.

ALLERGIC CONJUNCTIVITIS

This condition, which may be linked to allergic rhinitis, impacts 15–40% of the population. Conditions that are dry and windy tend to worsen the symptoms of allergic conjunctivitis.

ATOPIC DERMATITIS

The itchy skin lesions are caused by atopic dermatitis, an inflammatory skin condition that lasts for a long time and often goes hand in hand with allergic asthma and rhinoconjunctivitis. Most people with atopic dermatitis have tested positive for *Malassezia* sensitivity.

ALLERGIC FUNGAL SINUSITIS

An extreme kind of chronic rhinosinusitis, allergic fungal sinusitis, is marked by a powerful inflammatory reaction to fungi in the air. Pathogenesis in atopic individuals is defined by a fungal antigen-induced type I hypersensitivity reaction that is eosinophil predominant and persistent in the sinonasal tract mucosa.

ALLERGIC ASTHMA

It is distinguished by bronchial hyperresponsiveness and airflow restrictions. Fungal sensitization may be linked to severe asthma attacks that necessitate hospitalization. Although there is widespread agreement that fungi can act as an asthma trigger, the mechanisms by which this occurs remain unknown.

CHAPTER

34 Fungal Rhinosinusitis

INTRODUCTION

Infection of the nose and paranasal sinuses caused by fungi is known as fungal rhinosinusitis (FRS). Orbit and brain tissues being in close vicinity are among those that might be affected by the disease's potential to spread. Patients with healthy immune systems as well as those with impaired immune systems can experience this illness. Although many other types of fungi can cause this disease, the agents of mucormycosis and *Aspergillus* species are the most common culprits.

HISTORY

A soldier's maxillary sinus was characterized by Plaignaud in 1791 as having a "fungus tumor." The soldier was 22 years old. An *Aspergillus* species that caused sinusitis in a patient with an infection of the sphenoid sinus was identified by Oppe in 1897. Back in 1894, Mackenzie documented the initial instance of what seemed to be noninvasive fungal sinusitis. In 1957, Baker et al. initially documented a case of FRS, an invasive form of FRS caused by *Zygomycetes*, in patients with impaired immune systems. To try to reach a consensus on illness categorization and terminology, the International Society for Human and Animal Mycology (ISHAM) formed a working group. The classification of fungal sinusitis and causative fungi is given in **Table 34.1**.

Depending on whether the fungus invades the mucous membrane or not, FRS is classified as either invasive or noninvasive. Acute invasive (fulminant), granulomatous invasive, and chronic invasive are the three subtypes of invasive FRS. Eosinophil-related FRS (including allergic FRS and eosinophilic FRS), fungal ball (sinus mycetoma), and localized colonization are the subtypes of noninvasive FRS.

TABLE 34.1: Classification of fungal sinusitis.

Classification	*Subtype*	*Causative agents*
Noninvasive fungal rhinosinusitis	Allergic fungal rhinosinusitis (AFRS)	• *Aspergillus* species (e.g., *Aspergillus fumigatus*, *Aspergillus flavus*, *Aspergillus niger*) • *Curvularia* species • *Alternaria* species • *Penicillium* species • *Fusarium* species
	Eosinophilic fungal rhinosinusitis (EFRS)	• *Aspergillus* species (e.g., *A. fumigatus*) • *Curvularia* species • *Alternaria* species
	Localized colonization	• *Aspergillus* species (e.g., *A. niger*, *A. flavus*) • *Fusarium* species • *Penicillium* species
	Fungal ball (Mycetoma)	• *Aspergillus* species (e.g., *A. fumigatus*, *A. flavus*) • *Fusarium* species • *Curvularia* species

Continued

Continued

Classification	Subtype	Causative agents
Invasive fungal rhinosinusitis	Acute invasive rhinosinusitis (fulminant)	• *Aspergillus* species (e.g., *A. fumigatus, A. flavus*) • *Mucor* species (e.g., *Mucor* species, *Rhizopus* species) • *Fusarium* species
	Chronic invasive rhinosinusitis	• *Immunocompetent* • *Aspergillus* species (e.g., *A. niger, A. flavus*) • *Fusarium* species • *Curvularia* species • *Immunocompromised* • *Aspergillus* species (e.g., *A. fumigatus, A. flavus*) • *Mucor* species (e.g., *Mucor* species, *Rhizopus* species) • *Fusarium* species • *Histoplasma capsulatum*
	Granulomatous invasive rhinosinusitis	• *Aspergillus* species (e.g., *A. fumigatus*) • *Histoplasma capsulatum* • *Blastomyces dermatitidis* • *Sporothrix schenckii*

INVASIVE FUNGAL RHINOSINUSITIS

Acute Invasive (Fulminant) Fungal Rhinosinusitis

The disease is defined by vascular invasion and has a brief duration—typically a duration of 4 weeks or less. Nearby orbits are quickly infected. Brain tissue and the channels of the cavernous sinus vascular system are likely to be invaded. The fungus invades the body either directly or via the blood vessels, leading to clots in the blood vessels and tissue death. The fatality rate from acute invasive (fulminant) FRS (AIFRS) ranges between 50 and 80%.

This condition usually develops in immunocompromised people, such as those with impaired neutrophil function, aplastic anemia, hematologic malignancies, hemochromatosis, or who are undergoing immunosuppressive treatments such as chemotherapy or oral corticosteroids. It can also happen in people with acquired immunodeficiency syndrome (AIDS). Poorly controlled diabetes is an important risk factor. Blood sugar spikes and acidity promote fungal development and tissue invasion as ketoacidosis inhibits phagocytosis. An increase in number of patients with this condition was noted during COVID-19 pandemic.

The term "mucormycosis" is used for infections of paranasal sinuses caused by *Rhizopus, Absidia,* and other fungi of the Mucoraceae family (Zygomycetes order). Apart from these, *Aspergillus* species is the next most common fungus to cause infection of paranasal sinuses.

Based upon the extension of the disease, the following *clinical presentations* are seen:

Rhinomaxillary disease: The most common symptoms include a runny nose, headache, fever, facial pain, diplopia, hypesthesia, and periorbital and facial edema. Black eschar over skin, nasal mucosa, or the hard palate is are typically seen in mucormycosis.

Sino-orbital disease: Proptosis, ophthalmoplegia, chemosis, diplopia, decreased visual acuity, and blindness are possible symptoms that patients may experience when the disease spreads to the orbit. Necrosis of the cheeks and palates can occur when the disease spreads beyond the walls of the maxillary sinuses.

Rhino-orbito-cerebral disease: Thrombosis in the cavernous sinus, internal carotid artery, cranial nerve palsies, stroke, and acute subdural hematoma are all conditions that can be caused by extension across or through the base of the skull.

Radiological Findings

Unilateral nasal or sinus thickening and opacification, in part or in whole, is the most common feature. CT scans have shown bone degradation and thickening of the soft tissues. Perisinus infiltration and extra-sinus invasion are also noted. Magnetic resonance imaging (MRI) is the gold standard for identifying intracranial, intraorbital, and retroantral extension. "Black turbinate sign" refers to lack of contrast enhancement of nasal turbinates in angioinvasive fungal sinusitis on contrast-enhanced MRI. This is due to infarction caused by invasive fungi. Endoscopy of the nose would reveal a pale mucosa with ulcers and necrosis of the tissues.

Diagnosis

Acute necrotizing FRS is another name for this condition since necrotizing pathological reactions can happen even in people with modest inflammation.

Histopathology shows that there is vasculitis with thrombosis, vascular invasion, hemorrhage, tissue infarction, and acute neutrophilic infiltrates.

Microbiology

Potassium hydroxide (KOH) mount of biopsies taken from sinus tissues shows fungal hyphae. In zygomycetes, the hyphae are broad and nonseptate and of uneven thickness. Culture of the samples allows for a final diagnosis by identifying the fungus.

As for treatment, it may include a combination of vigorous surgical debridement, antifungal medication, and addressing the root causes of immunosuppression all at once.

Granulomatous Invasive Fungal Rhinosinusitis

Aspergillus flavus is the most common causative agent of this condition.

Signs and Symptoms

It is a slowly progressing lesion. This condition lasts for >12 weeks. It may take months or years for the development of the lesion. It affects immunocompetent hosts. The entity presents as mass in cheeks, orbits, nose, and paranasal sinuses. It may sometimes present with proptosis.

Diagnosis is done by biopsy and histopathology. There is significant fibrosis and a granulomatous response. On rare occasions, perivascular fibrosis, vascular proliferation, vasculitis, and noncaseating granulomas containing foreign bodies or Langhans' type giant cells may be seen. Rarely, hyphae may be seen in giant cells.

Molecular tests, such as in situ hybridization, can be useful.

Surgery followed by antifungals (voriconazole, itraconazole, or posaconazole) is the usual mode of treatment. Amphotericin B can also be given.

Although the United States has recorded a small number of instances, Sudan, India, Pakistan, and Saudi Arabia have been the main countries to report this condition.

Chronic Invasive Fungal Rhinosinusitis

Chronic invasive fungal infection, just like granulomatous invasive FRS (GIFRS), develops slowly over the course of months or even years (lasts > 12 weeks).

Tissue invasion, hyphae buildup, necrosis, and little inflammation characterize chronic invasive FRS (CIFRS). Any paranasal sinus could be affected, although the ethmoid and sphenoid sinuses are the most common.

Patients may be immunocompetent. Patients on corticosteroids or with diabetes mellitus may also suffer. Involvement of the orbit, leading to blurred or lost vision, occurs frequently.

A potentially deadly extension into the skull is more commonly observed in India and the Middle East than in the United States.

About half of the time, tissue cultures yield positive results. *Aspergillus fumigatus* is the most often agent.

Some researchers now consider CIFRS to be synonymous with GIFRS, and the boundary between the two is getting more and more blurry. The presence or absence of granulomas, fibrosis, vascular proliferation, fungal penetration into tissues, vascular invasion, and disease limits are likely to be the most essential distinguishing features. But there does not seem to be a clinicopathological distinction between the two groups. Both are highly involved in the orbit and have a lengthy journey. Additionally, this divergence does not affect prognosis or therapy in any way.

Clinical Features

The following symptoms may be present: Enlargements of the cheek, nose, paranasal sinuses, and orbit are the clinical hallmarks of *chronic invasive fungal sinusitis*. In addition, anosmia, epistaxis, sinus pain, and serosanguineous discharge from the nose with nasal polyposis may also be seen. Intracranial disease extension may cause neurological impairments, cranial nerve palsies, seizures, or migraines.

CT Findings

The collection of hyperattenuating soft tissues often involves one or more neighboring paranasal sinuses. Ethmoid and sphenoid involvement is prevalent.

The MRI shows a low to very low T2 signal and a low to normal T1 signal. Locations of extra-sinus extension are the orbit and brain. Cavernous sinus and internal carotid artery are other sites of infection. The degree of sinus involvement and biopsy tissue for culture can be examined using an endoscope. Biopsy shows dense accumulation of fungal hyphae, occasional invasion of blood vessels, and chronic or very little inflammation.

Treatment: The two most crucial procedures are (1) aeration and (2) sinus debridement. For *Aspergillus*, amphotericin B is advised. There have been reports that using itraconazole for long-term suppression at a dosage of 200 mg twice daily can lessen the likelihood of relapse.

Primary antifungal medications are voriconazole and posaconazole.

NONINVASIVE FUNGAL RHINOSINUSITIS

Localized Fungal Colonization (Saprobic Infestation)

Even in individuals who have had sinus surgery before, fungal infections can develop in the mucous crusts inside the nasal canal, often without any noticeable symptoms. A fungal ball may form if these infections spread more. Nonetheless, treatment might not be necessary in instances where the majority of people have a benign history.

Due to the lack of symptoms, it is frequently mistaken for something else. On the other hand, it could cause a foul smell to emanate from inside the nose.

Sinus Fungal Ball

The maxillary sinus is a common location for the development of fungal balls, which are dense clumps of fungal hyphae. There is less mucosal discomfort in this extramucosal variety, which is defined by an entangled mass of fungus. Additional sinuses or, in extremely unusual cases, multiple sinuses could be affected by the illness. This condition has other names, e.g., sinus mycetoma, nasal sinus aspergilloma, and chronic noninvasive granuloma; however, these names should be avoided.

Previously, these were known as *"Aspergillomas,"* after the most commonly encountered fungus *Aspergillus* species. However, other fungi have been implicated in the production of fungal balls, leading to the change in terminology to *"fungal ball."* Fungal ball occurs in immunocompetent, middle-aged persons, especially ladies. Previous surgery or injury to the mucosa may have played a role. Dental fillings and iatrogenic oroantral communication are two examples of dental treatments that might lead to maxillary fungal balls.

Clinical Features

Patients may be asymptomatic. The symptoms, if present, include headache, pain over the affected sinus on pressure, postnasal discharge, crusting in the nasal cavity, and change in smell sensation (cacosmia).

Sinus endoscopy: This allows visualization of the maxillary fungal ball. It also allows the collection of diagnostic material. The material is submitted for histopathology and microbiology. However, approximately 70% fungus ball specimens do not yield any growth.

Histopathology: It is helpful to confirm that the lesion is noninvasive.

Radiological findings (X-ray/CT): It is helpful to diagnose a fungus ball.

De Shazo et al. in 1997 have given five criteria considering clinical, endoscopic, radiological, and histopathological aspects to diagnose a fungus ball in sinus:

1. Radiological opacification of the sinus with or without calcification.
2. *Endoscopy:* Mucopurulent, cheesy, or clay-like materials inside the sinus.
3. *Histopathology*: Dense conglomerate of hyphae, separate but adjacent to the mucosa.
4. *Histopathology*: Chronic inflammation of the mucosa (lymphocytes, plasma cells, mast cells, and few eosinophils); no granuloma, no allergic mucin.
5. *Histopathology*: No histological evidence of fungal invasion of mucosa, blood vessels, or bone.

Eosinophil-related Fungal Rhinosinusitis

Fungal organisms can be identified. In the absence of a particular IgE response, typical observations include the presence of eosinophils and their breakdown products as mucus, as well as Charcot–Leiden crystals.

Allergic Fungal Rhinosinusitis

Allergic fungal rhinosinusitis is likely the most prevalent kind of fungal sinus infection. First identified in the 1970s, allergic bronchopulmonary aspergillosis (ABPA) and allergic rhinitis syndrome (AFRS) share mucus characteristics.

Young patients (aged 21–33 years) who have a normal immune system are more likely to have AFRS. People who have atopy, asthma, and allergic rhinitis are more prone to get AFRS. Prolonged swelling, stagnation of secretions, and superinfection with microorganisms of the sinuses are seen. Nasal polyps are also seen.

Signs and Symptoms

Signs and symptoms of chronic nasal airway blockage and congestion include nasal crusting, postnasal drip, rhinorrhea, and headache. Traditional antihistamine treatment is ineffective for these patients. The southern United States, countries in the Middle East, and warm, humid regions such as India are more prone to AFRS. With 56–57% of all cases, it is by far the most common type of FRS in India.

Inhaled fungus triggers type I and type III hypersensitivity reactions, which in turn promote inflammation and, most significantly, the creation of mucus, specifically referred to as "eosinophilic" mucin. This is thick, light tan to brown to dark green discharge of mucus. It has "peanut butter-like" consistency and looks like cement or rubber. Characteristics of this mucin are eosinophilic inflammatory cells and "Charcot-Leyden" crystals. When eosinophils break down, they leave behind these crystals. AFRS can be caused by *Aspergillus, Fusarium, Scedosporium, Curvularia,* or *Bipolaris.*

Radiological Findings

While AFRS usually affects both sides, it might affect just one side of the sinuses. The ethmoid sinus is the most typical site of involvement.

Computed tomography scan shows a centrally hyperdense (often serpiginous) area with hypodense periphery. Bony erosion, thinning of the sinus wall, and expansion of the affected sinus are seen.

MRI shows that hypointensity of T1WI and T2WI is the most common finding.

Diagnosis

The differential diagnosis of AFRS encompasses a range of viral, neoplastic, and inflammatory disorders that can induce sinusitis.

The current gold standard for diagnosis was laid out by Bent and Kuhn in 1994. These are:

- Type I hypersensitivity to fungi
- Nasal polyposis
- Radiological finding of the serpiginous areas of high attenuation of affected sinuses
- Eosinophilic mucin
- Positive fungal stain or culture

Geographical Distribution

The incidence of AFRS and GIFRS is believed to be significantly affected by one's geographical location.

Some regions of the United States, such as the Mississippi basin and the Southeast and Southwest, India, North Africa, and the Middle East have a higher prevalence of *AFRS.*

The United States has reported very few cases of *GIFRS,* while Sudan, India, and Pakistan are the only countries where it has been observed.

Since most reports of *sinus fungal ball* entities have come from France, Italy, and Taiwan, it is possible that this phenomenon is geographically limited.

Age and Sex Distribution

Fungal sinusitis is more common in men than in women. Nobody knows for sure what triggers this tendency. However, sinus fungal balls tend to affect women in their middle years or later in life.

Older adults have a higher risk of AIFRS, which may be attributable to the higher prevalence of diabetes and cancer chemotherapy.

In an immunocompromised host, if the fungi such as *Aspergillus* and *Zygomycetes* are inhaled, they can get past the host's defenses and invade sinonasal tissue, creating an acidotic necrosis area perfect for the fungal growth to flourish. Another important factor in the disease's alarming rise in incidence is the extensive usage of steroids. The steroid promotes hyperglycemia and also inhibits normal inflammatory cell responses.

Zygomycetes are the most prevalent fungi responsible for acute invasive rhinosinusitis, the most common of which is *Rhizopus oryzae*. Septate fungi, especially *A. fumigatus* and *A. flavus,* are the leading causes of AIFRS in patients with weak immune systems. Most often implicated dematiaceous fungi were *Alternaria alternata, Bipolaris* species, *Drechslera* species, and *Curvularia lunata.*

Aspergillus flavus has been detected in almost 80% of AFRS patients in India, regardless of region. When it comes to GIFRS, *A. flavus* is the most often found pathogen. Conversely, most cases of CIFRS are caused by *A. fumigatus.* Direct microscopy reveals fungus in most sinus fungal ball biopsy samples, which otherwise seem sterile. The fungus responsible for the disease, usually *A. fumigatus* or *A. flavus* (with the exception of *Pseudallescheria boydii*), only grows in 30–50% of these cultures.

LABORATORY DIAGNOSIS OF FUNGAL RHINOSINUSITIS

A biopsy sample is collected for microbial diagnosis.

Microscopy

In acute invasive FRS: Fungal components are shown by the KOH mount. The hyphae of mucormycosis look like ribbons and are wide, aseptate, or sparsely septate. Septate hyphae with dichotomous branching are characteristic of *Aspergillus* species.

Allergic FRS: A typical inflammatory infiltration consisting of eosinophils, lymphocytes, plasma cells, and eosinophilic breakdown products, i.e., Charcot–Leyden crystals, can be seen in a hematoxylin and eosin (H&E)-stained picture of mucin. Although there may be some swelling and enlargement of the mucosa, no signs of invasion, giant cells, granulomas, or necrosis should be present.

Fungal Stains

One notable characteristic of fungal components is their capacity to absorb silver. Several silver stains, such as Grocott–Gomori methenamine silver (GMS) stains, which transform fungus into black or dark brown, are based on this feature. Fungal staining is a crucial step in the identification process since it supplements the results of the initial H&E stain.

Both periodic acid–Schiff (PAS) and the Fontana–Masson stains are further options. Since melanin and the organism are quite similar, the Fontana–Masson stain can differentiate between hyaline fungi and phaeoid fungi.

Fungal Culture

Conventional media are usually favorable environments for the growth of sinusitis-causing fungi. Sabouraud Dextrose Agar is inoculated with antibiotics or a biopsy at 25°C with cycloheximide and 37°C without it. Prior to the cultures being deemed sterile, they should be inspected daily during the initial week and subsequently twice weekly for a duration of 4 months. Although fungal cultures can help in the diagnosis and treatment of AFRS, they should only be used with caution due to the wide range of yields (64–100%).

Recently, molecular techniques are used in many laboratories.

TREATMENT OF FUNGAL SINUSITIS

Surgical debridement and extensive aeration of diseased sinuses are the primary aims of the procedure, which also provides specimens for microbiological and histological analysis. All allergic mucus, polyps, and fungal debris must be surgically removed as part of surgical therapy in order to decrease the antigenic burden. For noninvasive types, surgery might be the only necessary procedure. The majority of medical professionals feel that a combination of medical treatment and surgery can effectively prevent the recurrence and advancement of invasive diseases.

Systemic amphotericin B is strongly recommended as an antifungal medication. Liposomal amphotericin B allows for substantially higher doses than free amphotericin B due to its reduced toxicity. Combining amphotericin with 5-fluorocystosine is recommended by Arroyo et al. due to the fact that 5-fluorocystosine is efficient against certain dematiaceous fungi.

It has also been reported that amphotericin B can be applied topically through intraoperative sinus irrigation or by repeatedly packing the antral cavity with gauze saturated with the medication.

Alternative treatment with azoles, especially itraconazole, has become important due to the recognized toxicity of amphotericin B.

Oral itraconazole was prescribed by Rone Jones and Moore-Gillon alongside surgical intervention for individuals suffering from damaging noninvasive fungal sinusitis. To help reduce polyps and mucosal edema and to aid in the identification of surgical landmarks, systemic corticosteroids can be given 7 days before surgery in the form of oral prednisolone at a dose of 0.5–1 mg/kg/day. Most cases involve a super-additive bacterial infection, which necessitates the use of concurrent antibiotics. One week before surgery, patients are prescribed nasal decongestants.

A successful surgical outcome is achieved in equal measure by postoperative care. A 10-days antibiotic treatment is recommended. The patient is instructed to self-administer saline nasal washes following the removal of the sinus packs. Following surgery, patients have weekly checkups for 4 weeks, then biannually for 1 year, and quarterly thereafter.

CHAPTER

35 Mycotoxins

INTRODUCTION

Mycotoxins are harmful byproducts of fungal metabolism. They can have a devastating effect on human and animal health. In addition to short-term acute impacts, these mycotoxins can induce chronic, long-term health problems, such as cancer.

Some important mycotoxins are found in food:

- Aflatoxins (AFB1, B2, G1, G2, etc.)
- Fumonisins (Groups A, B, C, P, etc.)
- Trichothecenes (Deoxynivalenol/Nivalenol, etc.)
- Ochratoxin-A
- Ergot
- Cyclopiazonic acid (CPA)
- Patulin
- Citrinin
- Zearalenone

Diseases caused by consumption of these mycotoxins are called mycotoxicoses (singular = mycotoxicosis). Some fungi of Basidiomycetes, referred to as mushrooms are edible. But there are some poisonous mushrooms. On ingestion of these fungi a person may suffer from a condition called 'mycetism'. Both these aspects are covered in this chapter. Some fungi are plant pathogens. Fungi in the fields infect crops prior to harvest. After harvest, during storage fungi emerge and are responsible for mycotoxin production.

Some fungi commonly found in fields include those that cause disease to plants (such as *Fusarium graminearum*), those that thrive when plants are under stress (such as *Aspergillus flavus* and *Fusarium moniliforme*), and those that can contaminate crops with mycotoxins (such as *Penicillium verrucosum* and *A. flavus*). Inadequate sanitation during shipping and storage, along with hot temperatures, high humidity, and heavy rain, create an ideal environment for mycotoxin development.

Mycotoxins are ubiquitous poisons that can be found in a wide range of materials, such as soil, animal products, human meals, and animal feed. They are commonly found in maize, sorghum (*jowar*), wheat, peanuts, peanut butter, sesame, and sunflower seeds. Among animal feeds, they are most often found in wheat bran, pea hulls, and corn grain. Pets such as poultry, ducklings, turkeys, pigs, and calves if consume such aflatoxin-containing feed (low dose) over a prolonged period may not suffer but store aflatoxin in their meat and eggs. Milk, eggs, and meat of such animals are a source of aflatoxin to humans.

It should be noted that aflatoxins can be found in any grain crop. Spores of the aflatoxigenic fungus can be transmitted by insects. Temperate and tropical areas are more prone to *preharvest* contamination and colonization by mycotoxin-producing fungi. Stressed (due to drought) plant seeds are especially at risk. Storage facilities that provide an ideal environment (warm and humid) for the growth of aflatoxigenic fungus pose a threat of *postharvest* contamination.

FACTORS AFFECTING MYCOTOXIN PRODUCTION AND CONTAMINATION

Various factors influence mycotoxin production and contamination in foods and feeds. These factors can be categorized as follows:

- *Physical factors*: These include environmental conditions conducive to fungal colonization and mycotoxin production, such as warm climate, high humidity, and insect infestation which promote mycotoxin production. Frequent droughts contribute to high mycotoxin production.
- *Chemical factors:* (1) Factors such as the use of fungicides will reduce mycotoxin production. (2) Balanced use of nitrogen-, zinc-, potassium-, phosphate-based, and compost fertilizers reduce mycotoxin production. (3) Over-fertilization by nitrogen fertilizers increases deoxynivalenol and zearalenone in maize kernels.

TABLE 35.1: Features of some important mycotoxins.

Mycotoxin group	*Fungi producing toxins*	*Types of mycotoxins*	*Associated commodities*	*Health effects*
Aflatoxins	*Aspergillus flavus*	B1, B2, G1, G2	Cotton, peanuts, spices, maize, pistachios	Carcinogenic (especially aflatoxin B1)
Fumonisins	*Fusarium verticillioides*	A, B1, B2, B3, C, P	Sorghum, maize	Cancer of esophagus humans; hepatotoxicity, carcinogenesis, pulmonary edema, hydrothorax in animals
Trichothecenes	*Myrothecium, Trichoderma, Stachybotrys, Phomopsis, Fusarium graminearum*	T2 toxin, DON, NIV, DAS	Barley, maize, rye, safflower seeds, wheat	Rashes, vomiting, and gastrointestinal bleeding; alimentary toxic aleukia
Ochratoxin	*Aspergillus* species, *Penicillium* species	A, B, C	Rye, wheat, coffee beans, oats, and barley; wines	Nephrotoxic, a potential carcinogen, hepatotoxic, immunosuppressor
Ergot	*Claviceps* species	Alkaloid mixture clavinet, ergopeptine, ergotamine	Historically found in contaminated cereals	Causes ergotism in humans and animals
Cyclopiazonic acid (CPA)	*Penicillium* species, *Aspergillus* species	Related to ergolin	Groundnuts, maize, other millets, cheese	Kodua poisoning
Patulin	*Penicillium* species, *Aspergillus species,*	–	Moldy fruits and vegetables, apples and figs	Damages the immune system in animals
Citrinin	*Penicillium* species, *Aspergillus* species	–	Grains, cheese, sake, miso, soy sauce	Nephrotoxin, uncertain significance
Zearalenone	*Fusarium* species	Zearalenone – F-2 toxin	Many cereals	Mimics estrogen action

(DAS: diacetoxyscirpenol; DON: deoxynivalenol; NIV: nivalenol)

- *Biological factors:* The interaction between toxigenic fungal species and their substrate plays a crucial role in mycotoxin production and contamination. Sugars are a common substrate for all fungi. However, though sugars favor growth, their effect on mycotoxin production may be different depending on the pH, temperature, and composition of the sugar.

Understanding these factors is essential for assessing and mitigating mycotoxin contamination in food products.

Features of some important mycotoxins are given in **Table 35.1**.

CONTROL OF MYCOTOXIN PROBLEMS

Control measures for mycotoxin contamination are crucial for both public health and economic development. Several strategies have been employed worldwide, including in African countries:

- *Prevention of mold and fungus growth:*
  - *Hygienic precautions*: Strict hygiene measures during harvesting, storage, and processing of crops and feedstuffs are essential.
  - *Early harvesting*: Early harvesting of crops, such as groundnuts, can result in lower aflatoxin levels.
  - Proper drying and storage
- *Decontamination of contaminated feeds/foods:*
  - *Physical approaches*: Methods such as sorting, washing, crushing, and dehulling of grains have been effective in removing aflatoxins and fumonisins.
  - *Chemical approaches*: The use of fungicides such as prochloraz, propiconazole, epoxyconazole, and others has been applied to reduce fumonisin and aflatoxin contamination.
  - *Biological approaches:* Introduction of atoxigenic strains of fungi that compete with toxigenic fungi in the environment has led to significant reductions in aflatoxin contamination, particularly in crops such as peanuts.
- *Continuous surveillance and awareness creation:*
  - *Surveillance*: Long-term intervention strategies involve continuous monitoring of mycotoxin levels in crops, animal feed, and human food. Regular food and feed inspections help ensure safety.

- *Awareness*: Creating awareness about the dangers of mycotoxins to human and animal health and productivity is crucial. This can be achieved through government initiatives, private organizations, national media networks, newspapers, magazines, seminars, workshops, and information exchange between researchers and the public.

A. MYCOTOXICOSIS

Aflatoxin

Aflatoxins are derivatives of difuranocoumarin. There are around 12 primary varieties, with B1, B2, G1, and G2 being the most common. The primary aflatoxin is B1. *A. flavus* and *Aspergillus parasiticus* are the primary toxin producers, while other species also create aflatoxins. *A. flavus* produces B1 and B2, while *A. parasiticus* produces G1 and G2. *Penicillium puberulum* also produces aflatoxins.

The metabolites that are light blue (B) or green (G) in thin layer chromatography are known as B1, B2, and G1, G2. The most common type of aflatoxin B1 is toxic and carcinogenic. Aflatoxin M1 (AFM1) is found in *A. parasiticus* fermentation broth, but AFMI and aflatoxin M2 are also created when AFB1 and AFB2 are metabolized in an infected liver. AFM1 can be passed on through milk. The liver is the major target organ, where the cytochrome P450 enzyme transforms aflatoxin to a reactive form capable of binding to proteins and deoxyribonucleic acid (DNA).

Some outbreaks of aflatoxicosis reported are as follows: Aflatoxin was identified in the 1960s in England as the causative agent of Turkey-x-disease, which resulted in the death of 100,000 birds due to the consumption of contaminated groundnuts in animal feed. In 1974, 100 people were killed in epidemics in Gujarat and Rajasthan caused by toxin poisoning in maize. Cancer is caused by aflatoxin metabolites when they intercalate into DNA and alkylate the bases using the epoxide group. Changes to the *p53* gene, which is necessary to halt cell cycle progression or signal programmed cell death (apoptosis), are caused by DNA mutations.

Histopathology

As far as organs are considered, aflatoxin poisoning mostly affects the liver. Aflatoxin overdose produces hepatocyte fatty alterations, acute hepatotoxicity (sudden hemorrhagic necrosis), and bile duct enlargement.

Hepatic architectural distortion and hepatocellular carcinoma (HCC) are possible outcomes of prolonged exposure to aflatoxin, which causes histopathologic cirrhosis symptoms such as fibrosis and nodular degeneration. Aflatoxin poisoning mostly impacts the liver. Aflatoxin toxicity causes bile duct development, sudden hemorrhagic necrosis, and fatty changes in hepatocytes in cases of acute hepatotoxicity.

Different Pathways of Pathogenesis

- The majority of aflatoxin exposure occurs through ingestion. When it enters the body, it is converted to a reactive epoxide intermediate by microsomal mixed-function oxidase (MFO) enzymes in the liver. The CYP450 enzyme family includes MFO. It is this epoxide intermediate (8,9-epoxide) that causes DNA mutations. Genomic analysis has revealed that the p53 tumor suppressor gene's GT transversion at codon 249 is the most prevalent mutation. This epoxide has the ability to disrupt cells by binding to ribonucleic acid (RNA) and proteins, among other macromolecules. The synthesis of DNA, RNA, and proteins is likewise halted.
- Glutathione depletion and consequent toxicity from reactive oxygen species is another route to toxicity.
- Other carcinogenesis routes, catalyzed by prostaglandin H (PGH) synthase and lipid peroxidase (LPO), are being investigated.
- Another method for aflatoxin metabolism is microsomal biotransformation of AFB1 by hydroxylation. It generates less harmful, nonpolar metabolites such as AFM1 and aflatoxin Q1 (AFQ1).
- Dialdehyde can also be generated by AFB1 by enzymatic and nonenzymatic activity. Aflatoxin dialdehyde is converted to dialcohol and eliminated in the urine by aflatoxin aldehyde reductase (AFAR). It is also capable of binding proteins, particularly albumin.

Acute toxicity results when someone consumes a high level of aflatoxins in a very short time. The most common signs and symptoms are nausea, yellowing of skin and sclera (icterus), itching, vomiting, bleeding, abdominal pain, lethargy, edema, convulsions, coma, and death.

Chronic toxicity occurs through consuming small amounts of aflatoxins over a prolonged period. Chronic exposure to aflatoxin can result in the following:

- Impaired growth and development, especially in children
- Immunosuppression
- Hepatocellular carcinoma (weight loss, abdominal mass, anorexia, vomiting, nausea, bleeding, psychosis, etc.)

Maternal exposure to aflatoxin is associated with a higher occurrence of preterm birth and late-term miscarriage.

Detection

Some popular methods to detect aflatoxin exposure in food and feed are:

- Thin-layer chromatography (TLC)
- High-performance liquid chromatography (HPLC)
- Liquid chromatography-mass spectroscopy (LCMS)
- Enzyme-linked immunosorbent assay (ELISA)

ELISA using AFB1-lysine (metabolite of AFB1) concentration in the patient's blood can help detect aflatoxin.

Other techniques are used to detect levels of aflatoxin in the human body.

The AFB-guanine adduct in urine is one indicator. Only exposures within the last 24 hours are considered by this method. This product's level may change as a result of dietary changes due to its variable half-life. This makes it unfit for use in determining the effects of chronic exposure. Another way to detect aflatoxin exposure over time is to measure the levels of AFB-albumin adducts in blood serum.

According to the International Agency for Research on Cancer, it is a Group 1 carcinogen. One of the main causes of HCC is a history of hepatitis B or C infection.

Patients exhibiting symptoms of encephalopathy and fatty degeneration of viscera may be presenting with Reye's syndrome, which is also believed to be an acute aflatoxicosis.

CYCLOPIAZONIC ACID

Tryptophan is the building block of indole tetramic acid, a chemical compound related to ergoline alkaloids. It is produced by *A. flavus, Aspergillus tamarii*, and various species of *Penicillium*, among others. Both groundnuts and maize contain this ATPase inhibitor. Loss of appetite, a decrease in body weight, weakness, nausea, vomiting, diarrhea, depression, seizures, and eventually death are all signs of toxicosis.

FUMONISINS

Since fumonisins disrupt sphingolipid metabolism, they have a wide range of effects on animals. They have a variety of harmful consequences, including hepatotoxicity, carcinogenesis, and pulmonary edema and hydrothorax in pigs, as well as leukoencephalomalacia (hole in the head syndrome) in horses and rabbits. It is possible that this is related to the development of esophageal cancer in humans. In Transkei (South Africa), northeast Italy, and China, fumonisin B1 is associated with an elevated risk of esophageal cancer.

Brief gastrointestinal (GI) pain, borborygmus, and diarrhea were reported in 27 villages in India after consuming moldy sorghum or maize bread, suggesting a potential case of acute fumonisin B1 exposure. Full recovery was achieved by those who were sick.

In animal studies, fumonisins have been associated with neural tube anomalies; in certain cases, this association may extend to humans as well. A cluster of anencephaly and spina bifida cases in southern Texas was allegedly caused by fumonisins found in maize products. After evaluating the potential carcinogenic effects on humans, the International Agency for Research on Cancer classified fumonisins as category 2B. Numerous poisons fall into the A, B, C, and P groups. B1, B2, and B3 are the most common and significant among BA. Ceramide synthetase is inhibited by toxins, preventing the conversion of sphingosine acetyl-CoA to ceramide. This toxin primarily affects maize crops.

PATULIN

While several molds can make patulin, it was *Penicillium patulum* (sometimes called *Penicillium griseofulvum*) that was initially identified in the 1940s as an antibacterial active component.

Even though it cannot withstand fermentation to produce cider products, patulin is frequently present in unfermented apple juice. High concentrations of patulin are lethal in a controlled laboratory setting, despite the fact that evidence for natural poisoning is indirect and inconclusive.

TRICHOTHECENES

Myrothecium, Trichoderma, Stachybotrys, Phomopsis, and F. graminearum are the fungi which produce this toxin.

Other fungi produce trichothecenes, a class of sesquiterpenoid metabolites. Ingesting mycotoxins, which are present in feed and food, can cause rashes, vomiting, and GI bleeding. Initiation, elongation, and termination stages of eukaryotic protein synthesis are all profoundly inhibited by trichothecenes. The Japanese people and their livestock have long been linked to moldy grain "intoxications" and illnesses caused by *Fusarium* mycotoxicosis.

Fusarium graminearum is often discovered on barley, oats, rye, and wheat. Akakabi toxicosis, or red mold disease, may be caused by it. One of the most prevalent mycotoxins discovered in cereals is deoxynivalenol. Pigs and other farm animals lose weight and refuse to eat at lower doses, while higher doses induce diarrhea, vomiting, and nausea. The reason why deoxynivalenol is often called vomitoxin or food rejection factor is because of this.

Many skin, GI, and neurological issues can be traced back to toxins. Diacetoxyscirpenol and T-2 may be related to the human disease known as alimentary toxic aleukia, according to one theory. Some symptoms of the illness include loss of hematopoietic tissues, vomiting, and skin irritation. Symptoms of the acute phase include problems with the central nervous system; bleeding from the mouth, nose, and vagina; and oral necrosis. The human illness known as alimentary toxic aleukia has been linked to T-2 and diacetoxyscirpenol, according to hypotheses. The disease manifests itself in a variety of ways, including skin soreness, nausea, and bleeding. Problems with the central nervous system and necrosis of the mouth, nose, and vagina are hallmarks of the acute phase.

A large portion of the people in the Orenburg region of the former Soviet Union contracted alimentary toxic aleukia during World War II (WWII). The overwintered grain that the sick patients had eaten was infected with *Fusarium sporotrichioides*. One famous example of how these compounds were linked to biological warfare is the purported yellow rain episode in Laos. The following countries have recorded cases of human toxicosis: India (Kashmir), China, Japan, and Korea.

OCHRATOXIN

Ochratoxin A, a metabolite of *Aspergillus ochraceus*, was found in 1965 during a screening for fungal metabolites that aimed to find new mycotoxins. Its isolation from a commercial maize sample in the United States led to its rapid discovery as a powerful nephrotoxin. *Aspergillus ochraceus* produced ochratoxin A, which was discovered in 1965.

The ochratoxin's most probable origin barley is contaminated. Some plants that have been found to contain it include rye, wheat, coffee beans, oats, and barley. It has also been brought to light that certain wines, especially those made from grapes infected with *Aspergillus carbonarius*, may contain ochratoxin. Out of all the toxins produced by *Aspergillus*, only ochratoxin has the potential to be as dangerous as aflatoxins. The kidney is the primary organ that gets targeted.

Being a nephrotoxin, ochratoxin A is lethal to humans and all other animals. Toxins hinder the metabolism of phenylalanine. Ochratoxin A is known to be a nephrotoxin, liver toxin, immunosuppressant, teratogen, and carcinogen, according to animal research.

Ochratoxin has been detected in several animal tissues, including blood, human milk, and others. Pork that is meant for human consumption often has it. Pork nephropathy, which has been studied extensively in Scandinavian countries, is believed to be caused by ochratoxin. Denmark has one of the highest incidences of porcine nephropathy due to the high prevalence of ochratoxin contamination in pig feed.

The human disease known as endemic Balkan nephropathy has sparked concern regarding the potential involvement of ochratoxins. This chronic, progressive kidney disease is more common in those who reside in areas close to the Danube River, such as those in Romania, Bulgaria, and the former Yugoslavia.

This peculiar illness has several possible causes, including exposure to ochratoxin, heavy metals, heredity, and even dormant pathogenic microbes. Several mycotoxin tests have definitively classified endemic Balkan nephropathy as an ochratoxicosis, but the exact cause remains a mystery. Some of the clinical symptoms include mild-to-severe fatigue, headaches, loss of appetite, pale skin, and signs of kidney failure. Furthermore, mycotic porcine nephropathy, a major disease in Denmark, has been linked to the toxin. There is evidence linking the disease to urinary tract cancers, according to American research. Ochratoxin is a substance that the International Agency for Research on Cancer has identified as a potential human carcinogen (type 2B).

ERGOT ALKALOIDS

The ergot alkaloid is produced by species of *Claviceps*. Rye, millet, and other grain flours could be contaminated with the toxin and end up in bread. The alkaloids found in ergot in nature are lysergic acid derivatives. It was not until 1934 that lysergic acid, structurally similar to other ergot alkaloids, was first isolated. The earliest known reference to ergot is in an Assyrian inscription from 600 BCE, which refers to a "noxious pustule in the ear of grain."

The human disease known as ergotism, or Saint Anthony's fire, is brought on by eating cereals that are infected with ergot sclerotia, the most prevalent of which is bread made from flour that is contaminated. There are two common ways that ergotism is categorized: Gangrenous and convulsive. While gangrenous ergotism impacts the circulation to the limbs, convulsive ergotism impacts the brain and spinal cord.

Clinical features of the gangrenous type include swelling, inflammation, paresthesia, and vasoconstriction in the limbs; this form can lead to amputations. The type that causes convulsions impacts the nervous system. According to Matossian, "bad food" is likely to blame for the "slow nervous fever" that eighteenth-century English physician Jon Huxham recorded, which could be another instance of human ergotism. Matossian has also proposed that the ergot alkaloids significantly affected the fertility rates of seventeenth and eighteenth centuries in England

and other European nations. There was a full-length book account of a supposed ergot poisoning in the French commune of Pont-Saint-Esprit in 1951 called The Day of St. Anthony's Fire.

Research on ergot alkaloids yielded the famous hallucinogen lysergic acid diethylamide (LSD) during the 1900s. A number of amines were combined with lysergic acid to form ergobasine, which is also called ergometrine and ergonovine. Then, by modifying the amino alcohol component, the methergine molecule was produced, which has been extensively utilized for decades to decrease postpartum hemorrhage. Sandoz tried to sell LSD to psychiatrists so they could treat schizophrenia, but it did not work. The American Central Intelligence Agency used LSD as a truth serum when questioning individuals suspected of being communists.

In recent times, migraines have been treated using pure ergotamine. When it comes to treating Parkinson's disease, cerebrovascular insufficiency, and prolactin, there are other ergot derivatives that are worth looking into.

ZEARALENONE (F-2 TOXIN)

Although zearalenone is biologically powerful, it is not toxic. Instead, it binds to estrogen receptors in mammalian target cells by suitably mimicking estradiol, the principal hormone produced by the human ovary. Mycoestrogens such as zearalenone, are a type of non-steroidal estrogen. One name for it is a phytoestrogen. The zearalenones are produced by *F. graminearum, Fusarium culmorum, Fusarium equiseti,* and *Fusarium crookwellense* through a polyketide route. Worldwide, cereal crops are frequently contaminated by all of these species.

Dietary zearalenone concentrations in pigs can elicit hyperestrogenic syndromes at as little as 1.0 ppm, and infertility and abortion at higher quantities. Research has also revealed that sheep and cattle can experience difficulties during pregnancy.

Oral contraceptives zearalenol and zearalenone have a history of helping women cope with the symptoms of menopause. It is widely known that endocrine (hormone) disrupters can lower male fertility in both animals and humans.

B. MTCETISM

Most mushrooms are basidiomycetes. Mushrooms are consumed as a food item all over the world. These are edible mushrooms. There are many "look-alike" mushrooms to these edible ones which are actually poisonous. The most prevalent cause of poisoning from mushrooms, which is also known as mycetism or mycetismus, is eating mushrooms that have been foraged and incorrectly recognized. The symptoms of poisoning from mushrooms can range from mild GI disruptions to hallucinations, delirium, cramping, and even death. These mushrooms contain different types of poisonous chemicals. Mushroom poisoning is referred to either with the name of the mushroom or the with the chemical responsible. Some of the important ones are described here.

List: Coprine, amanitin, orellanine, muscarine, gyromitrin, ibotenic acid, and muscimol.

Coprine poisoning: Coprinus atramentarius (C. atramentaria) is the poisonous mushroom—common ink cap—responsible for coprine poisoning.

Consuming "cream of butter sauce" (it contains this mushroom) followed by an alcoholic beverage causes coprine poisoning/syndrome. The following symptoms occur within 5–10 minutes of consuming alcohol: Facial flushing, metallic taste, palpitations, chest pain, headache, nausea, vomiting, vertigo, or disorientation. A week is the typical time frame for a natural healing process. A chemical analogous to disulfiram (Antabuse) is produced by converting coprine. Antabuse acts by blocking the oxidation of alcohol at acetaldehyde stage. Accumulation of acetaldehyde in the blood causes the unpleasant symptoms. This action is through blocking the enzyme aldehyde dehydrogenase (ALDH), which is usually innocuous unless the person is consuming alcohol at the same time.

Coprine poisoning occurs if alcohol is consumed within a few hours (in some cases even 5 days) after ingesting the mushrooms. In this particular situation, the alcohol cannot be metabolized in its entirety.

Amanitin (Amatoxins): The mushrooms of genus *Amanita,* especially *Amanita phalloides* (Green death Cap), as well as those of the genera *Pholiotina, Galerina,* and *Lepiota* produce the toxins called Amatoxins. Amatoxins are a group of cyclic peptides that inhibit RNA synthesis, thereby causing cell death.

During the latency of 6–24 hours, the toxin is absorbed from the GI tract and starts destroying the kidney and liver. After 24 hours, the patient starts vomiting, having cramps and bloody diarrhea. There is apparent recovery, but relapse occurs in which the patient may bleed severely due to destruction of clotting factors; kidneys and liver fail, leading to death.

Orellanine: Orellanine is a nephrotoxin produced by few species in the very large genus *Cortinarius.* It causes *delayed kidney damage.* This toxin generally causes no symptoms for 3–20 days after ingestion. After about 8 days, nausea and vomiting occur along with anorexia, lethargy, polyuria, and thirst. Typically, around day 11, the process of kidney failure begins and is usually symptomatic by day 20. Acute focal tubular damage and interstitial nephritis followed by fibrosis ensue. These changes are irreversible.

Amanita smithiana poisoning: This mushroom causes *prompt kidney damage*—within 3-11 hours. Symptoms start with GI distress, anxiety, chills, oliguria or polyuria, and kidney failure. Sometimes, it is confused with orellanine food poisoning. The exact poisonous moiety is not identified.

Muscarine: It is found in the mushrooms *Amanita muscaria, Inocybe* species, and *Clitocybe* species. Muscarine activates muscarinic receptors on nerve and muscle. Symptoms start after half an hour of consumption of the mushroom. Sweating, salivation, tears, impaired vision, palpitations, colicky pain, diarrhea, and, in large dosages, respiratory failure are all symptoms. Atropine is the specific antidote.

Gyromitrin: It is found in the mushroom of the genus *Gyromitra.* It causes stupor, delirium, muscular cramps, lack of coordination, tremors, and/or seizures by blocking the essential neurotransmitter gamma-aminobutyric acid (GABA). It irritates the GI tract severely, resulting in vomiting and diarrhea. GI disturbances occur after 5 hours of consuming the mushroom.

Liver and kidney damage has been documented in certain cases after about 2 days. It can also cause red blood cells to degrade, resulting in jaundice, renal failure, and anemia symptoms.

Ibotenic acid and muscimol: These are present in *Amanita muscaria* and *A. pantherina.* Upon ingestion, ibotenic acid undergoes decarboxylation to form muscimol. Muscimol causes nausea and vomiting. Bewilderment, elation, or drowsiness and deep sleep are all conceivable. Other possible symptoms include lack of muscular coordination, sweating, and chills. Delusions, intense emotions, or distorted vision affect certain people. Muscimol also induces hallucinations. Deaths have been documented; however, *A. pantherine* infections typically resolve on their own.

Apart from the mushrooms and their toxins mentioned here, there are many mushrooms that can cause mycetism. Some examples are *Omphalotus* species (nausea, vomiting, weakness, dizziness); *Clitocybe* species (erythromelalgia—increased blood flow to extremities); *Tricholoma* species, and *Russula* species (rhabdomyolysis—breakdown of muscle fiber, cardiomyopathy, kidney, and neurotoxicity); *Hapalopilus* (encephalopathy); Psilocybe (hallucinations).

Treatment: Gastric lavage may be helpful very early after consumption of the mushroom. It is mainly supportive—maintaining water and electrolyte balance. Hemodialysis might be helpful. Silibinin can be given; it blocks entry of amatoxins in hepatocytes. Antidotes are known only for few (Atropine for muscarine).

CHAPTER

36 Common Laboratory Contaminants

INTRODUCTION

As fungi are saprophytic and some of them require minimum growth requirement, they may contaminate the cultures. Some of them are associated with some diseases. It is crucial to distinguish the isolate as pathogen or contaminant.

Table 36.1 shows the list of common laboratory contaminants.

TABLE 36.1: List of common laboratory contaminants.

Group	Names
Mucoromycetes fungi	• *Cunninghamella* species • *Absidia (Lichtheimia)* species • *Mucor* species • *Rhizopus* species • *Syncephalastrum* species
Hyaline hypomycetes	• *Acremonium* species • *Aspergillus* species • *Penicillium* species • *Paecilomyces/Purpureocillium* species • *Scopulariopsis* species • *Trichoderma* species • *Trichothecium* species • *Verticillium* species
Phaeoid/Dematiaceous fungi	• *Alternaria* species • *Aureobasidium* species • *Bipolaris* species • *Chaetomium* species • *Cladosporium* species • *Curvularia* species • *Drechslera* species • *Epicoccum* species • *Helminthosporium* species • *Nigrospora* species • *Phoma* species • *Ulocladium* species
Yeast and yeast-like fungi	• *Geotrichum* species • *Rhodotorula* species • *Saccharomyces* species • *Trichosporon* species • *Ustilago* species
Others	• *Chrysosporium* species • *Malbranchea* species • *Sepedonium* species

A. MUCOROMYCETES FUNGI

Cunninghemella

It is possible for *Cunninghamella bertholletiae* to infect humans. The colony is expanding at a rapid rate. The entire Sabouraud dextrose agar (SDA) slant tube is filled with woolly colonies. At its very tip, the sporangiophore displays lateral branches. An enlarged vesicle is visible on every branch. In one stage of the life cycle, sporangioles (not sporangium, as in other Mucorales) contain spores.

Lichtheimia (Absidia)

Lichtheimia is a colony that looks like cotton wool and is developing quickly. Sporangiophores emerge from the internodal space. A prominent apophysis is present. The sporangia have branching.

Mucor

Colonies of this fast-growing fungal infection can be of any shade, from dull gray to brownish-gray. No rhizoids are found. Sporangiophores have several branches. Round or oval-shaped sporangia are seen.

Rhizopus

Colonies first appear white or light gray but eventually darken; the growth rate is rapid. The rhizoids emerge at the bases of the sporangiophores.

Sporangiophores are linear in shape and can be found singly or in clusters. Clusters of sporangia are round.

Syncephalastrum

The colonies start out cottony white and eventually turn gray. The merosporangia are tubular structures that contain chains of sporangia.

B. HYALINE HYPOMYCETES

Acremonium, Paecilomyces, Scopulariopsis, Chrysosporium, Trichoderma, and Penicillium species are discussed in the chapter hyalohyphomycosis.

Cylindrocarpon Species

Both soil and plants contain them. There are very few reports of this pathogen producing infections in neutropenic patients, dermatomycosis, or keratitis. There are no microconidia. Straight or slightly curved macroconidia with smooth walls are present.

Trichothecium

White, pink, or orange-pink colonies are common. Erect and unbranched conidiophores produce clusters of conidia at their tips. Structures with two cells are called conidia.

Verticillium

The colony's surface turns powdery and its color changes from white to yellow, green, or red. Groups of conidiophores with acute tips are seen. Phialides produce single-celled, oval-to-ellipsoid conidia, which can be found alone or in clusters as shown in **Figure 36.1**.

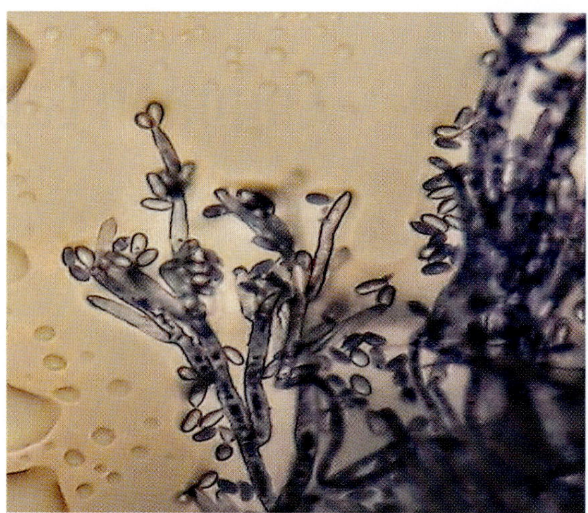

FIG. 36.1: LPCB mount of *Verticillium* species (400×). (LPCB: lactophenol cotton blue)

C. PHAEOID/DEMATIACEOUS OR MELANOGENIC FUNGI

Alternaria

The saprophytic *Alternaria* species fungi decompose plants and soil. You can find them in the air, on plants, and in the dirt. Not only is it a plant pathogen, but it also has clinical implications. In colonies, the hair might be suedelike or floccose, and the color can range from grayish black to black. In appearance, the conidiophore can be either flexuous or pale brown, and it can take the form of a straight, lengthy chain. Sympodial conidia are formed by conidiophores that are either short or long and simple or branched. The surface of the developing conidia is smooth. They have septa that run horizontally and vertically.

Aureobasidium

Mycotic keratitis and peritonitis are extremely rare complications that might occur in patients undergoing continuous ambulatory peritoneal dialysis (CAPD). The colonies start off smooth with a variety of cream to pink shades, but as they mature, they get coated in brown or black conidia.

Arthroconidia are chains of one- or two-celled, thick-walled, darkly pigmented organisms that develop from initially hyaline hyphae that turn dark brown with age. In reality, these arthroconidia are the *Scytalidium* form of *Aureobasidium.* Scar tissue or short denticles can develop conidia in clusters. The walls of conidia are smooth. They have one cell and can be any size or form, with an ellipsoidal shape and often an unclear hilum (a scar or mark where the cell attachment occurs).

Chaetomium

Onychomycosis, cutaneous lesions, peritonitis, and subcutaneous phaeohyphomycosis are the opportunistic infections caused by this extremely rare agent. Their perithecia have an aperture that allows ascospores to be released. There are black, robust hyphae that reach the perithecium. *Chaetomium globosa, Chaetomium strumarium,* and *Chaetomium atrobrunneum* are common species (cause brain abscess).

Cladosporium

The species that were previously known to be thermotolerant and truly harmful to humans have now moved to a different genus, *Cladophialophora.* As with the other species, *Cladosporium cladosporioides, Cladosporium herbarum, Cladosporium oxysporum,* and *Cladosporium sphaerospermum* were all considered medicinally significant. The colonies are fluffy and have a dark backside. Attachment scars are visible, and there is a chain of conidia.

Curvularia

The two most prevalent species are (1) *Curvularia lunata* and (2) *Curvularia geniculata.* Keratitis, sinusitis, phaeohyphomycosis, onychomycosis, and mycetoma are only some of the illnesses that can be caused by these common laboratory pollutants. Their colonies are floccose and black reverse, and they grow quickly. The conidia are arranged in a sympodial fashion, transversely septate, and with a bigger central cell.

Drechslera

It may cause allergic disease or rhinosinusitis. Colonies are rapidly expanding and can be either downy or suedelike, with a black reverse. Typically, spores have a club form, thick walls, and an incomplete transverse septum (pseudosepta). They might be straight or slightly bent. Germ tubes can develop in any part of the conidium. The absence of a protruding hilum and the presence of a flat scar inside the basal cell's base are diagnostic features that distinguish this genus from *Bipolaris.*

Epicoccum

The colonies which can range from downy to suedelike grow rapidly. Mutation from yellow to orange-brown is visible on the back. Under a microscope, it reveals clumps of conidiophores, or black sporodochia. The conidia have a wide attachment scar and a basal morphology resembling a funnel, and their sizes range from 15 to 25 µm. A basal cell is protruding. The outside surface has a bumpy texture.

Helminthosporium

Because of its reputation as a potential contaminant, *Helminthosporium* is rarely found in laboratory specimens. It has six or more cells, is big (9–40 µm), and has a club-shaped appearance. These cells accompany the conidiophores and, at their widest point, face the conidiophore itself. The formation of tall, parallel-walled conidiophores distinguishes this species from *Exserohilum, Drechslera,* and *Bipolaris.*

Nigrospora

Woolly colonies with reverse black emerge in 3–4 days. At the tip of each conidiogenous cell, there is one conidium that measures 14–20 µm in diameter. The conidia are tiny, single-celled, and black and feature a small equatorial germ slit. They are also somewhat flattened horizontally.

Phoma

This plant pathogen is often thought of as a common laboratory contaminant. There is fast colony growth, and the surface is turning gray to brown. A membranous globose structure with a tiny papilla is present; it is called a pycnidium. Conidia are formed by pycnidia, which emerge from pycnidia shaped like volcanoes.

Ulocladium

Colonies are rapidly growing, cottony, brownish, with black reverse.

Conidiophores are simple or branched with geniculate arranged conidia having vertical as well as transverse septae, and are narrowest at the base. Conidia of the genus *Alternaria* look similar but are more elongated.

D. YEAST AND YEAST-LIKE FUNGI

Geotrichum, Rhodotorula, and *Trichosporon* have been discussed in previous chapters.

Saccharomyces

This is called brewer's or baker's yeast. It can occasionally cause thrush, vulvovaginitis, and fungemia. Round-to-oval yeast cells show multilateral buds which is a characteristic finding. When sexual reproduction occurs, internally ascospores are seen.

Ustilago

Colonies are white, moist initially which become membranous to powdery. There are irregular, spindle-shaped yeast-like cells.

E. OTHERS

Chrysosporium

Colonies produced by this fungus are whitish and granular. Hyaline, one-celled conidia are produced directly on vegetative hyphae by nonspecialized conidiogenous cells. Conidia are pyriform to clavate with truncate bases. They may be intercalary (arthroconidia), laterally (often on pedicels), or terminally arranged conidia.

Malbranchea

This fungus is present in soil. It has similarity to *Coccidioides immitis.* The colonies are raised or flat; with or without furrows; and powdery, woolly, or cottony in texture. The color of the colony varies between white, orange, buff, tan, brown, and dark golden. Arthroconidia are one-celled, cylindrical, straight or curved, and truncate. Arthroconidia alternate with disjunctor (sterile and empty) cells. Liberated arthroconidia bear an annular frill. In doubtful situations when it resembles *C. immitis*, it is better to go for a molecular test.

Sepedonium

Colonies produced by this fungus are white to golden yellow and have suede-like or cottony texture. It shows warty macroconidia and microconidia. The differentiating point between this fungus and *Histoplasma* is that the projections present on the surface of macroconidia in it are blunt, while those of *Histoplasma* are sharp.

SECTION

7

Pseudofungal Infections

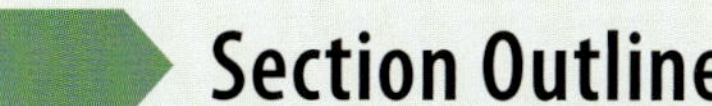

Section Outline

CHAPTER 37

Protothecosis and Chlorellosis

INTRODUCTION

The *Prototheca* genus causes diseases in animals and, rarely, in humans called protothecosis. These are achlorophyllous, algae-like organisms and can be found in nature on a regular basis. To distinguish them from true fungi, these algae cause illnesses that are called "pseudofungi." In animals, the organism causes bovine mastitis and visceral disease, while in humans, the skin, subcutaneous tissue, and lymph nodes are affected. Both immunocompetent and immunocompromised individuals can contract infections; however, those with impaired immune systems are at a higher risk of developing serious and potentially systemic illnesses. Forceful injection through trauma is the mode of spread of infection from environmental sources.

A number of *Prototheca* species, including *Prototheca ciferrii* (previously *Prototheca zopfii* genotype 1), *Prototheca bovis* (formerly *P. zopfii* genotype 2), *Prototheca wickerhamii, Prototheca blaschkeae, Prototheca cutis,* and *Prototheca miyajii,* infect both people and animals. Most of the animal and human infections are caused by *P. wickerhamii* and *P. zopfii*.

HISTORY

In 1894, Krüger found microalgae which he identified as fungi because they were similar to yeasts. He had retrieved the organism from the slime flux of trees. At that time, the pathogenic potential of *Prototheca* was not known. Both animal and human cases of *Prototheca* infection were initially documented in 1952 (Lerche) and 1964 (Davies et al.), respectively. The first human epidemic of protothecosis occurred in a tertiary care chemotherapy department in 2018, and the organism gained importance as a pathogen.

TAXONOMY

The green algae *Chlorella* species and the *Prototheca* microalgae are both members of the Chlorellaceae family, which is in turn part of the Chlorellales order and the Trebouxiophyceae class.

MYCOLOGY

The organism is a heterotroph which lacks chlorophyll and obtains its carbon, nitrogen, and thiamine from other sources. The two-layered cell wall and lack of chloroplasts are the defining characteristics which differentiate *Prototheca* from other types of algae, such as *Chlorella.* Differences between *Chlorella* and *Prototheca* are given in **Table 37.1**. The rRNA sequences showed that *Prototheca* has closer ties to plant life than fungal life.

Most species of *Prototheca* can be cultivated at 30°C for 72 hours, but the strains of *Prototheca* that cause mastitis can be cultured at about 35°C.

On the other hand, some strains do better at 25°C, and it can take up to 7 days for some slow-growing isolates to form noticeable colonies. Add 100 µg/mL of chloramphenicol to glucose-containing culture media (like Sabouraud dextrose agar) to limit bacterial growth.

Morphology of Tissue Forms

The forms seen in tissue are either unicellular endospores or multicellular sporangia which appear in clusters. Asexual reproduction is a feature of protothecosis. Endospores are produced when the cytoplasm is cleaved. Endospores enlarge as time passes and develop into sporangia. 2–20 endospores are produced inside sporangia. The sporangia are known as *morula*. Each

TABLE 37.1: Differences between various *Prototheca* and *Chlorella* species.

Features	*Prototheca species*	*Chlorella species*
Gross lesions (color)	Nonspecific yellowish discoloration or multinodular granulomatous reaction	Multinodular granulomatous reaction
Histopathology (H&E)	Granulomatous or pyogranulomatous chronic lesions with organisms inside	Almost the same as *Prototheca* species
Histochemistry, PAS, and GMS stains	Cell wall reacts positively; intracellular components are poorly stained	Cell wall positive; distinctive and strongly positive intracytoplasmic granules
Chloroplasts and starch bodies (TEM)	Absent	Present

(H&E: hematoxylin and eosin; GMS: Grocott–Gömöri's methenamine silver; PAS: periodic acid-Schiff; TEM: transmission electron microscopy)

morula has a central endospore surrounded by about five endospores.

As a rule, *P. zopfii* sporangia are 7–30 µm in diameter, while *P. wickerhamii* sporangia are 3–10 µm in diameter. The cells of *P. wickerhamii* are round, while the cells of *P. zopfii* are oval or cylindrical. The endospores of *P. wickerhamii* take on a symmetrical arrangement like a *daisy* in the *morula* form, also called *mulberry, spoke wheel,* or *daisy appearance.* Species such as *P. zopfii* do not produce sporangia with as many septa. The term "dauer cell" describes the nondividing and resting states of cells.

PATHOGENESIS

The infectivity of the organism is low. The low number of cases of protothecosis in cancer patients and human immunodeficiency virus (HIV) infection suggests that this group does not pose a significant threat. We know very little about the pathogenesis of protothecosis.

Many species of *Prototheca* may occur as colonizers on human body parts, including the skin, fingernails, lungs, and intestines. This *Prototheca* infection is usually not contagious, whether it is exogenous or endogenous. In humans, *Prototheca* species can spread by contaminated water or soil or through painful injections of the algae.

Surgical and orthopedic procedures have been associated with protothecosis infections in healthcare facilities. There are few situations in which chlorination fails to kill all dangerous microbes. Sewage water and household trash are home to many *Prototheca* species.

Deficiencies in neutrophil function, patients using immunosuppressant or steroid medication, those with a history of blood or solid-tissue cancer, or those with diabetes mellitus are at increased risk of developing endogenous infections. Those who are colonized and have preexisting conditions are more likely to develop endogenous infections.

The organism can be isolated from the environment, animals, and food. Some common habitats for the *Prototheca* species include trees, grass, water (both fresh and salt), animal waste (including that of dogs, deer, and cattle), stables, animal structures, and excrement. In the majority of instances, victims could not pinpoint when the trauma occurred. Incubation periods ranging from 10 days to 4 months have been verified in reports.

Infection in Animals

Not only has protothecosis been observed in bovine mastitis, but it has also been found in many other animal species, such as roe deer, dogs, cats, fruit bats, flying foxes. The identification of antiprotothecal antibodies in serum is used for the diagnosis of protothecal mastitis.

CLINICAL FEATURES

Skin Infection

The skin lesion may be polymorphic and take any form as an erythematous plaque, pustule, papule, nodule, verrucous lesion, vesicle, and ulcer.

Lesion types that are most common include vesicular and ulcerative. Infections typically manifest on the face and extremities. The wounds may drain slowly. Localized lesions are most common. However, those with impaired immune systems are more likely to experience the spread of such diseases.

Olecranon Bursitis

Injuries are the most common cause of subcutaneous olecranon bursa infections. Inflammation, reddening, and mild bursitis (a painful swelling of the bursa) manifest themselves weeks after the injury has occurred.

Systemic Infections

Patients receiving chemotherapy, a solid organ transplant, or an acquired immunodeficiency syndrome (AIDS) treatment are at an increased risk of developing disseminated protothecosis. Dissemination primarily impacts the following organs: Skin, subcutaneous tissue, intestines, peritoneum, blood, and spleen.

LABORATORY DIAGNOSIS

Microscopy

- *Potassium hydroxide (KOH) mount*: 8–20 µm sporangia are seen **(Fig. 37.1)**.
- On Gram staining, the sporangia look like *gram positive* **(Fig. 37.2)**.

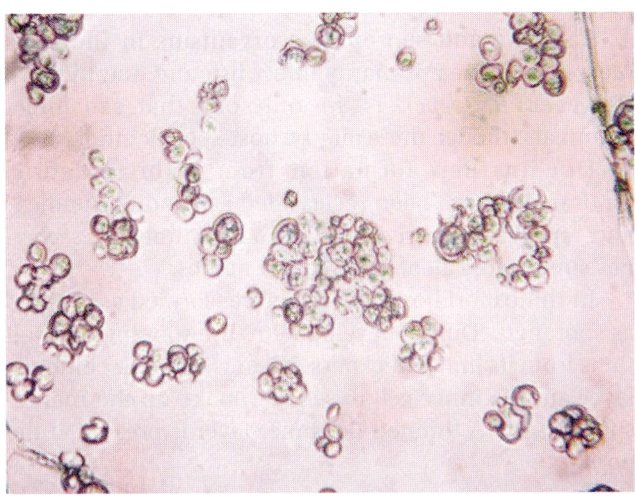

FIG. 37.1: LPCB mount of *Prototheca* species.
(LPCB: lactophenol cotton blue)

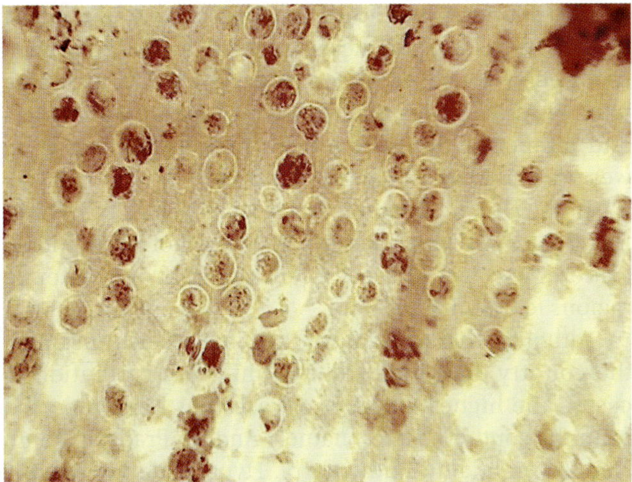

FIG. 37.2: Gram-stained smear of *Prototheca* species.

- For histopathological staining, GMS and PAS are used. The wall of the sporangium and the endospores are uniformly stained. Cells of *P. zopfii* are larger. The morula-like structures are evident in GMS and PAS staining.
- The sensitivity of direct examination is increased by using direct immunofluorescence (DIF).
- The organisms may be confused with spherules of coccidioidomycosis and rhinosporidiosis.

Culture

Sabouraud dextrose agar slants *without* cycloheximide are used for culture, and the yeasty, creamy, dull, or moist to mucoid colonies appear after 24–72 hours of incubation. On *HiCrome Candida agar*, the colonies may be easily confused with those of *Candida*. A lactophenol cotton blue (LPCB) mount will show the sporangia. Various biochemical tests are used for speciation of *Prototheca*.

Commercially available identification systems, such as *API20* and the *Vitek2* identification system, are useful for diagnosis. Matrix-assisted laser desorption ionization-time of flight mass spectrometry (*MALDI-TOF)* is also another option.

TREATMENT

Intravenous amphotericin B is currently considered the most effective treatment for human protothecal infections. Itraconazole and fluconazole have also shown cure or improvement. Intravenous amphotericin B is used for serious infections.

Chlorellosis

Chlorellosis is a very rare illness which is similar to protothecosis, and it is caused by unicellular green algae of the genus *Chlorella*. The organisms are unicellular, spherical or polygonal of size 4–5 µm, and reproduce by an asexual method (endosporulation), producing approximately 20 sporangiospores within sporangia. The wet mount of the specimen shows endosporulating cells with greenish refractile granules suggestive of chloroplasts. The staining methods used for the organism are PAS, GMS, and Gridley fungal stain. The algae grow on simple medium with greenish colonies. The lesions produced by the organisms are greenish in color. The treatment includes debridement. Amphotericin may be useful in the treatment of chlorellosis.

CHAPTER

38 Rhinosporidiosis

INTRODUCTION

Rhinosporidiosis is a granulomatous disease of the mucocutaneous tissue which is common in parts of Africa and the Indian subcontinent. The organism *Rhinosporidium seeberi* causes rhinosporidiosis. It is an aquatic protistan. In addition to the nasal cavity, other areas that may be affected include the nasopharynx, larynx, soft palate, skin, lacrimal sac, nasolacrimal duct, external urethral meatus, and bulbar and palpebral conjunctiva.

HISTORY

In 1812, Malbran was the first Argentinean to record the illness. In 1900, the protozoan parasite *R. seeberi* was discovered in Argentina by Guillermo Seeber as the culprit responsible for nasal polyps.

The causative agent was considered variously as a protozoan, fungus, or a cyanobacterium over the years. Currently, depending on 18S ribosomal DNA sequencing, it is placed in a group of fish pathogens called the DRIP (*Dermocystidium*, the Rosette agent, *Ichthyophonus*, and *Psorospermium*) clade. The DRIP clade is a part of Eukaryota which was formerly a member of the kingdom Protista.

In modern times, *R. seeberi* has superseded all of these earlier names.

The researchers analyzed 18S ribosomal DNA sequences through a phylogenetic analysis. Currently the agent has its taxonomic position as:

- Domain—Eukaryota
- Kingdom—Mesomycetozoea
- Class—Mesomycetozoea
- Order—Rhinosporidia
- Family—Rhinosporideacae
- Genus—Rhinosporidium
- Species—*R. seeberi*

Parasitic and saprophytic organisms in the class Mesomycetozoea primarily infect fish and amphibians. However, *R. seeberi* is the only one that can infect mammals (though there may be host-specific strains).

Due to their formation from cellular debris, "sporangia" have been reclassified as "nodular bodies" and "spores" in *R. seeberi*. In modern times, *R. seeberi* has superseded all of these earlier names.

In rhinosporidiosis, the structures formed are known as sporangia. During development, the sporangium wall thins from its initial thickness of 5 μm. An outer chitinous layer and an inner cellulose layer make up the mature sporangium. A thinned-out inner layer is present at the pore.

EPIDEMIOLOGY

Although it is most common and endemic in tropical and subtropical regions, reports have come in from more than 90 countries. India and Sri Lanka account for almost 90% of the cases. Sporadic cases of the disease have been reported in several countries across the globe, including parts of Africa, the southern United States, South Africa, and temperate South American regions, as well as in western and Middle Eastern countries.

In the United Kingdom, horses and ponies have been found to have several diseases. As a result of international trade and travel, diseases can spread from endemic regions to uninhabited land.

Although rhinosporidiosis is quite prevalent in India, the country does not exhibit a uniform distribution of cases. The highest number of cases has been reported from the southern states, namely Andhra Pradesh, Tamil Nadu, Kerala, and Puducherry. Hyperendemic regions of the disease include Tamil Nadu. Although humans are the most common hosts for rhinosporidiosis, other animals and birds such as horses, caprines, dogs, cats, waterfowl, swans, geese, and wild ducks have also been found to contract the disease. There have been cases of disease in fish as well.

For unknown causes, the disease is prevalent in the 20–40 year age bracket. In Sri Lanka and the southern region of India, this disease is endemic. With the exception of Delhi, Punjab, and Himachal Pradesh, the disease has expanded from its initial detection in Bihar to the following Indian states: Madhya Pradesh, Maharashtra, Odisha, Puducherry, Rajasthan, Uttar Pradesh, Haryana, Kerala, Tamil Nadu, and Chhattisgarh. An outbreak of rhinosporidiosis was detected in both humans and swans in 1990. In a similar vein, Serbia saw a human epidemic of rhinosporidiosis affecting the nose and eyes. Swans in Florida, United States, were also found to have an instance of ophthalmic and cutaneous rhinosporidiosis. Different blood types are associated with different diseases, according to several studies.

Although they are thought to live in soil and water, very little is known about their habitat. Recent research has shown that *R. seeberi* is prevalent in subterranean water sources.

TRANSMISSION

Living in contaminated water, *R. seeberi* is an inevitable part of the ecosystem. The majority of cases originate from communities located close to wetlands, where water pollution poses a threat of infection. Consequently, it was formerly thought of as a fungus that thrives in water. In stagnant water, *R. seeberi* and other aquatic microbes may work together to spread infection.

An interesting aspect of the disease's incidence is that, although hundreds of people in Sri Lanka and many in India take holy baths in stagnant waters, only a small number of people really get the progressive sickness. This could be because there are predisposing factors in the host.

Soil is also a likely natural source. The particles of dust contain spores. Thus, this illness can be spread by dust and contaminated water.

Spores of the agent can be transmitted from animals to humans by aerosols, dust, infected clothing, and swimming in stagnant, dirty water. However, there is no direct transfer between animals and humans.

Mode of Dissemination in the Body

"Autoinoculation" might account for the development of satellite lesions in close proximity to granulomas, especially in the upper respiratory regions, and for the spread of the disease beyond the initial site. Polyp endospore spillover after trauma or surgery is thought to be followed by "autoinoculation" into the surrounding epithelium.

Hematogenous Spread

There is proof that rhinosporidiosis can spread hematogenously to different parts of the body. One possible cause of subcutaneous granulomata in the limbs and other affected areas could be the spread through blood from a latent infection in the upper respiratory tract.

Lymphatic Spread

Nevertheless, the process of regional dissemination remains controversial. Despite the possibility of lymphatic propagation, lymphadenitis has not been seen in any histological examination of localized or disseminated rhinosporidiosis. In 2002, a case of disseminated rhinosporidiosis including the lower limbs was reported for the first time, along with inguinal lymphadenitis.

HISTOPATHOLOGY

Based on the organism's presence in most histological sections throughout its development, its "life cycle" has been speculated. The stroma, which can be fibrous or fibromyxomatous, contains chronic inflammatory cells, including lymphocytes and macrophages. Near the released endospores, there are many neutrophils.

Granulomatous tissue often contains giant cells, sporangia, and stroma. In places other than the lungs, fibrosis is common. Tissues from the same individual can exhibit vastly different stromal and cellular responses. There is a striking similarity between the histology of human and animal rhinosporidiosis. Particularly in areas other than the lungs, fibrosis is noticeable. The fact that stromal and cellular responses might vary widely, even within tissues from the same patient, is an interesting aspect. Veterinary rhinosporidiosis shares many similarities with human rhinosporidiosis in terms of histology.

Pitfalls in the Histopathological Diagnosis

There are, however, instances when confusion, misdiagnosis, or a false-negative diagnosis can be made on histopathology. Such instances were reviewed as follows:

- Rhinosporidial tissue, especially in nasopharyngeal rhinosporidiosis, in which rhinosporidial structures may be absent despite the presence of marked cell infiltrates; other portions of the polyp, however, may show rhinosporidial structures. Inappropriate selection of portions of such polyps for histology might result in a false-negative diagnosis.

- Sporangia with atypical walls in which the well-marked, bilamellar thick wall is absent.
- Only fragments of the sporangial wall are occasionally visible; and hence may be missed.
- Sporangia may be absent in some sections though sporangiospores are present. These could be missed unless stained by mucicarmine or PAS.

Differences from Similar Pathogens

Rhinosporidiosis may have to be differentiated from adiaspiromycosis. The walls of adiaconidia (size 200–400 μm) are substantially thicker in adiaspiromycosis. These adioconidia are enlarged single fungal cells; while rhinosporidiosis shows sporangia that are filled with sporangiospores. Another agent to be differentiated is *Coccidioides immitis*. *Coccidioides immitis* can be distinguished morphologically because it lacks electron-dense bodies (EDBs) by an electron microscope. The intrasporangial endospores of *R. seeberi* are bigger and more frequent, but the endospores of *C. immitis* are considerably smaller (2–5 μm). Rhinosporidiosis can be stained by mucicarmine stain, while *Coccidioides* cannot.

Other Features and Life Cycle of Rhinosporidiosis

When stained properly, cytodiagnosis on lump aspirates from rhinosporidial infections, surface secretion smears from accessible polyps, and fine-needle aspirates from lumps can reveal a variety of diagnostic characteristics.

In the nasopharynx in particular, endospores might be mistaken for epithelial cells. The PAS stain is used to differentiate between these two states. In contrast to the PAS-negative epithelial cells, the endospores are a vivid magenta color. Identification is made easier when EDBs are found in endospores.

Having a single nucleus in granular cytoplasm, the sporangium, initially, is thin walled and is 6–8 μm in size. As sporangia evolve from immature to intermediate to mature (50–400 μm), their wall thickness and lamination change, and the appearance of the nuclei around which the cytoplasm condenses to form endospores changes as well.

Round, thick-walled structures inside the sporangium with a diameter of 10–12 μm are the mature endospores. The most mature endospores along the inner wall of the sporangium or the sporangium itself are thought to be the origin of the endospores in the intermediate sporangia. Up to 20 spherical EDBs measuring 1-3 μm embedded within endospores are a distinguishing feature of the mature endospores. These are nutritional reserves made of protein, perhaps precursors of trophocytes.

Several stages of development occur in the sporangia, beginning with the thin-walled juvenile sporangia (15–40 μm, trophocytes) and progressing to the mature sporangia (containing hundreds of endospores embedded in a mucoid matrix).

The operculum is an opening in the mature sporangium that allows the endospores to be released. The many stages of fungal development can be easily discernible using specialized stains such as Grocott-Gömöri methenamine silver (GMS), Gridley's, and PAS stains.

A "capsule" of fibrils and a hazy, electron-dense substance is found to encase the walls of immature sporangia, making them unilamellar. In more mature sporangia, the "capsule" encases bilamellar walls, which consist of a thinner electron-dense outer wall and a thicker, see-through interior wall. Juvenile and intermediate sporangia have been described by multiple authors as having a nucleus complete with a nucleolus and nuclear membrane. Several writers have provided descriptions of "laminated (multilamellar) bodies" that are around 2 μm in diameter and consist of granular material surrounded by two or more rings that are electron dense. One distinguishing feature of sporangia is the sporangial wall, which is thickened around the opening through which the endospores are released into the surrounding tissues, thus concluding the "life cycle." It is believed that tissue pressure from sources external to the sporangia produced the ejection.

IMMUNITY

Although antirhinosporidial humoral and cell-mediated immune responses occur in human rhinosporidiosis, there is evidence that *R. seeberi* avoids particular immune responses via the methods listed below:

- *Sequestration of antigen*: The endospores' thick wall, which comprises chitin and cellulose, is impenetrable to the outflow of intraendosporial antigens and immune destruction. However, phagocytosis and the subsequent death of endospores may result in antigen release.
- *Antigenic variation*: A new antigen appears in the wall of sporangia.
- *Immune distraction*: There is a possibility that immune distraction by free antigen might conceivably contribute to immune evasion.

CLINICAL FEATURES

The organism affects mucocutaneous surfaces, and the clinical presentation is determined by the location, size, and extent of the lesion. The organism has a varied incubation time, and the disease lasts from 1 to 10 months.

Nasal Rhinosporidiosis

The nasal passages are the usual sites of rhinosporidiosis symptoms. Polypoid, friable lesions are visible that bleed easily. Raised bumps on the skin of lesions look like strawberries, raspberries, or cauliflower. The front of the nose is the most typical location for polypoid lesions. In rare cases, a polypoid tumor could develop in the nasopharynx.

A foreign body sensation, nasal obstruction, and epistaxis are present, yet the patient is not in pain. Sporangia, which appear as little white spots under the epithelium, can be seen upon close inspection.

Ocular Rhinosporidiosis

This site accounts for a significant portion of infections. The bulbar and palpebral conjunctiva show signs of lesions.

While most cases involve only one eye, there have been reports of binocular cases as well. Perceiving a foreign body is the result of the lesion. The lesions are known to bleed. It is quite unlikely to be the cause of keratitis.

Cutaneous Rhinosporidiosis

Lesions that resemble warts or are sessile can be discovered on the face and nose. It is common for subcutaneous nodules to develop ulcers.

Disseminated Rhinosporidiosis

Lymphatic or hematogenous dissemination can lead to the spread of disease. Any part of the body could be affected. Evidence from postmortem examinations suggests that the disease may have spread to several organs, including the skin, bones, liver, spleen, brain, and lungs.

Miscellaneous Manifestations

Instances of rhinosporidiosis in the penis, urethra, buccal cavity, vulva, and vagina are rare. The most often recognized route of infection for genitourinary infections is bathing in contaminated water, while sexual transmission is also a possibility. The scalp, larynx, lips, mouth, and rectum are uncommon sites of rhinosporidiosis infection. A painless polyp can protrude through the meatus and cause hematuria and intermittent bleeding when the urethra is involved. Anal lesions of rhinosporidiosis are comparable to hemorrhoids or condyloma.

Differential Diagnosis

Neoplasia, tuberculosis, syphilis, lepromatous leprosy, leishmaniasis, and rhinoscleroma are some differential diagnoses depending on the site of the lesion.

Histopathological differentiation from coccidioidomycosis and adiaspiromycosis should be performed. In comparison to *Coccidioides, R. seeberi* has a larger and thicker sporangium, but the spherule is thinner and smaller (30–60 µm). It has thinner walls than adiaspiromycosis.

LABORATORY DIAGNOSIS

Microscopy

Since it cannot be grown, the diagnosis is made based on histological findings. Samples can be obtained in a variety of ways, including fine needle aspiration, biopsies and nasal washes. It all starts with the potassium hydroxide (KOH) mount. KOH mount can show sporangia with endospores. For biopsy, FNAC other staining methods are Mayer's Mucicarmine stain, GMS, PAS, and hematoxylin and eosin (H&E) **(Fig. 38.1)**. One identifying feature is the presence of endospores inside the sporangia that measure 10–400 µm.

Mayer's mucicarmine stains mucopolysaccharide in the sporangium wall and on the outside of newly released endospores. It stains these structures red.

Culture

No artificial culture media have been found to be suitable for successfully cultivating the organism. Epithelial cancer

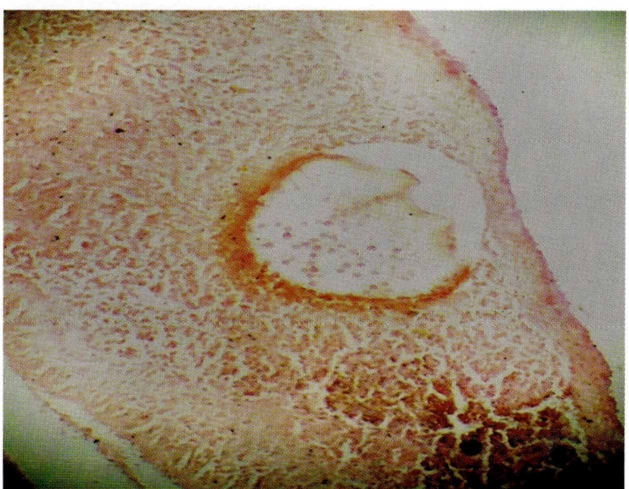

FIG. 38.1: Biopsy stained with H&E showing sporangium (400×). (H&E: hematoxylin and eosin)

cell lines may show some growth, but this expansion cannot be sustained.

Immunodiagnosis

Very little is known about the serodiagnosis of the disease. No diagnostic tests are available.

TREATMENT

Surgical procedures, electrocautery, laser therapy, and conventional medicine are all viable options for treatment. Recurrence is the issue after surgical resection. Electrocautery not only reduces bleeding, but also stops spores from being released and deposited on nearby tissues.

The antileprosy drug dapsone is now undergoing clinical trials for the treatment of skin lesions and the prevention of recurrence after surgery. Surgery using coblation is also utilized by some surgeons to treat rhinosporidiosis (Coblation technology uses a plasma field to precisely dissolve targeted tissue. It ensures maintaining the integrity of the surrounding tissue. Radiofrequency-based devices use high temperatures to cut and cauterize, while coblation technology uses lower temperatures, causing minimal damage to the surrounding tissue).

Additionally, the simultaneous irrigation with saline causes a constant cooling effect. Through the use of the coblation technique, it is possible to completely remove the lesion while minimizing blood loss and contamination and preserving the health of the surrounding tissue.

CHAPTER

39 Pythiosis

INTRODUCTION

Some of the free-living organisms capable of producing human infection are included in the group of hydrophilic organisms. One of them includes pseudofungi. *Pythium* and *Lagenidium* are the organisms which may occasionally produce human infections. The organisms are flagellated and have fungus-like filamentous morphology. The disease has many similarities with mucormycosis.

These oomycetous fungi can be found in soil and water all around the world. *Pythium* species are significant plant diseases that cause seed decay, pre- and postemergent damping off, seedling root rot, and rot of stored foods.

HISTORY

In 1901, Dutch researchers in Indonesia discovered the disease, which was previously known as hyphomycosis destruens equi.

The other names of the disease are equine phycomycosis, granular dermatitidis, leeches, swamp cancer, and summer sores. The disease was observed in horses from India and was called bursatee (from the vernacular name Burus which means rain sores).

Organism (*Pythium insidiosum*)

Due to coenocytic filamentous forms seen in the organism, the *Pythium* species was initially considered as fungus (water mold). Its cell wall composition is different; it has unique molecular and biochemical characteristics; it contains biflagellate zoospores (asexual reproduction); and it reproduces sexually via oogamic techniques. The cell wall contains cellulose and β-glucan instead of chitin. There is no ergosterol in the plasma membrane. It carries diploid nuclei. The organism is also differentiated from fungi by 18S rRNA studies. The infecting agent is now placed in the kingdom Protista.

The male sexual structures are known as antheridia, while female structures are known as oogonia. Sexual reproduction occurs by oogamy, and it results in the production of sexual spores known as oospores. Asexual reproduction occurs by the formation of zoospores in sporangia. The zoospores are motile due to the presence of two flagella, and they have diploid nuclei.

Many different media are suitable for *Pythium insidiosum* growth. Submerged colonies with short aerial filaments and a gently radiating pattern can be found on cornmeal agar. The colonies can range in color from white to colorless. A hypha's diameter ranges from 4 to 10 µm, and its lateral branches are angled at right angles to one another. In contrast to their abundance in mature, viable hyphae, cross-septa are extremely rare in immature hyphae. Many different-sized appressoria and hyphae are present.

To attach themselves to host plants and animals, zoospores secrete an amorphus sticky material. As a potential virulence factor, this molecule—which may be a glycoprotein—has been associated with infection initiation.

TAXONOMY

Pythium insidiosum is included in the family Pythiaceae of order Pythiales in the class Oomycetes of phylum Oomycota in the kingdom Stramenopila.

LIFE CYCLE

Pythium insidiosum can be found in both water and land. A plant host, neutral pH, and low ion concentrations are necessary for sporangia generation and zoospore release. Zoospores are able to attach to the surface of their hosts because they are encased in an amorphous material that has adhesive properties. They shed their flagella, attach to a sticky substance, and germinate upon arrival at the host, developing hyphae and a germ tube. Hyphae reassert themselves inside the host tissue.

EPIDEMIOLOGY

Compost, water, and decomposing organic matter are all potential breeding grounds. There may be infection of livestock, pets, and crops. Its prevalence increases during the wetter months, leading some to refer to this veterinary disease as "swamp cancer." Infectious agents can be found in many plant species, including water lilies. Transmission from animal to animal or animal to human is not observed. Infectious zoospores can penetrate through tiny wounds. Drinking of contaminated water may rarely transmit the disease. The majority of cases have been reported from Thailand, and thalassemia has been found to be the most common underlying condition. Cases have been documented in several countries, including Thailand, India, Indonesia, Japan, Australia, New Zealand, South and North America, and North Korea.

IMMUNITY

In terms of immune response, the fungus can activate either antibody-mediated or cell-mediated mechanisms. Two important antigens are the (1) one found in culture filtrate and (2) second found in sonicated hyphae.

PATHOGENESIS AND PATHOLOGY

Infectious forms are zoospores. Tissue infection can also occur through other structures, such as hyphae and dormant spores. When white blood cells attack zoospores, degranulation happens. The presence of eosinophil precipitate surrounding the hyphae is the culprit behind the Splendore-Hoeppli (S-P) phenomenon. The histopathology report shows eosinophilic granular, stony masses of necrotic tissue with hyphae and eosinophils within hyphae, called "kunkars" (occur in animals). The organism is angioinvasive. Arteritis, thrombosis, and the development of aneurysms are all outcomes of the agent's angioinvasive nature. The differences between this fungus and other fungi with aseptate hyphae are shown in **Table 39.1**.

CLINICAL FEATURES

A comparison of pythiosis with mucormycosis and entomophthoromycosis is given in **Table 39.1**. Though human infection is rare, but if not treated, it may result in a fatal disease. There are four types of infections caused by the organism which include:

1. Cutaneous–subcutaneous disease
2. Ocular disease
3. Vascular–systemic disease
4. Disseminated disease

Cutaneous and Subcutaneous Infection

Lesions include cellulitis, ulcerative granulomatous lesion, and nodules under the skin. All parts of the body are affected, including the head and neck, face, limbs, perineum (which contains the genitalia and anus), and periorbital region (which includes the face, nose, lip, and oral cavity). The lesions may open outside by the formation of sinus tracts.

Ocular Infection

Keratitis, orbital cellulitis, or corneal ulcers accompany cases of ocular pythiosis. Redness and swelling around the eyes and nose can be signs of cellulitis.

It could take anything from 2 days to over a month for clinical ocular pythiosis to emerge. The formation of grayish-white stromal infiltrates with feathery margins

TABLE 39.1: Comparative clinical and related features of pythiosis, mucormycosis, and entomophthoromycosis.

Features	*Pythiosis*	*Mucormycosis*	*Entomophthoromycosis*
Status of host	Host is apparently normal; thalassemic patients are more prone and disease has a protracted course	Compromised, particularly with underlying diabetes, rapidly progressive	Host normal; slow progress
Inflammatory response	Granulomatous response occurs, and Splendore–Hoeppli phenomenon is seen; angioinvasion is seen	Suppurative response; angioinvasion is seen	Granulomatous response marked; Splendore–Hoeppli phenomenon and angioinvasion are rare
Angioinvasion	Common	Very common	Unusual
Size of hyphae in the infected tissue	Approximately 3–10 μm diameter; uniform in size; nonseptate	Approximately 10–15 μm diameter; nonseptate	Approximately 7–20 μm diameter; nonseptate; ribbon

on slit-lamp biomicroscopy is a characteristic clinical sign. In untreated cases, enucleation or evisceration is required.

Vascular and Systemic Infection

Myelodysplasia, thalassemia, aplastic anemia, paroxysmal hemoglobinuria, idiopathic thrombocytopenic purpura, leukemia, and, to a lesser degree, alcoholism, malnutrition, immunosuppression, human immunodeficiency virus (HIV) infection, cancer, and neutropenia are the underlying predisposing conditions.

Arteritis with gradual ascent is present in the legs. Infection of a medium- to large-sized artery (arteritis) is a common complication of vascular pythiosis, leading to inflammation of the surrounding tissues, thickening of the arterial wall, formation of aneurysms, blockage of the vascular lumen (such as thrombosis), and gangrenous tissue. Arteries can experience blood loss. When the renal artery, aorta, and common iliac and femoral arteries are implicated, the prognosis is not good. The patient usually succumbs to a systemic disease within 2 weeks. Surgical treatment is the sole alternative since antifungal drugs do not alleviate this condition.

Disseminated Infection

It is common for multiple organs to be engaged in the diagnosis process. After the condition progresses, it involves the arteries.

Differential Diagnosis

Pythiosis, like infections with *Conidiobolus* and *Basidiobolus,* causes an eosinophilic granuloma. Aspergillosis and mucormycosis are two possible manifestations of the angioinvasive infections.

LABORATORY DIAGNOSIS

It is easy to mistake this illness for mucormycosis since most microbiologists are unaware of it. The importance of early diagnosis cannot be overstated, as the illness has the potential to be lethal. The diagnosis is made by collecting pus exudate and biopsy samples.

Microscopy

Hyphae are aseptate or sparsely septate, with a width of 3–10 µm and a branching angle of almost 90°. Mucormycosis cases have broad, hyphae which are 10–15 µm in diameter.

Histopathological Examination

When stained with hematoxylin and eosin (H&E), hyphae appear irregularly stained. Because of this, we advise using Grocott's-Gömöri methenamine silver (GMS) and periodic acid-Schiff (PAS) stains. Encircling the hyphae is where you can observe the S-P phenomenon is present surrounding the hyphae.

Yellow masses with foci of coagulative necrosis containing neutrophils, eosinophils, occasional giant cells, and hyphae are characteristic histopathological findings. Because *Aspergillus, Fusarium,* and *Scedosporium* hyphae exhibit narrow-angle dichotomous branching, this type of hypha is easily distinguishable.

Direct immunofluorescence test can be useful for the diagnosis of *P. insidiosum.*

Culture

Various media can be utilized, including Sabouraud dextrose agar (SDA), blood agar, brain heart infusion agar, and others, which are incubated at temperatures of 25 and 37°C, respectively. Colonies are formed during incubation for around 24–48 hours; they are flat, glabrous, and initially yellowish white but eventually turn cream or light brown. At 25°C, the organism stops growing.

A cultured lactophenol cotton blue (LPCB) mount reveals hyphae that are aseptate and have granular cytoplasm. Extensive branching and terminal swelling are observed in several of the hyphae.

The histopathological finding of the presence of eosinophilic inflammatory response is used to differentiate the cases of pythiosis from mucormycosis.

Induction of Sporulation

It is not always the case that the isolate will show spores when grown on regular media. The *P. insidiosum* growth is covered with a few sterile grass leaves and left to incubate at 37°C for 24 hours. Under a microscope, sporangium that contains zoospores can be observed along the border of the leaf. Take the grass leaves into a beaker containing a mild salt solution and let them sit at 37°C for 2 or 3 hours. The leaf is carefully studied under a microscope. Zoospores that are motile and have flagella will serve as a diagnostic tool.

Serological Tests

The antigen is tested by reacting it with antisera that have been generated in animals in an immunodiffusion test that uses culture filtrate antigen.

Despite its modest sensitivity, the test has a high specificity. Due to this, alternative methods such as complement fixation test (CFT), enzyme-linked immunosorbent assay (ELISA), and Western blotting are employed.

One sensitive method for prognosis monitoring is the ELISA that uses soluble antigen from damaged hyphae. The disease can be detected at an early stage with its help.

Keratitis is diagnosed via molecular assays, specifically DNA sequence analysis. Reverse transcriptase polymerase chain reaction (RT-PCR) is a great tool for diagnosis as well. Matrix-assisted laser desorption ionization-time of flight mass spectrometry (MALDI-TOF MS) may quickly and cheaply identify the pathogen. A DNA probe is also developed for the diagnosis.

TREATMENT

Some of the treatment options include immunotherapy, surgical debridement, and antimicrobial medications. The lack of ergosterol as the principal sterol in the cytoplasmic membrane of the agent renders antifungal medicines ineffective. A course of itraconazole with terbinafine for 1 year was effective in treating arteritis in certain patients. In cases of subcutaneous infections, a solution of saturated potassium iodide is administered to the patient. The best course of treatment is surgery. Radical removal of diseased tissue is necessary for a localized lesion. In order to treat keratitis, a keratoplasty operation is performed.

Vaccines

Antigens are derived from the infectious pathogen and used to create vaccines. Animals are treated with them. The antigen used to make Mendoza's soluble concentrated antigen vaccine is extracted from culture filtrate. Another choice is the sonicated hyphal antigens used in Miller's cell mass immunization. Immunotherapy was used to treat one human case. A year after receiving two doses of the *P. insidiosum* vaccine at 2-week intervals, the child showed signs of improvement.

LAGENIDIOSIS

The disease was officially recognized as distinct in 2003. In the United States, it was found in canines suffering from an invasive cutaneous infection. The mosquito larvae are infested with the parasite *Lagenidium giganteum*. Its infectious zoospores are biflagellate. Mosquitoes may carry these spores on their cuticles. Multiple tissues are engaged, including those on the surface, under the skin, and in the subcutaneous layer. Like pythiosis, this organism is an oomycete. Infection develops when environmental zoospores penetrate wounds that are exposed to the skin. No record exists of the transmission from one to the other. The United States, and more especially the states of North and South Carolina, is the site of the vast majority of mammalian infections.

The important species of the genus *Lagenidium* are *L. giganteum, Lagenidium ajelloi, Lagenidium albertoi,* and *Lagenidium vilelae.*

Clinical Features

Dogs can get oomycotic infections all over their bodies, including their limbs, mammary gland, perineum, and trunk, which manifest as cutaneous and subcutaneous sores. Cellulitis and sinus formation, most commonly on the extremities, are symptoms in humans.

Ulcers may form from nodules. Aneurysms can form in animals when lymph nodes and large blood arteries are affected. Death occurred when the aneurysms ruptured.

Giemsa staining of the specimens shows extensive hyphae with branches.

In order to diagnose and assess prognosis, antibodies are detected by the use of ELISA and Western blotting.

Many species of *Lagenidium* are easily cultured. Rapid colony growth occurs at 37°C for this species. Wide aseptate hyphae with spherical features are visible under the microscope. Colonies of various sizes are produced by incubating the peptone yeast extract agar culture at 30°C for 3 days.

Treatment

The treatment is similar to that of pythiosis. Early surgery followed by itraconazole is successful.

SECTION

8

Annexures

Section Outline

ANNEXURE

1 Culture Media

INTRODUCTION

The selection of the proper medium is a crucial step in diagnostic medical mycology laboratories, as it plays a significant role in the isolation, identification, and maintenance of fungal strains. The choice of medium depends on the expertise of the mycologist and the fungi typically found in a particular geographic region. Several culture media are commonly used in mycology, but one of the most prominent is *Sabouraud dextrose agar (SDA).*

BASAL MEDIA

Basal media are essential for isolating, growing, and maintaining common fungal pathogens. One of the most widely used basal media in mycology is *SDA.*

Sabouraud Dextrose Agar

Sabouraud dextrose agar is one of the primary media used for isolating fungi from clinical samples, subculturing, and short-term maintenance of fungal isolates. Originally developed in 1892 by the French dermatologist and mycologist *Raymond Jacques Adrien Sabouraud,* it is now a standard in diagnostic mycology laboratories. It is particularly useful for isolating dermatophytes and other pathogenic fungi, as it supports fungal growth while inhibiting contaminating bacteria due to its acidic pH.

Key Features of Sabouraud Dextrose Agar

- *Composition*: Peptones (source of nitrogen), 4% dextrose (carbon and energy source), and agar
- *pH*: Acidic (around 5.6), which supports fungal growth but can inhibit bacterial growth
- *Usage*: Primarily used for studying colony morphology of fungi, especially dermatophytes
- *Dextrose (glucose)*: Carbon source for fungal growth
- *Peptones*: Provide nitrogen and essential nutrients
- *Agar*: Acts as a solidifying agent
- *Mixing*: Combine ingredients
- *Boiling*: Bring to a boil
- *pH adjustment*: Adjust pH to 5.5–6.0
- *Dispensing*: Pour approximately 7.0 mL into large test tubes
- *Autoclaving*: Sterilize for 10 minutes at 15 psi
- *Solidification*: Allow tubed media to solidify in a slanted position
- *Storage*: Keep at 4°C
- *Shelf life*: 30 days in test tubes and 14 days in Petri dishes
- *Quality control*:
    - Sterility check
    - Color examination
    - Performance test: Good growth of *Aspergillus flavus* at 30°C
    - Additional notes:
        - SDA can be dispensed into sterile Petri dishes, available commercially with preparation following the manufacturer's instructions.
        - pH 5.5–6.0 inhibits bacterial contaminants and enhances dermatophyte pigmentation.
        - pH 7.0 is optimal for isolating systemic organisms.

Sabouraud Dextrose Agar with Antibiotics

Contents

- *Peptone*: 10.0 g
- *Glucose*: 10.0 g
- *Cycloheximide*: 0.5 g
- *Chloramphenicol*: 0.05 g

- *Agar*: 15.0 g
- *Distilled water*: 1.0 L

Preparation

- Dissolve cycloheximide in 10.0 mL of acetone.
- Dissolve chloramphenicol in 10.0 mL of 95% ethanol.
- Mix all ingredients.
- Bring to a boil. Adjust pH to 6.8–7.0.
- Dispense approximately 7.0 mL in large test tubes.
- Autoclave for 10 minutes at 15 psi.
- Slant test tubes.
- *Storage*: 4°C.
- *Shelf life*: 30 days in test tubes, 14 days in Petri dishes.

Quality Control

- Sterility
- Color
- Performance (see below)

Fungus Incubation Results

- *Trichophyton mentagrophytes* 30°C: Good growth
- *A flavus* 30°C: No growth

Variants

Sabouraud dextrose agar with antibiotics: SDA can be supplemented with antibiotics such as cycloheximide or benomyl to selectively inhibit bacterial or saprophytic fungal growth, making it more effective for the selective cultivation of pathogenic fungi.

Neutral Sabouraud Dextrose Agar (Emmons' Modification)

Neutral SDA, also known as *Emmons' modification*, is a modified version of the traditional SDA that was developed by *Chester W Emmons*. The modification involves two key changes:

1. *Lower glucose concentration*: The dextrose content is reduced from 40 to 20 g/L, bringing the concentration down to 2%.
2. *pH closer to neutral*: The pH is adjusted to 6.8–7.0, which is more neutral compared to the original acidic formulation.

This modification was made to improve the isolation of certain fungi, particularly *opportunistic* and *dimorphic fungi*, which may not thrive in the more acidic environment of traditional SDA. For example, *Blastomyces dermatitidis* is better recovered using this neutral medium. Neutral SDA is also widely used for the *maintenance of clinical fungal isolates*.

Composition of Neutral Sabouraud Dextrose Agar (Emmons' Modification)

- *Neopeptone*: 10 g
- *Dextrose*: 20 g
- *Agar*: 20 g
- *Distilled water*: 1,000 mL
- *Final pH*: 6.8–7.0

Preparation Procedure

1. *Combine* the ingredients (neopeptone, dextrose, and agar) with distilled water.
2. *Adjust the pH* of the medium to 6.8–7.0.
3. *Sterilize* the medium by autoclaving at 121°C for 15 minutes.
4. *Pour* the medium into sterile Petri dishes or test tubes, allowing it to solidify.
5. *Store* the prepared plates at 4°C until use.

This neutral SDA is favored in diagnostic mycology laboratories for the *primary isolation* of various fungi and is a reliable medium for the growth of opportunistic pathogens that might not grow well on traditional acidic SDA.

ENRICHED MEDIA

Enriched media are designed to support the growth of fastidious or pathogenic fungi by providing additional nutrients. They are especially useful for isolating fungi from clinical specimens and may include selective agents to inhibit contaminants. The following enriched media are commonly used:

- *Brain heart infusion agar (BHIA)*:
  - *Purpose*: Used for growing fastidious fungi and for the in vitro conversion of mycelial to yeast forms of dimorphic fungi (M↔Y)
  - *Ingredients*:
    - Brain heart infusion: 37 g
    - Glucose: 20 g
    - L-Cysteine hydrochloride: 1 g
    - Agar: 20 g
    - Distilled water: 900 mL
  - *Preparation*:
    - Dissolve the ingredients by boiling.
    - Dispense into screw-cap tubes and autoclave at 121°C for 15 minutes.
    - Adjust pH to 6.7.
    - Cool in a slanted position with a 1-inch butt.
    - Store in the refrigerator.

Note: Antibiotics such as cycloheximide, chloramphenicol, and gentamicin can be added to inhibit unwanted organisms.

- *Cystine heart and hemoglobin agar (CHHA)*:
    - *Purpose*: Alternative to BHIA for primary isolation and in vitro conversion of dimorphic fungi (M↔Y)
    - *Ingredients*:
        - Dehydrated cystine heart agar: 10.2 g
        - Hemoglobin: 2.0 g
        - Distilled water: 100 mL
    - *Preparation*:
        - Dissolve the ingredients.
        - Autoclave the medium.
        - Add antibiotics if necessary.
        - Store in the refrigerator.
- *Biphasic medium*:
    - *Purpose*: Used for recovering fungi from blood; it combines an agar medium with broth.
    - *Ingredients:*
        - *BHIA*: Sterilized and slanted
        - *BHI broth:* Added aseptically
    - *Preparation*:
        - Sterilize BHIA and keep it slanted.
        - Aseptically add BHI broth to cover approximately 40% of the agar in the standing position.
        - It can be used with or without antibiotics.

NUTRITIONALLY DEFICIENT MEDIA

Nutritionally deficient media are designed to suppress vegetative growth and stimulate sporulation in fungi. They are also useful for the preservation of fungi as stock cultures. Some commonly used nutritionally deficient media are as follows:

- *Cornmeal agar (CMA)*:
    - *Purpose*: Stimulates chlamydospore formation in yeasts and is used for morphological examinations
    - *Ingredients*:
        - Cornmeal: 8 g
        - Agar: 4 g
        - Distilled water: 200 mL
        - Tween 80 (1%): 2 mL
    - *Preparation*:
        - Heat cornmeal and water at 60°C for 1 hour.
        - Filter the mixture through filter paper.
        - Add distilled water to make up to 200 mL and then add agar.
        - Autoclave at 121°C for 15 minutes.
        - Pour into Petri plates.

Notes:

- Zein, a protein extracted from corn, can be used as an alternative to cornmeal (Zein 40 g/100 mL).
- Cornmeal Tween agar can be prepared by adding Tween 80 before autoclaving. Tween 80 decreases surface tension, aiding in chlamydospore production.
- To examine yeast morphology, streak a heavy inoculum of yeast across the plate and cover with a coverslip. Incubate for 24–48 hours at 25°C. Observe under low-power microscopy at the edge of the coverslip, where aerobic and anaerobic conditions meet.
- Chlamydospores are best observed at this junction. Trypan blue, a vital dye, can be added to the medium to enhance the visibility of chlamydospores.
- Chlamydospores are rarely produced at 37°C.
- *Rice starch agar (RSA)*:
    - *Purpose*: Used to induce faster chlamydospore formation in *Candida albicans* and *Candida dubliniensis* compared to CMA.
    - *Ingredients*:
        - Cream of rice: 2 g
        - Tween 80: 2 mL
        - Agar: 4 g
        - Distilled water: 200 mL
    - *Preparation*:
        - Add cream of rice to boiling water and boil for 30 seconds.
        - Filter through a cotton tampon and adjust the volume to 1 L with water.
        - Add agar and Tween 80 and then dissolve while heating.
        - Autoclave at 121°C for 15 minutes.
        - Pour into a cylinder and leave overnight in a water bath at 60°C.
        - Decant the clear portion, refilter through cotton, and autoclave again at 121°C for 15 minutes.
        - Adjust pH to 6.2 and pour into Petri plates.

These media are critical for observing specific fungal characteristics and aiding in the identification of fungi based on their sporulation patterns.

SELECTIVE MEDIA

- *Bird seed agar (BSA)*:
    - *Purpose*: Used for the primary isolation of *Cryptococcus* species. The medium helps in the presumptive identification of this genus by its brownish pigmentation due to melanin production.
    - *Ingredients*:
        - Niger seed extract: 200 mL
        - Glucose: 1 g
        - Diphenyl solution: 10 mL
        - Agar: 20 g
        - Distilled water: 800 mL
    - *Preparation*:
        - Autoclave at 121°C for 15 minutes.
        - Dispense into tubes.

Notes:

- Diphenyl inhibits saprotrophic fungi.
- After inoculation, incubate at 37°C for up to 2 weeks. Examine periodically for brown-colored, mucoid colonies that turn black or brown.
- An SDA control should be inoculated simultaneously to ensure that the colonies are not naturally pigmented.
- *Sunflower seed agar (SSA)*:
  - *Purpose*: Used for the primary isolation of *Cryptococcus* species, similar to bird seed agar.
  - *Ingredients*:
    - Pulverized sunflower seed: 45 g
    - Chloramphenicol: 100 mg
    - Agar: 20 g
    - Distilled water: 1,000 mL
  - *Preparation*:
    - Autoclave at 121°C for 15 minutes.
    - Dispense into plates.

Notes:

- Adjust the pH to 5.6.
- Incubate at 30°C after inoculation.
- *Dichloran Rose Bengal Chloramphenicol (DRBC) agar:*
  - *Purpose*: Used for selective isolation of yeasts and molds, especially in food samples
  - *Ingredients*:
    - Rose Bengal: Xanthene dye used for color
    - Dichloran: Additional component
    - Chloramphenicol: Inhibits bacterial growth
  - *Preparation*:
    - Suspend 31.6 g in 1,000 mL distilled water.
    - Heat to boiling to dissolve.
    - Sterilize by autoclaving at 15 lbs pressure (121°C) for 15 minutes.
    - Mix well and pour into sterile Petri plates.

Note: An improved DRBC medium (DRBCm) can be prepared with *Guizotia abyssinica* seeds and creatinine for better recovery of *Cryptococcus neoformans.*

- *Blood agar*:
  - *Purpose*: Used to isolate *Histoplasma capsulatum* and *B. dermatitidis* from clinical specimens
  - *Ingredients*:
    - Agar base: 40 g
    - Sheep blood: 50 mL
    - Distilled water: 1,000 mL
- *Lowenstein-Jensen medium*:
  - *Purpose*: Primarily used for isolation and cultivation of *Mycobacterium tuberculosis* but can also be used for isolating *Madurella* and *Nocardia* species
  - *Ingredients*:
    - Coagulated hen's egg
    - Mineral salt solution
    - Asparagine
    - Malachite green: Acts as a selective agent
- *Dermatophyte test medium (DTM)*:
  - *Purpose*: Used for presumptive identification of dermatophytes in hair, nail, and skin specimens. Produces a red color due to a pH change.
  - *Ingredients*:
    - Phyton: 10 g
    - Dextrose: 10 g
    - Phenol red solution: 40 mL
    - 8 N HCl: 6 mL
    - Actidione: 500 mg
    - Gentamicin: 100 mg
    - Agar: 20 g
    - Distilled water: 1,000 mL
  - *Preparation*:
    - Final pH is 5.5 ± 0.4.
    - Incubate at 25°C. Color change occurs within 3–6 days.
- *Dermatophyte identification medium (DIM)*:
  - *Purpose*: Used for presumptive identification of dermatophytes and can also be used for primary isolation of dimorphic fungi
  - *Ingredients*:
    - Dextrose: 20 mg/mL
    - Neopeptone: 10 mg/mL
    - Cycloheximide: 4 mg/mL
    - Penicillin: 20 U/mL
    - Streptomycin: 40 U/mL
    - Bromocresol purple: 1.6 mg/mL
  - *Preparation*: Incubate at 37°C. Color changes from greenish blue to purple within 24–48 hours.
- *Czapek-Dox agar*:
  - *Purpose*: Synthetic medium recommended for subculturing filamentous fungi, useful for identifying *Aspergillus* and *Penicillium* species.
  - *Ingredients*:
    - $NaNO_3$: 3.0 g
    - K_2HPO_4: 1.0 g
    - KCl: 0.5 g
    - $MgSO_4 \cdot 7H_2O$: 0.5 g
    - $FeSO_4 \cdot 7H_2O$: 0.01 g
    - Glucose: 30 g
    - Agar: 15 g
    - Distilled water: 1,000 mL
- *Peptone yeast extract glucose (PYG) agar medium:*
  - *Purpose*: Contains peptone, yeast extract, and glucose. It is useful for cultivating fungi.
  - *Ingredients*:
    - Bactopeptone: 5 g
    - Yeast extract: 5 g
    - Glucose: 20 g
  - *Preparation:* Adjust pH to 7.2.

- *Malt extract agar*:
  - *Purpose*: Used for early growth and sporulation of fungi and for maintenance. It can be acidified for purifying bacterial contaminants.
  - *Ingredients*:
    - Malt extract: 20 g
    - Peptone: 1 g
    - Glucose: 20 g
    - Agar: 15 g
    - Distilled water: 1,000 mL
- *Oatmeal agar*:
  - *Purpose*: Enhances sporulation in phaeoid fungi
  - *Ingredients*:
    - Tomato paste: 10 g
    - Oatmeal: 10 g
    - Magnesium sulfate: 1 g
    - Potassium phosphate: 1 g
    - Sodium nitrate: 1 g
    - Agar: 15 g
    - Distilled water: 1,000 mL
  - *Preparation*: Adjust pH to 5.6.
- *Potato dextrose agar (PDA)*:
  - *Purpose*: Stimulates sporulation and helps in maintaining stock cultures. It is used for primary isolation and morphological description.
  - *Ingredients*:
    - Potatoes: 250 g
    - Dextrose: 20 g
    - Agar: 20 g
  - *Preparation*: Scrub, slice, and boil potatoes in distilled water. Filter and add agar and dextrose.
- *Modified Dixon agar*:
  - *Purpose*: Used for growth of *Malassezia* species
  - *Ingredients*:
    - Malt extract: 3.6%
    - Mycological peptone: 0.6%
    - Ox bile: 2%
    - Tween 40: 1%
    - Oleic acid: 0.2%
    - Glycerol: 0.2%
    - Agar: 1.2%
    - Chloramphenicol: 0.5%
    - Cycloheximide: 1 g/L
- *Leeming and Notman agar*:
  - *Purpose*: Provides better recovery of *Malassezia* species and has a longer shelf life.
  - *Ingredients*:
    - Peptone: 1.0 g
    - Glucose: 1.0 g
    - Yeast extract: 0.2 g
    - Ox bile: 0.8 g
    - Glycerol: 1.0 mL
    - Glycerol monostearate: 0.05 g
    - Tween 60: 0.5 mL
    - Olive oil: 2.0 mL
    - Agar: 1.5 g

MEDIA USED FOR BIOCHEMICAL TESTS

In a diagnostic mycology laboratory, various media are employed for biochemical testing to differentiate and identify fungi. A summary of some key media used for these purposes is as follows:

- *Carbohydrate fermentation media*:
  - *Purpose*: Determines the ability of fungi to ferment various carbohydrates
  - *Ingredients*:
    - Peptone: 1%
    - NaCl: 0.5%
    - Andrade's indicator: 0.005%
    - Carbohydrates (e.g., dextrose, lactose, maltose, sucrose): 2%
    - Inverted Durham tube for gas detection
  - *Preparation*:
    - Mix peptone, NaCl, Andrade's indicator, and carbohydrates in distilled water.
    - Autoclave at 10 lbs pressure.
  - *Incubation*: At 37°C for 24–48 hours
  - *Observations*: Production of acid and gas
- *Carbohydrate assimilation media*:
  - *Purpose*: Tests the ability of yeasts and yeast-like fungi to assimilate specific carbohydrates.
  - *Ingredients*:
    - Carbohydrate-free medium
    - Carbohydrate-containing filter paper disks
    - Glucose (internal control)
  - *Procedure*:
    i. Inoculate on carbohydrate-free medium.
    ii. Add carbohydrate-containing disks.
    iii. Growth around the disk indicates positive assimilation.
  - *Components*:
    - Sugar disks (10% concentration)
    - Extra pure agar: 2%
    - KNO_3 disk: 4%
    - Yeast carbon base (YCB): 1.17%
    - Yeast nitrogen base (YNB): 6.7%
- *Tetrazolium reduction medium (TRM)*:
  - *Purpose*: Differentiates various *Candida* species based on their ability to reduce tetrazolium.
  - *Ingredients*:
    - Peptone: 1 g
    - Glucose: 4 g
    - Beef extract: 0.1 g
    - Tetrazolium: 20 mg

    - Neomycin: 50 mg
    - Distilled water: 100 mL
  - *Preparation*:
    - Autoclave all ingredients except tetrazolium and neomycin.
    - Add tetrazolium and neomycin after autoclaving.
    - Adjust pH to 5.6–6.2.
  - *Results*:
    - *Candida albicans*: Pale pink
    - *Candida tropicalis*: Orange pink
    - *Candida pseudotropicalis*: Salmon pink
    - *Candida parapsilosis*: Rose pink
    - *Candida guilliermondii*: Pink and pasty
    - *Candida krusei*: Pink and dry
    - *Candida glabrata*: Pale pink
- *Urease medium*:
  - *Purpose*: Detects urease production in yeasts
  - *Ingredients*:
    - Peptic digest: 1.0 g
    - Dextrose: 1.5 g
    - NaCl: 5.0 g
    - Disodium phosphate: 1.2 g
    - Monopotassium phosphate: 0.8 g
    - Phenol red: 0.012 g
    - Agar: 15.0 g
    - Distilled water: 950 mL
  - *Preparation*:
    - Mix all ingredients in distilled water.
    - Autoclave at 121°C for 15 minutes.
    - Adjust pH to 6.8 ± 0.2.
    - Add 50 mL of 40% filter sterilizes urea solution to autoclaved and cooled (50°C) basal medium.
  - *Results*: Color changes from amber to pinkish red, when test is positive.
- *Rapid urease test*:
  - *Purpose*: Provides quick results for urease production.
  - *Procedure*:
    i. Inoculate a sterile swab with yeast colony.
    ii. Dip in Christensen's urea agar base.
    iii. Place swab in a tube with three drops of 1% benzalkonium chloride and plug with cotton.
    iv. Incubate at 45°C and check for color change from yellow to purple.
  - *Results*: It indicates urease production by *Cryptococcus* species.
- *CHROMagar Candida medium*:
  - *Purpose*: Selective and differential medium for identifying various *Candida* species and other yeast-like organisms
  - *Ingredients*: Chromogenic substrates for enzyme detection
  - *Preparation*:
    - Prepare medium and pour into plates, as per manufacturer's instructions.
    - Incubate at 30°C for 48–72 hours.
  - *Results*:
    - *Candida albicans*: Light green
    - *Candida dubliniensis*: Dark green
    - *Candida glabrata*: Pink to purple
    - *Candida krusei*: Pink
    - *Candida parapsilosis*: Cream to pale pink
    - *Candida tropicalis*: Blue with pink halo
    - *Prototheca*: Cream-colored colonies, smaller than *C. parapsilosis*
- *Canavanine glycine bromothymol blue (CGB) agar*:
  - *Purpose*: Differentiates *Cryptococcus gattii* from other *Cryptococcus* species
  - *Components*:
    - *Solution A*:
      - Glycine: 10 g
      - KH_2PO_4: 1 g
      - $MgSO_4$: 1 g
      - L-Canavanine sulfate: 30 mg
      - Thiamine hydrochloride: 1 mg
      - Distilled water: 100 mL
    - *Solution B*:
      - Sodium bromothymol blue: 0.4 g
      - NaOH (0.01 M): 64 mL
      - Distilled water: 36 mL
  - *Preparation*:
    - Prepare and sterilize both solutions.
    - Mix and prepare the medium with agar.
    - Pour into tubes to make slants.
  - *Testing*:
    - Inoculate and incubate at 37°C for 1–5 days.
    - *Cryptococcus gattii* will turn the medium cobalt blue; others remain yellow to light green.

ANNEXURE

2 Mycology Stains

CLASSIFICATION OF STAINS IN DIAGNOSTIC MYCOLOGY

Clearing Agents

Preparation of Potassium Hydroxide Solution

- *Standard potassium hydroxide (KOH) solution (10%)*:
  - KOH: 10 g
  - Glycerol: 10 mL
  - Distilled water: 80 mL
- *Enhanced KOH solution with dimethyl sulfoxide (DMSO)*:
  - KOH: 20 g
  - DMSO: 40 mL
  - Distilled water: 60 mL

Note: DMSO allows for immediate examination without waiting for dissolution.

Procedure

1. *Slide KOH preparation*:
   - *Specimen*: Place epidermal scales, skin scrapings, nail clippings, or homogenized biopsy tissue on a clean glass slide. For suspected mucormycosis, place tissue without homogenization to preserve morphology.
   - *Application*: Add a drop of KOH (10%) on the specimen and cover with a coverslip. Press lightly to create a monolayer and remove excess fluid.
   - *Heating*: Gently warm the slide using a flame or slide warmer to speed up the clearing process. Avoid excessive heating to prevent KOH crystallization. With DMSO, heating is not required.
   - *Observation*: Let the slide sit for 5–30 minutes at room temperature and then examine under a microscope. If the specimen is not adequately dissolved, it can be kept in a wet Petri dish and examined later.
   - *Enhancement*: For better visualization, especially of *Malassezia* species, mix KOH (20%) with an equal part of Parker ink. Alternatively, add a drop of acridine orange (0.01%) for fluorescent microscopy.
2. *Tube KOH preparation*:
   - *Application*: For biopsy specimens or materials that dissolve slowly, dissolve the homogenized specimen in KOH (10%) and incubate at 37°C overnight. After incubation, prepare a slide mount for examination.
   - *Concentration*: For difficult specimens such as nail clippings or skin biopsies, increase KOH concentration up to 40%.

Examination

- *Microscopy*: Examine the wet preparations under 10×, 20×, and 40× magnification. Thoroughly search the smear for fungal elements such as hyphae, yeast cells, pseudohyphae, spherules, or sclerotic bodies.
- *Reporting*: If no fungal elements are seen, report as "no fungal element seen." Distinguish between artifacts and actual fungi and confirm findings with additional wet mounts and differential stains.

Notes:

- *Sensitivity*: The KOH wet mount is a simple and cost-effective method for fungal diagnosis. Adding fluorescent brighteners such as calcofluor white (CFW) enhances sensitivity.
- *Identification*: Experienced technicians can differentiate between yeast and mycelial forms (septate/nonseptate) and between dermatophyte and nondermatophyte fungi.
- *Culture correlation*: If KOH mount is negative but fungal growth is observed in cultures, repeat the culture. The presence of the same fungal growth in subsequent cultures confirms its significance.

Alternatives

Sodium hydroxide (NaOH): It can be used instead of KOH but tends to crystallize faster.

Negative Stains

- *India ink stain*:
  - *Purpose*: Visualizes encapsulated fungi such as *Cryptococcus* species by creating a contrast between the clear halo around the fungus and a black background.
  - *Ingredients*:
    - India ink: 150 mL
    - Merthiolate (1:1,000): 3 mL
    - Tween 80 (1:10,000): 0.1 mL
  - *Modification*: Add 2% chromium mercury for enhanced detail
- *Nigrosin stain*:
  - *Purpose*: Alternative negative stain to India ink, used to visualize encapsulated fungi
  - *Ingredients*:
    - Nigrosin granules: 10 g
    - Formalin (10%): 100 mL
- *Procedure for both*: Mix clinical material with stain on a slide, cover with a coverslip, and examine under a microscope.

Note: Nigrosin has a longer shelf life and reduces infection risk compared to India ink.

Fluorescent Stains

Overview

Calcofluor white is a fluorescent dye used to visualize fungal cell walls by binding to chitin and cellulose. It enhances the sensitivity of fungal detection compared to conventional methods such as KOH wet mounts. CFW fluoresces light blue under UV light, making it useful for identifying fungi in clinical specimens and mixed infections.

Preparation

- *CFW solution*:
  - Reagents:
    - CFW M2R: 100 mg
    - *Evans blue*: 50 mg
    - *Distilled water*: 100 mL
  - *Procedure*:
    i. Dissolve CFW powder in distilled water to a final concentration of 0.1%.
    ii. Add Evans blue (0.1%) to reduce nonspecific background fluorescence.
    iii. Mix well and store in a refrigerator.
- Procedure:
  i. Prepare a slide with a specimen and KOH solution, add CFW solution, and observe under a fluorescent microscope.
  ii. *Fluorescence*: Fungi fluoresce apple-green under UV light.

  Note: It is useful for mixed infections and various fungi, including *Pneumocystis* and *Microsporidium*.

Advantages

- *Higher sensitivity*: CFW is more sensitive than KOH wet mounts, making it easier to detect fungal elements.
- *Mixed infections*: CFW allows better visualization of mixed fungal infections.
- *Nontoxic*: CFW is a nontoxic biological marker that fluoresces bright apple green.

Limitations

- *Artifacts*: Artifacts may appear if the stain is not freshly prepared or properly filtered.
- *Equipment*: It requires a fluorescent microscope, which may not be available in all laboratories.

Alternatives

Blankophor (1%): An alternative to CFW, giving less artifacts and not precipitating with KOH. It is useful for diagnosing fungi, including *Pneumocystis* and *Microsporidium* species, as well as nonfungal agents such as free-living amoebae and larvae of *Dirofilaria*.

Lactophenol Cotton Blue Stain

Overview

Lactophenol cotton blue (LCB) is used to study the morphological features of fungal isolates from culture media. It helps visualize the external and internal structures of fungi.

Types and Preparation

- *Plain LCB*:
  - *Ingredients*:
    - Melted phenol: 20 mL
    - Lactic acid: 20 mL
    - Glycerol: 40 mL
    - Cotton blue: 0.05 g
    - Distilled water: 20 mL

- *Procedure*:
  i. Dissolve cotton blue in distilled water.
  ii. Mix with melted phenol, lactic acid, and glycerol.
  ii. Store the solution properly.
- *LCB with polyvinyl alcohol (PVA)*:
  - *Ingredients*:
    - PVA powder: 15 g
    - Distilled water: 100 mL
    - Melted phenol: 22 mL
    - Lactic acid: 22 mL
    - Cotton blue: 0.05 g
  - *Procedure*:
    i. Prepare PVA stock solution by dissolving PVA powder in hot distilled water.
    ii. Mix PVA stock with melted phenol, lactic acid, and cotton blue.
    iii. Warm gently to dissolve.
  - *Alternative stain*: Safranine can replace cotton blue.

Procedure

1. *Mount preparation*:
   - For yeasts, use a round loop; for molds, use an L-shaped loop to take a small fragment of fungal culture.
   - Add a drop of LCB stain to the slide.
   - Tease apart the culture using two needles or a transparent tape method.
   - Place a coverslip and seal edges with nail polish, if needed.
2. *Microscopy*: Examine under a light microscope to study morphological details.

Advantages

- *Morphological detail*: It provides excellent detail of fungal structures, useful for identifying and differentiating fungal species.
- *Permanent mounts*: PVA allows for permanent preservation of mounts.

Limitation

Artifact identification: The preparation requires careful handling to avoid artifacts.

PHOL Stain

Overview

PHOL stain is used for the examination of fungal isolates and *Prototheca* species. This is an alternative stain to LCB with few modifications. It uses formalin instead of phenol and methylene blue instead of cotton blue.

Preparation

Reagents:
- *Formalin*: Replaces phenol
- *Methylene blue*: Replaces cotton blue

Procedure

The procedure is similar to LCB.

Advantage

Morphological analysis: It is useful for fungal and algal differentiation.

Neutral Red Stain

Overview

Neutral red is a vital stain used to assess the viability of fungal elements. It penetrates viable cells and is stored in lysosomes.

Procedure

Application:
- Apply neutral red stain to the specimen.
- Viable cells will take up the dye, which is useful for differentiating live cells from nonviable ones.

Advantages

Viability testing: It measures the effect of test substances on fungal viability, particularly in dermatophytes and *Candida* species.

Diazonium Blue B Stain

Diazonium blue B (DBB) is used to differentiate between *Trichosporon* (basidiomycetous) and *Geotrichum* (ascomycetous) species based on their pigmentation reaction.

Procedure

- *Reagent*: Alkali-ethanol DBB solution
- *Application*:
  - Inoculate the sample and perform the DBB reaction by adding 1–2 drops of DBB solution directly on the colonies and observe color that usually develops within 2 minutes.

- Observe color changes: Pink to violet indicates *Trichosporon*; no color change indicates *Geotrichum*.

Advantages

Differentiation: It helps distinguish between morphologically similar genera based on pigment production.

Limitations

Reproducibility: The molecular basis is not fully understood, but the reaction is reliable and empirical.

DIFFERENTIAL STAINS

Several stains are used to identify fungal elements in clinical specimens, either routinely or as special stains when fungal infections are suspected. The commonly used stains for fungal detection are given in the following text.

Gram Stain

Gram stain was developed by Hans Christian Gram in 1882; this method distinguishes bacterial species as *gram-positive* or *gram-negative* based on their cell wall properties. Fungi also appear *gram-positive* and stain violet in Gram-stained smears.

Routine Gram stain procedure:

1. Fix the smear by passing it through a flame.
2. Apply 0.5% aqueous *crystal violet* solution for 20 seconds.
3. Rinse with tap water.
4. Apply *Gram's iodine* for 20 seconds and rinse again.
5. *Decolorize* with a solution of acetone and ethanol (1:1), followed by a quick water rinse.
6. Counterstain with 0.5% aqueous *safranin* for 10 seconds.
7. Rinse, air dry, and examine under a microscope.

Modifications:

- *Weigert's modification*: It uses *carbol gentian violet* as the primary stain, *Gram's iodine* as a mordant, and *aniline-xylol* as the decolorizer. This method stains *Pneumocystis* cysts.
- *Brown and Brenn modification*: It stains *Nocardia*, *Actinomyces*, and *Microsporidium* species in tissues. It is preferred for sections over smears.

Observations:

- *Gram-positive organisms*: Violet
- *Gram-negative organisms*: Red
- *Nuclei*: Red
- *Background*: Light pink or colorless

Modified Acid-fast Stain

This stain is particularly useful for detecting *aerobic actinomycetes* like *Nocardia*, which are *weakly acid-fast* and appear pink or red. It also stains fungal species such as *Pichia anomala* and *Saccharomyces cerevisiae*.

Procedure (modified Ziehl-Neelsen):

1. Fix the smear by passing it over a flame.
2. Flood the slide with 1% *carbol fuchsin*, applying intermittent heat.
3. Rinse and decolorize with 1% aqueous sulfuric acid.
4. Counterstain with 0.3% *methylene blue* for 1 minute.
5. Rinse, dry, and examine.

In the *cold acid-fast staining (Kinyoun method)*, the phenol concentration is increased, allowing for the stain to penetrate without heating. This method also stains *Coccidian protozoa* (e.g., *Cryptosporidium*, *Cyclospora*, *and Cystoisospora*).

Hematoxylin and Eosin (H&E) Stain

H&E staining is a basic method in diagnostic pathology, used to observe *nuclei* and *tissue structures*. It serves as a background stain for suspected fungal elements, which may be confirmed using special stains such as periodic acid-Schiff (*PAS*) or Grocott-Gömöri's methenamine silver (*GMS*).

Staining procedure:

- *Hematoxylin* stains nuclei *blue* or *purple*.
- *Eosin* counterstains cytoplasm and various tissue components *red* or *pink*.

Observations:

- *Nuclei and fungi*: Blue to purple
- *Muscle and keratin*: Deep pink/bright red
- *Collagen and reticulin*: Pink
- *Red blood cells*: Reddish orange

May–Grunwald Giemsa (MGG) Stain

This compound stain, which results from the interaction of *methylene blue* and *eosin*, is especially useful for detecting *intracellular yeast cells* such as *Histoplasma capsulatum*.

Staining procedure:

1. Fix smears in *methanol* for 5–10 minutes.
2. Stain with *May-Grunwald* for 10 minutes and then with *Giemsa* for 15 minutes.
3. Wash, differentiate in water, and air dry.

Observations:
- *Nuclei*: Purple
- *Cytoplasm*: Blue to mauve
- *Red blood cells*: Pink

Diff-Quik Stain

Diff-Quik is a differential stain primarily used for blood and vaginal smears. It provides rapid staining and differentiation and is based on a modification of the Wright stain pioneered by Bernard Witlin in 1970. The stain is widely used for its ability to provide quick results, reducing a 4-minute process into a simplified 15–50 seconds operation. It allows selective increased eosinophilic or basophilic staining depending on the time the smear is left in the solutions.

Solutions required:
- *Fixative (fast green in methanol)*—pale green
- *Stain solution 1 (eosin G in phosphate buffer)*—red
- *Stain solution 2 (thiazine dye in phosphate buffer)*—blue

Staining procedure:
1. Fix smear by immersing the slide in Diff-Quik fixative for 10 seconds. Blot edges.
2. Stain by immersing the fixed slide in Diff-Quik solution 1 for 20 seconds. Blot edges.
3. Counterstain by immersing the slide in Diff-Quik solution 2 for 20 seconds. Blot edges.
4. Rinse the slide gently in distilled water. Blot and allow to dry.
5. Examine under low power and then under oil immersion for detailed observation.

Observations:
- Yeasts, bacteria, and squames generally stain blue.
- Inflammatory cells stain similar to Romanowsky stains.

Periodic Acid-Schiff Stain

The PAS stain highlights polysaccharides in the fungus and bacterial cell walls by oxidizing them to aldehydes, which then react with Schiff's reagent to produce a magenta or deep pink color. This stain is especially useful for demonstrating fungi in tissue.

Solutions required:
- Periodic acid (1% aqueous)
- *Schiff's reagent:*
  - Basic fuchsin: 1 g
  - Potassium/sodium metabisulfite: 2 g
  - Concentrated hydrochloric acid: 2 mL
  - Activated charcoal: 2 g
  - Distilled water: 200 mL

Staining procedure:
1. Oxidize sections with periodic acid solution for 5 minutes.
2. Rinse well with distilled water.
3. Treat with Schiff's reagent for 15 minutes.
4. Wash in running tap water for 5–10 minutes to intensify the color reaction.
5. Stain nuclei with hematoxylin, then dehydrate, clear, and mount.

Observations:
- PAS-positive substances stain *magenta/deep pink.*
- Nuclei stain *blue.*

Gridley's Fungal Stain

This stain, uses chromic acid as an oxidizing agent to stain fungi purplish-red. It is advantageous for revealing more internal structures of fungi but can also stain elastic fibers and mucins, complicating fungal identification.

Solutions required:
- Chromium trioxide (4% aqueous)
- Schiff's reagent
- Aldehyde fuchsin solution
- Tartrazine solution

Staining procedure:
1. Oxidize with chromic acid for 1 hour and then wash.
2. Treat with Schiff's reagent for 15 minutes.
3. Treat with sulfurous acid for 6 minutes.
4. Wash thoroughly and then treat with aldehyde fuchsin for 20–30 minutes.
5. Stain with tartrazine and then wash and mount.

Observations:
- Fungi, elastic tissue, and mucins stain *purple.*
- Background stains *yellow.*

Grocott–Gömöri's Methenamine Silver Stain

Grocott–Gömöri's methenamine silver (GMS) stain is a staining technique primarily used to demonstrate fungal organisms and certain bacteria in tissue sections. It works on the principle of aldehyde group liberation, where aldehydes reduce the methenamine silver nitrate complex, resulting in the deposition of reduced silver in the fungal cell walls, causing them to appear brown-black.

Key features and applications:
- *Used for demonstrating fungi* in tissue, such as *P. jirovecii* and various filamentous bacteria (e.g., *Actinomyces, Nocardia*)
- *Stains both live and dead fungi*, unlike the PAS stain, which stains only live fungi
- Stains fungal elements *black*, mucopolysaccharides *dark gray*, cytoplasm *old rose*, and tissue *pale green*

Advantages:
- GMS is a more reliable method for visualizing both fungi and filamentous bacteria.
- It can stain certain bacteria, such as actinomycetes, which are not stained by other fungal staining methods.

Disadvantages:
- The tissue reaction is not clearly visible with GMS stain alone. Therefore, it is sometimes combined with H&E staining to simultaneously visualize fungi and the tissue reaction.
- Overimpregnation can lead to the blackening of connective tissues, making fungal identification more difficult.

Staining solutions:
- Chromium trioxide (chromic acid) solution (4% aqueous)
- Methenamine solution (3% aqueous)
- Silver nitrate stock solution (5%)
- Borax solution (5%)
- Ferric chloride solution (0.1% aqueous)
- Sodium metabisulfite solution (1% aqueous)
- Sodium thiosulfate solution (5% aqueous)
- Light green stock solution (used for counterstaining)

Staining procedure:
1. *Prepare tissue sections* and bring them to water.
2. *Oxidize* in 5% chromic acid solution for 1 hour. Wash in water.
3. Bleach in metabisulfite solution for 1 minute.
4. After silver impregnation in GMS staining, the tissue sections can sometimes develop excess background silver or unwanted dark precipitates.
5. Sodium metabisulfite acts as a mild reducing/bleaching agent to remove this background without stripping the silver from fungal walls.
6. This improves contrast between fungi (black) and background (pale green).
7. Then wash in tap water (5–10 minutes) and four changes of distilled water.
8. Long washing removes residual chemicals that could cause non-specific staining or continue reacting.
9. Using distilled water in multiple changes ensures no mineral contamination that could precipitate with silver later in the procedure.
10. *Preheat* the working hexamine silver solution to 56°C for 1 hour in a Coplin jar using a water bath:
    - *Treat sections* with the hexamine silver solution at 56°C. Examine the sections at 10–20-minute intervals until fungi appear black and the background remains clear.
    - *Tone* in 0.1% aqueous ferric chloride for 3 minutes.
    - *Fix* in sodium thiosulfate for 5 minutes and then wash.
    - *Counterstain* with light green for 1–2 minutes. Wash, dehydrate, clear, and mount the tissue sections.

Results: *Fungi, chitin, P. jirovecii, amoebae, some mucins, melanin, glycogen, and starch* will stain black in a green background.

This stain is highly effective for diagnosing fungal infections, particularly in lung tissues where *P. jirovecii* infections are common, such as in immunocompromised patients.

Mayer's Mucicarmine Stain

Mayer's mucicarmine stain is primarily used to demonstrate mucin, and it is especially valuable for detecting *Cryptococcus* and *Rhinosporidium* species.

Staining solution: Carmine, alcohol, aluminum hydroxide, and anhydrous aluminum chloride mixture.

Staining procedure:
1. Stain nuclei with hematoxylin.
2. Stain with mucicarmine for 20 minutes.
3. Wash and mount.

Observations:
- Mucins stain *red*.
- Nuclei stain *blue*.

Masson–Fontana Stain

The *Masson-Fontana silver staining (MFSS)* is used to detect melanin-containing phaeoid (dematiaceous) fungi in tissues or smears. It is also known as the *Fontana-Masson stain*. This stain is effective for identifying *melanin*, which directly reduces silver to metallic silver without the need for an external reducer.

Key features:
- *Application*: It is used to detect melanin in phaeoid fungi and other substances such as argentaffin and chromaffin granules.
- *Mechanism*: Melanin binds to silver and reduces it to metallic silver, causing the stained elements to appear black.

- *Comparison with GMS*: While *GMS* stains all fungal elements black with a greenish background, *Masson–Fontana* specifically stains phaeoid fungi black against a brownish background.

Advantages:
- It is useful for detecting fungi with *melanin* in their cell walls, such as *phaeoid fungi.*
- It is a simple technique and effective for histological studies of fungal infections.

Limitations:
- It may stain nonphaeoid fungi, making it less specific for phaeoid fungi.
- It should be used selectively, keeping in mind that the stain can produce false positives with nonphaeoid organisms.

Staining solutions:
- *Silver solution*: Ammoniacal silver solution prepared with 10% silver nitrate and strong ammonia
- *Sodium thiosulfate* (0.5% aqueous)
- *Neutral red* (1% aqueous)

Staining procedure:
1. Bring sections to distilled water.
2. Treat with ammoniacal silver solution in a dark container (e.g., black-painted Coplin jar) for 20–40 minutes at 56°C or overnight at room temperature.
3. Wash well in distilled water.
4. Treat with 0.5% sodium thiosulfate for 2 minutes.
5. Wash and then counterstain with neutral red for 3–5 minutes.
6. Dehydrate, clear, and mount.

Results:
- *Melanin*, argentaffin granules, chromaffin, and some lipofuscin pigment stain *black.*
- *Nuclei* stain *red.*

Schmorl's Melanin Stain

Schmorl's melanin stain is another method for detecting melanin and other reducing substances in tissue, such as *argentaffin granules, lipofuscin, and chromaffin cells.* It is commonly used to identify *phaeoid fungi* by highlighting the melanin in their cell walls.

Key features:
- Based on melanin's reducing properties, which convert ferricyanide to ferrocyanide, producing *Prussian blue* in the presence of ferric ions
- Stains melanin granules *bluish-green* as opposed to the *black* color in the Masson–Fontana stain

Staining solutions:
- Ferric chloride (1% aqueous)
- Potassium ferricyanide (1% aqueous)
- Distilled water

Staining procedure:
1. Immerse sections in the ferric chloride and potassium ferricyanide solution in a Coplin jar.
2. Examine microscopically at 30-second intervals for up to 5 minutes.
3. Wash in running tap water.
4. Treat with 1% acetic acid for 5 minutes.
5. Counterstain with *nuclear fast red* for 5 minutes.
6. Wash, dehydrate, clear, and mount.

Results:
- *Melanin* and other reducing substances stain *bluish-green.*
- *Nuclei* stain *pinkish-red*, and cytoplasm appears *pale pink.*

Toluidine Blue O Stain

Toluidine blue O stain is a rapid and easy method for detecting *P. jirovecii* in lung biopsies, imprint smears, and bronchoalveolar lavage (BAL) fluid.

Key features:
- Stains *P. jirovecii cysts* as reddish-blue or dark purple, while tissue remnants and debris stain light blue.
- The cysts typically appear clumped and crescent-shaped.

Staining procedure:
1. Place air-dried slides in *sulfation reagent* (45 mL glacial acetic acid mixed with 15 mL concentrated sulfuric acid) for 10 minutes.
2. Rinse in cold water for 5 minutes and then drain.
3. Stain with *toluidine blue O* (0.3 g in 60 mL water) for 3 minutes.
4. Rinse in 95% ethanol, followed by absolute ethanol and xylene.
5. Dry the slide and observe under oil immersion.

Results:
- *P. jirovecii cysts* stain *purple.*
- *Tissue remnants and debris* stain *blue.*
- *Trophozoites* are not discernible.

Limitations: This stain only reveals the cyst form of *P. jirovecii*, and the background material can sometimes obscure identification. For more accurate results, other stains such as *GMS*, monoclonal antibodies, or CFW stains are preferred.

Acridine Orange Stain

Acridine orange stain is a fluorescent dye primarily used for detecting *nucleic acids* in cells, commonly applied in *bacteriology* and *oncology*. It differentiates between RNA and DNA by fluorescing in different colors when viewed under *ultraviolet light*.

Key features:
- *RNA* stains *orange-red*.
- *DNA* stains *yellow-green*.
- It is used for identifying rapidly growing cells, such as *malignant cells*, which have increased cytoplasmic RNA content.

Application: This stain has been widely used in the study of *exfoliative material* from the female reproductive tract due to the high clarity of RNA fluorescence. Although its popularity has decreased because of the impermanence of preparations and the need for experienced interpretation, especially in diagnosing squamous carcinoma cells, it remains useful for differentiating nucleic acids.

Fixation:
- *Alcohol* is the fixative of choice for this stain.
- Formalin-fixed material and material fixed in Bouin's solution do not stain satisfactorily.

Staining solution:
- *Acridine orange solution*:
  - Prepare 0.1% aqueous acridine orange solution.
  - Dilute 1 part stain with 10 parts of phosphate buffer (pH 6.0) to make a 0.01% working solution.
- *Phosphate buffer (pH 6.0)*
- *Differentiator*: Calcium chloride (0.1 M)

Staining procedure:
1. Fix smears in alcohol and then bring them to distilled water.
2. Rinse in 1% acetic acid for a few seconds.
3. Transfer through two changes of distilled water over 1 minute.
4. Stain in the diluted acridine orange solution for 3 minutes.
5. Rinse in pH 6.0 phosphate buffer for 1 minute.
6. Differentiate in 0.1 M calcium chloride for 30 seconds.
7. Wash in phosphate buffer and mount in the same solution.
8. Examine under a *fluorescence microscope*.

Observations:
- *DNA* fluoresces *yellow-green*.
- *RNA* and *mucins* fluoresce *red*.

Fluorescent Antibody Stain

The fluorescent-antibody stain (FAS) is used for detecting *fungal antigens* in clinical materials such as *pus, blood, cerebrospinal fluid (CSF)*, tissue impression smears, and *paraffin sections* of formalin-fixed tissue. It is less effective for sputum specimens but has shown efficacy in detecting antibody-coated fungal organisms in urine, such as *Candida* cells.

Key features:
- Used for detecting fungal *antigens* with the help of *fluorescent-labeled antibodies*
- Effective for samples with a *scanty number of organisms*
- Limited by the availability of specific antisera for different fungi

Application:
- Primarily used for detecting *pathogenic fungi* in clinical samples where organisms are scarce
- Laboratories such as the Centers for Disease Control and Prevention (CDC) have developed sensitive and specific *immunofluorescence reagents* for fungal detection and identification.

Fluorescent antibody staining helps clinicians detect fungi in complex tissue samples and body fluids, often assisting in the diagnosis of fungal infections even when other staining methods fail due to low organism counts.

ANNEXURE 3

Mycology Techniques

YEAST IDENTIFICATION

Germ Tube Test

The *germ tube test* is a rapid screening method used for the presumptive identification of *Candida albicans*. The test assesses the ability of *C. albicans* and *Candida dubliniensis* to produce germ tubes within 2 hours in serum. Germ tubes are short, hyphal outgrowths formed by yeast cells that are characteristic of these species.

Procedure

1. *Starting culture*: Use a fresh growth from a pure yeast culture.
2. *Suspension*: Prepare a very light suspension of the yeast in 0.5 mL of sterile serum (pooled human serum or fetal calf serum). The optimal concentration of yeast cells is between 10^5 and 10^6 cells/mL.
3. *Incubation*: Incubate the suspension at 37°C for exactly 2 hours.
4. *Microscopy*: After incubation, place one drop of the serum on a microscopic slide, cover it with a coverslip, and examine under the microscope for the presence of germ tubes. Germ tubes are distinguished by their parallel walls at the point of origin without any constriction.
5. *Positive result*: A positive test is indicated when about 30% of the cells produce germ tubes.
6. *Controls*: Use known *C. albicans* strains as positive controls with each new batch of serum to validate the results.

Notes:

- *Influencing factors*: The medium, inoculum size, incubation temperature, and the presence of simple carbohydrates affect germ tube formation.
- *Optimal inoculum*: Too few cells → May not detect germ tube production (false negative). Too many cells → Crowding and nutrient depletion can inhibit germ tube formation. The "light suspension" described in most protocols visually looks like slightly turbid serum (often compared to 0.5 McFarland or less).
- *pH*: A neutral pH of 7.4 is ideal for maximum germ tube formation.
- *Contamination*: Bacterial contamination may interfere with germ tube production.
- *Interference*: Antimicrobial agents in the isolation medium or inhibitory substances in human serum (such as ferritin) may suppress germ tube formation.
- *Controls*: *C. albicans* should be used as a positive control, while *Candida tropicalis* serves as a negative control to ensure reliable results **(Figs. 1A and B)**.

Morphological Characters on Cornmeal Agar (Dalmau Plate)

Cornmeal agar (CMA) with 1% Tween 80 is used to observe the microscopic morphology of *Candida* and other yeast species. The medium induces the development of specific structures such as pseudohyphae, hyphae, chlamydospores, and blastospores, aiding in the identification of different species **(Table 1)**.

Procedure

1. *Preparation of CMA plates:*
   - Prepare CMA with 1% Tween 80 in a 90-mm Petri dish.
   - Divide the plate into four quadrants and label each quadrant.
2. *Inoculation:*
   - Using a sterile needle or straight wire, lightly touch the yeast colony.
   - Make two to three streaks about 3.5–4 cm long and spaced 1.2 cm apart in each quadrant.
3. *Coverslip placement:*
   - Flame sterilize and cool a 22-mm square cover glass.

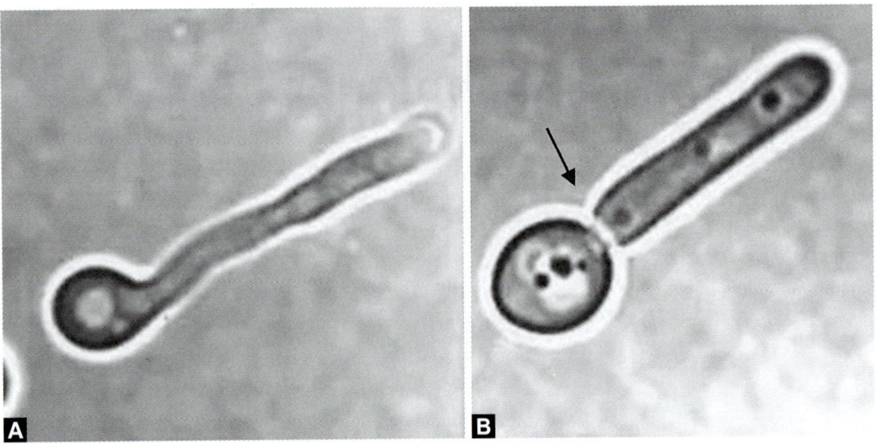

FIGS. 1A AND B: (A) Germ tube formation in *Candida albicans*; (B) *Candida tropicalis* blastoconidial germination with constriction.

TABLE 1: Morphological features of yeasts on cornmeal agar with Tween 80.

Morphological features	*Species*
Terminal chlamydoconidia	*Candida albicans, Candida dubliniensis*
Abundant pseudohyphae, pine forest arrangement, and blastoconidia formed at or in between septa	*Candida tropicalis*
Elongated yeasts, abundant pseudohyphae (matchstick-like appearance)	*Candida krusei*
Giant hyphae, blastospores at nodes	*Candida parapsilosis*
Scant pseudohyphae with chains of blastoconidia	*Candida guilliermondii*
Yeasts only	*Candida glabrata, Candida famata, Pichia anomala, Pichia angusta,* and *Cryptococcus neoformans*
Short, distinctly curved pseudohyphae with occasional blastoconidia at septa	*Candida lusitaniae*
Arthroconidia with blastoconidia	*Trichosporon*
Arthroconidia without blastoconidia	*Geotrichum*

- Place the cover glass over the control streak to provide a microaerophilic environment at the margins.

4. *Incubation*: Incubate the plate at 25°C for 3–5 days.
5. *Microscopic examination:*
    - After incubation, remove the lid of the Petri plate and place the plate on the microscope stage.
    - Observe the edge of the cover glass using the low power objective (10×) and then switch to high power (40×).
    - Note the morphological features such as hyphae, pseudohyphae, blastospores, ascospores, chlamydospores, basidiospores, or sporangia.

Ascospore Production and Detection Test

The ability of yeast to form ascospores is an important identification feature. The test involves using specific media that promote ascospore formation and examining the yeast cultures for these structures.

Media Used

- *Malt extract agar (MEA)*: It contains 5% malt extract and 2% agar.
- *Acetate agar*: It contains 0.5% sodium acetate trihydrate and 2% agar, pH 6.5–7.0.
- *V-8 juice agar*: It is commercially available.

Procedure

1. *Inoculation*: Inoculate the yeast onto the selected ascospores-producing agar plates.
2. *Incubation*: Incubate the plates aerobically at 25°C.
3. *Examination*: Examine the cultures at 3–5 days and weekly thereafter for up to 3 weeks.
4. *Wet mount preparation*: Prepare a wet mount of the yeast in distilled water.
5. *Microscopic examination*: Examine the wet mount under an oil immersion objective.

TABLE 2: Ascospore morphology on malt extract agar (2–5 days' growth).

Ascospore morphology	*Species*
1–4 hat-shaped ascospores in asci	*Pichia anomala, Pichia norvegensis, Candida utilis,* and *Candida ciferrii*
1–4 spherical or short ellipsoidal ascospores	*Saccharomyces cerevisiae*
1–2 ascospores per ascus, spherical with warts	*Candida famata*
4 ascospores per ascus, ellipsoidal with slimy sheath	*Blastoschizomyces capitatus*
1–2 ascospores per ascus, spherical	*Candida krusei*
1–4 ascospores per ascus, spherical to hat-shaped, protuberances on one or two edges	*Candida lipolytica*
1–4 ascospores per ascus, clavate	*Candida lusitaniae*

6. *Observation*: Observe for ascospores' form, surface topography, size, color, brims, and the number of ascospores per ascus.
7. *Modified acid-fast stain (if ascospores are not visible)*: Perform a modified acid-fast stain since ascospores are often acid-fast.
8. *Control*: Include *Saccharomyces cerevisiae* as a positive control for both production on media and staining procedures **(Table 2)**.

Ballistospore Formation

Ballistoconidia formation is crucial for distinguishing between *Sporobolomyces* and *Rhodotorula*. The presence of satellite conidia on the agar plate indicates the formation of ballistoconidia.

Procedure

1. *Plate preparation*: Pour a thin layer of MEA or yeast extract agar onto the top and bottom of the Petri plate.
2. *Inoculation:*
    - Inoculate the bottom part of the plate with the yeast culture.
    - Cover the inoculated bottom layer with the top layer of agar.
3. *Incubation*: Incubate the plate at 25°C for 2–3 days, ensuring the inoculated surface is on the top.
4. *Observation*: Formation of ballistospores is indicated by new growth on the uninoculated bottom surface, resembling a mirror image of the original colony.

Sugar Fermentation

This test helps determine the ability of yeast to ferment different sugars, indicated by acid and gas production.

Procedure

1. *Medium preparation*:
    - Prepare a liquid fermentation medium with:
        - Peptone (1%)
        - Sodium chloride (0.5%)
        - Andrade's indicator (0.005%)
    - Sterilize by autoclaving at 120°C for 15 minutes at 15 pounds pressure.
2. *Adding sugar*:
    - After sterilization, add filter-sterilized sugar to achieve a 2% concentration.
    - Pour the medium into sterile test tubes (approximately 5 mL).
    - Place a sterile Durham's tube in each test tube.
3. *Sealing*: Plug the tubes with color-coded cotton plugs.
4. *Inoculation*:
    - Prepare a heavy inoculum from yeast grown on a sugar-free medium.
    - Inoculate each carbohydrate broth with approximately 0.1 mL of the yeast inoculum.
5. *Incubation*:
    - Incubate the tubes at 25°C for up to 1 week.
    - Examine the tubes every 48–72 hours for the production of acid (indicated by a pink color) and gas (in the Durham's tube).
6. *Interpretation*:
    - Acid and gas production = Heterolactic fermentation
    - Acid production only but no gas = Homolactic fermentation

Sugar Assimilation Test (Auxanographic Technique)

This method helps in determining the yeast's ability to assimilate different sugars. The disk impregnation method, based on Wickerham's technique, is practical and effective.

Preparation of Yeast Nitrogen Base

Ingredients

- Potassium dihydrogen orthophosphate (KH_2PO_4)—1.0 g
- Magnesium sulfate ($MgSO_4$)—0.5 g
- Ammonium sulfate $(NH_4)_2SO_4$—5.0 g
- Noble agar—25.0 g
- Distilled water—1 L

Method

- Dissolve all ingredients in distilled water.
- Autoclave at 115°C for 15 minutes.

Procedure

1. *Preparation of yeast suspension*: From a 24 to 48-hour old culture, prepare a heavy yeast suspension in 2 mL of YNB.
2. *Mixing with agar*:
   - Add this suspension to 18 mL of molten agar (cooled to 45°C) and mix well.
   - Pour the mixture into a 90-mm Petri plate and let it solidify at room temperature.
3. *Application of sugar disks:*
   - Place various carbohydrate-impregnated disks on the agar surface.
   - *Disk preparation:*
     - Punch 6 mm diameter disks from Whatman No. 1 filter paper.
     - Sterilize the disks by heating in a hot air oven at 160°C for 1 hour.
     - Add a drop of 10% filter-sterilized sugar solution to each disk.
     - Dry the disks at 37°C and store in an airtight container at 4°C.
4. *Incubation*: Incubate the plates at 37°C for 3–4 days.
5. *Observation:*
   - Growth around the disks indicates positive assimilation of the specific carbohydrate.
   - Record growth around the glucose disk first as a positive control for yeast viability.

Nitrate Assimilation Test (Auxanographic Technique)

This test assesses the yeast's ability to assimilate nitrate.

Preparation of Yeast Carbon Base

Ingredients

- KH_2PO_4—1.0 g
- $MgSO_4$—0.5 g
- Glucose—20.0 g
- Noble agar—25.0 g
- Distilled water—1 L

Method

Mix the ingredients and autoclave at 121°C for 15 minutes.

Procedure

1. *Preparation of yeast suspension*: From a 24 to 48-hour culture, prepare a suspension equivalent to McFarland No. 1 standard in 2 mL of YCB.
2. *Mixing with agar*: Add the yeast suspension to 18 mL of molten agar (cooled to 45°C), mix well, and pour into 90-mm Petri plates. Allow the agar to solidify at room temperature.
3. *Application of nitrate and peptone disks:*
   - Divide the plate into two halves and label.
   - Place potassium nitrate (KNO_3) disks on one half and peptone disks on the other.
   - *Disk preparation*:
     - Prepare KNO_3 disks: Saturate 6-mm disks punched from Whatman no. 1 filter paper with a 30 g/L KNO_3 solution. Dry and store at 4°C.
     - Prepare peptone disks similarly using a 30 g/L peptone solution.
4. *Incubation*: Incubate the plates at 37°C for 7 days.
5. *Observation:*
   - The test is valid if there is growth around the peptone disk (indicating yeast viability).
   - Positive for nitrate assimilation if there is growth around the KNO_3 disk.

BactiCard Candida® (Remel Laboratories, Lenexa, KS)

- *Time required*: 5 minutes
- *Principle*:
  - It measures N-acetylgalactosaminidase and L-proline aminopeptidase activity using chromogenic substrates.
  - *C. albicans* produces both enzymes, and the colorimetric reactions are read visually.

Trehalase Test for Rapid *Candida glabrata*

- *Time required*: 20 minutes
- *Principle*: Although trehalase is present in other yeast species, this test is based on the speed with which the *C. glabrata* enzyme hydrolyzes trehalose.

Rapid Urease Test for *Cryptococcus neoformans*

- *Time required*: 15 minutes
- *Principle*:
  - Urease produced by the fungus splits urea, producing ammonia, which causes a pH increase.
  - The pH indicator changes from pale yellow to bright magenta.

- *Procedure*:
    i. Cotton-tipped medicine applicator sticks soaked in 5× Christensen's urea agar base are frozen and lyophilized.
    ii. The lyophilized applicator sticks are brushed over two to three colonies of the yeast suspected to be *Cryptococcus neoformans*.
    iii. The applicator stick is transferred to a test tube containing a few drops of 1% benzalkonium chloride (aids in releasing urease from the yeast cell), previously adjusted to pH 4.86.
    iv. Swirling the applicator stick into the broth transfers the yeast growth.
    v. The cotton swab is removed, the tube is capped, and it is incubated at 45°C.
- *Result*: Ninety-nine percent of *C. neoformans* cultures produce a color change from colorless to purple within 15 minutes of incubation.

Christensen's Urea Agar

- *Time required*: 18–24 hours
- *Composition*: Commercial powder
- *Forms*:
    - Broth
    - With 1.5% agar

Procedure

- *Constitution*: Constituted from commercial powder
- *Usage*:
    - It can be used as broth or with 1.5% agar.
    - Once seeded with an unknown yeast, urea agar takes longer than the rapid urease test to indicate a color change.
- *Indication of color change*:
    - *Trichosporon* species and *Rhodotorula* species also produce the magenta color.
    - Differentiation is done by microscopic morphology and/or colony color on standard laboratory media.
- *Additional use*: Urea agar is also used to differentiate molds such as the dermatophytes *Trichophyton rubrum* and *Trichophyton interdigitale* (urease positive).

Birdseed (Niger Seed) Agar Test for *Cryptococcus neoformans*

- *Time required*: 2–24 hours
- *Principle*:
    - Niger seed (*Guizotia abyssinica*) contains melanin precursors.
    - When planted on Birdseed Agar, *C. neoformans* (but not *Candida* species or *Cryptococcus albidus*) will produce melanin pigment, causing the "brown colony effect."
    - Other yeast species colonies produce a cream to beige color.
- *Usefulness*:
    - It is useful for presumptive identification of *C. neoformans* isolated from blood or cerebrospinal fluid (CSF).
    - It detects a few colonies of *C. neoformans* among a larger number of *Candida* species colonies, as is sometimes observed in the urine of persons living with acquired immunodeficiency syndrome (AIDS) and cryptococcosis.
- *Color development time*: The time necessary to produce detectable brown color can vary from 2 to 24 hours at 25°C.

Glucose–Salts–3,4-Dihydroxyphenylalanine Medium for *Cryptococcus neoformans*

- *Usage*:
    - This medium is used for the isolation and identification of *Cryptococcus* species.
    - Yeasts suspected of being *Cryptococcus* species are streaked for isolation on the medium.
- *Incubation*: Petri plates are incubated in the dark at 30°C.
- *Inspection*: The plates are inspected daily for the production of melanin pigment.
- *Substitution for Birdseed Agar*:
    - Glucose-salts media containing caffeic acid or dihydroxyphenylalanine [1 mM, d,l-3,4-dihydroxyphenylalanine (DOPA)] can be substituted for Birdseed Agar.
    - Glucose-salts-DOPA medium is preferred over dihydroxyphenylalanine because it is stable to ordinary daylight.

CHROMagar Candida® for Yeast Identification

- *Manufacturer*: BD Diagnostic Systems, Sparks, MD
- Time *required*: 24–48 hours
- *Usage*:
    - Primary culture medium
    - Differential and selective medium
- *Advantages*:
    - Demonstrates the presence of a mixed yeast infection
    - Nearly 100% sensitive and specific for *C. albicans*

- *Disadvantage*: As a primary medium, recoveries may not be as complete as with Sabouraud dextrose agar (SDA)-Emmons.
- *Identification*: Colonies of different yeast species exhibit distinct colors:
  - *C. albicans*: Green
  - *C. tropicalis*: Blue
  - *C. glabrata*: Dark purple (after 3–4 days)
- *Definitive identification*: A germ tube test is recommended for more definitive identification, especially if a *C. albicans* isolate does not turn green.
- *Principle*: Chromogenic substrates in the agar change from colorless to colored, indicating specific enzyme activities (β-N-acetylhexosaminidase and phosphatase).
- *Application*: Very useful in identifying mixed cultures of yeast in specimens from human immunodeficiency virus (HIV)-positive patients and other patients.

Canavanine Glycine Bromothymol Blue Agar

- *Purpose*: Specialized agar to differentiate between *C. neoformans* (no growth, no color change) and *Cryptococcus gattii* (growth, color change from yellow to blue)
- *Principle*:
  - *C. gattii* (serotypes B and C) can detoxify L-canavanine and grow in media containing this compound.
  - Glycine (1%) serves as the sole source of carbon and nitrogen, utilized by *C. gattii*, leading to increased pH and a color change.

Preparation of Canavanine Glycine Bromothymol Blue Medium

Solution A (Glycine-L-Canavanine Solution)

- *Ingredients*:
  - 10 g of glycine
  - 1 g of KH_2PO_4
  - 1 g of $MgSO_4$
  - 1 mg of thiamine HCl
  - 30 mg of L-canavanine sulfate
  - 100 mL of distilled water
- pH is adjusted to 5.6, and the solution is filter sterilized.

Solution B: Bromothymol Blue and Agar

Sterilize by autoclaving. Mix solution A and B in specific proportions.

- *Usage*: Specifically designed for the differentiation of *Cryptococcus* species
- *Result interpretation*:
  - *C. neoformans*:
    - No growth
    - No color change
  - *C. gattii*:
    - Growth
    - Color change from yellow to blue.
- *Application*: It provides a selective environment for the growth of *C. gattii* based on its ability to detoxify canavanine.

COMMERCIAL YEAST IDENTIFICATION SYSTEMS

API 20C Yeast Identification System

Procedure

1. *Preparation*:
   - Melt the basal broth medium in the ampoules by autoclaving or boiling in a water bath.
   - Cool to 48–50°C.
2. *Inoculation*:
   - Use a squeeze bottle to dispense 20 mL of water into an incubation tray.
   - Open the ampoule and inoculate the molten medium with a sterile applicator stick.
   - Adjust the density to <1+ on a Wickerham card.
   - Inoculate 0.2 mL of yeast suspension into the 20 capsules using a Pasteur pipette.
3. *Incubation*:
   - Incubate at 28–30°C for 72 hours.
   - Read the results after 24, 48, and 72 hours.

Vitek Yeast Identification System

Procedure

1. *Preparation*: Prepare a yeast suspension in tubes containing 1.8 mL of saline and adjust to McFarland no. 2 standard using a Vitek colorimeter.
2. *Inoculation*:
   - Label the yeast cards and place them in a filling stand.
   - Inoculate the card using the filling tube with the yeast suspension.
   - Seal the card and incubate at 30°C for 18–24 hours, depending on the instrument's recommendations.
3. *Reading*: Results are obtained usually after 24 hours, with some isolates requiring additional incubation.

Notes:

- *API 20C*:
  - Does not include rhamnose and urea tests.

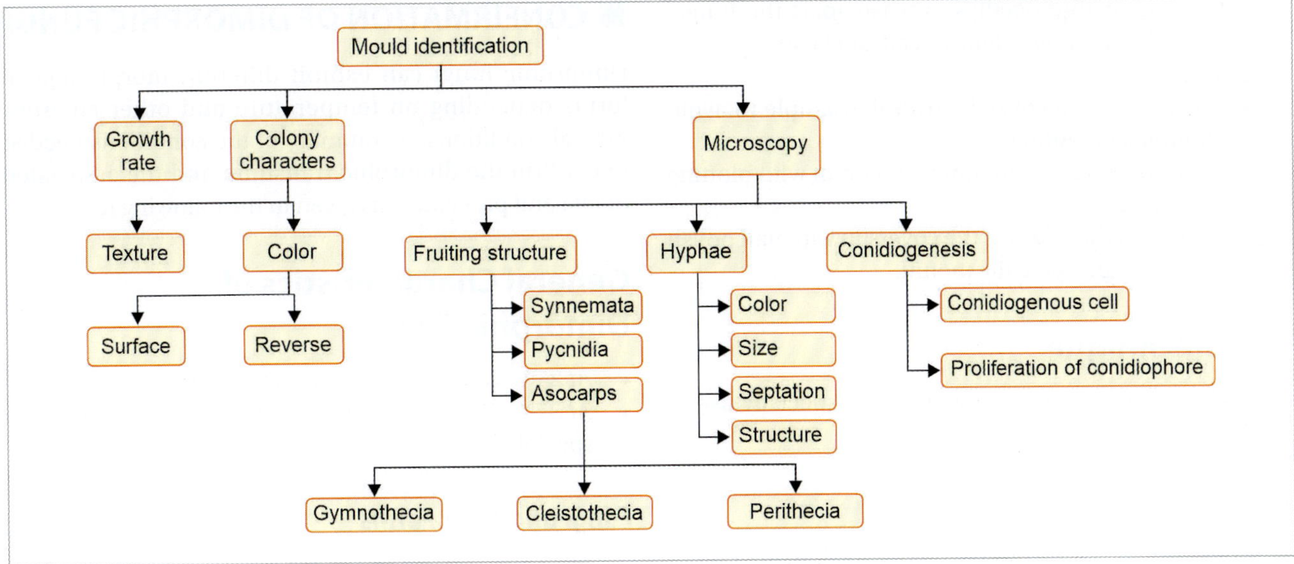

FLOWCHART 1: Techniques used for identification of molds.

- Germ tube test and morphological studies should be included.
- May give one to three different identifications for a single isolate.
- Results are available in 3 days.

- *Vitek*:
  - Yeasts with abundant capsules or extensive mycelial growth may be difficult to suspend.
  - Additional morphological studies may be needed for ambiguous results.
  - Results are typically available after 24 hours, with some strains requiring longer incubation (**Flowchart 1**).

TECHNIQUES FOR STUDYING FUNGAL MORPHOLOGY AND MICROSCOPY

Colony Characteristics

For examining colony morphology, the following media are commonly used:

- SDA
- MEA
- Potato dextrose agar (PDA)
- Czapek–Dox agar

Parameters to Note

- *Growth rate*: Fast or slow
- *Color*: Hue and intensity
- *Texture*: Smooth, rough, or wrinkled
- *Diffusible pigment*: Pigment production in the agar
- *Exudates*: Any secretions or fluid produced
- *Aerial and submerged hyphae*: Structures above and below the surface of the medium
- *Colony topography*: Surface appearance (e.g., raised and flat)

Special Structures

- Ascocarps: Sexual fruiting bodies
- *Pycnidia*: Asexual fruiting bodies
- *Sclerotia*: Hardened masses of mycelium
- *Sporodochia*: Conidial heads
- *Synnemata*: Branched, conidial structures

Dissecting Microscope

It is useful for detailed examination of these structures.

Tease Mount

It is a quick method for mounting fungi for microscopic examination. Note that this method may lead to dislodgement of spores or conidia.

Standard Tease Mount Procedure

1. *Preparation*: Place a small drop of lactophenol cotton blue (LCB) (mounting medium) on a clean slide.
2. *Sampling*: Remove a small portion of fungal growth from midway between the colony center and edge.
3. *Mounting*:
   - Place the fungal sample on the drop of mounting medium.

- Use dissecting needles to tease apart the fungal sample, creating a thin, spread-out layer.

4. *Coverslip*:
   - Gently place a coverslip over the sample to avoid trapping air bubbles.
   - Wipe away excess mounting medium with blotting paper if necessary.
5. *Sealing*: Seal the edges of the coverslip with nail polish or varnish to preserve the mount.

Tape Technique

This is an alternative mounting method, especially useful for delicate fungi.

Procedure

1. *Preparation*: Place a drop of mounting fluid on a slide.
2. *Sampling*:
   - Take a 2-cm long piece of tape and attach one end to a stick or forceps.
   - Lightly touch the tape to the fungal colony.
3. *Mounting*:
   - Lay the tape with the fungal side facing down into the mounting fluid on the slide.
   - Detach the tape from the stick.
4. *Examination*: Examine the mount directly.

Note: The teased preparation may dislodge conidia and conidiophores, making identification difficult. The tape touch method is a low-distortion alternative, resulting in high-quality mounts.

Mounting Zygomycetes and Fruiting Structures

These fungi often trap air bubbles, making mounting challenging. Use the following techniques to improve clarity.

Procedure

1. *Wetting agents*: Place a drop of 95% ethanol, ethyl acetate, or water with 0.05% Tween 80 on a slide. These agents help prevent air bubble formation.
2. *Sampling*: Transfer a portion of the fungal culture to the drop of fluid on the slide.
3. *Mounting*:
   - Add a drop of mounting fluid to the sample.
   - Examine using the standard microscopy technique.

CONFIRMATION OF DIMORPHIC FUNGI

Dimorphic fungi can exhibit different morphological forms depending on temperature and other environmental conditions. A summary of the conditions needed to confirm the dimorphic transition and the associated media and procedures is given in the following text.

General Characteristics of Dimorphic Fungi

- *At 25°C*: Grow as molds on routine media
- *At 37°C*: Convert to yeasts or spherules in tissue or on special media

Fungi and Their Forms

- *Blastomyces dermatitidis*: Yeast form at 37°C; resembles *Chrysosporium* species at 25°C.
- *Histoplasma capsulatum*: Yeast form at 37°C; resembles *Sepedonium* species at 25°C.
- *Paracoccidioides brasiliensis*: Yeast form at 37°C; resembles *Chrysosporium* species at 25°C.
- *P. marneffei*: Yeast form at 37°C; resembles other *Penicillium* species at 25°C.
- *Sporothrix schenckii*: Yeast form at 37°C; resembles *Acrodontium* species at 25°C.
- *Coccidioides immitis*: Forms spherules and endospores at 37°C; resembles various fungi such as *Malbranchea* species at 25°C.

Media and Conditions for Mold to Tissue Form Conversion

- *B. dermatitidis*:
  - *Media*: Kelley's agar, KT medium
  - *Conditions*: Incubate at 37°C
  - *Similar at 25°C*: *Chrysosporium* species
- *C. immitis*:
  - *Media*: Modified converse medium
  - *Conditions*: Incubate at 40°C with 5–10% CO_2
  - *Similar at 25°C*: *Malbranchea* species, *Uncinocarpus* species, *Auxarthron* species, and *Arachniotus* species
- *H. capsulatum*:
  - *Media*: Brain heart infusion agar (BHIA) with glutamine, Pine's agar medium
  - *Conditions*: Incubate at 37°C
  - *Similar at 25°C*: *Sepedonium* species

- *P. brasiliensis*:
    - *Media*: BHIA
    - *Conditions*: Incubate at 37°C
    - *Similar at 25°C*: *Chrysosporium* species
- *S. schenckii*:
    - *Media*: BHIA
    - *Conditions*: Incubate at 37°C with 5–10% CO_2
    - *Similar at 25°C*: *Acrodontium* species
- *P. marneffei*:
    - *Media*: 5% sheep blood agar (BA), BHIA
    - *Conditions*: Incubate at 37°C
    - *Similar at 25°C*: *Penicillium* species other than *T. marneffei*

Procedures for Confirmation

- *Safety*: Carry out all procedures within a biological safety cabinet.
- *Slide cultures*: Do not set up slide cultures for dimorphic fungi.
- *Quality control*: Use a known culture to check for conversion conditions.

Techniques for Observation

- *Direct microscopy*: Examine cultures under a microscope to observe the morphological forms at different temperatures.
- *Special media*: Use specific media tailored to each dimorphic fungus for accurate results.

CYCLOHEXIMIDE RESISTANCE

Cycloheximide is an antifungal agent that inhibits protein synthesis in fungi. It is commonly used to differentiate fungi based on their resistance or susceptibility to this compound.

- *Resistant to cycloheximide at 30°C (i.e., they grow in the presence of cycloheximide)*:
    - *Blastomyces dermatitidis*
    - *S. schenckii*
    - *C. immitis*
    - *H. capsulatum*
    - *P. brasiliensis*
    - Most dermatophytes
- *Inhibited by cycloheximide*:
    - *Absidia*
    - *Rhizopus*
    - *Scedosporium*
    - Some strains of *Candida* and *Aspergillus*
    - *Mucor*
    - *Cryptococcus*

Temperature Tolerance

Thermotolerance helps in identifying medically important molds based on their ability to grow at high temperatures **(Table 3)**.

TECHNIQUES FOR IDENTIFICATION OF FUNGI (TABLE 4)

Techniques to Enhance Sporulation in Molds

Slide Culture Technique

Slide cultures are useful for examining fungal morphology when tease mounts are insufficient. A step-by-step guide for setting up and processing slide cultures is as follows:

1. *Preparing the setup*:
    - *Materials*: 100 mm glass Petri dish, filter paper, V-shaped glass rod, microscopic slide, and coverslip.
    - *Sterilization*: Autoclave the setup at 121°C for 15 minutes.
    - *Storage*: Store the setups in a Petri dish canister for up to 2 weeks.
2. *Procedure*:
    - *Agar blocks*: Cut 1-cm square blocks of CMA or PDA.
    - *Inoculation*: Place the agar block onto the slide in the setup. Transfer a small amount of the fungal colony to each side of the agar block.
    - *Covering*: Place the coverslip on the inoculated agar block.
    - *Humidity*: Add 1–1.5 mL of sterile water to the Petri dish to maintain a humid environment. Optionally, add 5–20% glycerine to prevent condensation.
    - *Incubation*: Place the slide culture in a Petri dish canister and incubate in the dark until mature conidia or spores are observed.

TABLE 3: Thermotolerance of some medically important fungi.

Fungus	*Upper growth limit (°C)*
Aspergillus fumigatus	48–50
Cladophialophora bantiana	42–43
Cladophialophora carrionii	35–36
Fonsecaea pedrosoi	38
Rhizomucor pusillus	50–55
Trichophyton mentagrophytes	37
Exophiala dermatitidis	40

TABLE 4: Techniques for identifying fungi.

Suspected mold	Technique utilized/recommended
Aspergillus fumigatus	Temperature tolerance at 48°C
Blastomyces dermatitidis	Exoantigen test, mold to yeast conversion, Gen-Probe technique
Basidiobolus species	Forcibly ejected sporangiola
Cladophialophora carrionii	Temperature tolerance at 35°C
Conidiobolus species	Forcibly ejected conidia
Histoplasma capsulatum	Exoantigen test, mold-to-yeast conversion, Gen-Probe technique
Paracoccidioides brasiliensis	Mold-to-yeast conversion
Rhizomucor pusillus	Temperature tolerance at 55°C
Sepedonium species	Morphology and negative exoantigen for *Histoplasma*
Sporobolomyces	Forcibly ejected conidia
Exophiala dermatitidis	Temperature tolerance at 40°C
Cladophialophora	Temperature tolerance at 42°C

3. *Taking down the slide culture*:
    - *Mounting medium*: Place a small drop of LCB on a clean slide.
    - *Removing coverslip*: Carefully remove the coverslip from the agar block with forceps. Avoid pushing or pulling the coverslip.
    - *Heat fixation*: Quickly pass the coverslip through a blue portion of a flame to heat fix the fungus and its spores. Be cautious to avoid overheating, which can collapse hyphae.
    - *Mounting*: Place the coverslip onto the mounting medium, avoiding air bubbles. Seal edges with nail polish.
    - *Additional mounts*: Prepare a second mount by placing the agar block on a microscope slide with a drop of lactophenol. Seal with nail polish.
    - *Preservation*: Soak the colony in 95% alcohol or ethyl acetate to avoid air bubbles before applying lactophenol. The agar block can be placed back on suitable media to maintain the fungus.

Microculture Technique

- *Purpose*: It is a simplified method to enhance sporulation.
- *Procedure*:
    i. Use a nutrient-deficient medium. Cut three to four small blocks from the medium.
    ii. Place blocks on a Petri plate and inoculate each with the fungus.
    iii. Cover each block with a coverslip, seal the plate, and incubate at 25°C.
    iv. Examine frequently for sporulation over a period of a week to a month.

Water Agar Technique

- *Purpose*: It is especially useful for Mucorales.
- *Procedure*:
    i. Pour 18–20 mL of distilled water (with or without 0.2 mL of 10% yeast extract) into a sterile Petri plate.
    ii. Place four to five blocks of fungal growth in the water, ensuring growth is on the obverse side.
    iii. Seal the plate with parafilm and incubate at 25°C.
    iv. After 1 week, if there is extensive growth above the water, prepare an LCB mount. If sporulation is insufficient, incubate for an additional week.

Hair Perforation Test

- *Purpose*: It differentiates dermatophytes such as *Trichophyton mentagrophytes* and *T. rubrum*, as well as *Microsporum canis* and *Microsporum equinum*.
- *Procedure*:
    i. Place a sterile filter paper strip at the bottom of a sterile Petri dish.
    ii. Cover the filter paper with sterile distilled water.
    iii. Add small portions of sterilized prepubertal or infant hair into the water.
    iv. Add five to six drops of 10% yeast extract to enhance the reaction.
    v. Inoculate the fungal colony directly onto the hair.
    vi. Incubate at 25°C for 4 weeks.
    vii. Examine the hair by making a wet smear or LCB mount to check for conical perforations of the hair shaft.
- *Results*:
    - *Positive*: *T. mentagrophytes* and *M. canis* (shows perforation)
    - *Negative*: *T. rubrum* and *M. equinum* (no perforation)

Hair Bait Technique

- *Purpose*: It is used to isolate keratinophilic fungi from soil.
- *Procedure*:
    i. Place the soil sample in a sterile Petri dish.
    ii. Spread about 30 pieces of 1 inch long, preferably horse's hair on the soil. The hair should be sterilized by autoclaving.

iii. Wet the surface of the soil with sterile distilled water, ensuring the soil is moist but not flooded.
iv. Add more water and incubate at 30°C.
v. When white to brown fungal growth appears around the hair, transfer pieces of hair with fungal growth to the surface of SDA plates.
vi. Scatter about three to four pieces of hair on each agar plate. Bury one end of the hair under the agar surface.
vii. Examine the hair with the growth under LCB mount.
viii. Transfer fungal colonies to separate SDA plates for further identification.

Adhesive Tape Technique

- *Purpose*: To make direct smears from superficial lesions or cultural isolates for examination of fungal structures.
- *Procedure*:
  i. Apply a piece of Scotch tape (6–8 cm long × 1–2 cm wide) to the infected area or fungal colony.
  ii. Immediately adhere the tape (glue side) to a clean slide.
  iii. Raise one edge of the tape and place a small drop of KOH between the tape and the slide.
  iv. Press gently with cotton or gauze to distribute the dye evenly and remove excess.
  v. For cultural isolates, the same procedure can be used for making LCB mounts from the colony material.
- *Uses*:
  - Superficial fungal infections caused by *Malassezia* species or dermatophytes
  - Subcutaneous infections such as chromoblastomycosis
  - Cutaneous manifestations of systemic infections such as paracoccidioidomycosis

ANNEXURE 4

Antifungal Susceptibility Tests: Key Points

DEFINITION

An antifungal susceptibility (AFS) test is an in vitro laboratory test designed to determine the minimum inhibitory concentration (MIC) of an antifungal drug against a clinical isolate of a pathogenic fungus.

NATIONAL AND INTERNATIONAL STANDARDS

- The Subcommittee on Antifungal Susceptibility Testing of the Clinical and Laboratory Standards Institute (CLSI) in the United States and the European Committee on Antimicrobial Susceptibility Testing (EUCAST) internationally developed standard operating procedures for AFS tests.
- Commercial test procedure methods are available in the package inserts for such tests.

CLINICAL INDICATIONS FOR ANTIFUNGAL SUSCEPTIBILITY TESTING

Antifungal susceptibility testing is crucial when:

- The isolated yeast or mold is from a sterile site, such as the bloodstream:
    - For yeasts, AFS is determined after species identification.
    - For molds, AFS may be determined before definitive identification due to slow growth.
- The patient fails to respond to primary therapy or becomes intolerant to the drugs of choice.
- The fungus involved has a wide range of susceptibilities or is known to be refractory to antifungal agents.
- A new class or member of an existing class of antifungal agents is being considered for use.
- An outbreak of a fungal disease requires treatment for a group of patients.

Safety Note

Technologists should perform AFS ONLY in a Class II, Type A2 Biosafety Cabinet (BSC), wear personal protective equipment (PPE), and follow Clinical Laboratory Improvement Amendments (CLIA)-approved standard operating procedures to minimize the risk of aerosol generation during AFS tests.

Correlation between in vitro Minimum Inhibitory Concentration and Clinical Efficacy

The clinical efficacy of antifungal drug therapy is influenced by various host factors, including:

- *Contaminated indwelling medical devices*: Yeast embedded in biofilms coating indwelling medical devices are less susceptible to killing than free-floating yeast.
- *Dosage regimen*: The prescribed dosage of antifungal drugs affects clinical outcomes.
- *Drug interactions*: Interactions between antifungal drugs and other medications may alter therapy availability.
- *Immune and endocrine functions*: Immunocompromised or neutropenic patients may have altered responses.
- *Other medical problems*: The overall clinical status of the patient, as indicated by factors such as the Acute Physiology and Chronic Health Evaluation II (APACHE II) score.
- *Patient's age*: Very young (neonates) and elderly patients are at a higher risk.

- *Drug absorption*: Monitoring itraconazole (ITC) blood concentration is essential for proper absorption.
- *Patient compliance*: Adherence to the prescribed drug regimen is crucial.
- *Timeliness of therapeutic intervention*: Prompt diagnosis is key, especially for high fungal burdens.

Microbial factors, such as differences in pathogenic potential within a fungal species, also influence the clinical course.

Despite in vitro AFS tests, there is a disparity between in vitro and in vivo results. The "90/60 rule" predicts clinical outcomes based on MIC values:

- Infections caused by isolates with susceptible MICs respond favorably approximately 90% of the time.
- Infections caused by isolates with resistant MICs respond favorably approximately 60% of the time, suggesting a need for better drug selection based on AFS profiles.

Support for the rule exists for susceptible *Candida* species isolates. For isolates with high MICs (≥64 µg/mL), only 42% of patient-episode-isolate events were successfully treated with fluconazole (FLC).

Clinical correlations for molds have been problematic, but successful correlations exist, especially in immunocompromised patients. For example, patients with hematologic diseases treated by myeloablative chemotherapy and stem cell transplants developed invasive aspergillosis, where in vitro resistance was the only parameter correlating with clinical outcome.

Determination of "Susceptible" or "Resistant"

The conditions of "susceptible" or "resistant" in AFS testing are determined by interpretive "breakpoints" or drug concentrations. Committees such as the CLSI and the EUCAST establish these breakpoints based on the performance of the drug in a population of patients. Breakpoints represent discriminatory antimicrobial concentrations used to interpret AFS test results.

What are breakpoints?

Breakpoints are specific antimicrobial concentrations (expressed in µg/mL) that help interpret AFS test results, categorizing isolates as "susceptible (S)," "intermediate (I)" [susceptible-dose dependent (S-DD)], or "resistant (R)." The S-DD category emphasizes the importance of reaching maximal drug concentrations for isolates with higher MICs, suggesting that a higher dose may lead to a good response.

For yeast susceptibility tests, breakpoints are established for various antifungal agents. The expectation is that a good clinical response to infection occurs with a "susceptible" yeast isolate at a typical dosage regimen. If the MIC is in the "S-DD" range, a higher dose may result in a good response. However, if the MIC is in the "resistant" range, a good response is unlikely at any dose.

Examples of breakpoints for yeast susceptibility tests (µg/mL):

- *FLC*:
  - Susceptible (S): ≤2
  - S-DD: 4
  - Resistant (R): ≥8
- *ITC*:
  - Susceptible (S): ≤0.125
  - S-DD: 0.25–0.5
  - Resistant (R): ≥1
- *Amphotericin B (AmB)*:
  - Susceptible (S): ≤1
  - Resistant (R): ≥2
- *Voriconazole (VRC)*:
  - Susceptible (S): ≤1
  - S-DD: 2
  - Resistant (R): ≥4
- *Echinocandins*:
  - Susceptible (S): ≤0.25
  - S-DD: 0.5
  - Resistant (R): ≥1

OBJECTIVE OF ANTIFUNGAL SUSCEPTIBILITY TESTS

The primary objective of AFS testing is to predict the clinical efficacy of drug therapy for a patient's mycotic disease.

Minimum Inhibitory Concentration Defined

- The MIC is the minimum concentration of an antifungal agent (expressed in µg/mL) required to prevent the in vitro growth of a yeast or mold.
- For yeasts the MIC for AmB is the lowest drug concentration resulting in the absence of growth after 48 hours of incubation.
- For yeasts and azole antifungal agents, the MIC is the lowest drug concentration resulting in a ≥50% reduction in the growth when tested by the broth microdilution (BMD) method.
- When azoles are tested by the broth macrodilution method (as per CLSI M27 standard for yeasts), the MIC is the lowest drug concentration resulting in an 80% reduction in the growth.
- The distinction in computing the MIC for AmB and azole antifungal agents is based on the fungicidal nature of AmB and the fungistatic nature of azole drugs.

MIC50 and MIC90

- *MIC50*: The lowest concentration of an antifungal agent inhibiting the growth of 50% of the population of clinical isolates of a fungal species
- *MIC90*: The lowest concentration inhibiting growth in 90% of that population

Broth Microdilution Method

- Developed by CLSI, it tests a range of drug concentrations.
- Two variations include the following:
  i. *BMD method*: Conducted in a 96-well microtitration plate
  ii. *Broth macrodilution*: Conducted in test tubes but has fallen out of favor due to being slow and awkward compared to BMD

YEAST: BROTH DILUTION ANTIFUNGAL SUSCEPTIBILITY TESTING

Overview

- This method tests yeasts such as *Candida* species and *Cryptococcus neoformans* from invasive infections.
- It is not used for dimorphic fungi's yeast form.
- It follows the CLSI M27/A3 protocol to test for antifungal agents such as AmB, FLC, ITC, and echinocandins.

Antifungal Agents

- *Source*: Obtain pure antifungal reference powders from reputable sources, not from pharmacy stock.
- *Storage*: Store powders at –20°C or below in a desiccator. Allow them to reach at room temperature before opening.

Weighing antifungal powders: Use analytical balances and ensure accuracy by compensating for potency variations using the following formulas:

$$\text{Weight (mg)} = \frac{\text{Volume (mL)} \times \text{Concentration } (\mu\text{g/mL})}{\text{Assay potency } (\mu\text{g/mg})}$$

(Formula 1)

Or

$$\text{Volume (mL)} = \frac{\text{Weight (mg)} \times \text{Assay potency } (\mu\text{g/mg})}{\text{Concentration } (\mu\text{g/mL})}$$

(Formula 2)

Preparing stock solutions:

- Prepare stock solutions at ≥1,280 µg/mL or 10× the highest concentration.
- Solvents such as dimethyl sulfoxide (DMSO), ethanol, and polyethylene glycol are used for water-insoluble drugs.

Filtration and storage:

- Filter stock solutions if sterility is required.
- Store solutions at –60°C or below for 6 months.

Ranges for antifungals:

- *AmB*: 0.0313–16 µg/mL
- *FLC*: 0.125–64 µg/mL
- *Echinocandins*: 0.0313–16 µg/mL

Test Procedures

Broth medium:

- Use RPMI 1640 with glutamine, without bicarbonate, buffered to pH 7.0 ± 0.1 using 3-(N-morpholino) propanesulfonic acid (MOPS) buffer.
- Avoid buffers such as Tris that antagonize antifungal agents.

Dilution procedures:

- Prepare antifungal dilutions according to specific solubility instructions.
- *Common solvents for drugs:*
  - AmB, ITC: DMSO
  - FLC, caspofungin (CASF): Water

Key Points for Broth Dilution Testing

- Use RPMI 1640 broth for testing and prepare stock solutions as described.
- Ensure each concentration tested includes appropriate controls.
- Perform MIC performance checks using quality control (QC) organisms.

Water-soluble antifungal agents:

- *Dilution preparation*: Twofold dilutions are prepared volumetrically in broth, and 0.1 mL of each antifungal dilution is used for each test. The antifungal solutions used are 10 times more concentrated than the final concentration to account for dilution with inoculum.
- *Adjusting ratios*: While 1:10 dilutions are common, a 1:11 ratio may be used when pipettes deliver only specific volumes. The final test volume can vary between 1.0 and 1.1 mL.

Water-insoluble antifungal agents:

- *Preparation*: Water-insoluble antifungals (e.g., ketoconazole and AmB) require a solvent such as DMSO for stock preparation at 100 times the final strength. They are diluted 10-fold in RPMI 1640 broth.

- *Dilution example*: To achieve a final concentration range of 16–0.0313 μg/mL, prepare an initial stock solution of 1,600 μg/mL in DMSO and perform serial dilutions using RPMI 1640 medium.
    - Prepare stock solution
    - Make stock 100× the highest final concentration.
    - Highest final conc = 16 μg/mL → 100× = 1,600 μg/mL.
    - Dissolve drug in DMSO to reach 1,600 μg/mL.
    - First dilution:
        - Take the DMSO stock and dilute 10-fold into RPMI 1640 broth to reduce DMSO concentration (too much DMSO can inhibit fungal growth).
        - Now you have 160 μg/mL working solution.
        - Prepare twofold serial dilutions in RPMI 1640 to cover the range: 160 → 80 → 40 → 20 → 10 → 5 → 2.5 → ... until you reach 0.0313 μg/mL.
        - Inoculate with fungal suspension according to CLSI or EUCAST protocol.

Inoculum preparation:

- *Steps*: Organisms are cultured on Sabouraud dextrose agar or peptone dextrose agar, and a suspension is prepared by vortexing colonies. The suspension is adjusted to a specific cell density using a spectrophotometer.
- *Dilution*: A working suspension is made by diluting the stock suspension in RPMI 1640, ensuring a final concentration of 5.0×10^2 to 2.5×10^3 cells/mL.

Broth microdilution modifications:

Microdilution: Similar to broth macrodilution, the procedure is modified to fit a 96-well microdilution plate format. Drug dilutions are made, and inoculum is added to the wells. The plates are incubated, and results are read using a scoring system that evaluates turbidity.

Quality control:

Control measures: Growth, purity, and end point interpretation controls are crucial for test validity. QC organisms are tested alongside the isolates to ensure accurate results.

Reading results:

MIC: The lowest concentration that significantly inhibits growth is recorded as the MIC. Interpretation varies slightly based on the drug, with clear guidelines provided for AmB, azoles, and flucytosine.

Time and reading impact:

48- versus 24-hour readings: For most *Candida* species, readings at 24 and 48 hours are similar. However, for isolates with trailing growth, a 48-hour reading may present a higher MIC, and it is suggested that these isolates be categorized as susceptible based on 24-hour readings.

Minimum Effective Concentration

Echinocandins, such as CASF, exhibit activity against *Aspergillus* species both in vitro and in vivo. The determination of in vitro activity involves using an inverted microscope to assess the drug dilution at which there is an effect on the growing tips of hyphae. This effect results in the production of small, rounded, and compact microcolonies, and at higher magnification, the hyphae appear highly branched, short, and stubby. This concentration is referred to as the minimum effective concentration (MEC).

The MEC remains stable across time intervals, with variations less than MIC values at periods of measurement beyond 24 hours (usually measured at 48 hours). Readings are typically made at 24 hours for *Aspergillus* species and *Paecilomyces variotii*, 48 hours for *Fusarium* species, and 72 hours for *Scedosporium* species.

While the MEC provides valuable information about drug effectiveness, it is a more labor-intensive measurement compared to MIC, requiring experienced observers.

ANTIFUNGAL SUSCEPTIBILITY METHODS CURRENTLY AVAILABLE FOR USE IN THE CLINICAL LABORATORY

- *BMD method*: Microtitration plates are precoated with a panel of drugs in dilutions covering a broad range (e.g., YeastOne®, Clinical Sensititre®).
- *ETEST®*: The ETEST®, developed by bioMérieux, consists of plastic strips, each embedded with a drug gradient.
- *Disk diffusion method*: Similar to the Kirby–Bauer method used in antibacterial drug susceptibility tests, this method involves testing the susceptibility of fungi to antifungal drugs using disks.

Antifungal Disk Diffusion Susceptibility Testing for Yeasts (*Candida* Species)

The disk diffusion method is a standardized procedure specifically for *Candida* species. This method is based on the *CLSI M44/A2 protocol* and does not extend to other genera or dimorphic fungi. A breakdown of the steps and procedures involved in this method is given in the following text.

Reagents for the Disk Diffusion Test

Agar medium: Use *Mueller-Hinton Agar supplemented with 2% glucose and 0.5 µg/mL methylene blue dye* (GMB medium). This medium is optimal for routine susceptibility testing of yeasts.

pH of the medium: The pH of the prepared agar should be between *7.2 and 7.4* at room temperature after gelling. It can be checked by:

- Submerging a pH electrode in a macerated agar sample
- Using a calibrated surface electrode

Moisture on agar surface: Excess surface moisture should be removed by drying the plates in an incubator or laminar flow hood with the lids ajar for *10–30 minutes.*

Storage of Antimicrobial Disks

- *Refrigeration*: Store the disks at *8°C or below* or *freeze at –14°C or below.*
- *Equilibration*: Remove disks from the refrigerator or freezer *30–60 minutes before use* to allow them to reach at room temperature.
- *Desiccation*: Keep the disks in a desiccated container or a dispensing apparatus with an adequate desiccant.
- *Expiration*: Discard any disks after their expiration date.

Procedure for Performing the Disk Diffusion Test

Inoculum preparation (direct colony suspension method):

- Subculture organisms on *blood agar* or *Sabouraud dextrose agar.*
- Pick five colonies (~1 mm diameter) from a *24-hour-old Candida culture* and suspend them in *5 mL of sterile saline.*
- Vortex the suspension for *15 seconds* and adjust the turbidity to match a *0.5 McFarland standard* using a spectrophotometer (530 nm wavelength), which yields *1 × 10⁶ to 5 × 10⁶ cells/mL.*

Inoculation of test plates:

- Dip a sterile cotton swab into the adjusted suspension, remove excess fluid, and streak the *Mueller-Hinton + GMB agar plate* evenly.
- Allow plates to absorb surface moisture for *3–5 minutes* before applying the drug-impregnated disks.

Application of disks:

- Place antimicrobial disks onto the inoculated agar surface. Each disk should be *pressed down to ensure complete contact* with the agar. Ensure disks are spaced at least *24-mm apart* from center to center.
- Not more than *12 disks on a 150-mm plate* or *five disks on a 100-mm plate* should be used.
- Incubate the plates at *35°C (±2°C)* within *15 minutes* of applying the disks.

Reading Plates

- After *20–24 hours of incubation*, measure the zone diameters of inhibition to the nearest whole millimeter using reflected light and a black background.
- Pinpoint colonies or microcolonies should be ignored. If necessary, read at *48 hours* for insufficient growth.

Interpretation of Disk Diffusion Test Results

Interpretive categories are based on the size of the zone of inhibition as follows:

- *Susceptible (S)*: It implies that the strain can be treated effectively with the recommended dosage.
- *S-DD*: It indicates that higher dosages are needed for an effective response.
- *Intermediate (I)*: It suggests a borderline susceptibility, where treatment efficacy may vary.
- *Resistant (R)*: The strain is not inhibited by the antifungal agent at achievable dosages.
- *Nonsusceptible (NS)*: It indicates a lack of categorization for intermediate or resistant interpretations, often applied to new drugs.

Zone diameter interpretive criteria: Disk diffusion zone diameters are inversely correlated with MICs. Specific zone diameter interpretive criteria can be found in CLSI protocols and related tables.

Quality Control

Quality control ensures that the disk diffusion test for AFS consistently produces accurate and reliable results. This section outlines essential QC measures, including reference strains, testing frequency, corrective actions, and limitations.

Reference strains for quality control: To maintain the *precision* and *accuracy* of the test, the following reference strains should be obtained from reliable sources:

- *Candida albicans* ATCC 90028
- *Candida parapsilosis* ATCC 22019
- *Candida tropicalis* ATCC 750
- *Candida krusei* ATCC 6258

These strains are used to monitor the consistency and performance of the disk diffusion test.

Frequency of quality control testing:

- *Daily testing*: To test each day, the disk diffusion method is performed. For each antimicrobial agent/organism combination, 1 out of every 20 results may fall outside the acceptable range due to random variation (95% confidence limit). If >1 out of 20 tests is out of range, corrective action is required.
- *Weekly testing*: If the performance is satisfactory during daily testing for 20 consecutive days, weekly QC testing can be implemented. This includes testing one QC strain weekly and testing every time a reagent or disk lot is changed.

Implementing weekly quality control testing: Weekly QC testing may be implemented under the following conditions:

- Satisfactory daily test results for 20 consecutive days with no more than one out-of-range result.
- Perform weekly testing and additional testing when new reagents or disk lots are used.

If weekly QC results fall outside the acceptable range, revert to daily testing until the issue is resolved.

Corrective action: When QC test results fall outside the acceptable limits, corrective action is required.

- *Out-of-control due to an obvious error*: Examples include using the wrong disk, strain, or incubation conditions. Document the error and repeat the test immediately.
- *Out-of-control without an obvious error*: Immediate corrective action is required, including:
  - Testing the antimicrobial agent/organism combination for 5 consecutive days.
  - If all five zone diameters are within the acceptable range, no further action is needed.
  - If any of the five measurements are outside the range, additional corrective actions are required, such as checking materials, storage conditions, or strain quality.

Common sources of error:

- Incorrect zone diameter measurement or transcription
- Expired or improperly stored turbidity standards
- Expired or improperly stored materials (e.g., disks and agar plates)
- Incorrect incubation temperature or conditions
- Contaminated control strains or improper inoculum preparation

In case of persistent errors, obtaining a new control strain, testing materials from different manufacturers, or switching to an alternate method may be necessary.

Reporting patient results during quality control issues: During an out-of-control test, assess whether to report patient results based on the nature of the error. Options include:

- Suppressing individual agent results
- Retrospective review of patient data for unusual patterns
- Using an alternate test method or referring samples to a reference laboratory

Limitations of Disk Diffusion Methods

- *Organism-specific testing*: This method is standardized only for *Candida* species. For other yeast species, consultation with an infectious disease specialist is recommended. A reference dilution method or referral to a reference laboratory may be required for unusual species.
- *Verification of patient results*: Acceptable results for control strains do not guarantee accuracy for patient isolates. Always verify patient results by reviewing transcription errors, contamination, and previous results on the same patient's isolates. Retesting may be necessary for unusual or inconsistent results.

Standard method for antifungal susceptibility testing of yeasts: The standard BMD method (CLSI document M27-A3) is approved for testing *Candida* species and *C. neoformans*. The key parameters of this method include:

- *Medium*: RPMI 1640 medium, adjusted to pH 7.0
- *Inoculum*: Standardized using a spectrophotometer
- *Incubation*:
  - *Candida* species: 35°C for 24–48 hours. The 24-hour time point is used to exclude errors resulting from trailing growth in the presence of azoles.
  - *Cryptococcus* species: 35°C for 72 hours
- *Endpoint determination*:
  - Visual detection of 50% growth inhibition for azoles and flucytosine
  - 100% inhibition for AmB
- *QC strains*: These strains have defined MICs, providing internal standards for susceptibility and resistance determinations.

Minimum fungicidal concentration (MFC): The MFC is the minimum concentration of a substance required to kill the target fungal isolate, determined by subculture. It is an important parameter in evaluating the effectiveness of antifungal drugs.

Limitations of the M27-A susceptibility test method for yeasts:

- *Clinical correlations*: The correlation between in vitro susceptibility and clinical outcome may not always align. Clinical success is influenced by various factors.

- *Trailing growth phenomenon*: Trailing growth of *Candida* species isolates exposed to azole agents complicates endpoint determination. It is observed in *C. albicans* and *C. tropicalis* isolates with a low FLC MIC after 24 hours and a high MIC (>64 µg/mL) after 48 hours.
- *Mechanisms of trailing growth*:
  - *Activation of calcineurin*: Calcineurin, a protein phosphatase, is implicated in the survival of yeast under stress conditions, contributing to residual growth in the presence of high drug concentrations.
  - *Upregulation of ERG11*: The upregulation of the *ERG11* gene, which encodes lanosterol demethylase, is observed in response to azole exposure, affecting ergosterol synthesis.
  - *Incubation temperature*: Trailing growth at 35°C may be inhibited at 25°C and 42°C.
  - *Genotype clustering*: Certain genotypes, such as DST 140 in *C. tropicalis*, may be associated with both resistant and trailing growth phenotypes.

ETEST® (bioMérieux, Marcy-l'Etoile, France): The ETEST® is a plastic strip embedded with a gradient of the drug to be tested, and numbers on the scale correspond to drug concentrations on the strip (in µg/mL). The procedure involves plating the isolate as a "lawn" on agar medium in a Petri plate, and the ETEST® strip is then placed on the agar surface. This method can be used for both yeasts and molds.

Test conditions:
- *Medium*: RPMI + 2% glucose + MOPS + 1.5% Bacto agar
- *Inoculum*: Yeast suspension in saline is used to swab plates. For *Candida* species, 0.5 McFarland standard is used, and for *C. neoformans*, 1 McFarland is used.
- *Incubation*:
  - For *Candida* species: 35°C for 24–48 hours
  - For *C. neoformans*: 35°C for 48–72 hours

Reading the MIC end point:
- *AmB*: Read at the drug concentration resulting in complete inhibition of growth.
- *Flucytosine*: Read at almost complete (90%) growth inhibition.
- *Azoles*: Read at the first point of significant inhibition, marked by a decrease in growth density. The 80% inhibition principle is applied here.
- *Echinocandins*: Read the end point at the first visual point of significant inhibition, which corresponds to 80% inhibition.

Quality control: MIC limits for standard tester isolates (*C. krusei* ATCC 6258 and *C. parapsilosis* ATCC 22019) against AmB, flucytosine, azoles, and echinocandins are described in the ETEST® Technical Manual.

ETEST® for molds:
- *Medium*: RPMI + 2% glucose + MOPS agar. Alternatively, modified Casitone Agar is used for azoles. A chemically defined medium is preferable for QC.
- *Inoculum*: Suspension of conidia and hyphae in saline with Tween 80, adjusted to 0.5 McFarland standard for *Aspergillus* species and 1 McFarland for *Fusarium* and *Rhizopus* species.
- *Incubation*: Plates are incubated at 35°C for 24–72 hours, depending on the genus.

Quality control: ETEST® MIC limits for standard tester isolates (*Aspergillus flavus* ATCC 204304 and *Aspergillus fumigatus* ATCC 2043051) are described in the ETEST® Technical Manual.

MOLDS: BROTH DILUTION ANTIFUNGAL SUSCEPTIBILITY TESTING

This section details the procedures for broth dilution testing of filamentous fungi (molds) that cause both invasive and cutaneous fungal infections. The protocol aligns with standard procedures for AFS testing, including inoculum preparation and incubation conditions.

Procedure

Drug Concentrations

Test the following concentration ranges for nondermatophyte molds:
- *AmB*: 0.0313–16 µg/mL
- *Flucytosine*: 0.125–64 µg/mL
- *Ketoconazole, ITC, PSC, and VRC*: 0.0313–16 µg/mL
- *FLC*: 0.125–64 µg/mL
- Echinocandins *(anidulafungin, CASF, and micafungin)*: 0.0313–16 µg/mL

For dermatophytes, test the following ranges:
- *Ciclopirox, miconazole, and luliconazole*: 0.016–16 µg/mL
- *Griseofulvin*: 0.25–128 µg/mL
- *ITC, amorolfine, and VRC*: 0.0078–4 µg/mL
- *FLC*: 0.0625–32 µg/mL
- *Ketoconazole, clotrimazole, and naftifine*: 0.0312–16 µg/mL
- *Terbinafine and sertaconazole*: 0.0156–8 µg/mL

Inoculum Preparation

Nondermatophyte species:

- Use nongerminated conidial or sporangiospore suspensions at 0.4 × 10^4 to 5 × 10^4 CFU/mL for reproducible MIC data.
- Grow fungi on *potato dextrose agar* for 7 days at 35°C for sporulation. *Aspergillus* and *Mucorales* species may sporulate in 48 hours, while *Fusarium* species may take up to 7 days.
- Prepare conidial/sporangiospore suspensions using saline and optionally, one drop of Tween 20 for *Aspergillus* species.
- Transfer the homogeneous suspension, mix, and adjust to an optical density (OD) at 530 nm. Use different OD ranges for specific fungi (e.g., *Aspergillus* species: 0.09–0.13).

Dermatophyte species:

- Grow on *potato dextrose agar* or *oatmeal* agar (for *Trichophyton rubrum*). Incubate at 30°C for 4–5 days.
- Prepare conidial suspensions and adjust to 1 × 10^3 to 3 × 10^3 CFU/mL.

Inoculating RPMI-1640 Medium

Inoculate each well with 0.1 mL of the 2× concentrated inoculum suspension. Include growth control wells and test QC strains alongside patient isolates.

Incubation

- *Aspergillus species, Fusarium species, and Sporothrix schenckii*: Incubate at 35°C for 46–50 hours.
- *Rhizopus species*: Examine after 21–26 hours.
- *Scedosporium species*: Examine after 70–74 hours.
- *Echinocandins*: Examine after 21–26 hours for *Aspergillus* species and 46–72 hours for *Scedosporium* species.
- *Dermatophytes*: Evaluate after 4 days.

Minimum Inhibitory Concentration and Minimum Effective Concentration Reading Results

- *AmB*: MIC is the lowest concentration that inhibits 100% of growth.
- *FLC and ketoconazole*: MIC is defined by 50–80% growth reduction compared to the control.
- *ITC, PSC, and VRC*: MIC is the lowest concentration with 100% growth inhibition.
- *Echinocandins*: MEC is the lowest concentration that causes the growth of small, rounded, and compact hyphal forms.
- *Ciclopirox, griseofulvin, terbinafine, and naftifine:* MIC is defined by 80% or more growth reduction for nondermatophytes and 100% inhibition for dermatophytes.

Proceed with QC as previously mentioned and refer to established guidelines for interpreting the results.

Disk Diffusion Antifungal Susceptibility Testing for Molds

- *Selection of molds and preparation of inoculum*:
    - Various molds, including *Aspergillus, Mucorales, Fusarium, Scedosporium, Alternaria, Bipolaris,* and *Paecilomyces* species, are chosen for testing.
    - The molds are tested by both BMD and disk diffusion methods. Inoculum preparation involves suspending conidia and hyphae in saline for *Mucorales* and adjusting the suspension to a specific McFarland standard.
- *Disk diffusion method*:
    - The CLSI guideline for disk diffusion susceptibility testing of nondermatophyte molds (M51-AE) is followed.
    - Disks containing different antifungal drugs, including PSC, VRC, CASF, AmB, and ITC, are placed on the agar surface.
- *Incubation and reading zones*:
    - The Petri plates are incubated at a specified temperature and duration, with readings made at different time intervals depending on the species. Fast growers such as *Mucorales* are read after overnight incubation, while others are read at 48 or 72 hours.
    - The presence of inhibition zones around the disks is observed and measured.
- *Interpretation and breakpoints*:
    - Tentative in vitro breakpoints for disk diffusion tests are applied. Breakpoints are determined based on the diameter of the inhibition zone and are categorized as resistant (R), intermediate susceptibility, and susceptible (S).
    - Breakpoints for triazoles (e.g., VRC and ITC) and CASF are defined based on the specific zone diameters corresponding to MIC values.
- *QC and reproducibility*: QC measures are implemented to ensure the reliability of results. Zone diameters are reproducible, and good correlation is observed between zone diameters and MICs or MECs.

Automated System for Antifungal Susceptibility Testing

The VITEK 2 system by bioMérieux, France, is an automated platform that performs both microorganism identification and susceptibility testing.

- *Approved antifungal agents and tests*:
  - The system is approved for AFS with FLC.
  - It determines MICs for AmB, flucytosine, and VRC against *Candida* species.
  - MIC results obtained from the VITEK 2 system are compared with the reference method M27-A BMD to assess accuracy.
- *Reproducibility and speed*:
  - Results from the VITEK 2 system are highly reproducible and reliably predict MICs as determined by the reference M27-A BMD method.
  - The system provides rapid results, with a mean time to results ranging from 12 to 15 hours.
  - The use of spectrophotometry for determining MIC endpoints reduces observer subjectivity.
- *Flow cytometry in antifungal susceptibility testing*:
  - Flow cytometry is proposed as a method that measures killing of the target fungal cell, offering potential advantages in improved clinical correlations.
  - Dyes such as FUN-1 [2-chloro-4-(2,3-dihydro-3-methyl-(benzo-1,3-thiazol-2-yl)-methylidene)-1-phenylquinolinium iodide] or propidium iodide (PI) are commonly used in flow cytometry to differentiate and enumerate live and dead fungal cells, thereby providing reliable correlations in antifungal susceptibility testing.
  - The procedure involves treating a yeast cell suspension with serial dilutions of the antifungal agent, followed by incubation, washing, and staining with a fluorophore.
  - The flow cytometer then measures scattered light and fluorescence of individual cells, detecting the activity of the antifungal agent.
- *Interpretation and reporting*:
  - Flow cytometry results are expressed as percentages of positive cells showing high fluorescence for PI or as staining indices (SI) for FUN-1.
  - Susceptibility is defined based on the minimum concentration of the antifungal agent resulting in a SI above the control (>1) after drug treatment.
- *Clinical correlation*:
  - Clinical correlation studies have been conducted using flow cytometry for susceptibility testing.
  - In a study with *C. albicans* isolates, the agreement between the M27-A BMD test and flow cytometry methods ranged from 96 to 99%.
- *Application to A. fumigatus*:
  - Flow cytometry has been applied to *A. fumigatus* as a model mold for susceptibility testing.
  - Studies on *A. fumigatus* susceptibility to AmB, ITC, and VRC showed good overall agreement (93%) with the M38-A BMD reference method.
- *Advantages and potential*:
  - Flow cytometry is faster than traditional AFS tests.
  - The ability to detect and quantitate dead cells may offer closer clinical correlation than traditional MIC determination.
  - Heterogeneity in susceptibility within an isolate population can be observed through flow cytometer data.

BIBLIOGRAPHY

1. Adl SM, Simpson AGB, Lane CE, Lukeš J, Bass D, Bowser SS, et al. The revised classification of eukaryotes. J Eukaryot Microbiol. 2012;59(5): 429-93.
2. Ajello L, Threlkeld M, Alpert M. Phaeohyphomycosis: a new term for hyphomycosis caused by pigmented fungi. Mycologia. 1974;66(6): 1105-25.
3. Ajello L. Phaeohyphomycosis: definition and etiology. Mykosen. 1975;18(9):419-24.
4. Al-Sweih N, Khan Z, Ahmad S. Malassezia fungemia in a Kuwaiti hospital: a 10-year review. Diagn Microbiol Infect Dis. 2010;66(3):286-90.
5. Alviano DS, Franzen AJ, Travassos LR, Liebhard P, de Souza W, Alviano CS. Diversity of carbohydrates and glycoconjugates on the surface of fungal cells. FEMS Microbiol Rev. 2001;25(2):149-63.
6. Ameen M. Epidemiology of superficial fungal infections. Clin Dermatol. 2010;28(2):197-201.
7. Antimicrobial Resistance Surveillance and Research Network, Indian Council of Medical Research. Standard Operating Procedures for Fungal Identification and Detection of Antifungal Resistance, 2nd edition. New Delhi: Indian Council of Medical Research; 2019.
8. Arrillaga-Romany IC, Rex JH. Sporotrichosis. Infect Dis Clin North Am. 2007;21(3):685-701.
9. Arvanitis M, Anagnostou T, Sperry AR, Mylonakis E. Molecular methods for the diagnosis of invasive fungal infections. Future Microbiol. 2019;14:1-18.
10. Ashbee HR, Evans EG. Malassezia species. In: Richman DD, Whitley RJ, Hayden FG (Eds). Clinical Virology, 3rd edition. Washington, DC: ASM Press; 2009. pp. 1361-73.
11. Ashworth JH. On Rhinosporidium seeberi (Wernicke, 1903), with special reference to its sporulation and affinities. Earth Environ Sci Trans R Soc Edinb. 1924;53:301-42.
12. Assi MA, Wheat LJ, Gold JM, McKinsey DS, Chang CT, Cracunoiu N, et al. The spectrum of pulmonary histoplasmosis in immunocompetent adults. Chest. 2013;144(5):1629-34.
13. Badali H, de Hoog GS, Mendoza L, Bonifaz A, van den Ende AH, Gerrits van den Ende B, et al. Fonsecaea: taxonomy, ecology and molecular epidemiology of an important genus of human pathogenic fungi. Fungal Divers. 2010;43(1):123-63.
14. Baddley JW, McVay CS, Kheir F, Soong SJ, Morris M, Gathings R, et al. Progressive disseminated histoplasmosis in patients with AIDS: treatment with itraconazole and amphotericin B. Mycoses. 2002;45(3-4):124-9.
15. Barsok. Sur une nouvelle mycose cutanée produite par une Alternaria. Bull Soc Fr Dermatol Syphiligr. 1933;40:1240-5.
16. Batra R, Boekhout T, Guého E, Cabañes FJ, Dawson TL Jr, Guillot J, et al. Diversification of five Malassezia species as revealed by ribosomal DNA non-coding regions. FEMS Yeast Res. 2005;5(4-5):347-58.
17. Boekhout T, Fonseca A. The genus Trichosporon. In: Kurtzman CP, Fell JW, Boekhout T (Eds). The Yeasts: A Taxonomic Study, 5th edition. Amsterdam: Elsevier; 2011. pp. 1557-60.
18. Bonifaz A, Badali H, de Hoog GS, Meygandi M, Carrasco-Gerard E, Saúl A, et al. Chromoblastomycosis: a comprehensive review. J Fungi (Basel). 2021;7(8):671.
19. Bonifaz A, Paredes-Solis V, Saul A. Chromoblastomycosis. Clin Dermatol. 2004;22(1):4-8.
20. Bonifaz A, Tirado-Sánchez A, Calderón L, Saul A, Araiza J, Fernández-Fonts G. Actinomycetoma: experience of 18 consecutive cases in a referral center in Mexico. Int J Dermatol. 2007;46 (Suppl 5):23-7.
21. Bonifaz A, Vázquez-González D, Saúl A. Dermatofitosis y otras micosis superficiales. Clin Dermatol. 2009;27(1):13-21.
22. Bonifaz A, Vázquez-González D, Saúl A. Phaeohyphomycosis, chromoblastomycosis, and mycetoma. Clin Dermatol. 2010;28(2):170-5.
23. Bonifaz A, Vázquez-González D, Saúl A. White piedra: clinical, mycological, and therapeutic experience of 7 cases. Med Mycol. 2003;41(1):75-9.
24. Bonifaz A. Botryomycosis. Clin Dermatol. 2012;30(6):675-8.
25. Bowman SM, Free SJ. The fungal cell wall: structure, synthesis, and assembly. Curr Genet. 2006;49(3):157-72.
26. Butler G, O'Dwyer DN, Boland F, O'Mahony L, Fitzgerald NT, Shanahan F. Microbiome in asthma: a role for fungi. J Fungi (Basel). 2023;9(7):712.
27. Cafarchia C, Figueredo LA, Otranto D. Molecular identification of dermatophytes from animal ringworm cases in southern Italy. Mycoses. 2013;56(5):552-7.
28. Carlos IZ, Libório TI, Sacramento L. Host immunity to Sporothrix schenckii. Front Biosci (Elite Ed). 2015;7(1):137-48.
29. Carter HV. On a new and striking form of fungus disease principally affecting the foot and prevailing endemically in many parts of India. Trans Bombay Med Phys Soc. 1860;6:104-42.
30. Chakrabarti A, Das A, Sharma A, Panda N, Singh R, Behera B, et al. Clinicoepidemiology of sporotrichosis in India. Mycoses. 2015;58 (Suppl 1): 87-95.
31. Chakrabarti A, Denning DW, Ferguson BJ, Ponikau J, Buzina W, Kita H, et al. Fungal rhinosinusitis: a categorization and definitional scheme addressing current controversies. Laryngoscope. 2009;119(9):1809-18.
32. Chander J. Textbook of Medical Mycology, 4th edition. New Delhi: Jaypee Brothers Medical Publishers (P) Ltd.; 2018.

33. Chen TA, Billmyer S, Michaels J, Sebastian A, Horsley W, Goldberg L, et al. The mycobiome of the human scalp: a multiethnic study of Managementia restricta and Managementia globosa. Int J Cosmet Sci. 2018;40(5):481-8.
34. Chiller TM, Magill SS, Francisco S, Warnock DW. Laboratory biosafety in clinical mycology. Med Mycol. 2018;56 (Suppl 1):S86-92.
35. Chowdhary A, Sharma C, Meis JF. Candida auris: a rapidly emerging cause of hospital-acquired multidrug-resistant fungal infections globally. PLoS Pathog. 2017;13(5):e1006290.
36. Cole GT, Samson RA. Patterns of development in conidial fungi. London: Pitman; 1979.
37. Cortez KJ, Roilides E, Quiroz-Telles F, Farmakiotis D, Bilbao-Casaus R, Al-Aidaroos AY, et al. Infections caused by Scedosporium species. Clin Microbiol Rev. 2008;21(1):157-97.
38. Couppie P, Clyti E, Nacher M, Carme B. Disseminated histoplasmosis and AIDS. Med Mycol. 2006;44(8):757-60.
39. da Silva Pontes ZBV, Ramos AL, de Oliveira LE, de Lacerda GMF, Oliveira NMC, dos Santos JP. Clinical and mycological study of scalp white piedra in the State of Paraíba, Brazil. Mem Inst Oswaldo Cruz. 2002;97(5):747-50.
40. Dawson TL Jr. Malassezia globosa: a lipase secretor and major contributor to dandruff. J Investig Dermatol Symp Proc. 2007;12(2):15-9.
41. De Beurmann L, Gougerot H. The sporotrichoses. Br Med J. 1911;2(2653):1153-9.
42. De Hoog GS, Guarro J, Gené J, Figueras MJ. Atlas of Clinical Fungi, 3rd edition. Washington, DC: ASM Press; 2010.
43. de Lima Barros MB, de Almeida Paes R, Schubach AO. Sporothrix schenckii and sporotrichosis. Clin Microbiol Rev. 2011;24(4):633-54.
44. Deepe GS Jr. Immune responses to Histoplasma capsulatum. Clin Microbiol Rev. 2005;18(3):415-25.
45. Dixon DM, Walsh TJ, Merz WG, McGinnis MR. Concentrations of the pigment melanin in human pathogenic fungi. J Clin Microbiol. 1980;12(4):643-4.
46. Dixon DM, Walsh TJ, Merz WG, McGinnis MR. Isolation, identification, and characterization of Sporothrix schenckii. Curr Top Med Mycol. 1991;4:52-88.
47. Ely JW, Rosenfeld S, Cureton EL. Diagnosis and management of common tinea infections. Am Fam Physician. 2004;69(10):2595-602.
48. Emmons CW. Isolation of Histoplasma capsulatum from soil. Public Health Rep. 1949;64(44):1330-6.
49. Faergemann J, Mayser P. Pityriasis versicolor. Clin Dermatol. 2014;32(4):429-33.
50. Fahal AH, Hassan MA. Mycetoma. Br J Surg. 1992;79(11):1138-41.
51. Fahal AH, Mahgoub ES, El Hassan AM, Attiah EA, Rahman IA. Ultrasonographical imaging in mycetoma. Br J Surg. 1997;84(6):765-6.
52. Fahal AH. Mycetoma: a clinical and histopathological study. J Trop Med. 2004;2004(Pt 1):1-16.
53. Figueras MJ, Guarro J. Black piedra. Clin Microbiol Rev. 2021;35(1):e0020820.
54. Figueras MJ, Guarro J. Piedraia hortae: ultrastructure of the ascostroma and taxonomic implications. Mycol Res. 1997;101(7):833-8.
55. Fraser DW, Bérard T. Histoplasmosis. Am J Trop Med Hyg. 2021;105(1):9-14.
56. Frealle E, Favory R, Crewieux E, Chabasse D, Delhaes L. Exophiala dermatitidis and associated infections. Med Mycol. 2014;52(8):779-91.
57. Gaitanis G, Bassukas ID, Velegraki A. Malassezia species in atopic dermatitis. J Fungi (Basel). 2020;6(4):190.
58. Gerrits van den Ende B, de Hoog GS. Variability and molecular diagnostics of the neurotropic species Exophiala dermatitidis. Med Mycol. 1999;37(4):235-46.
59. Ginter-Hanselmayer G, Weger W, Menzinger-Seger L, Soyer HP, Smolle J. Epidemiology of tinea capitis in Graz, Austria. Mycoses. 2004;47(7):311-4.
60. Guého E, Improvisi L, de Hoog GS, Dupont B. Trichosporon on humans: a practical account. Mycoses. 1994;37(1-2):3-10.
61. Guého E, Midgley G, Guillot J. The genus Malassezia: a review. Med Mycol. 1998;36 (Suppl 1):1-8.
62. Gugnani HC. Black piedra: looking back and looking ahead. Med Mycol. 2018;56 (Suppl 1):S60-7.
63. Gupta AK, Ryder JE, Baran R. Onychomycosis: an update. Acta Derm Venereol. 2004;84(1):3-8.
64. Gupta AK, Stec N, Summerbell RC, Shear N, Piguet V, Tosti A, et al. Onychomycosis: identification of diagnostic methods and therapeutic strategies, 2019 update. J Drugs Dermatol. 2019;18(7):674-8.
65. Hagan RH, Messer SA, Pfaller MA. Laboratory diagnosis of fungal infections. In: Carroll KC, Pfaller MA, Landry ML, McAdam AJ (Eds). Manual of Clinical Microbiology, 12th edition. Washington, DC: ASM Press; 2019. pp. 1954-2001.
66. Hainer BL. Dermatophyte infections. Am Fam Physician. 2003;67(1):101-8.
67. Hald M, Arendrup MC, Svejgaard EL, Lindskov R, Foged EK, Saunte DML, et al. Evidence-based Danish guidelines for the treatment of Malassezia-related skin diseases. Acta Derm Venereol. 2015;95(1):12-9.
68. Harrington MS, Hofherr SE. Microscopy. In: Leber AL (Ed). Clinical Microbiology Procedures Handbook, 4th edition. Washington, DC: ASM Press; 2016.
69. Havlickova B, Czaika AH, Friedrich M. Epidemiological trends in skin mycoses worldwide. Mycoses. 2008;51 (Suppl 4):2-15.
70. Hawksworth DL. Naming fungi on one hand: unified nomenclatural system for fungi. Mycoscience. 2012;53(3):163-72.
71. Hay RJ. The management of onychomycosis: an update. J Eur Acad Dermatol Venereol. 2005;19 (Suppl 1):23-8.
72. Hazen KC. Ophiostomatales. In: Perfect JR, Casadevall A, Larsen RA, Pardoll D, Pirofski LA (Eds). Cryptococcus: From Human Pathogen to Model Yeast. Washington, DC: ASM Press; 2020.
73. Hektoen L, Perkins FF. Sporothrix schenckii, a new pathogenic fungus. A preliminary report. JAMA. 1900;35:836-8.
74. Hibbett DS, Binder M, Bischoff JF, Blackwell M, Cannon PF, Eriksson OE, et al. A higher-level phylogenetic classification of the fungi. Mycol Res. 2007;111(Pt 5):509-47.
75. Howard DH. Dimorphism in medically important fungi. Clin Microbiol Rev. 1999;12(3):328-52.
76. Inácio CP, Rocha AP, Barbosa RN, Oliveira NT, Silva JC, de Lima-Neto RG, et al. Experimental white piedra: a robust approach to ultrastructural analysis, scanning electron microscopy and etiological discoveries. Mycoses. 2016;59(1):41-9.
77. International Mycological Association. (2025). MycoBank. [online] Available from https://www.mycobank.org/. [Last accessed July, 2025].

78. Irinyi L, Serena C, Garcia-Hermoso D, Arabatzis M, Maurer E, Klaassen CHW, et al. International Society of Human and Animal Mycology (ISHAM) reference species for medical fungi. Med Mycol. 2015;53(6):555-90.
79. Isenberg HD. Clinical Microbiology Procedures Handbook, 3rd edition. Washington, DC: ASM Press; 2010.
80. Isenberg HD. Clinical Microbiology Procedures Handbook, 4th edition. Washington, DC: ASM Press; 2016.
81. Jenks JD, Eun-Kyung N, de Hoog Sebastian, Douglas DR, Kelly OS, Thomas PM, et al. Invasive fungal sinusitis: pathophysiology, microbiology, and diagnosis. Infect Drug Resist. 2021;14:217-38.
82. Jo JH, Kim HS, Park JK, Shokrollahzadeh S, Cho DH, Lee MH. Identification of Malassezia species isolated from patients with seborrheic dermatitis and pityriasis versicolor in Korea. Ann Dermatol. 2016;28(1):15-21.
83. Katkar A, Kar S, Pandey M, Khare P, Agarwal R, Muduli SK, et al. Histoplasmosis in India: an overview. Mycoses. 2021;64(2):126-37.
84. Kauffman CA, Bustamante B, Chapman SW, Pappas PG. Clinical practice guidelines for the management of sporotrichosis: 2007 update by the Infectious Diseases Society of America. Clin Infect Dis. 2007;45(10):1255-65.
85. Kauffman CA. Sporotrichosis. Clin Infect Dis. 1999;29(2):231-7.
86. Kemna ME, Elewski BE. A clinician's guide to the "minor" tineas. Arch Dermatol. 1996;132(9):1045-8.
87. Kidd S, Halliday C, Ellis D. Descriptions of Medical Fungi, 4th edition. Wallingford, UK: CABI; 2022.
88. Kirk PM, Cannon PF, Minter DW, Stalpers JA. Dictionary of the Fungi, 10th edition. Wallingford, UK: CABI; 2008.
89. Konopka JB. Yeast cell wall construction and morphogenesis. Curr Opin Microbiol. 2012;15(6):697-70.
90. Kwon-Chung KJ, Bennett JE. Medical Mycology. Philadelphia: Lea & Febiger; 1992.
91. Kwon-Chung KJ, Bennett JE. Piedra (tinea nodosa trichomycosis nodularis, trichomycosis nodosa, Beigel's disease, Chignon disease). In: Kwon-Chung KJ, Bennett JE (Eds). Medical Mycology. Philadelphia, PA: Lea & Febiger; 1992. pp. 183-90.
92. Lacaz CS, Porto E, Martins JE, Heins-Vaccari EM, Melo NT. Tratado de Micologia Médica, 9th edition. São Paulo: Sarvier; 2002.
93. Lackner M, Böhm A, Coelho C, Carleton A, Genlinger C, van den Ende BG, et al. Phylogeny of the fungal neurotrophic genus Cladophialophora (Chaetothyriales, Eurotiomycetes) with a focus on the pathogenic species C. bantiana. Fungal Genet Biol. 2014;62:32-48.
94. Lackner M, Teixeira MM, Barker BM, Hagen F, Boekhout T. Phylogeny and taxonomy of the Exophiala spinifera clade and the novel species Exophiala primulum and Exophiala lacus. Fungal Biol. 2013;117(10):711-23.
95. Lamoth F, Akan H, Pasqualotto AC, Herbrecht R. 1,3-β-D-Glucan in the diagnosis of invasive fungal infections. J Fungi (Basel). 2016;2(4):34.
96. Lane CG. Chromoblastomycosis. Report of a case originating in North Carolina. Arch Derm Syphilol. 1915;1:35.
97. Lange M, Lange N, Kranz W, Uhrlass S, Rimek D. Susceptibility of Malassezia species isolated from blood cultures to antifungal agents. Mycoses. 2012;55(1):48-54.
98. Latgé JP. The fungal cell wall: a protective shield against host defenses. Clin Microbiol Rev. 2009;22(2):387-408.
99. Laxmisha C, Rao R. Chromoblastomycosis: clinical manifestations, diagnosis and management. Indian J Dermatol Venereol Leprol. 2013;79(5):617-30.
100. LibreTexts™ Biology. (2025). Molds. [online] Available from https://bio.libretexts.org/Bookshelves/Microbiology/Microbiology_(Kaiser)/Unit_4%3A_Eukaryotic_Microorganisms_and_Viruses/08%3A_Fungi/8.3%3A_Molds. [Last accessed July, 2025].
101. LibreTexts™ Biology. (2025). Yeasts. [online] Available from https://bio.libretexts.org/Bookshelves/Microbiology/Microbiology_(Kaiser)/Unit_4%3A_Eukaryotic_Microorganisms_and_Viruses/08%3A_Fungi/8.2%3A_Yeasts. [Last accessed July, 2025].
102. Lopes-Bezerra LM, Schubach A, Costa RO. Sporothrix schenckii and sporotrichosis. An Acad Bras Cienc. 2006;78(2):293-308.
103. Louie JP, Hobson R, Ostrosky-Zeichner L. Serological assays for the diagnosis of invasive fungal infections. Curr Fungal Infect Rep. 2017;11(1):11-20.
104. Lutz A. Uma mycose arborescente (Molliolla) observada no homem; estudo de zoo-parasitologia comparada. Centralbl Bakteriol Parasitenkd Infektionskr Abt 1 Orig. 1908;46:660-8.
105. Madrid H, Cano J, Gené J, Castañeda Ruiz RF, Guarro J. Phylogenetic taxonomy of pathogenic Sporothrix species. Mycologia. 2013;105(6):1611-20.
106. Matsumoto T, Ajello L, Matsuda T, Szaniszlo PJ, Walsh TJ. Developments in hyalohyphomycosis and phaeohyphomycosis. J Med Vet Mycol. 1994;32 (Suppl 1):329-49.
107. Mayser P, Haze P, Pichlmeier U, Guidetti F, Rühl-Hörster B, Schmidt E, et al. Effects of lipophilic yeast products on inflammatory cytokine production by human keratinocytes. J Invest Dermatol. 2001;116(2):328-33.
108. Medlar EM. A new fungus, Phialophora verrucosa, pathogenic for man. Mycologia. 1915;7(4):200-3.
109. Mylonakis E, Clancy CJ, Ostrosky-Zeichner L, Pappas PG, Cunha CA, Venkatasubramanian RL, et al. T2 magnetic resonance assay for the rapid diagnosis of candidemia in whole blood: a clinical trial. Clin Infect Dis. 2015;60(6):892-9.
110. Nell AS, Kemmerling B. Malassezia-induced skin diseases: cellular and molecular mechanisms. Front Cell Infect Microbiol. 2020;10:108.
111. Nenoff P, Krüger C, Schaller J, Ginter-Hanselmayer G, Schulte-Beerbühl B, Tietz HJ. Mycology—an update. Part 1: dermatomycoses and onychomycoses. J Dtsch Dermatol Ges. 2014;12(3):188-209.
112. Nucci M, Marr KA, Herbrecht B, Quakyi I, Kartsonis N, Schlamm H, et al. Invasive infections caused by Scedosporium species in immunocompromised patients: clinical spectrum, diagnosis, and management. Clin Infect Dis. 2005;41(10):1458-64.
113. Odds FC. Candida and Candidosis: A Review and Bibliography, 2nd edition London: Baillière Tindall; 1988.
114. Orofino-Costa R, de Macedo PM, Rodrigues AM, Bernardes-Engemann AR. Sporotrichosis: an update on epidemiology, etiopathogenesis, laboratory and clinical therapeutics. An Bras Dermatol. 2017;92(5):606-20.
115. Ostrosky-Zeichner L, Walsh TJ, Bennett JE. Medical mycology. In: Bennett JE, Dolin R, Blaser MJ (Eds). Mandell Douglas and Bennetts Principles and Practice of Infectious Diseases, 9th edition. Philadelphia, PA: Elsevier; 2020. pp. 3376-402.
116. Paphitou NI, Ostrosky-Zeichner L, Rex JH. Trichosporon species, Malassezia species, and uncommon yeast infections in the era of new antifungal agents. Clin Infect Dis. 2003;37 (Suppl 3:)S199-205.

117. Pappas PG. Invasive Trichosporon infections. Clin Infect Dis. 2001;33(1):129-33.
118. Pinoy E. Actinomycoses et mycetomes. Bull Inst Pasteur. 1913;11:929-33.
119. Poster JN, Pfaller MA. Fungal culture media. In: Leber AL (Ed). Clinical Microbiology Procedures Handbook, 4th edition. Washington, DC: ASM Press; 2016.
120. Procop GW. Molecular diagnostics in medical mycology. Clin Infect Dis. 2007;45 (Suppl 6):S331-41.
121. Queiroz-Telles F, de Hoog GS, Santos DWCL, Salgado CG, Pasqualotto AC, Denning DW, et al. Chromoblastomycosis. Clin Microbiol Rev. 2017;30(1):233-76.
122. Queiroz-Telles F, Esterre P, Perez-Blanco M, Vitale RG, Salgado CG, Bonifaz A. Chromoblastomycosis: an overview of clinical manifestations, diagnosis and treatment. Med Mycol. 2009;47(1):3-15.
123. Redhead SA. The name of the anamorphic genus formerly linked to disciotis. Mycologia. 2014;106(4):823-4.
124. Reiss E, Shadomy HJ, Lyon GM III. Fundamental Medical Mycology. Hoboken (NJ): Wiley-Blackwell; 2012.
125. Relhan V, Agarwal P, Singh SK, Gupta R, Ramachandran V. Mycetoma: a review. Indian J Dermatol. 2017;62(3):332-40.
126. Revankar SG, Clemons KV, Hanson LH, Martinez KR, Stevens DA. In vitro activity of azoles, amphotericin B, and terbinafine against Ramichloridium mackenziei. Med Mycol. 1999;37(4):241-5.
127. Revankar SG, Kauffman CA. Sporotrichosis. Med Mycol. 2007;45(2):125-54.
128. Revankar SG, Sutton DA. Melanized fungi in human and veterinary medicine. Clin Microbiol Rev. 2010;23(2):884-928.
129. Rex JH, Walsh TJ, Anaissie JP, Chanock EP, Pizzo PA, Goldberg BW. Fungal reading panel. Candida species. Antimicrob Agents Chemother. 1994;38(8):1691-71.
130. Richardson M, Ellis M. Laboratory diagnosis of fungal infection. Curr Opin Infect Dis. 2005;18(2):131-6.
131. Richardson M, Warnock D. Fungal Infections: Diagnosis and Management, 4th edition. Chichester, UK: Wiley-Blackwell; 2012.
132. Rimek D, Uhrlass S. Malassezia bloodstream infections in neonates: a 12-year survey in Germany. Mycoses. 2010;53(1):51-5.
133. Rippon JW. Medical Mycology. The Pathogenic Fungi and the Pathogenic Actinomycetes, 3rd edition. Philadelphia: WB Saunders; 1988.
134. Rodrigues AM, de Hoog GS, de Albornoz MM, de Ataídes FS, Bezerra LC, da Silva MB, et al. Molecular phylogeny of the Gibellulopsis nigrescens complex and the newly established family Gibellulopsidaceae. Mycol Prog. 2016;15(2):1-12.
135. Rodríguez G, Sarmiento L. The asteroid bodies of sporotrichosis. Am J Dermatopathol. 1998;20(3):246-9.
136. Royal Botanic Gardens, Kew. Index Fungorum [Internet]. 2025 [cited 2025 Jul]. Available from: http://www.indexfungorum.org/
137. Rudolph M. Falle von Figueira (Chromophytose?). Ann Bras Med. 1914;6:376.
138. Saëz-Llorens X, Castaño E, McFarlane C, Gamez L, Arguèdas JA, Mayorga L. Association of white piedra and Trichosporon beigelii colonization with diarrheal syndromes in children. Pediatr Infect Dis J. 1991;10(4):319-24.
139. San-Blas G. Molecular mechanisms of fungal dimorphism. Arch Med Res. 2000;31(6):S75-8.
140. Santos DWCL, de Azevedo CMPES, Vicente VA, Queiroz-Telles F, Rodrigues MA, Hay R, et al. The global burden of chromoblastomycosis. PLoS Negl Trop Dis. 2021;15(8):e0009611.
141. Saunders CW, Scheynius A, Wolf R. Malassezia. In: Cellino MR (Ed). Microbiology Spectrum, 2nd edition. Washington, DC: ASM Press; 2014.
142. Schenck B. On the wort-mold, isolated from a human arm. Bull Johns Hopkins Hosp. 1898;9:286-9.
143. Schwartz RA. Superficial fungal infections. Lancet. 2004;364(9440):1173-82.
144. Sehgal VN, Kaviarasan PK. Majocchi's granuloma: concept revisited. Int J Dermatol. 2004;43(12):906-9.
145. Semelka RC, Kelekis NL, Sallah S. Gastrointestinal histoplasmosis: a difficult diagnosis with a wide range of manifestations. AJR Am J Roentgenol. 1999;173(4):949-53.
146. Sepúlveda VE, Rodrigues AM, de Hoog S, Sutton DA, Cano J, Caridad-Funcasta P, et al. Molecular taxonomy, phylogeny, and geographical distribution of the Histoplasma capsulatum species complex. PLoS Negl Trop Dis. 2017;11(6):e0005648.
147. Sigler L. Molecular evolution of ascomycetous yeasts: uncertain conservation of the genus Candida. In: Ruping L (Ed). Molecular identification of fungi. Berlin, Heidelberg: Springer-Verlag; 2001. pp. 171-87.
148. Singhal N, Kumar M, Singh P, Singh AK, Setia P, Singh A, et al. MALDI-TOF mass spectrometry: an emerging technology for microbial identification and diagnosis. Front Microbiol. 2015;6:897.
149. Singhal N, Yadav R, Kumar M, Asthana SP, Gautam T, Khan S, et al. White piedra: an uncommon yet significant hair shaft infection. Indian J Dermatol. 2014;59(5):521.
150. Siqueira AN, de Lima PB, da Silva Praserres J, de Siqueira W, de Souza JV, de Oliveira M, et al. Histoplasmosis: an endemic mycosis. Overview of epidemiology, clinical features, diagnosis, and treatment. Infectio. 2024;28(4):468-77.
151. Spatafora JW, Chang Y, James TY, Riley R, Ravinel KK, Rokas A, et al. A phylum-level phylogenetic classification of fungi derived from combined EF1alpha, RPB1, and RPB2 genes: trees as taxonomies. Mycologia. 2006;98(6):891-905.
152. Springer J, Morton P. Histopathology of fungal infections. In: Springer J, Morton P (Eds). Medical Mycology: Molecular and Clinical Approaches. Chichester, UK: John Wiley & Sons, Ltd.; 2010. pp. 93-104.
153. Taylor JW, Spatafora JW. Fungal taxonomy comes of age. Evol Biol. 2007;34(3-4):283-7.
154. Terra F, Torres M, de Area Leão AE, Christen J. Novo typo de mycose a blastosporos patogenicos (Chromoblastomycosis). Sci Med. 1922;1: 426-34.
155. Thomas J, Agarwal R, Woodworth MH, Glielmi C, Geddes-McAlister J. Malassezia atopic dermatitis. J Fungi (Basel). 2020;7(1):10.
156. Tobin EH, Jih WW. Histopathology of sporotrichosis. J Cutan Pathol. 2006;33 (Suppl 2):32-4.
157. Turland NJ, Wiersema JH, Barrie FR, Greuter W, Hawksworth DL, Herendeen PS. International Code of Nomenclature for Algae, Fungi, and Plants (Shenzhen Code) adopted by the Nineteenth International Botanical Congress Shenzhen, China, July 2017. Königstein: Koeltz Botanical Books; 2018.
158. University of North Carolina. Specimen collection [Internet]. 2025 [cited 2025 Jul]. Available from: https://www.med.unc.edu/micro/files/2018/08/Specimen-Collection.pdf

159. Vanbreuseghem R. Histoplasmose africaine (Histoplasma duboisii n. sp.). Bull Acad Natl Med. 1952;136(23-24):535-8.
160. Vasconcelos C, Lopes-Bezerra LM, Orofino-Costa R. Sporotrichosis: recent updates on molecular approaches to diagnosis and treatment. Expert Rev Anti Infect Ther. 2022;20(11):1381-92.
161. Velegraki A, Cafarchia C, Gaitanis G, Iatta R, Boekhout T. Malassezia infections in humans and animals: pathophysiology, detection, and treatment. PLoS Pathog. 2015;11(1):e1004523.
162. Walker L, Gow NA, Munro CA. Fungal dimorphism and virulence. Methods Mol Biol. 2014;1151:251-71.
163. Walther G, Wagner L, Forrest G, Koehler P, Fisher M, Scherlach K, et al. Lichtheimia species exhibit temperature-dependent growth differences that explain their variable association with human mucormycosis. Mycoses. 2013;56(4):441-52.
164. Weitzman I, Summerbell RC. The dermatophytes. Clin Microbiol Rev. 1995;8(2):240-59.
165. Welsh O, Vera-Cabrera ET, Salinas-Carmona RH. Mycetoma. Clin Dermatol. 2007;25(2):195-208.
166. Westblade LF, Burd EM, Lockhart SR, Procop GW. Larone's Medically Important Fungi: A Guide to Identification, 7th edition. Washington, DC: ASM Press; 2023.
167. Weston WL, Morelli JG. Majocchi's granuloma in children. Arch Pediatr Adolesc Med. 2000;154(6):627-8.
168. Wheat LJ, Kauffman CA. Histoplasmosis. Infect Dis Clin North Am. 2007;21(3):635-61.
169. Whittaker RH. New concepts of kingdoms of organisms. Evolutionary relations are at least as important as the divergence of physiological characteristics. Science. 1969;163(3863):150-60.
170. World Health Organization. (2025). Neglected tropical diseases. [online] Available from https://www.who.int/health-topics/neglected-tropical-diseases. [Last accessed July, 2025].
171. Yurayart C, Malichan P, Dampawan P, Chaiprasert A. Molecular identification of Trichosporon species isolated from clinical specimens in Thailand. Med Mycol. 2011;49(6):603-11.
172. Zijlstra EE, van de Sande WW, Welsh O, Goodfellow M, Musa A, Fahal AH. Mycetoma: from scientific fungus to neglected tropical disease. PLoS Negl Trop Dis. 2016;10(8):e0004398.

GLOSSARY

ABPA: Allergic bronchopulmonary aspergillosis.

Acervulus (plural: acervuli): A saucer-shaped asexual fruiting structure that produces conidia beneath the plant epidermis, eventually rupturing the surface; typical of coelomycetes.

Acicular: Needle-shaped, gradually narrowing toward the apex; descriptive of some fungal spores or crystals.

Acid Fast: A property of microbial cell walls where the primary stain resists decoloration after treatment with acid–alcohol.

Acrogenous (Gr., acros = highest, outermost): Conidia developing at the apex, borne at the tip.

Acropetal (Gr., acros = highest, outermost, L., petre = to seek): A chain of conidia growing at the tip, with the youngest conidium at the apex.

Actidione: Trade name for cycloheximide, an antibiotic produced by *Streptomyces griseus* that inhibits eukaryotic protein synthesis; used in culture media to suppress contaminating fungi.

Adamson's Fringe: The portion of the lower hair shaft at the junction of the living (mitotically active) hair bulb and the keratinized, nonliving hair shaft. Dermatophytes can infect hair only down to Adamson's fringe.

Adhesin: A surface molecule that promotes adhesion with other cells or extracellular matrix molecules (EMMs).

Adiaconidium (plural: adiaconidia): A large, globose, thick-walled structure of *Emmonsia* species that enlarges isotropically when lodged in host tissue.

Adiaspore (Gr., a = not + dia = across): Conidium of *Emmonsia* species, which enlarges without cell division when deposited in the lung.

Adventitious Sporulation: Sporulation occurring in an unusual location, such as tissue.

Aerial Hyphae/Mycelium: Hyphae growing above the colony surface.

Aerospora: The burden of fungal conidia and spores in the ambient air.

Aflatoxins: Toxic metabolites produced by certain fungi in or on food and feed, such as peanuts and corn.

AFRS: Allergic fungal rhinosinusitis, formerly known as allergic fungal sinusitis.

AFS: Antifungal susceptibility testing, determining the minimum inhibitory concentration of an antifungal agent against a fungal isolate.

Air Crescent Sign: A radiologic sign describing necrosis around a lung nodule with air filling the space between devitalized tissue and the surrounding parenchyma.

Aleurioconidium (Aleuriospore): A terminal or lateral conidium that develops as an expanded end of an undifferentiated hypha or short stalk, often detaching by lysis or fracture of the supporting cell wall.

ALL: Acute lymphocytic leukemia.

Allogeneic: Referring to a graft from an individual with a different human leukocyte antigen (HLA) haplotype.

Alopecia (Gr., alopex = fox): Balding, which may be temporary or permanent.

ALS: A family of *Candida albicans* surface adhesins.

AmB: Amphotericin B, a polyene macrolide antifungal agent.

Anamorph (L., ana = away, through, again + morph = form): The asexual state in the fungal life cycle.

Anergy: A state of unresponsiveness to antigenic stimulation, often seen in infectious diseases.

ANF: Anidulafungin.

Angioinvasive: Tending to invade blood vessel walls.

Ann Arbor Stage IVB: A lymphoma staging system.

Annellide (L., anellus = a little ring): A vase- or tube-shaped conidiogenous cell that elongates with each conidium release.

Annelloconidium (pl., -ia): A conidium produced by an annellide via enteroblastic conidiogenesis.

Annelloconidium (plural: annelloconidia): A conidium produced in succession by an annellide, leaving ring-like scars at the apex; conidia are typically rounded with a flat base.

Annellophore: The conidiophore or stalk supporting an annellide.

Annular Frill: The remnant of hyphal wall or disjunctor cell clinging to an arthroconidium released by cleavage.

Antheridium (plural: antheridia): The male gametangium in the sexual reproduction of certain fungi; fuses with the female gametangium (ascogonium or oogonium).

Anthropophilic: Dermatophytes that preferentially or exclusively infect humans.

Antler Hyphae: Repeatedly branching hyphal tip resembling an antler.

APACHE II Score: A severity of disease classification system used for patients in intensive care units.

Apophysis (Gr., apo = off + phyein = to grow): A bell-shaped or funnel-shaped swelling at the tip of a sporangiophore, below the sporangium.

Apothecium (plural: apothecia): A wide, open, cup- or saucer-shaped sexual fruiting body of some ascomycota, containing asci on its exposed surface.

Appressorium (plural: appressoria): A swollen, specialized cell formed at the tip of a germ tube or hypha that facilitates attachment to and penetration of a host surface, often via turgor pressure.

ARDS: Adult respiratory distress syndrome.

ART: Antiretroviral therapy.

Arthroconidium (plural: arthroconidia): An asexual spore formed by the fragmentation of hyphae at septal junctions. May involve modification of the hyphal cell and formation of a double septum. Common in dermatophytes and *Coccidioides* species.

Ascocarp (plural: ascocarps): The general term for the fruiting body of Ascomycota fungi, containing asci and ascospores. Synonym: Ascoma. Forms include cleistothecium, perithecium, and apothecium.

Ascoma (plural: ascomata): The entire fruiting body of an ascomycete, containing asci; taxonomic term often interchangeable with ascocarp.

Ascospore (plural: ascospores): A haploid sexual spore produced inside an ascus following karyogamy and meiosis; usually eight per ascus.

Ascus (plural: asci): A sac-like structure in Ascomycota in which ascospores develop after sexual reproduction.

Aseptate (synonym: coenocytic): Lacking septa (cross-walls) between hyphal cells; characteristic of some early-diverging fungi such as *Mucor* and *Rhizopus*.

Asexual: Reproduction without the union of two nuclei.

Aspergilloma: A fungus ball composed of hyphae, fibrin, and debris, usually forming within a pre-existing lung cavity; most often caused by *Aspergillus fumigatus*.

Assimilation: The aerobic process wherein carbon and nitrogen compounds are utilized with oxygen as the final electron acceptor.

Asteroid Body: A star-like eosinophilic antigen–antibody complex surrounding yeast forms in tissue; classically associated with *Sporothrix schenckii* infection.

Atopy: A genetic predisposition to produce IgE antibodies in response to common environmental antigens, including fungal allergens.

AUC (Area Under the Curve): Pharmacokinetic term representing the total drug exposure over time, based on plasma concentration versus time curves.

Autochthonous: Organism originating in the same area where it is found.

Autospore: Daughter cells formed within the covering of *Prototheca* species.

Autotrophic: Capable of growing without an organic source of energy, as seen in algae and plants.

BA (Blood Agar): A nutrient-rich medium containing blood, used for growing bacteria and fungi.

Bactrim (Cotrimoxazole): A combination antibiotic containing trimethoprim and sulfamethoxazole.

BAL (Bronchoalveolar Lavage): A procedure that collects samples from the lungs for diagnostic purposes.

Ballistoconidium: A conidium formed on a spine-like outgrowth of a cell, forcibly discharged by a droplet mechanism.

Ballistospore: A spore that is actively ejected at maturity, as in the *Entomophthorales*.

Balloon Cell: An enlarged globose microconidium formed by some dermatophytes, particularly characteristic of *Trichophyton tonsurans* in culture.

Basal Ascomycetes (Archiascomycetes): A group of fungi originating near the evolutionary divergence between ascomycetes and basidiomycetes.

Basidiocarp: A fruiting body seen in Basidiomycota, which produces basidia.

Basidiospore: A haploid sexual spore formed on the upper surface of a basidium following karyogamy and meiosis; characteristic of Basidiomycota.

Basidium (pl., Basidia): A club-shaped sexual cell that gives rise to external basidiospores, characteristic of the phylum Basidiomycota.

Basipetal: A form of conidiogenesis where the youngest conidium is at the base of a chain, as seen in *Aspergillus* and *Scopulariopsis* species.

BGC Agar (blood–glucose–cysteine agar): A medium to maintain yeast forms of dimorphic fungi.

BHI (Brain Heart Infusion): An agar medium, sometimes supplemented with 5% defibrinated sheep blood.

Biofilm: A fungal or bacterial community encased in an extracellular matrix, commonly found on indwelling medical devices.

Biomaterial: Synthetic materials used in medical devices, such as catheters and implants.

Bird Seed Agar: A selective medium for isolating *Cryptococcus neoformans*, which forms dark colonies due to melanin production.

Biseriate: An arrangement of conidiogenous cells where a row of phialides is supported by metulae, as in *Aspergillus flavus*.

BLAST: Basic Local Alignment Search Tool used to find regions of similarity between sequences.

Blastic: A mode of conidiogenesis where a cell swells and produces conidia before septum formation.

Blastoconidium/Blastospore: A conidium formed through a budding process, typically seen in yeasts.

BMBL5: Biosafety in Microbiological and Biomedical Laboratories, 5th edition, available online.

BMT (Bone Marrow Transplant): Now referred to as a hematopoietic stem cell transplant (SCT).

Botryomycosis: A bacterial infection that was once thought to be fungal, characterized by granulomatous masses.

Breakpoint: The drug concentration considered effective or ineffective based on in vitro testing, determined by committees such as the Clinical and Laboratory Standards Institute (CLSI).

Brown and Brenn Stain: A tissue Gram stain.

BSC (Biological Safety Cabinet): A containment device used to handle infectious agents safely.

Bubo: An inflammatory swelling of a lymph gland, often in the axilla or groin.

Budding: Asexual reproduction in yeasts where small outgrowths form daughter cells.

Bullous: A blister larger than 5 mm, typically filled with fluid.

Calcofluor White: A fluorescent stain that binds to fungal, bacterial, and plant cell walls.

Candidemia: A bloodstream infection caused by *Candida* species.

CAPD (Continuous Ambulatory Peritoneal Dialysis): A form of dialysis where fluid exchanges occur continuously.

Capilloconidia: Minor conidia formed in *Basidiobolus ranarum*, often with an adhesive tip.

Capsule: A hyaline polysaccharide sheath surrounding a cell, such as in *Cryptococcus neoformans*.

Carryover: Substances carried over from the inoculum or original culture medium to new media.

CASF: Caspofungin, an antifungal drug.

Catenulate: Conidia arranged in chains of two or three.

CBP (Calcium-Binding Protein): A protein that binds calcium, often involved in cellular signaling or structure.

CDC: US Centers for Disease Control and Prevention.

Cellulitis: An infection of skin and subcutaneous tissues.

CFU (Colony-Forming Unit): A measure of viable fungal or bacterial cells that can form colonies.

CGB Medium (Canavanine–Glycine–Bromothymol Blue Medium): A differential agar to distinguish *Cryptococcus neoformans* from *Cryptococcus gattii*.

CGD (Chronic Granulomatous Disease): A genetic disorder where white blood cells cannot kill certain bacteria and fungi.

Charcot–Leyden Crystals: Eosinophilic crystals formed from the breakdown of eosinophils, seen in conditions like asthma.

Chlamydospore: A thick-walled resting conidium that serves as a survival propagule, commonly seen in *Candida albicans*.

CHROMagar Candida®: A selective agar for differentiating *Candida* species based on colony color.

Circinate: Coiled in a ring or partly so.

Clade: A taxonomic group consisting of a common ancestor and all its descendants.

Cladogram: A diagram showing evolutionary relationships between organisms.

Clamp Connection: A hook-like structure in basidiomycetes ensuring the equal distribution of nuclei between new cells.

Clavate: Club shaped.

Cleistothecium (pl., Cleistothecia): A closed fruiting body of ascomycetes containing randomly dispersed asci.

CLIA: Clinical Laboratory Improvement Amendments; establishes quality standards for laboratory testing.

CLSI: Clinical Laboratory Standards Institute, which sets standards for antimicrobial susceptibility testing.

CLT (Clotrimazole): An antifungal drug used for treating yeast infections.

CMA (Cornmeal Agar): Used to promote sporulation in molds and to induce pseudohyphae in yeasts like *Candida*.

C_{max}: Peak plasma concentration of a drug.

CMC (Chronic Mucocutaneous Candidiasis): A condition where persistent fungal infections occur on skin and mucous membranes.

CMI (Cell-Mediated Immunity): The immune response primarily involving T cells.

CMV (Cytomegalovirus): A type of herpesvirus that can cause infections in immunocompromised individuals.

CNS (Central Nervous System): Includes the brain and spinal cord.

Coccidioidin: A skin test antigen for detecting exposure to *Coccidioides* species.

Coccidioidoma: A residual granulomatous lesion in the lung following coccidioidomycosis.

Coenocytic: Hyphae without septa, characteristic of certain fungal groups like mucormycetes.

Collarette: A small ring of cell wall material at the tip of a phialide or base of a sporangium.

Columella (pl., Columellae): A sterile dome-shaped expansion at the apex of a sporangiophore in *Mucorales*.

Commensalism: A relationship where two organisms live in close association, where one benefits, but the other is neither harmed nor helped.

Conidiogenous: Describes a cell specialized for producing conidia.

Conidiophore: A specialized hyphal structure that bears conidiogenous cells.

Conidium (pl., Conidia): Asexual reproductive propagule formed by fungi, often released by detachment from a conidiogenous cell.

COPD (Chronic Obstructive Pulmonary Disease): A lung disease that makes it difficult to breathe.

Copper Pennies: Refers to muriform cells seen in chromoblastomycosis, named for their pigmentation.

Cording Effect: The linear chain of nodules tracing lymphatic drainage in sporotrichosis.

Coremium (pl., Coremia): A column of combined filaments forming spore-bearing structures.

Corymbiform: Flat-topped clusters of fruiting branches with branchlets arising at different points.

Crozier: A hook-shaped structure in ascomycetes, formed before ascus development.

Cryptic Species: Morphologically identical but genetically distinct species, often identified by molecular sequencing.

Cryptococcoma: A cyst-like granuloma containing cryptococci, often found in the brain or lungs.

CSF (Cerebrospinal Fluid): The fluid surrounding the brain and spinal cord.

CT (Computed Tomography): A medical imaging technique, sometimes referred to as HRCT (high-resolution CT).

Cuticle: The outermost layer of a hair shaft, acting as a protective barrier.

CXR (Chest X-ray): An imaging technique used to view the lungs and chest structures.

Cyst: A sac-like structure in tissues or, in fungal terms, an ascus in *Pneumocystis jirovecii.*

Czapek–Dox Medium/Agar: A defined medium for the growth of fungi such as *Aspergillus* and *Penicillium* species.

Dalmau Plate: A pattern of inoculation on nutritionally deficient medium. Corn meal agar is seeded with a suspected colony of *Candida albicans* or other yeast. A light inoculum is cut into, but not through, the agar forming a #- shape in the center of the agar plate.

Deep-seated (Systemic): Refers to an infection that has developed in an internal organ of the body.

Dehiscent (L., dehiscere = to split open): Opening of a structure to permit the escape of spores; the separation of spores from the structure that produced them.

Deliquescence (L., deliquescere = to melt, dissolve): Dissolution of the fungal cell wall, such as in *Rhizopus oryzae* when sporangiospores are released from the sporangium.

Dematiaceous: Melanized, having brown to black conidia and/or hyphal cell walls, also referred to as "phaeoid" fungi.

Dendrogram: A tree-like diagram used to illustrate clusters produced by a clustering algorithm, often used in computational biology.

Denticle: Small tooth-like projection from which conidia develop, seen in *Sporothrix schenckii* and *Schizophyllum commune.*

Denture stomatitis: Inflammation of the gums beneath dentures, characterized by erythema without an adherent white membrane.

Dermatomycosis: Fungal disease of the skin, hair, or nails caused by nondermatophytic molds and yeasts.

Dermatophyte: A pathogenic fungus of the genera *Microsporum*, *Trichophyton*, or *Epidermophyton* that causes cutaneous infections of the stratum corneum, hair, or nails.

Dermatophyte Test Medium (DTM): A medium used to identify dermatophytes by a color change to red due to pH shifts caused by fungal growth.

Dermatophytosis: Fungal infection of the stratum corneum, hair, or nails caused by *Microsporum*, *Trichophyton*, or *Epidermophyton*.

Desert Rheumatism: Joint pain caused by inflammatory response to infection with *Coccidioides* species.

DHN Melanin: Dihydroxynaphthalene melanin synthesized by the polyketide pathway. Common in melanized fungi like *Cryptococcus neoformans*.

Diaper Rash: A common skin issue in infants, often caused by *Candida albicans*, leading to red rashes and small bumps.

DIC (Differential Interference Contrast): A type of microscopy that provides a pseudo-three-dimensional appearance by splitting light into two beams, creating high-contrast images.

Dichotomous Branching: A type of branching in fungi where two branches are approximately equal in size, seen in *Aspergillus* species.

Dikaryon: A stage in fungal cells where two genetically dissimilar unfused nuclei coexist and divide synchronously, seen in *Ascomycota* and *Basidiomycota*.

Dimorphic: Fungi with two distinct morphologies (yeast and mold forms), often dependent on temperature, seen in species such as *Candida albicans* and dimorphic pathogens like *Histoplasma*.

Disjunctor Cell: A cell that promotes the disarticulation of conidia, seen in *Coccidioides* and *Malbranchea* species.

Disk Diffusion: An antifungal susceptibility test where paper disks impregnated with antifungal agents are placed on fungal lawns to measure zones of inhibition.

Disseminated: Refers to an infection distributed across multiple organ systems or the scattering of conidia/spores upon release.

Dolipore: A septal structure in Basidiomycota fungi, featuring a swollen septum and pore cap structure (parenthesome) that allows cytoplasm but not organelles to pass between cells.

Downy: A description of colonies covered with short, fine hyphae.

Dysgonic: Refers to organisms that grow with difficulty on artificial media.

Echinulate (L., echinus = hedgehog): Covered with small spines or rough projections.

ECM (Extracellular Matrix): The extracellular matrix produced by fungal biofilms, consisting of macromolecules like ß-(1→3)–D-glucan.

Ectothrix: A pattern of sporulation in dermatophytosis where hyphae grow in the hair shaft and arthroconidia form a sheath outside the hair shaft.

EIA (Enzyme Immunoassay): A method for detecting specific antigens or antibodies in a sample using enzyme-labeled antigens or antibodies.

Endemic: A disease found prevalently in limited geographical areas, with a consistent presence in the population.

Endogenous: Originating from within the body.

Endospore: An asexual spore produced within a spherule, commonly seen in *Coccidioides* species.

Endothrix: A pattern of sporulation in dermatophytosis where hyphae fragment into arthroconidia inside the hair shaft.

Enteroblastic: A type of conidiogenesis where a new conidium forms from within a conidiogenous cell and pushes through the outer cell wall, seen in *Aspergillus*.

Epidemiology: The study of patterns, causes, and transmission of diseases within populations, aiming to improve public health interventions.

Epizootic: A disease that affects many animals in a region simultaneously.

Erythema Multiforme: Target-like lesions and oral involvement associated with acute pulmonary coccidioidomycosis.

Erythema Nodosum: Tender subcutaneous red nodules, often developing in acute pulmonary coccidioidomycosis.

Exogenous: Originating from outside the body, such as environmental sources of infection.

Favus: A type of dermatophytosis characterized by the formation of crusts or "scutula" along the hair shaft, associated with *Trichophyton schoenleinii*.

Fomite: An inanimate object that can harbor and transmit infectious microbes.

Fungus Ball: A mass of fungal mycelium and cellular debris found in body cavities such as the lung, often associated with *Aspergillus* infections.

Floccose: A texture description for colonies that are fluffy or woolly.

Fungi Imperfecti: An archaic term for mitosporic fungi with no known sexual stage.

Fungus: Eukaryotic organisms with chitin-containing cell walls that grow as molds or yeasts, capable of sexual and asexual reproduction.

Fusiform (L., fusus = spindle): Spindle shaped, narrowing toward both ends.

Genus (Genera): A taxonomic rank below family and above species. It is used in binomial nomenclature to denote the generic name of a species, often combined with a Latin or Latinized specific epithet.

Geophilic: Describes fungi that primarily inhabit soil, such as *Microsporum gypseum*.

Germ Tube: The initial hyphal outgrowth from a yeast cell, conidium, or spore, characterized by a lack of constriction at the point of origin. Commonly used in presumptive identification of *Candida albicans*.

Giant Cell: A large multinucleated cell formed by the fusion of macrophages, often seen in granulomatous inflammation due to infection or foreign body reactions.

Glabrous: Smooth-surfaced colony morphology lacking aerial mycelia; appears waxy or shiny.

Globose: Spherical or nearly round in shape.

Granular: Having a coarse or particulate appearance or texture.

Granule: A compact aggregation of fungal or actinomycotic elements formed in vivo, characteristic of mycetoma.

Graphium: An anamorphic genus of *Ascomycota*, producing synnemata as its reproductive structure.

Gymnothecium (Gymnothecia): A type of fruiting body (ascoma) composed of loosely interwoven hyphae, enclosing asci without a protective peridium.

Halophilic: Capable of growing in environments with high salt concentrations.

Haploid: A nuclear state in which each nucleus contains a single complete set of chromosomes (n), common in many fungal life stages.

Herbarium: A curated collection of preserved plant specimens. In mycology, a similar concept is a fungal culture collection.

Heterokaryon: A fungal cell or mycelium containing genetically distinct nuclei within a shared cytoplasm.

Heterothallic: Refers to fungi that are self-sterile and require interaction between two compatible mating types (thalli) for sexual reproduction.

Hilum (Hila): The scar or attachment site at the base of a conidium where it was previously attached to the conidiogenous cell.

Holomorph: The complete fungal organism, encompassing its sexual (teleomorph), asexual (anamorph), and additional asexual forms (synanamorphs).

Holothallic: A mode of conidial development where all cell wall layers of the conidiogenous or sporogenous cell are involved in forming the conidium.

Homothallic: Self-fertile fungal species capable of completing sexual reproduction within a single thallus.

Hülle Cells: Thick-walled vegetative cells, often associated with cleistothecia in certain *Aspergillus* species (e.g., *Aspergillus nidulans* and *Aspergillus versicolor*), containing pores in their walls.

Hyalo-: A prefix indicating hyaline, light-colored, or colorless characteristics.

Hyaline: Transparent or colorless, commonly used to describe fungal hyphae or conidia that lack pigmentation.

Hyperendemic: Refers to diseases caused by fungi that are consistently present at high prevalence within a specific geographic region (e.g., coccidioidomycosis, sporotrichosis, and rhinosporidiosis).

Hypha (Hyphae): Filamentous fungal structures, 2–10 µm in diameter, which may be septate or aseptate. They form the basic unit of fungal growth and compose vegetative and aerial mycelia.

Hypopyon: Accumulation of pus in the anterior chamber of the eye, often associated with fungal keratitis.

Id Reaction: Hypersensitivity manifestations secondary to fungal infections, such as dermatophytid and candidid reactions.

Imperfect Fungi: Fungi that reproduce solely through asexual means (anamorph) and lack a known sexual (teleomorph) stage.

Indeterminate: Describes a conidiogenous cell that continues to elongate during or between successive conidial formations, characteristic of annellides.

Indurated: Describes tissue that has become hardened, often due to inflammation or chronic infection.

Intercalary: Refers to a structure formed between two adjacent cells or within a hyphal segment; commonly used to describe chlamydospores not formed at the terminal end.

Internodal: The hyphal region between two successive nodes (junctions or branches).

Keratinophilic: Describing fungi that possess the enzymatic ability to degrade keratin; includes dermatophytes which infect skin, hair, and nails.

Keratitis: Inflammation of the cornea, which may be of infectious, traumatic, or autoimmune origin.

Keratomycosis: Fungal infection of the cornea, frequently associated with trauma or contact lens use; common etiological agents include *Fusarium*, *Aspergillus*, and *Candida* species.

Kerion: A severe, suppurative inflammatory response to dermatophyte infection of the scalp (tinea capitis), characterized by painful nodules, boggy swelling, and alopecia.

KOH Mount (Potassium Hydroxide Preparation): A microscopic diagnostic technique in which potassium hydroxide is applied to clinical specimens to dissolve cellular debris, enhancing visibility of fungal elements such as hyphae or yeasts.

Lanose: Describes a woolly colony texture composed of dense, long, and uniform aerial mycelia.

Lyophilization: A preservation method in which fungal cultures are freeze-dried under vacuum for long-term storage without loss of viability.

mAb: Monoclonal antibody.

Macroconidium: The larger of the two types of conidia produced by a fungus, usually multicellular.

Macule: A small, flat, circumscribed change in skin color <10 mm in diameter.

Mannan: Soluble outer layer of *Candida* cell walls, an antigenic peptidopolysaccharide.

"m" Antigen: Catalase enzyme from *Histoplasma capsulatum*; anti-m-antibodies indicate acute pulmonary histoplasmosis.

MCF: Micafungin.

MEC: Minimum effective concentration (µg/mL) for echinocandins, observed as clubbing at hyphal tips.

Meiosporangium: Sporangium where meiosis occurs.

Meiosporic: Related to meiosis or sexual reproduction.

Melanized: Blackish brown-pigmented, synonym for phaeoid or dematiaceous fungi.

Meristematic: Continuous increase in fungal biomass and septum formation.

Merosporangium: Cylindrical sporangium producing sporangiospores in a single row, as seen in *Syncephalastrum*.

Metula: Specialized sterile branch in *Aspergillus* and *Penicillium* supporting phialides.

MIC: Minimum inhibitory concentration (µg/mL) needed to prevent yeast or mold growth.

Microbiome: Total microbial population in a defined environment, usually in humans.

Microbiota: Microbial population in a healthy individual.

Microconidium: Smaller, asexually produced conidia formed on aerial hyphae.

Middlebrook's 7H10 Agar: Medium for cultivating mycobacteria, stimulates *Blastomyces dermatitidis* conversion to yeast form.

Mitosporangium: Sporangium where mitosis occurs.

Mitosporic: Asexual reproduction phase of fungi.

MLST: Multilocus sequence typing, a genotyping method assessing partial sequences of seven gene loci.

"Moccasin" Tinea Pedis: Ringworm of the foot extending up the sides, often caused by *Trichophyton rubrum*.

Mold: Filamentous fungus, can be meiosporic or mitosporic.

Molluscum-like Lesions: Soft nodules similar to molluscum contagiosum, seen mainly in children and sexually transmitted in adults.

Moniliform: Hyphae with regular swellings resembling a string of beads.

Monomorphic: Growth exclusively in one form, either as mold or yeast.

Monophyletic: A group of organisms with a single common ancestor and all its descendants.

Morphogenesis: Development or change in an organism's form.

MRI: Magnetic resonance imaging.

MSM: Men who have sex with men.

Mucicarmine: Histologic stain producing a red color on *Cryptococcus neoformans* capsules.

Mucoromycotina: Subphylum of molds with aseptate or pauciseptate hyphae, reproducing via sporangia.

MUD: Matched-unrelated donor in stem cell transplantation.

Muriform: Fungal cells with both vertical and horizontal cross-walls, as in chromoblastomycosis.

Mycelium: Network of intertwined hyphae forming the body of a fungus.

Mycetoma: Chronic subcutaneous fungal or bacterial disease characterized by swelling and draining sinuses.

Mycosel (Mycobiotic) Agar: Medium used to isolate pathogenic fungi, contains cycloheximide and chloramphenicol.

Neutropenia: Decreased number of polymorphonuclear neutrophilic granulocytes (PMNs) in the blood; profound neutropenia when <100/µL.

NICU: Neonatal intensive care unit.

Nosocomial: Pertaining to infections acquired in hospital settings.

NYT: Nystatin.

Obclavate: Club shaped with thickening at the outer end.

Obovoid: Inverted egg-shaped conidium with the broad end up.

OD: Optical density.

Onychia (Onychomycosis): Fungal infection of the nails causing opacity, thickening, or brittleness.

Onygenales: Order of *Ascomycota* producing ascospores in gymnothecia or cleistothecia; includes dermatophytes and some dimorphic fungi.

OPC: Oropharyngeal candidiasis.

Opportunistic Infection: Infection occurring in debilitated or immunocompromised individuals.

Ostiole: Pore or opening in a reproductive structure through which spores escape.

Ovoid: Egg-shaped conidium with the broad end down and narrow end up.

PAMP: Pathogen-associated molecular pattern. Structures shared by pathogens but absent on host cells, recognized by the innate immune system early in the immune response and trigger inflammation (e.g., fungal mannans).

PaO_2: The partial pressure of oxygen in arterial blood.

Papanicolaou: A cytologic stain used for smears of various body secretions, including fungi, which acquire a pink coloration.

Papilla: Nipple-shaped elevation or small rounded process.

Papule: A small, solid, rounded bump rising from the skin, usually <10 mm in diameter.

Parafungal: Mycelial and unicellular organisms not classified within the kingdom fungi, such as *Pythium*, *Rhinosporidium*, and *Prototheca* species, which cause infections with features resembling those produced by fungi. Also called pseudofungal organisms.

Paraphyletic: In phylogenetics, a group of organisms that contains the most recent common ancestor but not all descendants of that ancestor.

Paraphysis: Sterile hypha growing up between asci in the hymenium of many ascomycetes.

Parasexual: A nuclear cycle resulting in recombinant haploid genotypes without meiosis, involving heterokaryosis, karyogamy to produce heterozygous diploid nuclei, and mitotic crossing over and/or nondisjunction and aneuploidy.

Parasexual Cycle: Method of recombining genes in which haploid nuclei of a fungal heterokaryon fuse, enabling mitotic recombination without meiosis.

Parenteral: Administration of medication or nutrition not through the alimentary tract but via subcutaneous, intramuscular, or intravenous injection.

Paronychia: A fungal infection involving the periungual tissue (the skin surrounding the nail), often caused by *Candida* species.

PAS (Periodic Acid-Schiff): A stain used in fungal histopathology that stains the fungal cell wall pink-red.

Pathogenicity: Ability to cause disease.

Pathognomonic: A sign or symptom so characteristic of a disease that it makes the diagnosis.

Pauciseptate: Sparse septations in the hyphae.

PCP: Pneumocystis pneumonia.

PDA: Potato dextrose agar. Medium used to stimulate conidia production in slide cultures.

Pectinate: Hyphal ends with protuberances resembling the teeth of a comb.

Penicillate: Having a tuft of fine hairs resembling a brush, as seen in *Penicillium* conidiophores.

Percurrent: Conidiogenous cell growth where a new axis grows through the previous apex, as seen in *Malassezia* species.

Perfect (teleomorph) state: The sexual (meiosporic) state of a fungus.

Perfect Fungi: Capable of sexual reproduction; part of the life cycle where spores are formed after nuclear fusion. Synonymous with teleomorph.

Peridium: The outer wall of a sporangium or an ascoma, composed of hyphae.

Perithecium: A usually flask-shaped ascoma with asci arranged as a fertile layer at the base; asci or ascospores are expelled through an ostiole at the apex.

Perleche: Angular cheilitis, an inflammatory lesion at the corners of the mouth caused by *Candida albicans*, other pathogens, or a nutritional deficiency.

Peronosporomycetes: Pseudofungal organisms belonging to the class Oomycetes under phylum Stramenopila, like *Pythium* species.

Phaeo-: Prefix meaning dark-colored and associated with melanized fungi.

Phaeohyphomycosis: Disease caused by melanized fungi with darkly pigmented hyphal or yeast-like tissue forms.

Phaeoid: Darkly pigmented, formerly dematiaceous.

Phagocytosis: The process of engulfing large particles or infectious agents by immune cells.

Phialide: A tube- or vase-shaped conidiogenous cell that produces successive conidia from a fixed point of origin.

Phialoconidium: A conidium produced by a flask-shaped conidiogenous cell termed a phialide, as seen in *Aspergillus* or *Phialophora* species.

Phore: Suffix used for a bearing structure.

Phragmoconidia: Conidia with three or more transverse septa, as seen in *Curvularia* species.

Phylogenetic: The study of evolutionary relatedness among various groups of organisms.

Phylogenetic systematic: Evolutionary tree.

Phylogeny: Evolutionary history of an organism or group.

Phylum (phyla): A taxon above class and below kingdom. In plants, equivalent to division.

Pityriasis Versicolor: A superficial cutaneous mycosis caused by lipophilic yeasts of the *Malasseziales*, resulting in hypo- or hyperpigmentation of superficial skin lesions.

Planktonic: Please see Biofilm.

Pleocytosis: Greater than normal number of cells in a body fluid such as cerebrospinal fluid.

Pleomorphic:

i. Displaying more than one form of asexual sporulation.
ii. In dermatophyte mycology, refers to the change from a wild-type mycelial growth to a sterile mycelial form.

PMN (syn., neutrophil): Polymorphonuclear neutrophilic granulocyte.

Polymorphic: Fungal species using more than one type of conidiation process.

Polyphyletic: Descended or derived from more than one ancestral stock or source.

Polyphyletic: A taxonomic group based on morphologic similarity that does not share a common ancestry when analyzed cladistically.

Polyploid: Having more than two sets of homologous chromosomes.

Poroconidia: Conidia formed apically through a pore, as seen in *Curvularia* species.

Poroconidium: A type of holoblastic conidiogenesis in which a multicelled conidium grows out of a pore in the hyphal cell.

Potassium Hydroxide: See KOH.

PPD: Purified protein derivative of tuberculin used in the tuberculosis skin test.

PPE: Personal protective equipment.

Preemptive Therapy: Early treatment of an infection using clinical, laboratory, or radiologic markers before clinical signs and symptoms appear.

Prevalence: Number of cases of a disease existing in a given population at a specific time.

Probe: Specific nucleic acid sequence used to detect a complementary sequence in an unknown fungus.

Propagule: A reproductive unit, or any part of an organism, that is capable of giving rise to a new individual through propagation (e.g., spores, conidia, or vegetative fragments).

Proteinaceous: Protein like.

Proteinase (Extracellular): Microbial secreted enzymes that digest host proteins, such as aspartyl proteinases of *Candida albicans*.

PRRs: Pattern recognition receptors that recognize pathogen-associated molecular patterns (PAMPs) and facilitate innate immune responses.

Pruritus: Severe itching.

PSC: Posaconazole.

Pseudo-: Prefix meaning false, indicating deceptive resemblance to the following element of the word.

Pseudofungal: Mycelial and unicellular organisms not classified in the kingdom Fungi, such as *Pythium, Rhinosporidium*, and *Prototheca* species, that cause infections with features resembling those produced by fungi. Also called parafungal organisms.

Pseudohypha: Fragile chain of cells, usually yeasts, elongated by budding and attached to adjacent cells with characteristics intermediate between yeast cells and hyphae.

Pseudomycelium: Mass of pseudohyphae.

Pusillus: Tiny.

Pycnidiospore: Spore/conidia formed within a pycnidium.

Pycnidium (pycnidia): Spherical to flask-shaped enclosed structure with an apical opening (ostiole) inside which conidia are formed, i.e., coelomycetes.

Pyriform: Pear- or teardrop shaped.

Rachis (Rachides): The terminal, often elongated portion of a conidiogenous cell or conidiophore, along which conidia are borne in succession.

Racquet (Racket) hyphae: Hyphal elements composed of a series of cells swollen at one end, resembling tennis rackets; observed in older or degenerating cultures, particularly in dermatophytes.

Rhexolytic cleavage: A mechanism of conidial release characterized by lysis and breakdown of the intervening cell wall, leaving behind residual wall fragments; exemplified by arthroconidium formation in *Coccidioides* species.

Rhizoid: A root-like hyphal outgrowth that penetrates the substrate, serving an anchoring function; characteristic of certain zygomycetes, particularly *Rhizopus* species.

Ringworm: A colloquial term for dermatophytosis, derived from the annular (ring-shaped) configuration of lesions and the historical belief in a worm etiology.

Rugose: Describes a colony surface that is deeply wrinkled, grooved, or folded; commonly seen in cultures of *Aspergillus niger* and other filamentous fungi.

SABHI: A combined agar medium consisting of Sabouraud dextrose agar (SDA) and brain heart infusion (BHI) for stimulating the growth of dimorphic fungal pathogens. It may be supplemented with cycloheximide, chloramphenicol, and defibrinated sheep blood.

Sabouraud Dextrose Agar (SDA): A widely used medium for cultivating yeasts and molds. It contains dextrose (glucose) and peptone, with a final pH of 5.5–5.6 to favor fungal growth while suppressing many bacteria. High dextrose concentration (40 g/L) may inhibit sporulation, and antibiotics can be added to control bacterial contamination.

SDA-Emmons: An Emmons' modification of SDA with half the glucose concentration (20 g/L) and a final pH of 6.8–7.0 to improve fungal sporulation.

Sandwich EIA: An antigen capture enzyme immunoassay where a capture antibody is affixed to a solid surface, an antigen is added and bound, and then an indicator antibody is used to develop color in the presence of a chromogenic substrate.

Saprobe: An organism that obtains nourishment from dead and decaying organic matter.

Saprotrophic: An organism that feeds on dead organic matter, a term replacing "saprophyte" to avoid plant connotations.

Scissiparity: Reproduction by fission.

Sclerotic Bodies: Also known as muriform cells, these are histopathological structures seen in chromoblastomycosis, consisting of dark brown, subglobose, multicellular bodies that divide along septal planes.

Sclerotium (Sclerotia): A resistant, hardened mass of hyphae that remains dormant during unfavorable conditions. It can germinate when conditions improve.

Scutulum: A compact mass of hyphae, keratinous material, and hair seen in favus.

Sensu Lato (s.l.): Latin phrase indicating a species complex in a broad sense.

Sensu Stricto (s.s.): Latin phrase indicating a taxon used in the narrow sense, consistent with the original description.

Septate: Hyphae containing cross-walls (septa).

Septum (Septa): A cross-wall in hyphae, conidiophores, conidia, or spores.

Sequela: A condition or pathology resulting from a disease.

Sessile: (i) A conidium arising directly from the surface of a hypha without an intervening conidiophore and (ii) attached directly to the substrate.

Settle Plate: A Petri plate exposed to the environment for a specified time to capture airborne fungi, which are then cultured and enumerated.

Shield Cell: A conidium with a shield or "V" shape, usually seen in melanized fungi like *Cladosporium*.

Slide Culture: A method for studying microscopic morphology and conidiogenesis by placing agar medium on a microscope slide, seeding with the mold, and covering with a coverslip.

Snowstorm Appearance: A radiographic image showing multiple nodules in lung fields, characteristic of acute pulmonary histoplasmosis.

SNP: Single nucleotide polymorphism.

SOT: Solid organ transplant.

Spathulate: Spoon shaped.

Spherule: A closed, thick-walled spherical structure containing endospores, produced by *Coccidioides* species during growth in vivo.

Spinose: Covered with small spines.

Spinous Cell Layer: The layer between the stratum granulosum and stratum basale of the epidermis, characterized by polygonal cells that synthesize keratin.

Splendore–Hoeppli Reaction: Eosinophilic pseudomycotic structures composed of necrotic debris and immunoglobulin, often associated with botryomycosis and various fungi.

Sporangiole: A small, usually spherical sporangium containing one or two sporangiospores, characteristic of *Cunninghamella*.

Sporangiophore: The specialized hypha that produces a sporangium in *Mucoromycotina*.

Sporangiospore: An asexual spore produced within a sporangium, characteristic of *Mucoromycotina*.

Sporangium (pl. sporangia): A sac-like structure in which spores are formed; characteristic of the *Mucorales*.

Spore: A reproductive propagule in fungi, produced by either sexual or asexual reproduction.

Sporodochium: A cushion-shaped stroma covered with conidiophores bearing conidia, seen in *Fusarium* and *Epicoccum* species.

Sporophore: Specialized hyphae that produce spores.

Sporulation: The process of spore production.

Stellate: Star shaped; arranged in rosettes.

Sterigma (pl. sterigmata): A thin, spine-like outgrowth of a cell supporting a conidium or spore.

Stipe: The stem or stalk of agarics, boletes, and other mushrooms, or the stalk of conidiophores in *Aspergillus* species.

Stolon: A horizontal hypha that grows along the surface of the substrate, bearing rhizoids and sporangiophores.

Stratum Corneum: The outermost layer of the epidermis, composed of flat, dead cells filled with keratin.

Subclavate: Somewhat club shaped.

Subglobose: Almost round.

Superficial Mycosis: Fungal infections affecting the hair or stratum corneum, with minimal pathology, caused by fungi other than dermatophytes.

Susceptible (Dose-dependent): A breakpoint indicating an intermediate level of susceptibility to an antifungal agent, with improved patient outcomes if higher doses are used.

Symbiont: An organism living in a symbiotic relationship with another organism.

Symbiosis: A partnership between two living organisms.

Sympodial: Conidial arrangement where new growing points form just beneath the apex of the previous one, resulting in a zigzag appearance.

Synanamorph: Any of the multiple asexual reproductive structures formed by the same fungus.

Synnema (pl. synnemata): A bundle of compact conidiophores forming an erect fascicle, resembling a stalk of wheat.

Systemic Mycosis: Fungal disease affecting deep tissues or organs of the body.

Spheroid: Large, round structure containing endospores, seen in *Coccidioides* species.

Spiral Hyphae: Vegetative hyphae with coiled or corkscrew-like turns.

Suspensor: Hyphal element supporting a zygospore.

Synonym: Another name for a species or taxonomic group.

Teleomorph: Sexual reproductive state of a fungus; also termed the "perfect" state.

Thallic: A mode of conidiogenesis where a conidium is formed by the transformation of an entire preexisting hyphal cell or when a conidium forms directly from the side or tip of a hypha.

Thallus: The entire body of a fungus consisting of both vegetative and reproductive structures.

Thrush: Mucosal candidiasis affecting the oral (oral thrush) or vulvovaginal (vaginal thrush) mucosae.

Tinea: General name for ringworm or dermatophytosis.

Tinea Gladiatorum: Dermatophytosis among high school and college wrestlers caused by *Trichophyton tonsurans*.

Tinea Versicolor: Also known as pityriasis versicolor.

TLR: Toll-like receptor, a pattern recognition receptor linked to inflammation.

TNF-α: Tumor necrosis factor-α, a cytokine involved in inflammation and immune response.

TPN: Total parenteral nutrition.

TRB: Terbinafine.

Trichophyton Agar: Media vitamin test agars to detect dermatophyte vitamin requirements.

Trophic Form: Asexual haploid cell in pneumocystosis that may divide by fission.

Truncate: Describes the base of a conidiogenous cell that appears flat, as if cut abruptly.

Tuberculate: Wart-like, spiny, or finger-like projections on the surface of conidia.

Uniseriate: Describes a single layer of phialides formed directly on the vesicle in *Aspergillus*.

Urea Agar: Medium used to differentiate *Candida* species from *Cryptococcus* species through urease testing.

Urease Test: Test for the enzyme urease, used to differentiate certain fungi.

URL: Uniform resource locator.

Valley Fever: Refers to coccidioidomycosis, a disease endemic to the Central Valley of California.

Vd ss: The volume of distribution at steady state.

Velutinous: Velvety.

Verrucous: Having many warts; cauliflower like.

Verticil: A group of conidiogenous cells whose bases are attached in a whorl around a conidiophore.

Vesicle: Swollen apex of a conidiophore or swollen end of a sporangiophore; also a small membrane-bound organelle in cell biology.

VF Titer: Endpoint serum dilution in the complement fixation test with coccidioidin in valley fever.

Villous: Covered with soft long hair.

Volume of Distribution (Vd): The amount of drug in the body divided by the concentration in the blood.

VRC: Voriconazole.

VVC: Vulvovaginal candidiasis.

WBC: White blood cell—leukocyte.

Western Blot: An enzyme-linked immunoelectrotransfer blot to demonstrate protein antigens.

Wood's Light or Wood's Lamp: A lamp producing ultraviolet radiation to inspect for certain fungal infections.

Woronin Body: A round, membrane-bound, granular vesicle in *Ascomycota* hyphae.

Yeast: A unicellular fungus that reproduces by budding or fission.

Yeast like: Soft, pasty, smooth colony usually without filamentous growth.

Zoophilic: Describing a dermatophyte growing preferentially on lower animals rather than on humans or in the soil.

Zygomycetes: Fungi that undergo sexual reproduction in a single enlarged cell (zygospore).

Zygospore: A thick-walled resting sexual spore formed from the fusion of two genetically compatible cells.

INDEX

Page numbers followed by *b* refer to box, *f* refer to figure, *fc* refer to flowchart, and *t* refer to table.

A

B

C

D

E

F

G

H

I

N

O

P

Q

R

S

T

U

V

W

X

Y

Z